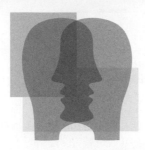

Assessment for Counselors

BRADLEY T. ERFORD

Loyola College in Maryland

Lahaska Press
Houghton Mifflin Company
Boston ▪ New York

Dedication

This effort is dedicated to The One: the Giver of energy, passion, and understanding; who makes life worth living and endeavors worth pursuing and accomplishing; the Teacher of love and forgiveness.

Publisher, Lahaska Press: Barry Fetterolf
Senior Editor, Lahaska Press: Mary Falcon
Editorial Assistant: Evangeline Bermas
Senior Project Editor: Kimberly Gavrilles
Art and Design Manager: Gary Crespo
Composition Buyer: Chuck Dutton
Associate Manufacturing Buyer: Brian Pieragostini
Director of Sales and Marketing, Lahaska Press: Heather Murray

Cover image © Mark Stephen/theispot.com

For instructors who want more information about Lahaska Press books and teaching aids, contact the Houghton Mifflin Faculty Services Center at
  Tel: 800-733-1717, x4034
  Fax: 800-733-1810

Or visit us on the Web at **www.lahaskapress.com**.

Printed in the U.S.A.

Library of Congress Control Number: 2006923762

ISBN-10: 0-618-49291-7
ISBN-13: 978-0-618-49291-6

456789-MP-10 09 08

CONTENTS

PREFACE

Assessment is counseling and counseling is assessment! The evolving profession of counseling has entered the age of accountability, regardless of specialization or practice venue. Managed care and school reform have become important forces driving decision making in contemporary society. Given this context, the more a professional counselor knows about formal and informal assessment procedures, the more informed, effective, and efficient the professional counselor's treatment of clients and students can be.

A second driving force comes from within the counseling profession itself. After many years of identity exploration and discussion, the counseling profession has agreed to a basic core of education and training standards that all professional counselors should meet. This book is designed to address the core curricular assessment requirements of the Council for Accreditation of Counseling and Related Educational Programs (CACREP), thereby providing state-of-the-art information on assessment and tests that professional counselors need to know. But what makes *Assessment for Counselors* different from other books is that it is written by professional counselors for professional counselors.

The first half of *Assessment for Counselors* provides important general information about assessment, including basic concepts, historical developments, ethical and legal implications, diversity issues, reliability, validity, test construction, and the selection, administration, scoring, and interpretation of assessment instruments. The second half of this book provides in-depth explorations of the major areas of assessment that professional counselors either provide or of which they must be aware. Embedded within these domains of counseling specialty, this text includes reviews of more than 100 commonly used tests in the areas of clinical, personality, behavioral, intelligence, aptitude, achievement, career, and couples and family assessment. In short, *Assessment for Counselors* is the most comprehensive introductory assessment text ever written specifically for professional counselors.

ACKNOWLEDGMENTS

The editor would like to thank Kami McNinch, Lauren Klein, Katie Hall, and Megan Earl for their tireless assistance in the preparation of the original manuscript. All of the contributing authors are to be commended for lending their expertise in the various topical areas or on the various tests reviewed in this volume. As always, Barry Fetterolf, publisher, and Mary Falcon, senior editor of Lahaska Press, have been wonderfully responsive and supportive. Finally, special thanks go to three outside accuracy reviewers who carefully scrutinized the entire manuscript and whose comments led to substantive improvement in the final product: Gerald Chandler, University of Central Oklahoma; Darcy Haag Granello, The Ohio State University; and Joshua C. Watson, Mississippi State University, Meridian.

ABOUT THE AUTHORS

THE EDITOR

Bradley T. Erford, Ph.D., is director of the School Counseling Program and a professor in the Education Department at Loyola College in Maryland. He is the recipient of the American Counseling Association's (ACA) Professional Development Award, ACA Research Award, and the ACA Carl Perkins Government Relations Award, and is an ACA Fellow. He has received the Association for Counselor Education and Supervision's Robert O. Stripling Award for Excellence in Standards, the Association for Assessment in Counseling and Education/Measurement and Evaluation in Counseling and Development Research Award, the Maryland Association for Counseling and Development's Maryland Counselor of the Year, Professional Development, Counselor Visibility, and Counselor Advocacy Awards. His research specialization is primarily in development and technical analysis of psychoeducational tests and has resulted in the publication of numerous books, journal articles, book chapters, and psychoeducational tests.

He is past chair of the American Counseling Association–Southern (U.S.) Region; past president of the Association for Assessment in Counseling and Education; past president of the Maryland Association for Counseling and Development; past president of the Maryland Association for Counselor Education and Supervision; past president of the Maryland Association for Mental Health Counselors; and president of the Maryland Association for Measurement and Evaluation. Dr. Erford is the past chair of ACA's Task Force on High Stakes Testing; past chair of ACA's Task Force on Standards for Test Users; past chair of ACA's Public Awareness and Support Committee; and past chair of ACA's Interprofessional Committee. Dr. Erford is a licensed clinical professional counselor, licensed professional counselor, nationally certified counselor, licensed psychologist, and licensed school psychologist. He teaches courses primarily in the areas of assessment, human development, school counseling, and stress management.

THE CONTRIBUTING AUTHORS

Alan Basham, M.A., is a counselor educator at Eastern Washington University, where he teaches (among other subjects) advanced appraisal for CACREP programs in school counseling and mental health counseling. He is past president of the Association for Spiritual, Ethical and Religious Values in Counseling and of the Washington Counseling Association. He drafted ACA's Code of Leadership and served on the task forces that wrote ACA's position papers on test user qualifications and high-stakes testing. He also provides leadership and teamwork training for Washington State's Critical Incident Management teams. He lives near, and often roams with his dog Chinook through, the woods surrounding the Spokane River.

Jon-Michael Brasfield, M.A., NCC, is a recent graduate of Wake Forest University's counseling program. He is a professional school counselor at R.J. Reynolds High School in Winston-Salem, North Carolina. Jon plans to pursue further training in educational research methods and statistics in the near future.

Carey Davis is obtaining her educational specialist degree in school psychology from Mississippi State University. Her areas of interest include academic assessment and intervention and group contingencies.

Dimiter Dimitrov has a Ph.D. degree in mathematics education from the University of Sofia, Bulgaria and a Ph.D. degree in educational psychology from Southern Illinois University, Carbondale. Currently, he is an associate professor of educational measurement and statistics in the Graduate School of Education at George Mason University, Fairfax, Virginia. He is also editor of the professional journal *Measurement and Evaluation in Counseling and Development*. Dr. Dimitrov's areas of expertise and teaching experience include classical and modern measurement theory, generalizability theory, and quantitative research methods. His recent research interests focus on validations of cognitive operations and processes using tools of item response theory and structural equation modeling, and on latent trait modeling for measurement of change.

R. Anthony Doggett, Ph.D., is an assistant professor in the school psychology program at Mississippi State University. Dr. Doggett received his doctorate in school psychology from the University of Southern Mississippi. He completed a predoctoral internship and a postdoctoral fellowship in behavioral pediatrics at the Munroe-Meyer Institute for Genetics and Rehabilitation in Omaha, Nebraska. His professional interests include applied behavior analysis, functional behavioral assessment, behavioral consultation, parent training, instructional interventions, and behavioral pediatrics.

Susan H. Eaves is a doctoral student in counselor education at Mississippi State University. Her research interests center around Borderline Personality Disorder, Conduct Disorder, and marital infidelity. She holds national certification and is a licensed professional counselor.

Catherine Flemming, M.A., NCC, is the director of Lay Ministry at Centenary United Methodist Church in Winston-Salem, North Carolina. As part of her church ministry, she places members in service opportunities appropriate for their gifts and interests. In addition, she provides individual, marital, premarital, and group counseling. She is a trained *PREPARE/ENRICH* administrator.

Kathleen Hall completed her master's degree in the School Counseling Program of the Education Department at Loyola College in Maryland. She is currently a professional school counselor in Florida.

Lauren Klein completed her master's degree in the School Counseling Program of the Education Department at Loyola College in Maryland. She is currently a high school counselor in Harford County Public Schools, Maryland.

Lynn Linde is an assistant professor of education and the director of Clinical Programs in the School Counseling Program at Loyola College in Maryland. She received a master's degree in school counseling and a doctorate in counseling from George Washington University. Dr. Linde was previously chief of the Student Services and Alternative Programs Branch at the Maryland State Department of Education, the Maryland State specialist for school counseling, a local school system counseling supervisor, a middle and high school counselor, and a special education teacher. She has made numerous presentations on ethics and legal issues for counselors, and public policy and legislation over the span of her career. Dr. Linde is the recipient of the ACA Carl Perkins Award, the Association for Counselor Education and Supervision's Program Supervisor Award, and the Southern Association for Counselor Education and Supervision's Program Supervisor Award, as well as numerous awards from the Maryland Association for Counseling and Development and from the state of Maryland for her work in student services and youth suicide prevention.

Kathleen McNinch completed her master's degree in the School Counseling Program of the Education Department at Loyola College in Maryland. She is currently a high school counselor in Howard County Public Schools, Maryland.

Michael D. Mong received a B.S. degree in psychology from Louisiana State University and is currently a Ph.D. student in school psychology at Mississippi State University. His research interests include language acquisition, behavior disorders, standardized versus nonstandardized testing procedures, and selective mutism. He is currently employed as a behavioral specialist with Head Start programs and is primarily responsible for student observations and assessments of both academics and behavioral concern.

Cheryl Moore-Thomas received her Ph.D. degree in counselor education from the University of Maryland. She is a national certified counselor. Currently, Dr. Moore-Thomas is an assistant professor of education in the school counseling program at Loyola College in Maryland. Over her professional career, she has published and presented in the areas of multicultural counseling competence, racial identity development of children and adolescents, and accountability in school counseling programs.

Deborah Newsome, Ph.D., LPC, NCC, is an assistant professor of counseling at Wake Forest University, North Carolina, where she teaches courses in career counseling, appraisal procedures, and statistics and supervises master's degree students in their field experiences. In addition to teaching and supervising, Dr. Newsome counsels children, adolescents, and families at a nonprofit mental health organization in Winston-Salem, North Carolina.

Masanori Ota is a graduate student pursuing an educational specialist degree in school psychology at Mississippi State University and is from Tokyo, Japan. Her research interests are functional behavioral assessment, functional behavioral analysis, and behavioral consultation in schools.

Carol Salisbury is a doctoral student in the Pastoral Counseling Department at Loyola College in Maryland. Her research interests include exploring the positive aspects of anger as a recuperative and useful emotion.

Carl J. Sheperis, Ph.D., NCC, LPC, is an assistant professor in the Department of Counseling, Educational Psychology, and Special Education at Mississippi State University. Dr. Sheperis's areas of specialization include assessment and treatment of behavioral disorders and psychopathology. He is co-owner of Behavioral Research, Assessment, and Training Services LLC, a psychological corporation primarily serving Head Start organizations.

CHAPTER 1

Basic Assessment Concepts

by Bradley T. Erford

This initial chapter provides a whirlwind tour through the critical terminology, purposes, and standards related to assessment. Assessment is sometimes viewed as having a language all its own, so professional counselors are well advised to learn this language in order to communicate with other professionals, and to advocate for, and make decisions in the best interests of, the clients and students they serve.

ASSESSMENT AND COUNSELING

Welcome to the world of counseling: a world of wonder, mystery, and fulfillment; a world where highly trained professional counselors attempt to understand and help people encountering trauma and challenges or adjusting to life circumstances; a world of clients and students (i.e., clients served by professional school counselors or college counselors) trying to get back on track. By nature, human beings are complex creatures made up of unique genetic structures and even more unique personal and psychosocial experiences. In the clinical sense, these factors combine to create clients and students who think, feel, and behave in individualistic ways—so individualistic that no clinician, no matter how skilled, can ever predict the client's actions with 100% accuracy. In this sense, people are somewhat like puzzles—some simpler to understand and solve than others, but all with pieces that never quite seem to fit, or are even missing. Nevertheless, the more professional counselors know about a client or student, the better they can understand and predict how the individual will react under certain circumstances.

This is what assessment is all about. It is integral to the counseling process; the professional counselor is *always* assessing. When a professional counselor first meets a student or client, the process of assessment for understanding begins. This process may be informal, formal, or somewhere in between; it may be structured, unstructured, or somewhere in between. The point is, assessment begins from the moment the professional counselor meets the student or client: Data are collected, impressions are formed, and pieces of the puzzle are collected, analyzed, and fitted. Assessment continues as the professional counselor helps the student or client to select therapeutic objectives and treatments. Assessment culminates in an evaluation of treatment outcomes to determine therapeutic success, or to obtain feedback indicating that other treatment methods are needed. Assessment *is* counseling, and counseling *is* assessment. Indeed, assessment is integral to every stage in the counseling process (Whiston, 2005).

We emphasize the interrelationship of assessment and counseling on the very first pages of this book because students new to the profession often show little excitement for a course in measurement or assessment. Unfortunately, counselor-educators who teach counseling assessment sometimes report that counseling students rate it low (close to research and statistics courses) on the "exciting courses scale." So please make the connection between assessment and counseling early in the course and your career: Assessment is the quickest way to understand students and clients. The better one understands clients or students, the better and faster one will be able to help them. Assessment saves the client time, money, and (most importantly) social and emotional pain. The more efficient a professional counselor becomes in knowing a student or client, the more effective and respected the counselor will become.

The purpose of this book is to help professional counselors to understand the most efficient and effective means for discovering, analyzing, and fitting the puzzle pieces together to understand and help students and clients. The reader will no doubt discover that some of the methods described are faster, more effective, technically more superior, and personally more appealing than others. There is wonderful diversity in how the puzzle pieces can be acquired and configured. Indeed, many clinicians assessing the same client through different methods may arrive at varying conclusions because of personal perspectives. Thus, in many ways this course, at its core, is about who you will become as a professional counselor. How will you discern the pieces of your developing professional identity, your strengths and weaknesses? How will you cope with the challenging coursework and its applications to clinical settings? What cognitive abilities, behavioral patterns, and personality dispositions will become barriers? Which will provide the resiliency needed to succeed? Let the assessment begin!

WHAT IS ASSESSMENT?

For all intents and purposes, and especially from a professional point of view, the terms *assessment* and *appraisal* are synonymous. In this book, we use the term **assessment** (or *psychological assessment*) consistently throughout. *Assessment* was defined in

Standards for Educational and Psychological Testing (AERA/APA/NCME, 1999, p. 3) as "a process that integrates test information with information from other sources (e.g., information from the individual's social, educational, employment, or psychological history)." Note that the preceding definition distinguishes *assessment* from *test, instrument,* or *inventory* in that assessment includes testing as only part of its process. Many authoritative sources differ slightly in their definitions of what comprises a psychological **test**. An often-cited definition of a **psychological test** is that provided by Anastasi and Urbina (1997, p. 4): "an objective and standardized measure of a sample of behavior." Assessment integrates tests in a way that helps a professional counselor to better understand clients and make decisions in their best interests.

Often overlooked, but implicit in the foregoing definition of a psychological test is the word *measure. Measure* implies that a quantity of some construct or concept will be determined: how much anxiety, intelligence, math skill, introversion, suicidal ideation, alcohol use, artistic interest, antisocial tendency, etc. The purpose of an assessment is to give the professional counselor valuable information regarding "how much" of a given characteristic the student or client possesses. Knowing how much helps to predict client behaviors, strengths, and weaknesses, thus facilitating important treatment or life decisions.

Second, assessments measure a *sample of behavior*. **Behavior** is what humans do, whether the "doing" be overt physical acts, emotional or affective displays, or cognitions that are conveyed to others. **Sampling** is key to understanding any psychological phenomenon. If a professional school counselor observes a student's activity level during different activities (e.g., physical education class, independent in-seat class work time, lecture presentation, lunchtime), these different samples of behavior will often lead to different observable data and subsequent conclusions. Likewise, in a clinical setting, professional counselors usually see clients only under fairly specific conditions (i.e., in an office), again leading to a specific sample of behavior. Samples of behavior assessed under various conditions are critical to understanding the student or client. These measures and observations allow professional counselors to make *inferences* about how clients will behave or perform under normal and unusual circumstances. Such inferences are indispensable to the client's insight and self-understanding, as well as to the insight of the professional counselor charged with the responsibility of helping the client to develop goals and an effective treatment plan.

When assessing a sample of behavior, it is important that the sample faithfully represent the total domain of behavior under study. For example, when assessing single-plus-single-digit addition without regrouping (i.e., 4 + 3, not 8 + 7), the test developer needs to determine how many problems of this type are required to assess a student's mastery of the behavioral domain—that is, how many of the 57 possible single-plus-single-digit-addition-without-regrouping problems would a child need to successfully perform before the examiner could have confidence the student had *mastered* this type of addition? One? Two? Five? All 57? Efficient sampling of behavior is crucial to effective assessment.

Sometimes the professional counselor is also interested in the perspectives of others (i.e., teacher, parent, spouse) who have observed a sample of the client's behaviors under various conditions. These more indirect methods help professional counselors to provide insights into student or client behavior in other environments not easily accessed by the clinician. The common factor here is that the data collection, analysis, and judgment of professional counselors are influenced by tangible observations of behavioral samples. But what if two professional counselors observe the same sample of behavior only to reach different conclusions?

As a final piece of the definition of a psychological test, the terms *standardized* and *objective* are meant to work hand in hand to address counselor judgment as a potential source of error. **Standardization** refers to the systematic collection and analysis of data. Cronbach (1984) provided a comprehensive definition of *standardization* when he referred to a standardized test as one in which exact devices, materials, verbal (or nonverbal) prompts, and scoring procedures have been fixed so that scores collected at various places and times and by different examiners are fully equivalent. **Objective** tests have scoring or observation criteria structured to such an extent that different examiners (e.g., trained judges, interviewers) have a very high likelihood of independently agreeing on a client's score on a given sample of performance behavior. To be sure, psychological assessments have varying degrees of standardization and objectivity. For example, on a multiple-choice test of written expression for a 5th-grade student, different examiners may easily agree that answer choice b is correct, but when asked to determine the maturity of written expression in this student's essay, less agreement is likely, because the scoring of essays often involves more **subjective** (less objective) scoring criteria. Of course, the more standardized the written-expression assessment procedures and the more objective the scoring procedures, the greater is the likelihood of examiner agreement.

Test developers strive to develop high-quality, accurate standardized and objective tests (samples of behavior), and professional counselors strive to administer these instruments according to standardized procedures and to score each according to objective criteria. Sounds like a perfect way to collect information about, and understand, a client, right? Unfortunately, even the best standardized and objective psychological assessments can lead to inaccurate conclusions. For example, the *Reynolds Adolescent Depression Scale—Second Edition* (*RADS-2*) (Reynolds, 2002), which will be discussed in Chapter 7, is incredibly easy to administer and score using the standardized procedures, and is very objective. However, if students or clients do not want a professional counselor to think they are depressed, they need only to "fake good" on their test responses, and the test score will not indicate significant levels of depression. Thus, an unsuspecting professional counselor may not reach the appropriate conclusion and may therefore not develop the most effective treatment plan for the client.

Test developers and assessment specialists have developed countermeasures to help detect dishonesty and inaccurate responses—for example, some clinical, personality, and behavioral inventories include *validity scales*. Also, professional counselors are trained to understand that all clients present information from their own point of view, and thus the counselor will seek validation of client perceptions from various sources of information (i.e., tests, inventories, rating scales, observations, interviews, questionnaires) and respondents (i.e., spouses, parents, teachers, peers) as possible and appropriate. These issues involve the reliability and validity of scores and the decisions based on those scores and will be addressed throughout the remainder of this book. But prior to entering that realm, one must understand the multiple purposes for which professional counselors use assessment.

The Purpose of Assessment

At least four purposes of assessment have been identified in the extant literature (Erford, 2006; Gregory, 1999; Sattler, 2001): screening, diagnosis, treatment planning and goal identification, and progress evaluation.

Screening

Screening is a quick procedure, usually involving a single measure, done for the purpose of determining whether deeper diagnostic assessment is necessary or warranted. A screening process is by no means comprehensive, and the instruments used for this purpose are sometimes held to lower standards of psychometric accuracy, although this is not always a desirable practice. Accuracy in screening is just as critical as accuracy in diagnosis because both procedures, done correctly, save students and clients emotional pain, time, and money. In all instances, professional counselors strive to use procedures that will maximize accurate decisions and minimize inaccurate decisions. For example, when conducting a screening procedure for depression, a professional counselor will frequently use a self-report inventory of depression with a predetermined cutoff to determine clinical significance. A client scoring above that cutoff score would be referred for further (diagnostic) assessment. Or, when a professional school counselor conducts a screening to determine which students are at risk for reading difficulties, students scoring below the predetermined level (perhaps ≤ 25th percentile) will subsequently be referred for deeper-level assessments to further diagnose any reading difficulties and develop an effective treatment plan. Screening is an efficient first step in an assessment process because not every student or client needs diagnostic assessment. Diagnostic assessment tends to be more expensive and more time consuming than screening and requires a greater level of skill to conduct, but there is a worthwhile trade-off in terms of efficiency and accuracy.

Anastasi and Urbina (1997) referred to accurate identification decisions (sometimes called *hits*) as *true positives* (clients who have a condition are identified by the screening test as having the condition) and *true negatives* (clients who do not have the condition are identified by the screening test as not having the condition). Inaccurate decisions (sometimes called *misses*) were referred to as *false positives* (clients who do not really have the condition are identified as having it) and *false negatives* (clients who really do have the condition are not identified as having it). (A graphic of these concepts can be found in Figure 4.2.) In screening procedures, professional counselors are most concerned with maximizing hits and minimizing misses, particularly false negatives, because these clients have the problem of concern but do not receive further diagnostic assessment to address the problem. They "slip through the cracks."

Diagnosis

Diagnosis entails "a detailed analysis of an individual's strengths and weaknesses, with the general goal of arriving at a classification decision" (Erford, 2006, p. 2). Diagnosis always involves more than one measure and often includes a *battery* of tests. Such a battery is usually composed of a series of tests that are integrated to yield specific information or identification decisions. For example, the *Wechsler Intelligence Scale for Children—Fourth Edition* (*WISC-IV*) (Wechsler, 2001a) and the *Woodcock-Johnson: Tests of Achievement—Third Edition* (*WJ-III ACH*) (Woodcock, Mather, & McGrew, 2001) are frequently used in conjunction to determine the existence and extent of learning disabilities in school-aged children. In some cases, diagnostic assessment can be used to enhance normal development, as when a client presents for career counseling and the professional counselor wants to assess the individual's interests, competencies, values, and interpersonal strengths and weaknesses to help the person to arrive at an acceptable career goal, educational plan, or vocational strategy. Similarly, in premarital counseling, which is currently becoming more popular, marriage and family counselors use diagnostic assessments to aid in leading couples to interpersonal and intrapersonal insights that will strengthen the bonds of the relationship and help the couple to predict and navigate the challenges of marriage and family life.

In general, diagnosis in counseling can be construed as trying to understand what is happening with a client, what the problem is, what causes or maintains the problem, and what strengths the client may harness to overcome the problem. However, in clinical contexts, diagnostic assessment has classification or diagnosis as its goal. This process generally requires the use of a classification system, and most professional counselors in clinical practice use the *Diagnostic and Statistical Manual of Mental Disorders—Fourth Edition—Text Revision* (*DSM-IV-TR*) (APA, 2000). The *DSM-IV-TR* provides clinicians from all mental health professions (e.g., professional counselors, psychiatrists, psychologists, social workers) with a standardized set of criteria upon which to base a diagnosis (i.e., a clinical description) of a client's presenting condition. Such a system facilitates accurate, reliable decisions and helps to inform the professional counselor of appropriate treatment strategies. The *DSM* is to mental health practitioners what the *International Classification of Diseases* (*ICD*) is to physicians and to mental health workers in most other countries that do not use the *DSM*. However, there is disagreement in the counseling profession regarding the helpfulness of diagnosis to clients, as it frequently results in *labeling* of a client that may lead to a plethora of unintended and undesirable consequences (see Sattler, 2001).

Treatment Planning and Goal Identification

Helping clients and students is what counseling is all about. Assessment helps clients and students to understand where they are and where they want to go, a key facet of developing a client's goals and objectives for counseling. A counseling process that does not have well-defined and measurable goals has no focus or direction, nor does it allow the client and professional counselor to know when the goals of counseling have been achieved. Thus, a primary purpose of assessment in counseling is to help establish counseling goals, often through a combination of assessment methods, including interviewing and standardized testing.

In addition, the information garnered from an initial assessment can be helpful in planning a client's treatment. Frequently, student or client strengths, weaknesses, challenges, and resiliency factors and resources are confirmed or better understood through assessment procedures. "Treatment planning must flow logically from assessment results, fit the given environmental context of the client, and be individualized to mesh with the client's strengths and weaknesses" (Erford, 2006, p. 3). After the client and professional counselor agree on the goals and objectives to be pursued through counseling, the counselor must consider the most effective treatment options to obtain the desired outcomes. Thus a primary focus of the initial assessment is to uncover student or client strengths and resources in order to plan for the most effective treatment. Of course, counseling would be incredibly simplified if specific test scores or client responses directly implied specific treatments or interventions. Unfortunately, the complexity of client problems rarely leads to such simplistic remedies. Important sources of information to help professional counselors with treatment planning are the outcomes research literature found in professional journals and compendiums of this research (e.g., Sexton, Whiston, Bleuer, & Walz, 1997; Whiston, 2003a). As a final note, treatment planning usually gets easier with experience and, to some, may be more akin to art than science. In some employment settings, professional counselors often approach treatment of client problems from a theoretical paradigm that they are proficient in or comfortable with. When it comes to treatment planning, assessment often informs the professional counselor's practice.

Progress Evaluation

Once goals for counseling have been agreed on and treatment has begun, it is a professional counselor's responsibility to ensure that the treatment is helpful to a client (and, even more important, not harmful). This process is referred to as *progress evaluation* or *outcomes evaluation* and, unfortunately, is frequently minimized in, or eliminated from, a treatment regimen. Failure to periodically evaluate treatment progress is unethical and unprofessional, not to mention inefficient. If a treatment is having no positive effects and a professional counselor is not assessing its impact, the client is wasting time and money while continuing to experience the discomfort and emotional pain that brought the client to counseling. Tests and inventories can be very helpful aids in assessing treatment outcomes.

The first step in evaluating progress is to establish a baseline measure of the student's or client's condition. This evaluation is generally done during an intake interview and initial assessment but can also be done at the time a counseling goal is established. Progress evaluation can be done formally or informally, subjectively or objectively. For example, an informal, subjective method would be to ask clients to rate their own feelings of anxiety (disorganization, depression, distractibility, etc.) on a scale from 0 to 10, with 0 being the total absence of anxiety and 10 being intense anxiety. If the client self-rates as a 9, this score becomes a baseline for comparison in future similar assessments, perhaps conducted at the beginning of each session over the following weeks. A more formal, objective method might involve a test such as the *Beck Anxiety Inventory* (*BAI*) (Beck, 1993). The client's initial score would serve as the baseline, and the counselor would periodically readminister the *BAI* to assess whether the client's anxious symptoms have declined. Furthermore, given the client's baseline score, it is possible to establish a goal of a certain score on the *BAI* as a target to determine when the anxiety has subsided to a substantial enough degree that termination of counseling can be considered.

The four purposes reviewed above provide a framework for the general use of assessment, but assessment is best applied to the practical aspects of counseling when fully integrated into the counseling process. The next section presents this fully integrated model.

HOW IS ASSESSMENT USED IN COUNSELING?

As mentioned previously, assessment is counseling, and counseling is assessment. Assessment is totally integrated into the counseling process. Whiston (2005) reported that most counseling processes delineate at least the following four steps: (1) assessing client problems, (2) conceptualizing and defining client problems, (3) selecting and implementing effective treatments, and (4) evaluating counseling effectiveness.

In the first stage, professional counselors engage in *screening and diagnostic assessment procedures to understand student or client concerns, issues, and problems.* It is particularly important that professional counselors conduct a comprehensive interview and administer appropriate tests and inventories to assess for broad functioning in the interest of "leaving no stone unturned." Incomplete assessments lead to incomplete and ineffective treatment plans. It is best practice to ask these broad questions and conduct formalized assessments in the beginning of counseling rather than not ask, thus risking an underestimation of the scope of a problem or missing it altogether. The type of formal assessment used is often dependent on the nature of the setting and on the training and experience of the professional counselor. Elmore, Ekstrom, Diamond, and Whittaker (1993) reported that nearly three-quarters of the professional counselors surveyed indicated that assessments and tests were either important or very important in their work setting. Predictably, the work of professional school counselors most frequently involved contact with achievement, intelligence, aptitude, and career or vocational measures (Elmore et al.; Giordano & Schweibert, 1997), while the work of community and mental health counselors most frequently involved contact with clinical diagnostic, personality, intelligence, and vocational inventories (Bubenzer, Zimpfer, & Mahrle, 1990; Frauenhoffer, Ross, Gfeller, Searight, & Piotrowski, 1998).

During the second stage of the counseling process, *conceptualizing and defining problems,* incomplete information will again limit a professional counselor's effectiveness (Mohr, 1995). Professional counselors must continuously assess their understanding of client concerns during the process of constructing a working definition of a client's problem. Counselors at this point must reciprocally rule in and rule out diagnostic categorizations and determine the frequency and severity of client concerns. Again, attention to comprehensiveness and detail at this stage will lead to a more effective treatment outcome.

Treatment selection and implementation relies on an analysis of the results of assessments conducted during the first two stages of the counseling process. Again, the professional counselor questions the comprehensiveness of previous assessments and conducts additional assessment as required. Most importantly, process evaluation begins at this time; it is the duty of the professional counselor to continuously assess the impact of the treatment strategies implemented. In evaluation parlance, this is referred to as *formative assessment* and allows for midcourse adjustments in treatment implementation to provide the most effective treatment possible. Formative assessment helps determine whether or not progress is being made toward treatment goals.

Finally, during the fourth stage of counseling, *evaluation,* determinations must be made regarding the overall effectiveness of treatment—a process that evaluation specialists refer to as *summative evaluation* or *outcomes assessment.* One of the reasons a baseline measurement is so highly recommended in counseling is that it provides a starting point for treatment and evaluation. Evaluation at the end of counseling provides another point of comparison that allows professional counselors to demonstrate to clients, students, and other stakeholders (i.e., employers, parents, insurance companies) that substantive, measurable gains have been noted, counseling goals have been met, and counseling services have been effective.

By now the meaning of the statement "assessment is counseling, and counseling is assessment" should be amply clear. Indeed, there was a time, during the 1930s and 1940s, when assessment and counseling were viewed synonymously (Hood & Johnson, 2002). Assessment is an essential, integrated part of an effective counseling process.

ASSESSMENT COMPETENCE AND PROFESSIONAL COUNSELORS

Professional counselors have a professional responsibility to become competent in the effective use of assessment procedures. A number of professional associations, scholars, and accreditation organizations have taken the lead in specifying what professional counselors need to know and be able to do in order to demonstrate assessment competence, while others have focused on the question of why assessment competence is intrinsic to effective counseling. This section explores the why, while the section that follows focuses on the what (i.e., the training standards for professional counselors).

Whiston (2005) provided six reasons why professional counselors must become proficient in the use of assessment procedures. Assessment proficiency is a *professional expectation.* The American Counseling Association's *Code of Ethics* (ACA, 2005a) dedicated an entire section to an explanation of ethical uses of tests, and the Council for Accreditation of Counseling and Related Educational Programs (CACREP), an organization that accredits university counselor education programs, dedicated one of its eight core curricular areas to the study of assessment. As a result, the public expects professional counselors to be proficient in the use and interpretation of tests. In fact, the use of formalized assessment can frequently lead to a perception of *enhanced credibility* on the part of clients (Goodyear, 1990; Sexton et al., 1997). Efficient *identification of problems* usually results from the competent use of tests (Anastasi & Urbina, 1997; Duckworth, 1990), and this efficiency is normally increased when professional counselors use multimethod assessment batteries (Meyer et al., 2001) rather than general interviewing procedures. Likewise, multimethod and multirespondent assessment methods usually help professional counselors uncover *diverse, even unique, client information* (Meyer et al.) and even lead to client or student insight and learning (Campbell, 2000; Sax, 1997). In addition, assessment helps *identify strengths and weaknesses* of clients and students, and professional counselors use this information to *facilitate decision making* (Drummond, 2000; Sax). Frequently, clients who "see" objective testing results documenting their interpersonal and intrapersonal strengths and weaknesses develop the motivation to make life decisions and to adjust their life course accordingly. Insightful realizations and details of conversations that occur during the course of counseling are sometimes forgotten or minimized as time goes on. Assessment results provide a concrete, visual record that can be referred to time and again to bring the counseling back on course and to show measurable progress. Now that we have addressed the why of assessment in counseling, let us turn our attention to the "what."

Training Standards for Professional Counselors

The Council for Accreditation of Counseling and Related Educational Programs (CACREP) is the national organization, affiliated with the American Counseling Association, that accredits universities with counseling programs meeting rigorous professional and curricular standards. CACREP offers accreditation for master's-level specialty counseling programs in the areas of career counseling; college counseling; community counseling; marital, couple, and family counseling and therapy; mental health counseling; school counseling; student affairs counseling; and doctoral programs in counselor education and supervision. The specific standard addressing the curricular requirements for assessment is Section II.K.7, found in Table 1.1. The reader will note that these standards align very well with the content of this book.

Professional Counseling Organizations and Assessment

Numerous professional counseling organizations and licensing or certification boards exist to promote best practices and develop policies and procedures that advocate for client or student needs and protect the public from harm. The American Counseling Association (www.counseling.org) serves as the parent or umbrella organization for all professional counselors and various professional counselor specialties in the United States. In this context, counseling specialties (called *divisions* within ACA's structure) are defined as counselor practitioner entities that have a guild or occupational presence in the counseling profession and job market. The fol-

Table 1.1   Assessment curriculum standard from section II.K.7
of the *CACREP 2001 Accreditation Manual*

7. ASSESSMENT—studies that provide an understanding of individual and group
approaches to assessment and evaluation, including all of the following:
    a. historical perspectives concerning the nature and meaning of assessment;
    b. basic concepts of standardized and nonstandardized testing and other assessment
    techniques including norm-referenced and criterion-referenced assessment,
    environmental assessment, performance assessment, individual and group test and
    inventory methods, behavioral observations, and computer-managed and computer-
    assisted methods;
    c. statistical concepts, including scales of measurement, measures of central tendency,
    indices of variability, shapes and types of distributions, and correlations;
    d. reliability (i.e., theory of measurement error, models of reliability, and the use of
    reliability information);
    e. validity (i.e., evidence of validity, types of validity, and the relationship between
    reliability and validity);
    f. age, gender, sexual orientation, ethnicity, language, disability, culture, spirituality, and
    other factors related to the assessment and evaluation of individuals, groups, and
    specific populations;
    g. strategies for selecting, administering, and interpreting assessment and evaluation
    instruments and techniques in counseling;
    h. an understanding of general principles and methods of case conceptualization,
    assessment, and/or diagnoses of mental and emotional status; and ethical and legal
    considerations.

lowing are among the current 19 ACA divisions (specialty areas) with special interests in the professional practice of assessment:

- American College Counseling Association (ACCA; www.collegecounseling.org)
- American Mental Health Counselors Association (AMHCA; www.amhca.org)
- American Rehabilitation Counseling Association (ARCA; www.arcaweb.org)
- American School Counselor Association (ASCA; www.schoolcounselor.org)
- Association for Assessment in Counseling and Education (AACE; http://aace.ncat.edu)
- Association for Counselor Education and Supervision (ACES; www.acesonline.net)
- International Association of Addiction and Offender Counselors (IAAOC; www.iaaoc.org)
- International Association of Marriage and Family Counselors (IAMFC; www.iamfc.com)
- National Career Development Association (NCDA; www.ncda.org)

All of these organizations' websites, mailing addresses, and phone number con-
tacts can be located through ACA's main website, www.counseling.org.

Think About It 1.1   Visit the ACA website at www.counseling.org or link to any of the websites individually listed above. Which professional organizations offer services and products helpful to your development as a professional counselor? Which are you interested in joining?

Another major influence in the counseling world is the American Psychological Association (APA; www.apa.org). APA serves as an umbrella organization for many other divisions dedicated to serving the public and the agenda of practitioner psychologists, some of whom are referred to as counseling psychologists. APA divisions serving specialties similar to ACA divisions include:

- Division 17—Society of Counseling Psychology (www.div17.org)
- Division 22—Rehabilitation Psychology (www.apa.org/divisions/div22)
- Division 28—Psychopharmacology and Substance Abuse (www.apa.org /divisions/div28)
- Division 29—Psychotherapy (www.divisionofpsychotherapy.org)
- Division 42—Psychologists in Independent Practice (www.division42.org)
- Division 43—Family Psychology (www.apa.org/divisions/div43)
- Division 50—Addictions (www.apa.org/divisions/div50)

A number of additional national associations exist that are not affiliated with ACA or APA, but which have substantial counselor and therapist memberships and legislative agendas, including:

- American Association for Marriage and Family Therapy (AAMFT; www .aamft.org)
- Association for Addiction Professionals (NAADAC; www.naadac.org)
- National Association of Social Workers (NASW; www.NASWDC.org)

Finally, all states have licensing boards that regulate the practice of psychology and/or counseling within their borders. Because laws and regulations vary substantially from state to state, necessary qualifications and what professional counselors can do when practicing within these states also vary. Add to this the turf wars between psychologist and professional counselor licensing boards and professional associations that flare up in various states around the country, and the whole issue of which assessments and tests professional counselors can administer and interpret, where, and when can become quite confusing. It is unlikely that this situation will change anytime soon. It is incumbent upon professional counselors to stay abreast of practice developments within their state.

Assessment Training Standards

The area of psychological assessment is perhaps among the most contentious and hard-fought battlegrounds in counseling. As this book goes to press, battles between psychologists and professional counselors over the right to use psychological tests in clinical practice are being fought in California, Indiana, Illinois, Louisiana, and Maryland. Organizations, including the ACA, AACE, Association of Test Publishers (ATP; www.testpublishers.org), and Fair Access Coalition on Testing (FACT; www.fairaccess.org), are leading a national effort to allow qualified psychologists and counselors access to psychological tests in clinical practice. An ongoing stumbling block to access has been forging agreement on the term *qualified*. ACA recently developed a position statement on test user qualifications with the goal that the document would serve as a consensus-building device (see Box 1.1).

Box 1.1   ACA Policy Statement on Test User Qualifications
Standards for Qualifications of Test Users

American Counseling Association

The professional qualifications essential to the use of tests in counseling arise from a synthesis of knowledge, skills, and ethics. While some professional groups are seeking to control and restrict the use of psychological tests,* the American Counseling Association believes firmly that one's right to use tests in counseling practice is directly related to competence. This competence is achieved through education, training, and experience in the field of testing. Thus, professional counselors with a master's degree or higher and appropriate coursework in appraisal/assessment, supervision, and experience are qualified to use objective tests. With additional training and experience, professional counselors are also able to administer projective tests, individual intelligence tests, and clinical diagnostic tests. This training may occur in graduate school, in post-grad professional development instruction, or in supervised training in use of the test. Professional counselors are qualified to use tests and assessments in counseling practice to the degree that they possess the appropriate knowledge and skills, including the following areas:

1. Skill in practice and knowledge of theory relevant to the testing context and type of counseling specialty.
Assessment and testing must be integrated into the context of the theory and knowledge of a specialty area, not as a separate act, role, or entity. In addition, professional counselors should be skilled in treatment practice with the population being served.

2. A thorough understanding of testing theory, techniques of test construction, and test reliability and validity.
Included in this knowledge base are methods of item selection, theories of human nature that underlie a given test, reliability, and validity. Knowledge of reliability includes, at a minimum: methods by which it is determined,

*For the purpose of this document, terms such as inventory, instrument, measure, and scale are encompassed by the terms test or assessment.

continued

Box 1.1 continued

such as domain sampling, test-retest, parallel forms, split-half, and inter-item consistency; the strengths and limitations of each of these methods; the standard error of measurement, which indicates how accurately a person's test score reflects their true score of the trait being measured; and true score theory, which defines a test score as an *estimate* of what is true. Knowledge of validity includes, at a minimum: types of validity, including content, criterion-related (both predictive and concurrent), and construct methods of assessing each type of validity, including the use of correlation; and the meaning and significance of standard error of estimate.

3. A working knowledge of sampling techniques, norms, and descriptive, correlational, and predictive statistics.

Important topics in sampling include sample size, sampling techniques, and the relationship between sampling and test accuracy. A working knowledge of descriptive statistics includes, at a minimum: probability theory; measures of central tendency; multi-modal and skewed distributions; measures of variability, including variance and standard deviation; and standard scores, including deviation IQ's, z-scores, T scores, percentile ranks, stanines/stens, normal curve equivalents, grade- and age-equivalents. Knowledge of correlation and prediction includes, at a minimum: the principle of least squares; the direction and magnitude of relationship between two sets of scores; deriving a regression equation; the relationship between regression and correlation; and the most common procedures and formulas used to calculate correlations.

4. Ability to review, select, and administer tests appropriate for clients or students and the context of the counseling practice.

Professional counselors using tests should be able to describe the purpose and use of different types of tests, including the most widely used tests for their setting and purposes. Professional counselors use their understanding of sampling, norms, test construction, validity, and reliability to accurately assess the strengths, limitations, and appropriate applications of a test for the clients being served. Professional counselors using tests also should be aware of the potential for error when relying on computer printouts of test interpretation. For accuracy of interpretation, technological resources must be augmented by a counselor's firsthand knowledge of the client and the test-taking context.

5. Skill in administration of tests and interpretation of test scores.

Competent test users implement appropriate and standardized administration procedures. This requirement enables professional counselors to provide consultation and training to others who assist with test administration and scoring. In addition to standardized procedures, test users provide testing environments that are comfortable and free of distraction. Skilled interpretation requires a strong working knowledge of the theory underlying the test,

test's purpose, statistical meaning of test scores, and norms used in test construction. Skilled interpretation also requires an understanding of the similarities and differences between the client or student and the norm samples used in test construction. Finally, it is essential that clear and accurate communication of test score meaning in oral or written form to clients, students, or appropriate others be provided.

6. Knowledge of the impact of diversity on testing accuracy, including age, gender, ethnicity, race, disability, and linguistic differences.
Professional counselors using tests should be committed to fairness in every aspect of testing. Information gained and decisions made about the client or student are valid only to the degree that the test accurately and fairly assesses the client's or student's characteristics. Test selection and interpretation are done with an awareness of the degree to which items may be culturally biased or the norming sample not reflective or inclusive of the client's or student's diversity. Test users understand that age and physical disability differences may impact the client's ability to perceive and respond to test items. Test scores are interpreted in light of the cultural, ethnic, disability, or linguistic factors that may impact an individual's score. These include visual, auditory, and mobility disabilities that may require appropriate accommodation in test administration and scoring. Test users understand that certain types of norms and test score interpretation may be inappropriate, depending on the nature and purpose of the testing.

7. Knowledge and skill in the professionally responsible use of assessment and evaluation practice.
Professional counselors who use tests act in accordance with the ACA's *Code of Ethics and Standards of Practice* (2005a); *Responsibilities of Users of Standardized Tests—Third Edition* (*RUST-3*) (AACE, 2003a); *Code of Fair Testing Practices in Education* (JCTP, 2002); *Rights and Responsibilities of Test Takers: Guidelines and Expectations* (JCTP, 2000); and *Standards for Educational and Psychological Testing* (AERA/APA/NCME, 1999). In addition, professional school counselors act in accordance with the American School Counselor Association's (ASCA's) *Ethical Standards for School Counselors* (ASCA, 1992). Test users should understand the legal and ethical principles and practices regarding test security, using copyrighted materials, and unsupervised use of assessment instruments that are not intended for self-administration. When using and supervising the use of tests, qualified test users demonstrate an acute understanding of the paramount importance of the well-being of clients and the confidentiality of test scores. Test users seek on-going educational and training opportunities to maintain competence and acquire new skills in assessment and evaluation.

continued

Box 1.1 continued

References

American Counseling Association. (2005a). *Code of Ethics and Standards of Practice.* Alexandria, VA: Author.

American Educational Research Association, American Psychological Association, National Council on Measurement in Education. (1999). *Standards for Educational and Psychological Testing.* Washington, DC: American Educational Research Association.

American School Counselor Association. (1992). *Ethical Standards for School Counselors.* Alexandria, VA: Author.

Association for Assessment in Counseling. (2003a). *Responsibilities of Users of Standardized Tests* (*RUST*). Alexandria, VA: Author.

Joint Committee on Testing Practices. (2000). *Rights and Responsibilities of Test Takers: Guidelines and Expectations.* Washington, DC: Author.

Joint Committee on Testing Practices. (2002). *Code of Fair Testing Practices in Education.* Washington, DC: Author.

Note: Approved by the American Counseling Association (ACA) Governing Council in March 2003, Anaheim, CA. The Standards for Test Use Task Force was an *ad hoc* committee of the American Counseling Association. The following counseling and education assessment professionals contributed to the drafting of this document: Dr. Bradley T. Erford (Chair), Mr. Alan Basham, Dr. Janet Wall, Dr. Craig S. Cashwell, and Dr. Gerald Juhnke.

The Association for Assessment in Counseling and Education's (AACE) *Responsibilities of Users of Standardized Tests—Third Edition* (*RUST-3*) (AACE, 2003a) statement is one of the most important documents speaking to standards for test users. The *RUST-3* statement addresses the issues of test user qualifications, technical knowledge, test selection, test administration, test scoring, interpreting test results, and communicating test results.

AACE is a division of ACA and has been collaborating with the *practitioner divisions* of ACA (i.e., divisions that serve employment groups, such as school, mental health, substance abuse, and marriage and family counselors) to develop training standards for each specialty area. The goal of this initiative is to standardize the assessment training within various counseling specialty areas so that all professional counselors emerging from a counselor education program will have the knowledge, skill, and training to use psychological tests relevant to their clinical practice. The documents shown in Exhibits 1.a and 1.b, obtained from the AACE/International Association for Addiction and Offender Counselors (IAAOCC) and the AACE/American School Counselor Association (ASCA), contain current assessment training standards for the specialty areas of substance abuse counseling and school counseling. Assessment standards for mental health counselors, career counselors, and marriage and family counselors are still under

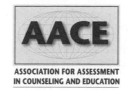

**ASSOCIATION FOR ASSESSMENT
IN COUNSELING AND EDUCATION**

Standards for Assessment in Substance Abuse Counseling

These training standards provide a description of the knowledge and skills needed by substance abuse counselors in the areas of assessment and evaluation. Because effectiveness in assessment and evaluation is critical to effective counseling, these training standards are important for substance abuse counselor education and practice. Consistent with existing Council for Accreditation of Counseling and Related Educational Programs (CACREP) standards for preparing counselors, they focus on standards for individual counselors and the content of counselor education programs. The standards, which represent aspirations for competent professional practice, can be used by counselor and assessment educators as a guide in the development and evaluation of substance abuse counselor preparation programs, workshops, in-services, and other continuing education opportunities. They may also be used by substance abuse counselors to evaluate their own professional development and continuing education needs.

During training, substance abuse counselors should meet each of the following assessment standards and have the specific skills listed under each standard.

Standard I. Substance abuse counselors are able to assess the effects and withdrawal symptoms of commonly abused drugs. Substance abuse counselors can:
1. Assess for and recognize acute intoxication syndromes for commonly abused chemicals (i.e., alcohol, benzodiazepines, marijuana, cocaine).
2. Assess for and recognize withdrawal complications (i.e., seizures, delirium tremens, hallucinations).
3. Assess for and recognize the effects of cross-addiction and dual addiction disorders.
4. Assess for and recognize symptoms of inhalant use (e.g. the smell of fuel on clothes, red eyes, runny nose, cough).

Standard II. Substance abuse counselors can assess the broad spectrum of concomitant disorders. Substance abuse counselors can:
1. Assess for other addictive disorders (i.e., gambling, food, sex).
2. Determine if a psychological disorder (i.e., anxiety, depression, panic, Post Traumatic Stress Disorder) was present prior to, or the result of, clients' substance use.
3. Assess for Attention-Deficit/Hyperactive Disorder (AD/HD).
4. Assess for suicidal or homicidal ideation.
5. Assess for the presence or possibility of domestic violence.
6. Use and interpret the results of adult and adolescent intelligence instruments.

Standard III. Substance abuse counselors are skilled in evaluating the technical quality and appropriateness of testing instruments. Substance abuse counselors can:
1. Identify acceptable reliability levels for instruments.
2. Identify appropriate types of validity for commonly-used instruments.
3. Evaluate the procedures used to validate commonly-used instruments.
4. Locate testing instruments and information about instruments for special populations (e.g. visually impaired, nonreaders).
5. Use computerized assessment instrument.
6. Articulate the limitations of commonly-used instruments within the substance abuse counseling field.

Standard IV. Substance abuse counselors are knowledgeable regarding qualitative assessment procedures including structured and semi-structured clinical interviews. Substance abuse counselors:
1. Are familiar with the advantages and disadvantages of structured and semi-structured clinical interviews.
2. Are familiar with qualitative assessment procedures (e.g. role playing, life line assessments, direct and indirect observations).
3. Understand the advantages and disadvantages of qualitative assessment procedures.
4. Understand the concepts of continuous assessment and wraparound services.

Exhibit 1.a Standards for Assessment in Substance Abuse Counseling

Source: Reprinted by permission of the Association for Assessment in Counseling/American Counseling Association.

Standard V. Substance abuse counselors employ multiple methods when assessing clients and monitoring the efficacy of treatment. Substance abuse counselors:
1. Use paper and pencil or computerized instruments and structured interviews, as appropriate.
2. Whenever possible, consult with and interview family, friends, and other corroborating sources of information, while always obtaining written consent to gather information from sources other than the client.
3. Monitor client progress throughout the counseling process.

Standard VI. Substance abuse counselors are skilled in interpreting assessment results with clients. Substance abuse counselors can:
1. Interpret assessment results in a helpful manner that emphasizes clients' strengths as well as possible problem areas.
2. Explain to clients the steps that are necessary to share testing results with others (e.g. informed consent).

Standard VII. Substance abuse counselors are skilled in using assessment results to develop and evaluate effective treatment interventions. Substance abuse counselors can:
1. Accurately score, analyze, and interpret the results of testing.
2. Create specific treatment plans based upon the results of testing.

Standard VIII. Substance abuse counselors are aware of the need for professional development within the assessment area. Substance abuse counselors:
1. Participate in training needed to keep abreast of new assessment instruments, procedures, and issues.
2. Keep up to date with advancements in the field of assessment by reading the appropriate professional journals, test manuals, and reports.
3. Join professional associations that provide relevant assessment and substance abuse information.

Standard IX. Substance abuse counselors are aware of the appropriate use of assessment instruments in research. Substance abuse counselors use assessment instruments:
1. To determine the efficacy of their interventions.
2. Appropriate for the intended population/clients.
3. In accordance with the American Counseling Association's Ethical Standards, Code of Fair Testing Practices, Standards for Educational and Psychological Testing, Responsibilities of Users of Standardized Tests, and Test Takers' Rights and Responsibilities.

Standard XI. Counselor educators and supervisors of substance abuse counselors-in-training are able to effectively train counselors in the area of substance abuse assessment. Counselor educators and supervisors:
1. Keep current with scholarship related to how to teach counselors-in-training how to best use assessment instruments in their work with clients.
2. Are knowledgeable in the selection, use, evaluation, and interpretation of assessment instruments.

Definitions of Terms
Assessment: active collection of information about individuals, populations, or treatment programs.
Instruments: standardized or nonstandardized tests, interviews, rating scales, inventories, or checklists used by mental health counselors to better understand the client; the client's past history; the client's current social, employment, physical or interpersonal environment; the client's intellectual functioning; the client's personality; or the client's presenting concerns.
Standards: minimal levels of skill, knowledge, or training.
Structured clinical interviews: clinical interviews with individuals, couples, families, or groups in which the mental health counselor asks questions precisely as directed by the instrument's author(s). Questions are posed in the order defined by the authors, and responses are recorded according to specific directions.
Unstructured clinical interviews: clinical interview in which the mental health counselor is free to pursue related lines of inquiry to gain needed or pertinent information.

Source: Reprinted with permission from the Association for Assessment in Counseling and Education. No further reproduction authorized without written permission from the Association for Assessment in Counseling and Education.

Note: These standards were developed as a joint effort between the Association for Assessment in Counseling and Education (AACE) and the International Association of Addictions and Offenders Counselors (IAAOC). The joint committee included Dr. Bradley T. Erford (Chair), Dr. Gerald Juhnke, Dr. Russell Curtis, Mr. Joe Jordan, Dr. Kenneth Coll.

Exhibit 1.a   continued

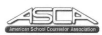

**Approved by the American School Counselor Association
on September 21, 1998,
and by the Association for Assessment in Counseling
on September 10, 1998[1]**

The purpose of these competencies is to provide a description of the knowledge and skills that school counselors need in the areas of assessment and evaluation. Because effectiveness in assessment and evaluation is critical to effective counseling, these competencies are important for school counselor education and practice. Although consistent with existing Council for Accreditation of Counseling and Related Educational Programs (CACREP) and National Association of State Directors of Teacher Education and Certification (NASDTEC) standards for preparing counselors, they focus on competencies of individual counselors rather than content of counselor education programs.

The competencies can be used by counselor and assessment educators as a guide in the development and evaluation of school counselor preparation programs, workshops, inservice, and other continuing education opportunities. They may also be used by school counselors to evaluate their own professional development and continuing education needs.

School counselors should meet each of the nine numbered competencies and have the specific skills listed under each competency.

Competency 1. School counselors are skilled in choosing assessment strategies.
  a. They can describe the nature and use of different types of formal and informal assessments, including questionnaires, checklists, interviews, inventories, tests, observations, surveys, and performance assessments, and work with individuals skilled in clinical assessment.
  b. They can specify the types of information most readily obtained from different assessment approaches.
  c. They are familiar with resources for critically evaluating each type of assessment and can use them in choosing appropriate assessment strategies.
  d. They are able to advise and assist others (e.g., a school district) in choosing appropriate assessment strategies.

Competency 2. School counselors can identify, access, and evaluate the most commonly used assessment instruments.
  a. They know which assessment instruments are most commonly used in school settings to assess intelligence, aptitude, achievement, personality, work values, and interests, including computer-assisted versions and other alternate formats.
  b. They know the dimensions along which assessment instruments should be evaluated, including purpose, validity, utility, norms, reliability and measurement error, score reporting method, and consequences of use.
  c. They can obtain and evaluate information about the quality of those assessment instruments.

Competency 3. School counselors are skilled in the techniques of administration and methods of scoring assessment instruments.
  a. They can implement appropriate administration procedures, including administration using computers.
  b. They can standardize administration of assessments when interpretation is in relation to external norms.
  c. They can modify administration of assessments to accommodate individual differences consistent with publisher recommendations and current statements of professional practice.
  d. They can provide consultation, information, and training to others who assist with administration and scoring.
  e. They know when it is necessary to obtain informed consent from parents or guardians before administering an assessment.

Competency 4. School counselors are skilled in interpreting and reporting assessment results.
  a. They can explain scores that are commonly reported, such as percentile ranks, standard scores, and grade equivalents. They can interpret a confidence interval for an individual score based on a standard error of measurement.
  b. They can evaluate the appropriateness of a norm group when interpreting the scores of an individual or a group.
  c. They are skilled in communicating assessment information to others, including teachers, administrators, students, parents, and the community. They are aware of the rights students and parents have to know assessment results and decisions made as a consequence of any assessment.
  d. They can evaluate their own strengths and limitations in the use of assessment instruments and in assessing students with disabilities or linguistic or cultural differences. They know how to identify professionals with appropriate training and experience for consultation.
  e. They know the legal and ethical principles about confidentiality and disclosure of assessment information and recognize the need to abide by district policy on retention and use of assessment information.

Source: Reprinted with permission from the Association for Assessment in Counseling and Education. No further reproduction authorized without written permission from the Association for Assessment in Counseling and Education.

[1]A joint committee of the American School Counselor Association (ASCA) and the Association for Assessment in Counseling (AAC) was appointed by the respective presidents in 1993 with the charge to draft a statement about school counselor preparation in assessment and evaluation. Committee members were Ruth Ekstrom (AAC), Patricia Elmore (AAC, Chair, 1997–1999), Daren Hutchinson (ASCA), Marjorie Mastie (AAC), Kathy O'Rourke (ASCA), William Schafer (AAC, Chair, 1993–1997), Thomas Trotter (ASCA), and Barbara Webster (ASCA).

Exhibit 1.b Competencies in Assessment and Evaluation for School Counselors

Competency 5.   School counselors are skilled in using assessment results in decision making.
   a. They recognize the limitations of using a single score in making an educational decision and know how to obtain multiple sources of information to improve such decisions.
   b. They can evaluate their own expertise for making decisions based on assessment results. They also can evaluate the limitations of conclusions provided by others, including the reliability and validity of computer-assisted assessment interpretations.
   c. They can evaluate whether the available evidence is adequate to support the intended use of an assessment result for decision making, particularly when that use has not been recommended by the developer of the assessment instrument.
   d. They can evaluate the rationale underlying the use of qualifying scores for placement in educational programs or courses of study.
   e. They can evaluate the consequences of assessment-related decisions and avoid actions that would have unintended negative consequences.

Competency 6.   School counselors are skilled in producing, interpreting, and presenting statistical information about assessment results.
   a. They can describe data (e.g., test scores, grades, demographic information) by forming frequency distributions, preparing tables, drawing graphs, and calculating descriptive indices of central tendency, variability, and relationship.
   b. They can compare a score from an assessment instrument with an existing distribution, describe the placement of a score within a normal distribution, and draw appropriate inferences.
   c. They can interpret statistics used to describe characteristics of assessment instruments, including difficulty and discrimination indices, reliability and validity coefficients, and standard errors of measurement.
   d. They can identify and interpret inferential statistics when comparing groups, making predictions, and drawing conclusions needed for educational planning and decisions.
   e. They can use computers for data management, statistical analysis, and production of tables and graphs for reporting and interpreting results.

Competency 7.   School counselors are skilled in conducting and interpreting evaluations of school counseling programs and counseling-related interventions.
   a. They understand and appreciate the role that evaluation plays in the program development process throughout the life of a program.
   b. They can describe the purposes of an evaluation and the types of decisions to be based on evaluation information.
   c. They can evaluate the degree to which information can justify conclusions and decisions about a program.
   d. They can evaluate the extent to which student outcome measures match program goals.
   e. They can identify and evaluate possibilities for unintended outcomes and possible impacts of one program on other programs.
   f. They can recognize potential conflicts of interest and other factors that may bias the results of evaluations.

Competency 8.   School counselors are skilled in adapting and using questionnaires, surveys, and other assessments to meet local needs.
   a. They can write specifications and questions for local assessments.
   b. They can assemble an assessment into a usable format and provide directions for its use.
   c. They can design and implement scoring processes and procedures for information feedback.

Competency 9.   School counselors know how to engage in professionally responsible assessment and evaluation practices.
   a. They understand how to act in accordance with ACA's Code of Ethics and Standards of Practice and ASCA's Ethical Standards for School Counselors.
   b. They can use professional codes and standards, including the Code of Fair Testing Practices in Education, Code of Professional Responsibilities in Educational Measurement, Responsibilities of Users of Standardized Tests, and Standards for Educational and Psychological Testing, to evaluate counseling practices using assessments.
   c. They understand test fairness and can avoid the selection of biased assessment instruments and biased uses of assessment instruments. They can evaluate the potential for unfairness when tests are used incorrectly and for possible bias in the interpretation of assessment results.
   d. They understand the legal and ethical principles and practices regarding test security, copying copyrighted materials, and unsupervised use of assessment instruments that are not intended for self-administration.
   e. They can obtain and maintain available credentialing that demonstrates their skills in assessment and evaluation.
   f. They know how to identify and participate in educational and training opportunities to maintain competence and acquire new skills in assessment and evaluation.

Definitions of Terms
Competencies describe skills or understandings that a school counselor should possess to perform assessment and evaluation activities effectively.
Assessment is the gathering of information for decision making about individuals, groups, programs, or processes. Assessment targets include abilities, achievements, personality variables, aptitudes, attitudes, preferences, interests, values, demographics, and other characteristics. Assessment procedures include but are not limited to standardized and unstandardized tests, questionnaires, inventories, checklists, observations, portfolios, performance assessments, rating scales, surveys, interviews, and other clinical measures.
Evaluation is the collection and interpretation of information to make judgments about individuals, programs, or processes that lead to decisions and future actions.

Exhibit 1.b   continued

development. Efforts such as these have the goal of standardizing and formalizing the education and training required for professional counselors in various specialty areas to effectively use psychological tests.

The right and responsibility to administer, score, and interpret psychological and educational tests involve the concerted efforts of professional counselors, legislators, state counseling board members, government bureaucrats, test publishers, advocates, professional associations and affiliates, and the public. Protection of this right to test must occur continuously on several fronts, including laws, regulations, ethics, professional training, and professional practice. Professional counselors are encouraged to join professional associations and become actively engaged in legislative and regulatory advocacy to benefit and protect the public safety and right to access quality, affordable counseling services.

ASSESSMENT TERMS AND CONCEPTS

The field of assessment contains many concepts that are essential to understand and remember. These concepts vary in degree of simplicity, familiarity, and abstractness. The list of terms and concepts presented in this section also serves as a way of classifying and describing most tests that professional counselors will encounter and use. One of the things that makes assessment such a challenging area of study is its new and unusual terminology, causing some professional counselors to suggest that assessment is a language unto itself. In that spirit, the reader is well advised to spend the time needed to master the concepts in the remainder of this chapter. These concepts are the building blocks for understanding the field of assessment and for comprehending the content in the remainder of this book and in the published test manuals one will encounter.

Standardized (Formal) and Nonstandardized (Informal) Tests

Standardized tests have specific conditions for administration, timing, and scoring. This systematic process ensures that no matter who the examiner or examinee, the test will be administered under strict, replicable conditions. Standardized procedures allow comparability of scores and interpretations across different examinees and for the same examinee across administration times. **Nonstandardized tests** and other informal measures do not provide systematic measurements, nor are the administration and scoring criteria fixed. Thus nonstandardized tests do not allow for comparability across examinees or administration times. In addition, standardized tests attempt to conform to rigorous test construction guidelines for establishing the reliability and validity of scores, whereas nonstandardized tests may not.

It is essential to understand that each method has advantages and disadvantages. For example, when interviewing, the professional counselor can use a *structured interview* (standardized), an *unstructured interview* (nonstandardized), or a *semi-structured interview* (standardized format with leeway for unstructured questioning). The advantage of the structured interview is that different professional counselors interviewing the same client will likely reach the same conclusion because they ask the same questions and will probably get the same answers. This enhances the reliability (and probably the validity) of the procedure. On the other hand, different professional counselors interviewing the same client using an unstructured interview will ask different questions, will likely get different results, and will possibly reach different conclusions. The use of nonstandardized procedures more frequently leads to variable results because of a lack of systematic methodology.

Norm-Referenced and Criterion-Referenced Tests

In most cases, standardized tests are administered to a representative sample of participants, called a *standardization sample,* to determine average performances for various subgroups of interest (e.g., age, grade, male, female). These subgroups are often called a *norm group.* A client's score on this **norm-referenced test** can then be compared to the standardization sample results to determine where the client's score falls within that distribution of scores (i.e., Average, Above Average, Below Average). Thus norm-referenced tests allow comparison of a person's score to the scores of a comparison group with like characteristics (e.g., sex, age) that has already taken the test. Norm-referenced tests are commonly used to assess intelligence, achievement, perceptual skills, personality, and behavior. Often the raw score obtained by a client is transformed into some type of standard score or percentile rank. Note that the client's score simply indicates the individual's position relative to others in the sample, not whether the client "passed" or "failed" the test or is diagnosed with some mental disorder. Such judgments require the use of a criterion.

Criterion-referenced tests compare a person's score to a predetermined standard or level of performance—a *criterion.* Often a criterion-referenced test is administered to a standardization sample to help establish the criterion scores. Criterion-referenced tests are common in education because most teacher-made tests and performance-based assessments have a standard for determining successful performance. For example, on a high-stakes state achievement test, a criterion for passing may be established at a cutoff score of 79; thus any student scoring at 79 or higher has "passed" the test; those below 79 did not. Likewise, on a depression screening test, a clinician may determine that scores of 20 and higher require further diagnostic evaluation, so a client receiving a score of 16 on the screening test would not meet the minimum criterion. Many *DSM-IV-TR* diagnostic checklists are set up to facilitate criterion-referenced decision making. For example, a diagnosis of Generalized Anxiety Disorder requires the documentation of three or more of the six specific listed diagnostic criteria to a significant degree.

While most tests are designed to be norm referenced or criterion referenced, some diagnostic, clinical, and research decisions are made by applying criterion-referenced standards to norm-referenced results. For example, it is widely believed that the prevalence of Attention-Deficit/Hyperactivity Disorder (AD/HD) in the childhood population is about 5%. The *Conners' Teacher Rating Scale—Revised* (*CTRS-R*) (Conners, 1997) is a norm-referenced behavior rating scale commonly used in assessing AD/HD. The *CTRS-R* yields a T score ($M = 50$; $SD = 10$). Applying the principles of the normal curve, it can be determined that a T score of 67 or higher would represent the highest 5% (most hyperactive, most distractible) of a school-aged population. Thus, even though the *CTRS-R* is a norm-referenced test, a clinician or researcher could use a criterion cut-score of $T \geq 67$ to identify children with AD/HD.

Individual and Group Tests and Inventories

Some tests and inventories are designed to be administered to only a single examinee at a time; others are designed for administration to groups of participants simultaneously. The advantages of **group tests** are speed and efficiency. At the same time, there are limitations in the type of group administration formats available, usually involving paper-and-pencil and response booklet or Scantron (bubble) formats. Professional school counselors most frequently use or encounter group assessments involving achievement, aptitude, and ability within large-scale testing programs (Gibson & Mitchell, 1999). A major drawback of group-administered assessment is the inability to observe all examinees and control the factors that sometimes influence student performance, the most important of which is student motivation.

Individual tests are often used for diagnostic decision making and generally require some interaction between the examiner and examinee. They allow the examiner to establish rapport, reduce anxiety, observe verbal and nonverbal behaviors, and pace the evaluation by providing breaks to decrease fatigue. Often the tasks administered in an individual test require special training, expertise, materials, and timing or scoring procedures that require individual attention. The individual administration format also gives the student or client the opportunity to demonstrate a deeper mastery of skill by allowing the examiner to query responses and provide instruction, and the examinee to clarify questions and task demands.

Objective and Subjective Tests

The terms *objective test* and *subjective test* refer to the method of scoring used in a given testing procedure. **Objective tests** leave no doubt as to the correctness of a given answer; correct answers are predetermined and require no judgment on the part of the examiner. As a result, regardless of who scores the test, the result will be the same. Multiple-choice, true-false items are examples of objectively scored questions. **Subjective tests** require the examiner to make a judgment on the quality of the response in scoring an item. Essay, constructed-response, and open-ended questions ordinarily require some judgment. Objective items help to control subjective bias in scoring procedures (i.e., help to improve interscorer reliability). Many client characteristics assessed by professional counselors can be determined by objective methods; other characteristics or issues in the lives of clients are more easily assessed through subjective methods.

Speed and Power Tests

Different tests have differing classifications of item difficulty and response rates. **Speeded tests** generally include a large number of simple items. The task is to measure how many of the simple items a person can complete within a certain amount of time. The test is structured so that very few, if any, examinees complete all of the items, and the score is simply the number of (correct) items completed within the time limit (i.e., a person's response rate). Tests of fluency and processing speed commonly use speeded procedures. For example, the Math Fluency subtest of the *WJ-III* (Woodcock, Mather, & McGrew, 2001) presents the examinee with 160 simple calculation problems (i.e., 2 + 4 = ?, 1 × 4 = ?) within a three-minute time limit. The examinee writes the number answer for each problem. The items are so simple that very few errors are made, and the person's raw score is the number of items correct. Obviously, the faster the examinee can compute and respond to simple math calculation problems, the higher the score.

A **power test** generally has fewer items, but they are of varying levels of difficulty, and there are no time limits. The examinee can take as much time as needed to work each problem, and the score is the number of items responded to correctly. In some instances, more difficult items may be worth more points than less difficult items. This kind of examination is called a power test because the score is an indicator of the skills or abilities possessed by the examinee, without the pressure of time limits. Generally, some items are so difficult that perfect scores are rare. When measuring math computation skill, the Math Calculation subtest from the *WJ-III* may be used. This subtest presents math calculation problems of varying difficulty levels (i.e., 3 + 4 = ?; 420 × 24 = ?; $^{3}/_{4}$ − $^{1}/_{4}$ = ?; 2x + 1 = 13, therefore x = ?), and the examinee's raw score is an indicator of the amount of math skill possessed. The items vary in difficulty, and most examinees eventually miss many items in a row (i.e., reach the ceiling level), at which time administration of the subtest ceases. The more proficient an examinee is in math calculation, the higher the person's score.

Interestingly, even though some tests are classified as pure speeded tests or pure power tests, many tests include both facets—that is, they are designed as power tests with varying item difficulties but are administered under time limits. Usually, these time limits are sufficient for the majority of test takers to complete the examination. However, slower (for whatever reason) test takers often run out of time. For example, the *Scholastic Assessment Test* (*SAT*), commonly used for college admissions decisions by American universities, is designed as a power test with items of widely varying difficulties, but it is administered under time-limited conditions. Importantly, time limit constraints frequently put disabled examinees at a distinct disadvantage, which is why many students and adults with documented learning disabilities or who receive accommodations under Section 504 of the U.S. Rehabilitation Act of 1973 petition for and receive extended time accommodations.

Verbal and Nonverbal Tests

Some **verbal tests** rely heavily on language usage, particularly oral or written responses. These verbal responses require an examinee first to understand or comprehend instructions, questions, and other task demands; then to verbally mediate and construct an appropriate response; and finally to deliver an oral or written response that passes the scoring criterion for the item. Even if a task does not require a verbal response, if the instructions are given orally, some verbal skill is required. Over the

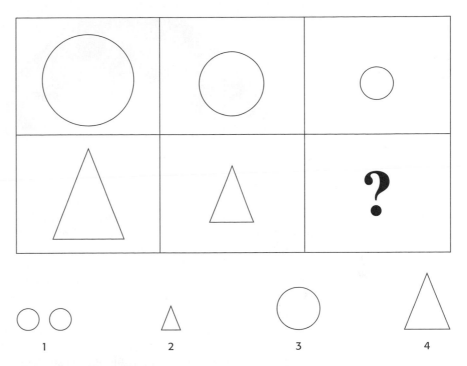

Figure 1.1   Matrix Design

past several decades, professional counselors have become acutely aware of the impact of culture on language development and usage, particularly with persons for whom English is not their primary language.

On the other hand, **nonverbal tests** require students and clients to solve and respond to problems without the use of language. Sometimes these tests are called *non-language tests,* or *performance tests.* (Note: The use of the term *performance* in the context of nonverbal assessment here differs somewhat from its use in the section on performance assessment later in this chapter.) For example, on a typical matrix analogy test, an examinee may be asked to look at several related designs and to select from among several choices the design that would either complete the pattern or predict which design would appear next in the sequence (see Figure 1.1). Or, with block pattern items, such as those found on the *Slosson Intelligence Test—Primary* (*SIT-P*) (Erford, Vitali, & Slosson, 1999) (see Figure 1.2), a client may be given several cubes (all black on two sides, all white on two sides, and half black–half white on the other two sides), shown a picture of the blocks making a certain design, then asked to put the blocks together so they look just like the picture. Such tasks minimize verbal input and require spatial, figural, or visual processing skills—all nonverbal intellectual processes.

It is easy to assume that someone who is very intelligent would excel at both verbal and nonverbal tasks, that someone with average intelligence would perform in an

Figure 1.2   Pattern Design

average capacity on verbal and nonverbal tasks, and that someone who is not very intelligent at all would do poorly on both types of tasks. Indeed, this is very frequently the case, though by no means always. An intelligent non-English-speaking client or a learning-disabled student may struggle tremendously on verbally laden tasks (as would be expected) while performing in an outstanding manner on the nonverbal tasks. Because culture influences language, examiners must take extra measures to ensure the fairness of the examination (i.e., be unbiased). On the other hand, individuals with some degree of brain damage or a visual processing disorder, or those who have an accelerated learning environment, may demonstrate verbal capabilities far superior to their nonverbal capabilities. Most tests have some verbal component, even if it is only some brief verbal or written instructions. It is the examiner's legal, ethical, and professional responsibility to ensure that examinees receive a fair, unbiased assessment that reflects the examinee's abilities to the greatest extent possible. In all instances, professional counselors must take into account the extent to which language and cultural influences may affect student or client results.

Cognitive and Affective Tests

Cognitive ability tests generally fall into three categories: intelligence, aptitude, and achievement. They all measure, to various degrees, perceptual, processing, memory, and reasoning capabilities. *Intelligence tests* measure a person's ability to learn, solve problems, and understand increasingly complex or abstract information. Commonly used tests of intelligence include the *Wechsler Adult Intelligence Scale—Third Edition* (*WAIS-III*) (Wechsler, 1997) and the *Stanford-Binet Intelligence Scale—Fifth Edition* (*SBIS-5*) (Roid, 2003). *Aptitude tests,* in general, predict a person's capacity to perform some skill or task in the future (e.g., college, a training program). Aptitude tests have broad educational and vocational applications. For example, the *SAT* has been used for decades by university admissions personnel to determine which college applicants are likely to do well in college (actually, the freshman year of college). Also, the *Differential Aptitude Tests* (*DAT*) (The Psychological Corporation, 1991a) are commonly used as part of a vocational assessment battery to help high school students understand the potential vocational strengths and weaknesses each possesses. *Achievement tests* are commonly used in education to measure knowledge students have acquired through instruction or training up to a certain point in their academic career. Achievement tests can be norm referenced (comparing the examinee with other students) or criterion referenced (comparing the examinee with a standard of mastery). Nearly all teacher-made, classroom-administered tests are achievement tests and are usually criterion referenced. However, many individually administered diagnostic- and screening-level tests have been developed, including the *WJ-III* (Woodcock, McGrew, & Mather, 2001); the *Wechsler Individual Achievement Test—Second Edition* (*WIAT-II*) (Wechsler, 2001b); and the *Peabody Individual Achievement Test—Revised* (*PIAT-R*) (Markwardt, 1998). Also, most states have mandated high-stakes achievement testing programs and contract with test publishers to develop standardized achievement tests that align with specific state educational standards.

Affective assessment is a broad category that, in general, assesses all noncognitive features of an individual, including temperament, clinical disposition, personality, attitudes, values, and interests. Both structured and unstructured assessments are commonly used in affective assessment. Professional counselors frequently use *structured (formal) personality inventories* for diagnostic purposes, hypothesis testing, treatment planning, and progress evaluation. Commonly used structured inventories include the *Minnesota Multiphasic Personality Inventory—II* (*MMPI-2*) (Butcher et al., 1992); the *Millon Clinical Multiaxial Inventory—III* (*MCMI-III*) (Millon, Davis, & Millon, 1997); and the *Strong Interest Inventory* (Harmon, Hansen, Borgen, & Hammer, 1994). *Unstructured (informal) assessment* often involves the use of projective techniques and qualitative methods. **Projective techniques** are based on psychoanalytic theory and normally present the client with unstructured, ambiguous stimuli, allowing the client to "project" thoughts and feelings onto the stimulus. Examples of ambiguous stimuli include inkblots, pictures, incomplete sentences, or even a single word. Such unstructured tasks give the client great latitude in how to respond or as to the content of the response, and it is incumbent upon the professional counselor to analyze and interpret the responses to yield insights into a client's motivation, personality, values, and so forth. An advantage of a projective technique is that because it is ambiguous and there are no right or wrong answers, it is difficult for clients to fake responses. Their responses were simply based on what came into their mind at the time they responded to the task. A disadvantage of projective techniques is that some of the tests require extensive education and training. Examples of projective tests include inkblot techniques such as the *Rorschach Inkblot Test* (Rorschach, 1969); picture-story techniques such as the *Thematic Apperception Test* (*TAT*) (Murray & Bellak, 1973) and *Robert's Apperception Test for Children* (McArthur & Roberts, 1994); drawing and query techniques such as the *House-Tree-Person* (*H-T-P*) (Van Hutton, 1994) and *Kinetic Drawing System for Family and School* (Knoff & Prout, 1985); and completion techniques such as incomplete sentences or word association.

Maximum and Typical Performance Measurement

In **maximum performance measurement,** the professional counselor strives to assess the best performance of which the examinee is capable. In this way, the examiner has a good estimate of the upper level of achievement or ability at which the client could be expected to perform. When conducting diagnostic assessment for the determination of a learning disability, the examiner strives to obtain maximum ability and achievement estimates because such decisions have important long-term implications.

In **typical performance measurement,** the professional counselor seeks to obtain a sample of the client's performance under normal circumstances, or on a "typical day." Professional counselors conducting clinical, personality, or vocational assessments often strive for typical performance estimates to understand the client's performance under normal circumstances. In this way, the professional counselor gets to know the client's habitual thoughts, feelings, interests, and behaviors.

Behavioral Observations

Unfortunately, many people view assessment only as the administration of tests. But assessment of any kind relies heavily on **behavioral observations,** observations that begin at the moment the professional counselor speaks to or meets the client or student for the first time. Observations can be conducted through either direct or indirect means. One common form of direct observation is *direct behavioral assessment,* in which the professional counselor is actually physically present in the same environment with the client and uses a data collection procedure to assess the frequency, duration, and/or magnitude of one or more target behaviors. For example, a professional school counselor may observe a 2nd-grade student referred for overactivity by using a time-on-task observation system. Briefly, such a procedure allows the counselor to observe the frequency of the target student's (the student suspected of being hyperactive) and of one or two control students' (students of the same sex, but not suspected to be substantially hyperactive) motor on-task behavior during classroom activities. Such observations allow the counselor to determine whether the target student is substantially more overactive than other children of the same age. *Anecdotal observations* are also commonly used and allow the observer to document in a narrative format what was observed during an observation period. The purpose of an anecdotal report is to describe client behaviors in some detail so that, over time, a rich understanding of the factors surrounding the behavior can be obtained. Often special training is required of observers to minimize bias and enhance inter-observer reliability (i.e., agreement between the observations or ratings of two or more observers).

Behaviors can also be assessed through *indirect observation,* usually using *behavior rating scales* or *checklists.* These instruments ask questions of people (e.g., spouse, parent, teacher, peer) in a good position to observe the typical behavior of a student or client and provide responses that give the professional counselor multiple perspectives and valuable clinical insights. Some behavioral disorders (e.g., AD/HD) require that problematic behaviors be observed in more than one setting, and behavior rating scales completed by parents or teachers help to verify student or client difficulties in a time-efficient manner.

Basals, Starting Points, and Ceilings

Many intelligence, aptitude, and achievement tests present items in order of increasing difficulty. For example, most subtests on the *Woodcock-Johnson: Tests of Achievement—Third Edition* (*WJ-III ACH*) (Woodcock, Mather, & McGrew, 2001) present items in approximate order from least difficult to most difficult. Likewise, the *Slosson Intelligence Test—Revised* (*SIT-R*) (Nicholson & Hipshman, 1990) presents 187 verbal ability items in an order that approximates least to most difficult. This hierarchical ordering allows administration procedures that substantially enhance efficiency and speed. Because the items are in approximate order from least difficult to most difficult, it is logical to assume that if a student gets item 11 correct, the odds are good that the student would also get items 1–10 correct, because each is easier than item 11. One can easily see how much faster administration would be if any examinee getting item 11 correct would not need to answer items 1–10. Of course, this is only an assumption, and exceptions do occur on a frequent basis. However, test developers have determined that the probability of violating this assumption diminishes tremendously when a series of consecutive items is used. A **basal series** is a predetermined number of consecutive, correct items that must be obtained by an examinee in order to eliminate the need to administer numerous easier items on the same test or subtest. For example, the *SIT-R* requires a basal series of 10 in a row correct, while many subtests on the *WJ-III ACH* require a basal of 6 in a row correct. Establishing a basal series gives the examiner confidence that, if the examinee were administered all the items preceding the basal, the examinee would get them all correct. Again this is an assumption, but one backed up by substantial statistical probability. The assumption is generally true in 95% or more of the cases, and when it is not true, the examinee almost never misses more that one or two of the easier items. Thus the examinees' scores ordinarily are not substantially inflated.

Of course, there is no need to establish a basal series if all examinees begin administration with item 1. That is why many test developers establish **starting points** for administration based on the age or grade of the examinee. For example, an 8-year-old being administered the 187-item *SIT-R* would ordinarily begin with item 55, a 13-year-old at item 105. These starting points are usually designated by determining the point at which nearly all (i.e., 95%) of 8-year-olds or 13-year-olds will get the first item correct and go on to obtain the required basal series of 10 in a row correct. For example, on the *SIT-R,* the examiner would begin administration to an 8-year-old with item 55, then continue until the basal series has been obtained. If the student gets item 55 correct and responds correctly to items 56–64, the basal series requirement has been met, and administration of the test items continues.

Different tests vary as to the proper procedure to follow if one of the items is missed during the attempt to establish the basal series. Some require the examiner to stop forward administration and administer the items in reverse order until the basal has been established. As an example, imagine that an 8-year-old student being administered the *SIT-R* answers items 55–60 correctly, then misses item 61. Because the *SIT-R* requires a basal of 10 items and the student has only 6 in a row correct, the professional counselor is required to return to item 54 and administer the items in reverse order until the student responds to 10 items correctly (i.e., 54, 53, 52, 51). At that point, having established the required basal series, the professional counselor returns to item 62 and administers the remaining items until a ceiling is reached. This example is provided in Figure 1.3.

A **ceiling series** is the number of incorrect items an examiner must obtain before test administration can be halted. The concept of a ceiling is based on the same

☑ SLOSSON

INDIVIDUAL TEST FORM

SIT-R
SLOSSON INTELLIGENCE TEST
Richard L. Slosson
Revised by: Charles L. Nicholson, Terry L. Hibpshman

Name _Johnson   Jack_____
          LAST   FIRST   MIDDLE

Address _____

School/Agency _____

Sex _M_ Grade _3_ Parent _____

Referred By _____
                    NAME   POSITION

Examiner _____
                    NAME   POSITION

Comments: _____

_____

Test Results:

Chronological Age (CA)...........	_8-2_ Yrs.-Mos.
Raw Score......................	_63_
Total Standard Score (TSS)........	_92_
Mean Age Equivalent (MAE).......	_8-3_
T-Score........................	_____
Normal Curve Equivalent (NCE)....	_____
Stanine Category..................	_____
Percentile Rank (PR)	_31_
Confidence Interval (95%) or 99%) ..	_92;84-100_
(circle interval used)	

Mark the questions with a (1) for passing or a (0) for failing. Begin testing where examinee can pass "10 in a row" without making a mistake. Continue testing until examinee misses "10 in a row." Refer to Manual for more complete directions.

NOTES

1.___	31.___	61.___ *Basal	91.___	121.___	151.___	181.___
2.___	32.___	62.___ Not Met, Go to #54	92.___	122.___	152.___	182.___
3.___	33.___	63._1_	93.___	123.___	153.___	183.___
4.___	34.___	64._0_	94.___	124.___	154.___	184.___
5.___	35.___	65._1_	95.___	125.___	155.___	185.___
6.___	36.___	66._0_	96.___	126.___	156.___	186.___
7.___	37.___	67._0_	97.___	127.___	157.___	187.___
8.___	38.___	68._0_	98.___	128.___	158.___	
9.___	39.___	69._0_	99.___	129.___	159.___	Basal Item _60_
10.___	40.___	70._0_	100.___	130.___	160.___	Questions
11.___	41.___	71._0_	101.___	131.___	161.___	passed after
12.___	42.___	72._0_	102.___	132.___	162.___	basal item + _3_
13.___	43.___	73._0_	103.___	133.___	163.___	
14.___	44.___	74._0_	104.___	134.___	164.___	Raw Score = _63_
15.___	45.___	75._0_ *ceiling	105.___	135.___	165.___	(total of above)
16.___	46.___	76.___	106.___	136.___	166.___	
17.___	47.___	77.___	107.___	137.___	167.___	Ceiling Item _____
18.___	48.___	78.___	108.___	138.___	168.___	
19.___	49.___	79.___	109.___	139.___	169.___	
20.___	50.___ Basal Met	80.___	110.___	140.___	170.___	
21.___	51._1_	81.___	111.___	141.___	171.___	
22.___	52._1_	82.___	112.___	142.___	172.___	
23.___	53._1_	83.___	113.___	143.___	173.___	
24.___	54._1_	84.___	114.___	144.___	174.___	
25.___	*55._1_ Start	85.___	115.___	145.___	175.___	
26.___	56._1_	86.___	116.___	146.___	176.___	
27.___	57._1_	87.___	117.___	147.___	177.___	
28.___	58._1_	88.___	118.___	148.___	178.___	
29.___	59._1_	89._1_	119.___	149.___	179.___	
30.___	60._1_	90.___	120.___	150.___	180.___	

Figure 1.3   Protocol for Slosson Intelligence Test–Revised

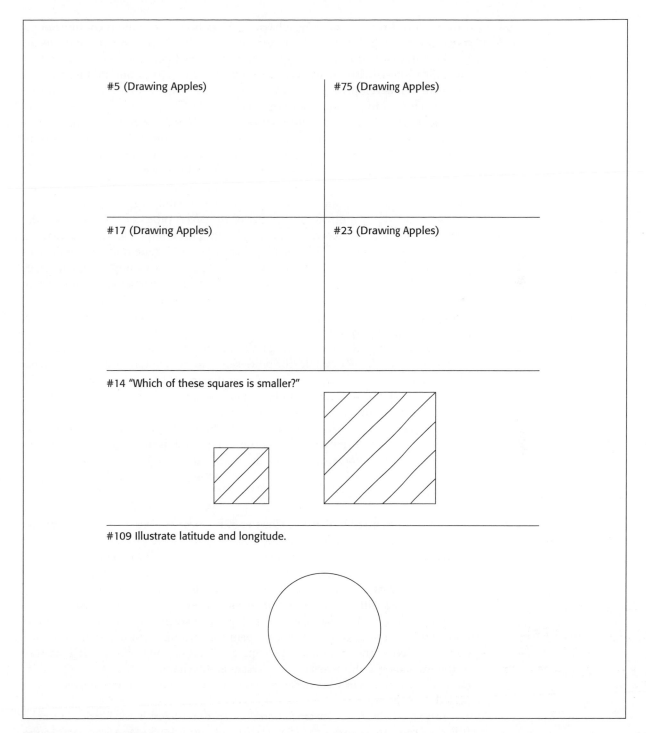

#5 (Drawing Apples)   #75 (Drawing Apples)

#17 (Drawing Apples)   #23 (Drawing Apples)

#14 "Which of these squares is smaller?"

#109 Illustrate latitude and longitude.

Figure 1.3 continued

assumptions as those underlying a basal—that is, because the items continue on in order of increasing difficulty, if a student misses item 60, there is a statistical likelihood that the individual would miss items 61 and above because these items are even more difficult. As with the basal series, the accuracy of that assumption is bolstered when the test developer specifies a certain number of items in a row that must be missed before administration can stop. The *WJ-III ACH* generally specifies a ceiling of 6 incorrect items to cease administration of a subtest. The *SIT-R* specifies a ceiling of 10 errors in a row. Continuing with our *SIT-R* example (see earlier discussion and Figure 1.3), suppose the student responds correctly to item 62 and 63, misses 64, gets 65 correct, but then misses items 66–75. Missing the last 10 items in a row fulfills the requirement of the ceiling series, so administration of the test ceases, and the student is given 0 points for all items above the ceiling series. The professional counselor can then complete the scoring of the *SIT-R* protocol and transform the raw score into standard scores and percentile ranks for interpretation. Note that the assumption is that missing 10 items in a row means the student is very unlikely to get any of the even more difficult items correct. Again, this assumption is almost always valid, but there is a negligible statistical probability that some examinees may get one or more additional items correct should the administration of items continue. Just as before, denying an examinee 1 or 2 additional raw score points probably will not substantially suppress an examinee's overall score.

One can easily see the timesaving efficiency and benefits of using basal and ceiling series. In our *SIT-R* example, the professional counselor administered only items 46–69. This means that a student's score was determined by administering only 24 of the 187 total items (about 13%). Basal and ceiling series can thus be tremendously time saving without compromising on accuracy and meaningfulness. In addition, these procedures save clients and students from having to endure the tedious administration of numerous items that are far too simple, and the emotional frustration of having to deal with numerous items that are far too difficult.

Reliability

Reliability is discussed in detail in Chapter 3. For now, it is important to know that *reliability means consistency*. If a client receives an IQ score of 70 one day and 130 the next, what helpful decision could a professional counselor make about a client's life? If a client's score cannot be consistently measured, it is of little use.

Reliability of scores can be determined through a variety of means, each of which assesses a different type of score error. For example, *test-retest reliability* involves determining the relationship (correlation) between scores on the administration of the same test to the same participants on two different occasions (e.g., one hour, two weeks, one month, one year apart). The resulting coefficient is a measure of the test scores' stability over time—essential information when trying to consistently track a client's or student's performance or response to treatment over a given period of time.

It is important to understand from the start that no test is reliable or unreliable. It is test scores that possess the characteristic of consistency. Most importantly, the reliability of test scores varies across samples of participants. For example, it is likely that the reliability coefficients derived from scores on a substance abuse inventory will vary substantially depending on whether clients who abuse substances or clients who do not abuse substances are used in the sample.

Validity

Validity means usefulness. Validity of scores can be determined through a variety of means, each of which provides evidence of a different type of usefulness. *Content-related validity* is a systematic examination of the items making up a test to determine the comprehensiveness of content coverage. This type of validity is particularly relevant for academic achievement tests because academic areas generally have a well-established domain of behavior, and sampling is critical to deriving useful generalizations from any derived score. For example, if a mathematics test is composed only of addition problems, the scores may be valid indicators of a person's addition skills but may be substantially less useful in predicting a person's overall mathematical abilities.

Criterion-related validity involves a test's ability to predict some criterion, either at the present time (*criterion concurrent*) or at some point in the future (*criterion predictive*). Many criteria are commonly used for comparison, and score validity is generally expressed as a specialized correlation coefficient known as a *validity coefficient.* If one is attempting to validate scores from a new anxiety inventory, one may choose criteria such as previously existing anxiety scales, behavioral observations, or diagnostic categorizations (i.e., previously diagnosed or currently diagnosable).

Construct validity helps determine what a test measures (the idea or construct) and how well it measures it. A construct is a relatively abstract idea that cannot be measured directly, but which can be inferred. Intelligence, depression, introversion, self-esteem, and locus of control are all examples of constructs. Constructs can be validated through a variety of methods, including factor analysis, correlations with other tests, and convergent or discriminant techniques. Chapter 4 covers in detail each of these classical methods for determining validity of scores, as well as decision-making strategies using these scores.

As with the concept of reliability, no test is valid or invalid. It is test scores that possess the characteristic of usefulness, and the validity of test scores varies across samples of participants and according to the various purposes that a test is intended to address. For example, it is likely that the validity of scores on a measure of self-esteem will vary substantially depending on the characteristics of the clients being assessed; such as when a more *homogeneous* sample of adolescent Hispanic females with eating disorders is studied, as opposed to a more *heterogeneous* sample of culturally diverse males and females without diagnosable pathology. Likewise, that same self-esteem scale may provide excellent, accurate predictions of academic self-esteem, but only moderately accurate predictions of academic performance (i.e., grades, test scores) and poor predictions of a client's degree of depressive symptoms. Different tests are designed for different purposes and for use with different populations. *Validity is the study of these uses and populations.*

Formative Versus Summative Evaluation

Tests are often used to evaluate curricular and treatment programs. When a test is administered during the course of treatment or instruction with the purpose of informing the evaluator as to the intervention's effectiveness, it is called a **formative evaluation**. Such a practice allows for midcourse adjustments and modifications to more effectively meet the final goal or objective. If an assessment is administered on completion of instruction or treatment, it is referred to as a **summative evaluation**. The purpose of summative evaluation is to determine whether a goal or objective has been met. How effective the assessment is in making this determination depends on the preciseness of the goal or objective, the alignment of the treatment with the goal, and the alignment of the assessment with both the goal and the treatment. For example, many counseling programs administer the *Counselor Preparation Comprehension Examination* (*CPCE*) (administered by the National Board of Certified Counselors [NBCC]) near the end of the program of study as a summative evaluation. The test is predicated on core educational areas (assessment, the topic of this text, is one of the more challenging core areas) and well-defined educational standards. The test is composed of items selected to accurately reflect the various domains of knowledge and the importance of each domain. Thus the *CPCE* is very well aligned with the standards it was designed to measure. Professional counselors participate in a graduate counseling program of study that prepares them for professional practice. Success on the exam is very much related to how closely the graduate program curriculum aligns with the test's standards, the skill of the instructors, factors listed in Table 7.1 (factors that affect student or client test performance), and the tenacity with which the students pursue and master the course contents. Stated another way, success on the *CPCE,* used as a summative evaluation, is enhanced by well-designed programs with good instruction and, even more importantly, motivated, competent students. Study hard!

Paper-and-Pencil Tests and Performance (Authentic) Assessments

A *paper-and-pencil test* requires examinees to mark an answer choice, either through the historically literal practice of using a pencil or through more recent computer-based innovations such as clicking the correct answer displayed on a computer screen. These tasks frequently rely heavily on verbal capabilities because they require reading and verbal comprehension.

Performance assessments, sometimes called *authentic* or *alternative assessments,* minimize verbal task demands but require the student or client to manipulate materials or to select visual stimuli without using language, or at least by substantially minimizing the use of language. There is a big difference between completing a multiple-choice test on how to rebuild car engines (a paper-and-pencil test) and actually rebuilding a car engine (a performance test). Performance assessment involves the evaluation of an examinee's product, action, or behavior. A strength of performance assessment is that it allows the individual to demonstrate a more comprehensive, real-life, hands-on understanding of a topic or dilemma. Performance assessments have been used for years in vocational training and gifted education programs, not to mention physical education, woodshop, metal shop, and home economics classes. Some state departments of education have implemented high-stakes performance assessment systems to assess students' depth of understanding by presenting them with a dilemma to be solved and the materials and time to solve it. Such procedures are expensive and time consuming but allow examiners to determine whether students develop necessary insights and follow desired procedures en route to solving complex problems. Performance assessment is sometimes done with less of an emphasis on reading and writing, thus minimizing the effects of verbal and linguistic capabilities. But this is not always the case. Some states use the manipulation of physical objects and props to solve a problem and then require the student to write a summary composition describing the various components of the performance task.

Professional training programs frequently use performance assessments. For example, counselors-in-training frequently present videotapes of counseling sessions for analysis and evaluation, and interns and practicum students are sometimes observed and evaluated in live counseling, consultation, or classroom sessions. Instructors or supervisors then observe the demonstrations, evaluate and judge each performance according to some scoring scheme (usually involving a scoring *rubric*), and provide feedback regarding the student's or intern's performance. A scoring rubric provides the rules to be followed when assessing the quality of a performance. Generally, the rubric is a rating scale or checklist of essential elements that must be included in the product. Point values are assigned according to the quality of each component.

Popham (1999) indicated that three components must underlie authentic performance assessments: (1) Multiple evaluative criteria must be used; (2) each of the evaluative criteria must be clearly articulated and defined prior to judging the performance; and (3) human judgments are necessary to determine the acceptability of performance responses. It is this final component that critics of performance assessment take issue with. The acknowledged weakness of performance assessment is the difficulty of establishing the reliability and validity of scores—which are critical regardless of the type of assessment undertaken. Because performance assessment is time consuming, it may be possible to complete only one or several problems (i.e., authentic science problems to be solved, perhaps even a single "experiment") over the course of a two-hour examination, whereas a student may be able to complete more than 100 multiple-choice problems during the same period. An important statistical concept within test development is that, all else being equal, the more items a test possesses, the more reliable the scores on that test (Anastasi & Urbina, 1997). Because human judgment (i.e., subjectivity) is required in performance assessment, *interscorer reliability* becomes an important issue. In nearly all circumstances, the multiple-choice test will be more reliable than the performance test, and test scores can be no more valid (useful) than they are reliable (consistent). Thus there is a trade-off in using paper-and-pencil and performance tests. Paper-and-pencil tests may be more efficient and psychometrically superior (i.e., have a higher reliability of scores), but performance assessments may get closer to the real-life circumstances for which a student is being prepared. These dilemmas are explored in detail in the chapter on high-stakes testing, which is available on the companion website for this text.

Practically speaking, as the owner of a car with a blown engine, who would you rather have working on your car: the mechanic who got more multiple-choice questions right or the one who rebuilt the engine in the quicker, more proficient manner? Perhaps a bit closer to home, who might a client prefer as a professional counselor: the one who received the higher score on the National Counselor Examination (NCE) or the one who performed better on the videotapes? If you said, "The one who did better (or well) on both," you can count yourself among a growing segment of professionals who see the benefits of both approaches. Breadth and depth are both critical elements of comprehensive assessment.

Portfolio Assessment

Portfolio assessment is a specific, and currently popular, type of performance assessment espoused by proponents of the philosophy that instruction and assessment are one and the same. A *portfolio* is a systematic and well-organized collection of work produced by an individual with the purpose of demonstrating that individual's skills and achievements. Portfolios have been used in the professions of art, architecture, modeling, journalism, and photography for years. In these professions, the individual selects exemplary works that demonstrate competence, style, talent, and versatility. In many counseling programs, counselors-in-training are required to develop a portfolio of exemplary works (e.g., counseling tapes or analyses, course papers or projects, events or lessons implemented, ancillary products developed). Portfolios are a wonderful way for interns to demonstrate for program faculty members the depth of their learning and understanding, and for potential employers the likely quality one could expect of the applicant if hired as an employee. However, portfolio assessment presents examiners with a couple of challenging problems: How does one go about evaluating the quality of a portfolio? Will the assessment lead to reliable and valid results?

By now, this problem should sound familiar, and the reader should have some ideas as to how to solve the dilemma. Because portfolio assessment is a type of performance assessment, rubrics and other issues discussed in the performance assessment section also apply here. What is critical is that evaluators of portfolios acknowledge that the assessment system devised must conform to the highest level of technical adequacy possible. If it does not, students and evaluators will waste much time and effort on an assessment process that is difficult (perhaps impossible) to evaluate. Such an assessment system could be perceived as burdensome, worthless, unfair, and even biased.

It is widely agreed that assessment of portfolios should involve both a self-assessment and an external assessment (Farr & Tone, 1994; Popham, 1999). In a *self-assessment*, the student provides evaluative commentary of the included works and how each meets certain requisite standards or demonstrates required mastery. The encouragement of self-evaluation is an important developmental skill in its own right and is a strength of the portfolio process. *External assessment* involves the process of obtaining judgments from professionals not related to the situation in which the works were created, but in a good position to evaluate those works. For example, in the example of a counselor-in-training's portfolio, it is likely that program faculty would be somewhat biased in their evaluation of student works. Indeed, studies have shown

Table 1.2   Advantages and disadvantages of portfolio (and performance) assessment

Advantages
1. Focuses on "doing."
2. Allows for demonstration of examinee strengths, flexibility, and adaptability.
3. Highlights improvements rather than comparisons.
4. Focuses on processes and products.
5. Provides self-assessment and analysis.
6. Assesses depth of understanding and application of instruction.
7. Integrates knowledge, skills, and abilities.
8. Allows diagnosis of strengths and weaknesses.
9. Provides concrete examples of application of skills.
10. Facilitates performance-based instruction.

Disadvantages
1. Evaluation process is time-intensive for students and evaluators.
2. Useful and accurate rubrics are difficult to create.
3. Interscorer reliability is low.
4. Judges require a lot of training.
5. Stakeholders often have difficulty understanding the results.
6. Performance tasks must be well crafted and meaningful.
7. Performance on one task is often unrelated to performance on other tasks.
8. Students are frequently unsure which products to include and why.
9. Performance tasks are difficult and frustrating for low-ability students.
10. Some cultural or socioeconomic groups may underperform on certain types of performance tasks (i.e., bias).

that teachers tend to be biased toward their own students' work (Popham, 1999). Thus it would be best to solicit volunteers from the professional community unrelated to the program or students.

Rubrics established for portfolio assessment must be specifically written and distributed to students well in advance so they can prepare *showcase* or *best-work portfolios* that will address the portfolio standards. Alternatively, students can be encouraged to develop portfolios that demonstrate growth and learning over time. Unfortunately, compared to most other types of assessments, portfolio assessment tends to be time consuming, expensive, and lacking in technical *rigor* (i.e., reliability and validity). All in all, the portfolio assessment process presents numerous difficult challenges, and "to date, the results of efforts to employ portfolios for accountability purposes have not been encouraging" (Popham, 1999). Table 1.2 presents a number of advantages and disadvantages of portfolio assessment.

> **Think About It 1.2**   Imagine that you are preparing for an employment interview. What kinds of "products" from your courses and clinical experiences would you include in your portfolio to demonstrate your effectiveness as a professional counselor?

Environmental Assessment

Environmental assessment moves the focus of assessment and evaluation from the individual to the environment in which the individual functions. In workplaces, relationships, and other social situations, clients often complain that they "don't fit in." Normally, the focus of counseling is on how clients can change to better adapt to their environment and circumstances. But what if the environment could be altered, or changed altogether? For example, clients with an alcohol dependency may benefit from an analysis of the "who," "where," and "what" related to their social activities. Such an analysis may point to factors that are actually barriers to recovery and abstinence. In schools, the contingencies in a classroom may become the primary focus of a behavioral observation and assessment to determine what environmental factors may account for the difficulties a student may be encountering. In families, professional counselors are keenly interested in the family environment so that systemic changes can be made to get a family moving in a more positive direction.

As a more specific example from the career realm, employees sometimes complain about workplace conditions, stress, and burnout but continue to work in such environments for years and years. Some researchers (e.g., Holland, Gottfredson) are addressing this problem by designing measures that assess the environmental context and the individual, using Holland's model, featured in the *Self-Directed Search* (*SDS*) (Holland, Fritzsche & Powell, 1994), to determine whether the client's interests and competencies actually match the demands of the work environment. In a simplistic extension, individuals who need to be physically active but who have a job that requires a lot of desk work may experience a "disconnect" and unhappiness. Likewise, a "people person" may be unhappy slogging away in a cubicle all day, or at least trying to survive until lunch or quitting time. In both of these circumstances, altering or changing the environment or work tasks within an environment may be the solution to client concerns. In some form or another, environmental assessment has been around for decades, but it appears currently to be experiencing a resurgence.

Computer-Managed, Assisted, and Adapted Assessment

Computers are in the process of revolutionizing psychological and educational assessment. As far back as the 1930s, technological innovations have helped make the process of assessment more efficient and accurate, usually by speeding up scoring procedures for large-scale test administrations. With the widespread availability of personal computers since the 1970s, test publishers have actively pursued the production of computer software that allows a clinician's computer to administer, score, and even interpret a client's protocol in the comfort and convenience of the clinician's own office. With easy access to the Internet through home and office computers and public venues such as libraries, the possibilities for computer-assisted assessment have become nearly unlimited. Of course, these wonderful access opportunities have arrived with a plethora of ethical and legal dilemmas.

Computer-managed assessment, also known as *computer-assisted assessment,* involves the harnessing of computers to administer, score, and interpret tests. Some software packages or Internet sites allow an integration of all three of these functions, while others may allow only one or two. Integrated functions are becoming more and more the standard. Today, computers can even store and accumulate test results for a single client or an entire school system in order to manage and compile summary reports. The implications of such computer-managed systems are phenomenal because such databases can facilitate everything from individual treatment plans to outcome assessment of an agency's clientele or the evaluation of an entire school system's curriculum.

Many historically paper-and-pencil tests are now available in online or personal computer versions. Using individualized computer-assisted assessment, the student or client generally completes the assessment at a personal computer on which specialized software has been installed, or on a computer linked to an Internet website offering the service. Responses are easily made by clicking the mouse on an appropriate answer space, using a touch screen, or typing a response. Frequently, tests can be automatically scored and an interpretive report printed out within seconds after completing the test. The comprehensiveness and quality of these reports vary substantially. For example, the computerized packages offered by Pearson to administer, score, and interpret the *MCMI-III* (Millon, Davis, & Millon, 1997) and the *MMPI*-2 (Butcher et al., 1992) include comprehensive, detailed narratives of likely examinee characteristics and behaviors as well as diagnostic and treatment implications—for about $20 a client. On the other hand, the *WISC-IV* and *WJ-III ACH* computer scoring programs, which come with the standard test kit package, provide only basic scoring and storage functions. When considering the purchase of assessment software or other scoring services, it is a good idea to ask the publisher for samples of reports to determine whether they will meet one's professional needs—at a reasonable price.

There are several advantages to computer-assisted assessment. Depending on the program, cost savings can be substantial, particularly given the speed of scoring and interpretive reports. Some tests and inventories may require hours to comprehensively score and interpret, whereas the computer program for the same test or inventory may require only seconds. Clients and students also have much greater control over the rate of response and interaction; thus individuals who desire a quicker or slower pace are accommodated by the computer. In addition, clients with special needs can sometimes be better accommodated by computer administration. Clients with visual handicaps or reading problems and who need to have items read orally may find auditory computer administration more user-friendly. Clients with writing disabilities may find the mouse or keyboard easier to manage than a pen or pencil. Students with visual processing disorders may find the auditory instruction capabilities and larger graphical displays of computers easier to adjust to, as opposed to a bubble form that may look like a jumbled mess. Clients with attentional problems may find the computer administration more engaging than a response booklet. The possibilities for accommodating clients with disabilities are substantial.

Computer-adapted assessment involves an interactive process between the examinee and the computerized assessment device. Computer-adapted assessment usually entails varying administration formats depending on the responses of the examinee to previous questions. For example, when taking the computer-adapted version of the *Graduate Record Exam* (*GRE*) administered by the Educational Testing Service (ETS), two examinees may be administered very different item sets depending on their abilities. On the paper-and-pencil administration of the *GRE,* all examinees respond to (virtually) the same set of questions, whether the student is of high or low ability. This leads to high-ability students answering questions that are mostly far too easy and lower-ability students answering questions that are mostly far too difficult. Computer-adapted testing solves this dilemma by establishing a bank of items for which the item difficulties and other technical item characteristics are already known. An examinee with strong ability will be administered an item of moderate difficulty, respond to it correctly, and receive an even harder question. The computer automatically scores the item, tracks performance, and is programmed to administer subsequent items until a very good estimate of the student's performance is obtained. Generally, students who respond correctly to an item continue to receive more and more difficult items until a plateau in performance occurs. At this point, the administration stops, and a final score is determined. Note that a higher-performing student never receives the easier items in the item bank, but continues to be administered items of ability-appropriate difficulty. For a student with lower ability, an incorrect response to the first moderately difficult item will be followed by an easier item. If this second item is missed, an easier item follows; if the response to this item is correct, a more difficult item follows. The process continues again until a plateau in performance is reached. Note that the lower-performing student is never administered the more difficult items that a higher-performing student receives, but continues to receive the more appropriate, less difficult items.

Many aptitude and achievement tests now offer a computer-adapted administration format. Generally, examinees complete computer-adapted assessments in less time than paper-and-pencil administrations, and the results are available instantaneously, rather than in the typical weeks-to-months wait time for mail-in scoring services. It is likely that computer-adaptive testing will eventually be used in other areas of assessment, particularly clinical, personality, and career assessment. For example, self-report during a computerized structured clinical interview protocol could allow clients to respond negatively to essential features of a major diagnostic category (e.g., "depressed mood or loss of interest or pleasure in normal activities") and subsequently skip all associated structured interview questions related to a disorder that is not applicable. The elimination of inappropriate items could yield a large time savings.

The advantages of using computers for assessment are many. Computers are not prone to bias; they do not discriminate on the basis of sex, race, ethnicity, sexual orientation, and so forth, as some clinicians may. It is also far easier to revise administration, scoring, and interpretive procedures when an examination is online, because the changes are instantaneous. These features offer a real advantage over paper-and-pencil administration, in which some professionals may continue to use older versions of a revised test simply because they have a stockpile of the older protocols they wish to use up, for economy's sake, before ordering newer materials. In addition, there is some evidence that clients may self-disclose sensitive information more honestly during computer administration, because of greater perceived anonymity, than during the face-to-face disclosures that occur during a typical interview (Davis, 1999; Joinson & Buchanan, 2001). Perhaps the most overlooked advantage of online assessment is the potential for access to quality services by professional counselors, clients, and students who are geographically isolated or in some other way unable to participate in more mainstream mental health services.

Important disadvantages of using computers for assessments relate to observation and comfort issues. Generally, when computerized assessments are used, the professional counselor is occupied elsewhere and not focused on observing the client or student engaged in the assessment process. Much helpful information can be lost when a client's assessment-related behaviors go unnoticed. To compound this issue, computer-generated interpretive reports are often accepted at face value by clinicians and imported wholeheartedly into reports and summaries. As is mentioned in the ethics discussion in Chapter 2, computerized interpretive reports are considered professional-to-professional consultations, and the burden of what to report and what not to report lies with the professional counselor charged with the care of the client. Computer-generated reports are meant to supplement a clinician's interpretation, not supplant it. Sampson, Purgar, and Shy (2003, p. 27) suggested that professional counselors should have, at a minimum, the following competencies to use computer-based test interpretation (CBTI) information effectively:

1. An understanding of the construct or behavior
2. An understanding of the test, including the theoretical basis (if any), item selection and scale construction, standardization, reliability, validity, and utility
3. An understanding of the test interpretation, including scale interpretations and recommended interventions based on scale scores
4. An understanding of the CBTI, including the equivalence of test forms (if interpretations from an original form are used) and the evidence of CBTI validity
5. Initial supervised experience in using the test and CBTI (with supervision provided by an appropriately qualified practitioner)

While computers are becoming more commonly used, tremendous diversity in use currently exists. People vary in their experience with and attitudes toward computers. While most people appear favorably disposed toward computers, group and individual differences have been noted. For example, Barak (2003) observed that uneasiness with technology led to lower performance tendencies in women in online assessments. While this empirical result has not been consistently verified, professional counselors are well advised to ensure computerized assessment technologies do not hold some groups at performance disadvantages.

Of course, the proliferation of computer-based assessment services is not without a cost. Frequently, online tests are not developed with the same attention to technical rigor as the print versions of standardized tests, and information on the reliability and validity of online scores is sometimes impossible to obtain. In addition, expert verification of rigor is more challenging because the testing experts may need to be familiar with sophisticated computer programming language in order to evaluate the interpretive procedures programmed into the software. The security and confidentiality of online assessments continue to be of major concern in the industry, although new encoding and encryption software shows promise in resolving these issues. With paper-and-pencil tests, the responsibility for the security of the tests and test results falls squarely on the professional counselor, who can frequently secure the information under lock and key. The issue of security and confidentiality becomes more complex when personal computers and Internet providers are involved, and professional counselors must take great care to ensure the security of the tests and the integrity of the assessment process. Finally, the *Standards for Educational and Psychological Tests and Manuals* (AERA/APA/NCME, 1999) specify that examinees offered a choice between computerized and paper-and-pencil tests should be educated about the features, characteristics, and pros and cons of each type of administration format.

Think About It 1.3   What are the ways you anticipate using computers in your practice as a professional counselor? Think about and seek out the type of training you will need.

SUMMARY/CONCLUSION

This chapter has addressed purposes, standards, and terminology related to professional use of assessment. Assessment has four purposes: screening, diagnosis, treatment planning and goal identification, and progress evaluation. Each contributes substantially to the overall counseling process. In addition, the counseling field has a number of sources intended to guide assessment education and practice. The Council for the Accreditation of Counseling and Related Educational Programs (CACREP) has established curricular requirements, and a number of professional organizations have developed standards to aid counselors in understanding good assessment practices. Finally, professional counselors need to be familiar with the terms and phrases essential to the field in order to communicate effectively with other professionals, to advocate for clients and students, and to make decisions in their best interests.

KEY TERMS

affective assessment
assessment
basal series
behavior
behavioral observations
ceiling series
cognitive ability test

computer-adapted assessment
computer-managed assessment
criterion-referenced test
diagnosis
environmental assessment
formative evaluation
group test

individual test
maximum performance measurement
nonstandardized test
nonverbal test
norm-referenced test
objective
objective test
performance assessment
portfolio assessment
power test
projective technique
psychological test
reliability

sampling
screening
speeded test
standardization
standardized test
starting point
subjective
subjective test
summative evaluation
test
typical performance measurement
validity
verbal test

CHAPTER 2

Foundations of Assessment: Historical, Legal, Ethical, and Diversity Perspectives

by Bradley T. Erford, Cheryl Moore-Thomas, and Lynn Linde

This chapter highlights the historical, legal, ethical, and diversity issues important to a professional counselor's understanding of assessment. From ancient times through modern day, assessment has been important to humankind's self-understanding, and a tool both for fairness and oppression, however intended. While many historical events were important to the evolution of assessment in general, this chapter explores events relevant to assessment in the more specialized areas of intelligence, achievement, career, and clinical and personality. Professional counselors are engaged in a variety of ways in ensuring that clients and students receive appropriate assessment in these areas. Therefore, a review of legal, ethical, and professional standards regarding assessment, diversity factors affecting assessment, and test bias is also provided. The chapter concludes with a discussion of strategies, counseling interventions, and recommendations to ensure fair testing.

THE HISTORY OF ASSESSMENT

Throughout recorded history, people have attempted to measure and assess human characteristics and traits. What follows is a brief exploration of these attempts over more than the past three millennia, segmented into three historical periods: ancient times, measurement in the laboratory, and modern clinical applications. A summary timeline of historic events in the field of assessment is included in Table 2.1.

Table 2.1   Assessment timeline

500 BCE	Greeks may have used assessments for educational purposes.
220 BCE	Chinese set up civil service exams to select mandarins.
AD 1219	English university administers first oral examination.
ca. 1510	Fiteherbert proposes first measure of mental ability (identification of one's age, counting 20 pence).
1540	Jesuit universities administer first written exams.
1575	Spanish physician Huarte defines intelligence in *Examen de Ingenius* (independent judgment, meek compliance when learning).
1599	Jesuits agree to rules for administering written exams.
1636	Oxford University requires oral exams for degree candidates.
1692	German philosopher Thomasius advocates for obtaining knowledge of the mind through objective, quantitative methods.
1799	In working with the "Wild Boy of Aveyron," Itard differentiates between normal and abnormal cognitive abilities.
1803	Oxford University introduces written exams.
1809	Gross develops theory of observational error.
1834	Weber, pioneer in the study of individual differences, studies awareness thresholds.
1835	Quetelet develops and studies normal probability curves.
1837	Seguin develops the *Seguin Form Board Test* and opens school for mentally retarded children.
1838	Esquirol advocates differences between mental retardation and mental illness, proposes that mental retardation has several levels of severity.
1869	Galton, founder of individual psychology, authors *Hereditary Genius,* sparking study of individual differences and cognitive heritability.
1879	Wundt establishes world's first psychological laboratory at the University of Leipzig in Germany.
1888	J. M. Cattell establishes assessment laboratory at the University of Pennsylvania, stimulating the study of mental measurements.
1890	Cattell coins the term *mental test.*
1897	Ebbinghaus develops and experiments with tests of sentence completion, short-term memory, and arithmetic.
1904	Spearman espouses two-dimensional theory of intelligence (g = general factor, s = specific factors). Pearson develops theory of correlation.
ca. 1905	E. L. Thorndike writes about test development principles and laws of learning and develops tests of handwriting, spelling, arithmetic, and language. He later introduces one of first textbooks on the use of measurement in education. First standardized group tests of achievement published. Jung's *Word Association Test* published.
1905	Binet and Simon introduce first "intelligence test," to screen French public schoolchildren for mental retardation.
1909	Goddard translates *Binet-Simon Scale* into English.
1912	Stern introduces term *mental quotient.*
1916	Terman publishes the *Stanford Revision and Extension of the Binet-Simon Intelligence Scale.*
1917	Yerkes and colleagues from the APA publish the *Army Alpha* and *Army Beta* tests, designed for the intellectual assessment and screening of U.S. military recruits.
1918	Otis publishes the *Absolute Point Scale,* a group intelligence test.
1919	Monroe and Buckingham publish the *Illinois Examination,* a group achievement test. *Woodworth Personal Data Sheet* published.
1921	Rorschach publishes his inkblot technique.
1923	Kelly, Ruch, and Terman publish the *Stanford Achievement Test.* *Kohs Block Design Test* measures nonverbal reasoning.

Table 2.1   continued

1924	Porteus publishes the *Porteus Maze Test*.
	Seashore Measures of Musical Talents published.
	Spearman publishes *Factors in Intelligence*.
1926	Goodenough publishes the *Draw-a-Man Test*.
1927	Spearman publishes *The Abilities of Man: Their Nature and Measurement*.
1928	Arthur publishes the *Point Scale of Performance Tests*.
1931	Stutsman publishes the *Merrill-Palmer Scale of Mental Tests*.
1933	Thurstone advocates that human abilities be approached using multiple-factor analysis.
	Tiegs and Clark publish the *Progressive Achievement Tests,* later called the *California Achievement Test*.
	Johnson develops a test scoring machine.
1935	Murray and Morgan develop the *Thematic Apperception Test*.
1936	Piaget publishes *Origins of Intelligence*.
	Lindquist publishes the *Iowa Every-Pupil Tests of Basic Skills,* later renamed the *Iowa Tests of Basic Skills*.
	Doll publishes the *Vineland Social Maturity Scale*.
1937	Terman and Merrill revise their earlier work (Terman, 1916) as the *Stanford-Binet Intelligence Scale*.
1938	Buros publishes first volume of the *Mental Measurements Yearbook*.
	Bender publishes the *Bender Visual-Motor Gestalt Test*.
	Gesell publishes the *Gesell Maturity Scale*.
1939	Wechsler introduces the *Wechsler-Bellevue Intelligence Scale*.
	Original *Kuder Preference Scale Record* published.
1940	Hathaway and McKinley publish the *Minnesota Multiphasic Personality Inventory* (*MMPI*).
	Psyche Cattell publishes the *Cattell Infant Intelligence Scale*.
1949	Wechsler publishes the *Wechsler Intelligence Scale for Children* (*WISC*).
	Graduate Record Exam (*GRE*) published.
1955	Wechsler revises the *Wechsler-Bellevue Intelligence Scale* as the *Wechsler Adult Intelligence Scale* (*WAIS*).
1956	Bloom publishes *Taxonomy of Educational Objectives*.
	Kuder Occupational Interest Survey published.
1957	Osgood designs the semantic differential scaling technique.
1959	Guilford proposes the structure of intellect model in his *The Nature of Human Intelligence*.
	Dunns publish the *Peabody Picture Vocabulary Test*.
	National Defense Education Act provides funding for career assessment screening and high school counselor positions.
1960	*Stanford-Binet Intelligence Scale* revised.
1961	Kirk and McCarthy publish the *Illinois Test of Psycholinguistic Ability*.
1963	R. B. Cattell introduces theory of crystallized and fluid intelligence.
1965	*Strong Vocational Interest Blank* published.
1966	AERA, APA, and NCME publish the *Standards for Educational and Psychological Testing*.
1967	Wechsler publishes the *Wechsler Preschool and Primary Scale of Intelligence* (*WPPSI*).
1969	Bayley publishes the *Bayley Scales of Infant Development*.
	National Assessment of Educational Progress program implemented.
	Jensen publishes controversial *How Much Can We Boost IQ and Scholastic Achievement?*
1972	Form L-M (3rd ed.) of *Stanford-Binet Intelligence Scale* released.
	McCarthy publishes *McCarthy Scales of Children's Abilities*.
1973	Marino publishes *Sociometric Techniques*.
1974	*Wechsler Intelligence Scale for Children—Revised* (*WISC-R*) published.
	Congress passes the Family Educational Rights and Privacy Act (FERPA).
1975	Congress passes Public Law 94-142, the Education for All Handicapped Children Act.
	Kuder's *General Interest Survey, Form E* published.

continued

Table 2.1   continued

1977	*System of Multicultural Pluralistic Assessment* (*SOMPA*) published.
1979	Federal judge Robert P. Peckham rules in *Larry P. v. Wilson Riles* that intelligence tests are culturally biased when used to determine African American children's eligibility for mental retardation services.
1979	*Leiter International Performance Scale,* a language-free test of nonverbal ability, published.
1980	In *Parents in Action on Special Education v. Joseph P. Hannon,* Illinois judge Grady concludes that intelligence tests do not discriminate against African American children due to cultural or racial bias.
	New York state legislators pass Truth in Testing Act.
1980s	Volumes 1–7 of *Test Critiques* published.
	High-speed computers begin to be used in large-scale testing programs.
	Computer-adaptive and computer-assisted testing developed.
1981	Wechsler publishes the *Wechsler Adult Intelligence Scale—Revised* (*WAIS-R*).
1983	Kaufman publishes the *Kaufman Assessment Battery for Children* (*K-ABC*).
1984	U.S. Employment Service publishes the *General Aptitude Test Battery.*
1985	Sparrow, Balla, and Cicchetti revise the *Vineland Adaptive Behavior Scales,* originally published by Doll (1936).
	AERA, APA, and NCME revise the *Standards for Educational and Psychological Testing.*
1986	*Stanford-Binet Intelligence Scale—Fourth Edition* (*SBIS-4*) published, as revised by Thorndike, Hagen, and Sattler.
1989	*Minnesota Multiphasic Personality Inventory—Second Edition* (*MMPI-2*) published.
	Wechsler Preschool and Primary Scales of Intelligence revised.
1990s	Authentic (performance) assessment and high-stakes testing rise to prominence.
	Volumes 11–13 of *Mental Measurements Yearbook* published.
	Volumes 8–10 of *Test Critiques* published.
1991	*Wechsler Intelligence Scale for Children—Third Edition* (*WISC-III*) published.
	Kuder's *Occupational Interest Survey, Form DD* published.
1992	*Wechsler Individual Achievement Test* (*WIAT*) published.
1997	*Wechsler Adult Intelligence Scale—Third Edition* (*WAIS-III*) published.
1999	AERA, APA, and NCME publish *Standards for Educational and Psychological Testing—Third Edition.*
	Volume 5 of *Tests in Print* published.
2000	Nader and Nairn publish *The Reign of ETS.*
2001	*Mental Measurements Yearbook* becomes available through an electronic retrieval system.
2002	Educational Testing Service revises its *Scholastic Assessment Test* (*SAT*).
	Wechsler Preschool and Primary Scales of Intelligence—Third Edition (*WPPSI-III*) published.
2003	*Wechsler Intelligence Scale for Children—Fourth Edition* (*WISC-IV*) published.
	Stanford-Binet Intelligence Scale—Fifth Edition (*SB-5*) published.

Ancient Times

Assessment has been used and documented in many civilizations throughout history. As far back as 220 BCE, and continuing for more than 2,000 years, the Chinese had an elaborate civil service examination system to select mandarins for public service (Dubois, 1966, 1970). Every third year, candidates would gather to undergo tests of skill in areas such as horsemanship, archery, and music. Essay tests were administered to assess a candidate's writing skills.

Knowledge was assessed in such areas as military competence, civil law, geography, and public and social ceremonies and rites. The Chinese strove to develop a fair and objective system by eliminating systematic bias when observed. For example, they used multiple judges to rate performance, rather than a single judge, and even had scribes copy written work in a standard handwriting format to focus judges on the ideas and content of a composition rather than on the differences in penmanship between candidates (Thorndike, 1997). Even in the early years, they went to great lengths to prevent cheating by isolating candidates during written and performance exams (Bowman, 1989). Many of these practices endure today. Such an elaborate system was deemed necessary in order to select the best candidates on merit, not patronage—and the failure rate often exceeded 90%. These grueling exams went on for 72 uninterrupted hours.

It is frequently hypothesized that the ancient Greeks, perhaps around 500 BCE, used testing in the educational processes of that day. Indeed, both Socrates and Plato are believed to have emphasized that efficient career choices should rely heavily on a student's demonstrated abilities and aptitudes. Unfortunately, much of the historical record for the next 2000 years was lost. In 1540, the Jesuits, a holy order of the Roman Catholic Church dedicated to education and scholarly pursuits, became early leaders in the establishment of assessment procedures at the university level by administering the first written examinations. As one can imagine, this was a somewhat controversial endeavor, followed by much debate over bias and fairness. Nearly 60 years later, the Jesuits issued agreed-upon rules for administration of written exams. This innovation was cautiously followed and implemented by other universities over the next several centuries.

Measurement in the Laboratory

A second "movement" in the history of assessment involved the use of testing in the emerging field of experimental psychology. This field sought to harness the emerging use of the scientific method to explore the psychological world of human beings. Prior to the use of the scientific method, mathematical models, such as those developed by Herbart, Weber, and Fechner were used to describe the effects of such concepts as stimulus intensity and psychological thresholds.

Charles Darwin is often credited with spurring the experimental interest in individual differences through publication of his book *On the Origin of Species by Means of Natural Selection* in 1859 (Cohen & Swerdlik, 1999). Darwin proposed that individual differences in adaptation and characteristics accounted for the survival of entire species and individuals within species. His theory of evolution was controversial and thought provoking. It was especially inspiring for Darwin's half-cousin, the English biologist Sir Francis Galton, who made tremendously influential contributions to the early attempts at measurement of individual differences and cognitive heritability (Forest, 1974).

Galton developed numerous techniques and instruments for measuring individual physical and psychological characteristics, and his methods inspired the precursors to modern-day rating scales and surveys. Overall, he inspired a whole generation of laboratory researchers to determine individuals' "deviation from average" (Galton, 1869, p.11) and to classify individuals "according to their natural gifts" (p. 1) through his studies of heritability on sweet peas. Galton's goal was to study human heredity by measuring the characteristics of related and unrelated individuals and showing that some characteristics made individuals more "fit for survival" than others. He was one of the first scholars to propose that intelligence could be measured through assessing sensory capabilities, for intelligence stems from information, and all information must pass through the senses. Thus the more acute and attuned one's senses, the greater the likelihood of information being passed through the senses and influencing intellectual judgments. In 1884 he opened an exhibit at the International Health Exhibition, which was later reestablished at University College, London, as the Anthropomorphic Laboratory. Here Galton measured human characteristics and abilities such as height, weight, arm span, muscular strength, reaction time, discrimination of color, and visual acuity. These initial attempts at measurement, while considered to be invalid measures of intelligence by today's standards, nonetheless created widespread excitement in the burgeoning field of psychological measurement. Galton also proposed the statistical concept of correlation, although it was the mathematician Karl Pearson—Galton's student, close friend, and biographer—who later provided the statistical formula for linear correlation (i.e., the Pearson product-moment correlation coefficient) that has endured to present day.

In 1879, Wilhem Wundt opened the world's first experimental psychology laboratory, at the University of Leipzig in Germany. He is widely regarded as the founder of the science of psychology (Hearst, 1979), and many of the early experimental psychologists, including Louis Leon Thurstone and James McKeen Cattell, studied at his lab. The hallmark of this era was the drive to rigorously control experimental conditions in order to standardize observations and collection of data.

Cattell, a U.S. psychologist, was inspired by Galton's writings to conduct his doctoral dissertation on individual differences in reaction time, a study that continued the momentum toward measurement of human characteristics. In 1890, Cattell was the first to use the term *mental test* to describe his efforts to measure intelligence. Kraepelin (1895) and his student Oehrn (1889), developed more sophisticated mental ability tests, including arithmetic, memory, and perceptual tasks. In addition, Ebbinghaus (1897) developed sentence completion, arithmetic, and short-term memory tasks. All of these early efforts to develop psychological tests continued the movement to the modern era of assessment.

Modern Clinical Applications of Assessment: Decision Making and Determination of Individual Differences

In any field of study it is important for the stage to be set with precursor events until a critical mass of knowledge has developed; historical events or social needs arise; and motivated, creative thinkers move the emerging field forward. In the field of assessment, many pioneers took the developing field in numerous directions quite quickly, leading to an explosion of assessment applications during the 20th century. These applications were primarily directed at identifying differences between and among individuals so that identification and diagnostic practices, as well as intrapersonal strengths and weaknesses, could be translated into remedial and treatment strategies.

At the core, these efforts were directed at helping clinicians and educators make better, more accurate decisions about human beings than could be made through other, less standardized methods of the day. Most notably, the field moved in four primary directions: intellectual assessment, achievement assessment, vocational and career assessment, and clinical and personality assessment.

Intellectual Assessment

Many individuals have contributed to the rise of testing with educational and clinical applications. In many ways, the work of Galton, Cattell, and Kraepelin laid the foundation for the proliferation of these tests during the 20th century. Early attempts at measuring **intelligence** stemmed from the need to develop procedures to identify students with mental and emotional deficiencies for remedial education. In the earliest recorded attempt, Seguin (1866/1907) in 1837 developed the *Seguin Form Board Test,* which in some ways resembles modern efforts to assess mental deficiencies.

In France, the minister of public instruction appointed physiologist and psychologist Alfred Binet to a commission tasked with determining efficient ways to identify children with mental retardation. Working with a French physician, Theodore Simon, Binet constructed the first practical intelligence test in 1905, the *Binet-Simon Scale.* This scale presented 30 brief tasks in approximate order of difficulty accompanied by relatively precise administration instructions. The original scale was administered under these standard conditions to a standardization sample of 50 children. With this comparison group, Binet could now determine any new child's score and evaluate or interpret it within some context. This revolutionary process, while crude by today's standards, allowed for a rudimentary decision-making process about a child's intellectual ability. In addition, Binet and Simon departed from the traditional focus on assessing sensory processes and focused item development more on reasoning and judgment. Unfortunately, the original scale derived no index or standardized score other than a raw score. Thus interpretations were limited primarily to descriptions of whether the child had basically normal intelligence or how far above or below normal the child's score appeared to fall. A further limitation of the original scale was the poor representativeness of the standardization sample to the overall population.

These limitations were addressed in the 1908 revision of the *Binet-Simon Scale,* which nearly doubled the number of items on the original scale. The standardization sample included more than 200 children and was more representative of the population the test was meant to assess. In addition, Binet introduced the concept of mental age, an important innovation at the time, which allowed the evaluator to determine performance in terms other than the raw score. Each scale task or item was evaluated to determine the average chronological age at which a child mastered the task. This helped to specify normal or average performance for each item according to an age equivalency, which became the item's "mental age." Thus a normal 7-year-old child would achieve a mental age of approximately 7 years, while a bright seven-year-old might have a mental age of 9 or 10 years. Conversely, a 7-year-old child with mental retardation might have a mental age closer to 4 or 5 years. The child's mental age (MA) and chronological age (CA) could be used to calculate a ratio intelligence quotient (IQ) using the formula [MA ÷ CA] × 100, a rudimentary form of the modern IQ score.

The *Binet-Simon Scale* received a minor revision again in 1911, but by this time the interest in assessing intelligence had caught on in a number of countries, including the United States. Lewis M. Terman of Stanford University translated the *Binet-Simon Scale* into English, adapting, revising, and adding many items and instructions in the process. In 1916, Terman released the *Stanford Revision and Extension of the Binet-Simon Intelligence Scale,* featuring a standardization sample of more than 1,000 people. In 1937, this test became the *Stanford-Binet Intelligence Scale* (*SBIS*), revised in 1960, 1972, and 1986. The *SBIS* is now in its fifth edition (Roid, 2003).

Terman's contribution was noteworthy in several ways, perhaps most importantly because it made the widespread assessment of intelligence possible. This was timely because around the same time that Terman released the *Stanford-Binet,* World War I broke out and the military had a tremendous need to screen soldiers in order to assign them to appropriate duties in an efficient manner. The army contacted Robert Yerkes, then president of the American Psychological Association, to seek the association's help in developing large-scale assessment instruments for selection and classification. Instruments of that time period were nearly all individual assessments, which were generally time-intensive and cost-prohibitive, requiring highly skilled evaluators—not the kind of efficient tools needed to screen thousands of military recruits each month. In 1917, Yerkes (1921) led a committee of many of that era's greatest measurement experts to produce two group-administered tests of ability: the *Army Alpha,* which required reading ability and comprehension, and the *Army Beta,* a nonverbal test used to assess the abilities of illiterate or non-English-speaking adults. These tests used a multiple-choice format, a recent innovation popularized by Arthur S. Otis. Although the tests were not completed in time to be of help in screening World War I recruits, these early efforts at developing individual and group-administered tests of intellectual ability fueled widespread optimism about the role assessment could play in society, especially in institutions such as education and the military.

Interestingly, the first tests of intelligence were produced with little thought given to theoretical underpinnings—that is, they were *atheoretical*. It was not until the late 1920s that discussions about the definition, makeup, and characteristics of intelligence were held by scholars. Spearman (1927) proposed that intelligence is displayed in two dimensions: one that helps an individual solve general tasks (*g*), and another that helps individuals solve specific tasks (*s*). Spearman's concept (*g*), perhaps the most famous, and infamous, in the field of intelligence testing, spurred a great deal of empirical study and philosophical and political discussion. For example, in contrast to Spearman, Thurstone argued that intelligence was not explained by one general (unidimensional) factor called intelligence, but was actually composed of seven primary mental abilities. Much more discussion on the topic of intellectual theories and models is presented in Chapter 10. Suffice it to say here that the early efforts by Binet, Spearman, Thurstone, and many others led to an explosion in modern-day intelligence and aptitude testing.

To be sure, there have been several periods of criticism associated with testing in general, and intelligence testing in particular. The first came during the 1930s, the time of the Great Depression, and stemmed from unclear expectations over the roles tests could and should play in measuring human experiences and abilities. Many challenges related to how to measure human abilities were raised during this time. Fortunately, social sciences took on these challenges with gusto, developing new assessment methods, tests, and more powerful statistical techniques to aid in analyzing test items and results.

Perhaps the most famous name in U.S. intelligence testing today is David Wechsler (Wechsler passed away in 1981). In 1939, Wechsler, at the time a clinical psychologist in New York City's Bellevue Hospital, published the *Wechsler-Bellevue Intelligence Scale.* This individually administered test of adult intelligence was designed to measure the "global capacity of the individual to act purposefully, to think rationally, and to deal effectively with his environment" (p. 3). In 1955, Wechsler revised the *Wechsler-Bellevue* and changed the name to the *Wechsler Adult Intelligence Scale (WAIS).* It was revised again in 1981 and 1997, and this most recent edition is known as the *Wechsler Adult Intelligence Scale—Third Edition (WAIS-III)* (Wechsler, 1997). Wechsler's adult test offered several innovations or practical facets that became industry standards over the years. First, his test was actually a series of "subtests," each measuring a different facet of intelligence. Each facet contributed to the overall (full-scale) intelligence quotient. Also, Wechsler was one of the first to use a standard deviation IQ, rather than the ratio IQ popularized by the *Stanford-Binet.* Finally, Wechsler took a very pragmatic view of intelligence, rather than a theoretical view. Basically, Wechsler chose what he believed to be the most efficient and useful measures of intelligence from previously developed measures and developed original items to create a particularly engaging and user-friendly format. Sources for his subtests included the *Army Alpha* (Information, Comprehension, and Picture Arrangement) and *Army Beta* (Coding); the 1916 *Stanford-Binet* (Vocabulary, Similarities, Comprehension, Digit Span, and Arithmetic); the *Healy Picture Completion Tests* (Picture Completion); and the *Kohs Block Design Test.* Importantly, Wechsler combined scores from each subtest to arrive at an estimate of general mental ability (g), not numerous primary mental abilities or specific facets of intelligence that others (e.g., Louis Leon Thurstone, Robert Sternberg, Howard Gardner) have described. The subtest format was simply a method for measuring general intelligence through multiple measures.

The success of the adult Wechsler scale led Wechsler to develop a version for use with school-aged children from 6 to 16 years. In 1949, Wechsler published the *Wechsler Intelligence Scale for Children (WISC).* The *WISC* was revised in 1974, 1991, and 2003. It is currently known as the *Wechsler Intelligence Scale for Children— Fourth Edition (WISC-IV)* (Wechsler, 2001a) and follows a subtest format similar to that of the adult version. It is the most commonly used individually administered intelligence test in the world. In order to address the recent increased need for assessing intelligence in the preschool population, Wechsler (1967) published the *Wechsler Preschool and Primary Scale of Intelligence (WPPSI),* again following a subtest format similar to that of the child and adult Wechsler versions. The *WPPSI* was revised in 1989 and again in 2002 and is currently known as the *Wechsler Preschool and Primary Scale of Intelligence—Third Edition* (*WPPSI-III*) (Wechsler, 2002). The Weschler series of intelligence tests has significantly influenced intelligence testing and the profession's conceptualization of intelligence, and is reviewed in more detail in Chapter 13.

A second period of intense social and political criticism developed during the 1960s and 1970s due to several societal factors, including the civil rights movement and congressional hearings into rights to privacy. This period was termed the Era of Discontent by Maloney and Ward (1976). Several influential books and court cases occurred during this period. Whyte (1956), in *Organization Man,* accused users of employment and other selection tests of choosing workers who fit the organization's structure, or status quo, rather than those who would do the best work or were most qualified. Houts (1977), in *The Myth of Measurability,* insisted that tests were instruments of oppression used by the privileged to control the poor. Houts maintained that tests punished creative individuals, caused irreparable damage to children through educational labeling, and generally were being used to make decisions the tests either were not meant to make or lacked the technical adequacy (e.g., reliability, validity) to make.

In 1967, in *Hobson v. Hansen,* a federal judge determined standardized group ability tests to be biased and discriminatory against minorities, rendering the tests unacceptable as placement tests for special education. In 1979, another federal judge made a similar ruling regarding individualized intelligence tests in *Larry P. v. Wilson Riles.* During the 1990s, New York State's Truth in Testing Act, ostensibly passed over concern about the possible misuse of *Scholastic Assessment Test* (*SAT*) test scores, requires the release of all questions used on the administration of the *SAT* after it has been conducted. While perhaps well intentioned, this law allows the public to view every question comprising recent versions of *SAT* administration, in effect making the items unavailable for further use. Such a practice drives up the cost to consumers (i.e., the parents of college-bound youth), because the College Board must spend a great deal of extra money to constantly create new items that have a one-time-only use.

During this period, many expressed concern over the widespread use of intelligence and personality tests in employment and school testing programs (Thorndike, 1997). Indeed, in 1972, the National Education Association actually called for an end to routine standardized achievement, aptitude, and intelligence testing. It was feared that such tests could be used, intentionally or unintentionally, to discriminate against people, particularly women and minorities. It was demonstrated that the content of some tests did, in fact, lead to discrimination in decision making, although not to the degree critics insisted was the case. However, as reported by Anastasi (1976), tests were already routinely being used to make decisions about college admissions, schoolchildren with learning difficulties, and adult populations with special needs. Often these test scores were used to make decisions that were beyond the test's technical specifications, leading to widespread criticism, disillusionment, and skepticism.

Again, test developers viewed these criticisms as challenges to be overcome through scientific study and developed procedures and methods to identify and correct biased test content. This process led to a movement to develop culturally fair and unbiased tests that is firmly implanted to this day. Nevertheless, in spite of efforts by the test publishing industry to address these issues and to allay public concerns, periodic legislation and court decisions occur that restrict the use of tests, because no test, no matter how well developed, is perfect. Furthermore, tests are interpreted by professionals with varying levels of training and expertise, and mistakes can and do occur. Of course, it is these mistakes that end up in legislative houses and court buildings, reported by the press, and concerning the public. A moderate amount of public wariness regarding testing can be expected to continue well into the future, and is probably helpful in keeping test developers and test users focused on best practices of test use. We further explore public concerns about testing later in this chapter.

Achievement Assessment

On the **achievement** testing front, a major shift in educational assessment occurred in 1845 when the Boston public school system opted for written essay exams over the traditional oral exams (Anastasi & Urbina, 1997). Interestingly, the arguments in favor of moving to this radical form of testing included broader content coverage, standardized conditions, standardized item selection, and reduced possibility of favoritism. If these criticisms of oral testing sound familiar, they should. Several were the same arguments later used to replace essay exams with the multiple-choice format.

Between 1897 and 1903 in the United States, Joseph Mayer Rice tested tens of thousands of students to create the first large-scale standardized tests of spelling, arithmetic, and language. Rice's work stimulated additional attempts at standardized test development by Edward L. Thorndike of Columbia University's Teachers College. During the early 20th century, the Teachers College became the hub of efforts to standardize educational tests, and Thorndike and the assessment specialists he trained were at the center of the revolution. It was at this time that issues of subjectivity of essay and extended-response items were explored. Test developers and users of this era were quick to notice that judges often did not agree on the "correctness" of a constructed answer. As a result, multiple-choice and other forced-choice item response formats were developed and came into prominence during the first several decades of the century. The advent of test scoring machines around the middle of the century made multiple-choice formats even more popular, as thousands of test protocols could be scored with ever-increasing efficiency (i.e., less time, greater accuracy, fewer scorers required).

In the first two decades of the 20th century, achievement was measured either by a single test combining several subject areas into a single score, or by a single test constructed to measure a single subject area score. In 1923, Truman L. Kelly, Giles M. Ruch, and Terman published the first edition of the *Stanford Achievement Test* (*SAT*—not to be confused with the *Scholastic Assessment Test*), which is currently in its 10th edition. The *Stanford Achievement Test* was the first standardized achievement battery and was designed to measure several subject areas simultaneously and to report each area score separately. In this way, a teacher could understand a student's separate performances in math, reading, and spelling through administration of a battery of achievement tests. Also, the *SAT* provided a national standard of comparison so that performance of students in one school could be compared to that of students in various other parts of the country. As normed, multiple-choice measures, standardized achievement tests had many advantages over teacher-administered and teacher-scored essay-based tests, which had previously dominated public and private school education. Standardized achievement tests were relatively easy to administer and score, objective (i.e., minimized favoritism), and less expensive; covered broader ranges of content; and gave a measure of student performance against that of others in the same grade. By the 1930s, standardized achievement tests were widely viewed as more reliable, meaningful, and fair than essay tests (Anastasi & Urbina, 1997).

Numerous group-administered achievement test batteries have been developed over the years. In 1936, Everett F. Lindquist published the *Iowa Every-Pupil Tests of Basic Skills,* an achievement battery known today as the *Iowa Tests of Basic Skills* (6th edition). Lindquist also later developed an electronic test scoring method that made mass scoring of multiple-choice questions quick and inexpensive. The *Metropolitan Achievement Test,* originally published in 1931, is now in its 8th edition. A recent arrival, *TerraNova 2*(CTB/McGraw-Hill, 2001), resulted from a merging of the most recent revisions of the *Comprehensive Test of Basic Skills* and the *California Achievement Test.* In 1969, the United States launched the National Assessment of Educational Progress program to determine the effectiveness of the country's educational system and track changes in student characteristics and performance over time. The program is still in operation today.

Perhaps the single most influential occurrence in educational testing was the passage of Public Law 94-142—The Education for All Handicapped Children Act (1975), which provided federal oversight and funding for special education programs across the country. Refunded in 1990 and now known as the Individuals with Disabilities Education Act (IDEA), this landmark legislation led to the widespread use of individualized intelligence and achievement tests in public schools. Public Law 94-142 resulted in educational services being provided to millions of students who have substantial learning problems, including learning disabilities, mental retardation, emotional disturbances, and visual, hearing, or orthopedic impairments.

Several important individual achievement batteries were developed in the late 1970s and 1980s to address the need for assessment of learning problems and were immediately put to use to assess the achievement of children and adolescents. These batteries included the *Woodcock-Johnson Tests of Achievement,* now in its third edition (*WJ-III ACH*) (Woodcock, Mather, & McGrew, 2001); the *Peabody Individual Achievement Test,* now in its revised edition (*PIAT-R*) (Markwardt, 1998); and the *Wechsler Individual Achievement Test* (1992), now in its second edition (*WIAT-II*) (Wechsler, 2001b).

At about the same time as Public Law 94-142, Congress passed the U.S. Rehabilitation Act of 1973. While the act was well known at the time for requiring wheelchair access ramps, curb cutting, and elevators in buildings and localities that accepted federal funds, some provisions went unnoticed until years later. Section 504 of this act required that any individual with a mental or medical impairment that affects occupational, learning, or social functioning (among others) is entitled to accommodations to facilitate success. Section 504 accommodations are commonly provided to students in schools today whose mental or medical conditions are not so severe as to qualify for services under IDEA.

During the 1980s and 1990s, many educators criticized the reliance on multiple-choice testing on the grounds that it does not allow assessment of students' understanding of depth of content or reasoning, their ability to integrate knowledge from various aspects of a discipline of knowledge, or their ability to explain complex thoughts and ideas, because they are only required to color-in a bubble, rather than to construct their own meaningful written response. This backlash led a large number of states and school systems to develop "authentic," or performance-based, assessment programs. Generally, these assessment programs present students with real-life problems to be solved, usually resulting in some constructed essay response. However, while multiple-choice questions present with strengths and limitations, so do performance-based tests. As explained in Chapter 1, one of the very important primary problems with performance-based assessment is its lower test score reliability. Many performance-based assessments do not reach a minimally acceptable standard of reliability to report an individual student's score. The passage of the No Child Left Behind Act of 2001 (NCLB) will likely reduce the use of performance-based tests because it requires that individual scores be reported in reading and math for students in grades 3 through 8. Still, many educators view portfolios and performance-based assessments as better indicators of student performance than multiple-choice tests (Muir & Tracy, 1999; Russo & Warren, 1999).

Vocational and Career Assessment

Although he never developed a standardized assessment of **vocational development**, Frank Parsons was a pioneer in the vocational guidance movement and has come to be known as a founder of the school guidance movement. He advocated for the understanding of the person and the world of work so that an individual could be matched with an appropriate occupation. Thus the specialized field of career assessment was born. Numerous applications and venues for **career assessment** have developed over the years, and career assessment often integrates knowledge of an individual's aptitudes, achievements, interests, competencies, values, and beliefs.

Around World War I, **aptitude** testing became critically important in the military (e.g., *Army Alpha* and *Army Beta*), followed by more specific applications to vocational choices. The gains made in the field of intelligence testing coupled with the realization that multiple abilities could be assessed (not just *g*) led to widespread applications in aptitude assessment. For example, scholastic aptitude tests were developed as far back as the 1920s to help identify students with the capabilities to meet the academic challenges of higher education.

During the 1920s and 1930s, the use of aptitude tests became common in industry for the selection and classification of employees. Specialized tests measuring mechanical and clerical aptitudes were particularly commonly used. Perhaps more important in the long run, several vocational interest inventories were developed, foreshadowing the importance vocational counseling would hold in the future.

During this time, Edward K. Strong published the *Strong Vocational Interest Blank* (today known as the *Strong Interest Inventory*), and Frederick Kuder published the *Kuder Preference Record—Vocational.*

During World War II, the armed services again had great need to identify recruits who could fulfill increasingly technical job responsibilities. This need, along with development and refinement of the statistical technique known as *factor analysis,* led to the further development of specialized aptitude tests and the general multiaptitude batteries. These multiaptitude batteries could help identify an individual's strengths and limitations, as well as predict performance in certain academic and vocational tasks. They still enjoy widespread popularity in many high school career assessment programs today because they can provide insights into intrapersonal strengths and weaknesses, thus helping to determine which higher education or vocational choices may make a good fit. These multiaptitude batteries, further described in Chapter 11, include the *General Aptitude Test Battery,* the *Differential Aptitude Test (DAT)*, and the *Armed Services Vocational Aptitude Battery (ASVAB).*

In 1959, in response to the successful Soviet launching of the first satellite, *Sputnik,* Congress passed the National Defense Education Act, funding school guidance counselor positions in high schools across the country with the express purpose of identifying students showing promise in the mathematical and science fields. Professional school counselors quickly learned to rely on career aptitude and interest inventories to help with this task. Numerous vocational interest, career values, and belief inventories have been published over the past 50 years, aiding counseling professionals in effectively addressing the critically important role career counseling plays in society today. In particular, career counselors, college counselors, and professional school counselors frequently use and encounter vocational aptitude and assessment instruments in their work.

Clinical and Personality Assessment

Clinical assessment pertains to the identification of mental disorders and related syndromes. **Personality assessment** is the applied area of psychology and counseling concerned with the measurement of nonintellectual affective characteristics. Importantly, many use the term *personality* in the broadest holistic sense and actually include the measure of intellect, aptitude, and achievement under a global category (Anastasi & Urbina, 1997). However, in the parlance of psychological and educational assessment, personality assessment is generally most concerned with attitudes, characteristics, motivations, and interpersonal and affective traits.

During World War I, the U.S. armed forces became interested in identifying recruits who were psychotic or otherwise not emotionally capable of military service. Asked to develop a personality inventory that could be efficiently administered to large groups of recruits, in 1919 Robert S. Woodworth developed the *Woodworth Personal Data Sheet,* basically a structured paper-and-pencil psychiatric evaluation. WWI ended without the original test ever being put into use. However, this protocol was later released for civilian use, and its creation spurred development of an entire generation of self-report personality and clinical inventories during the 1920s and 1930s. Unfortunately, these self-report tests assumed that respondents would answer truthfully and be of sound mind and judgment. Of course, those the test was meant to assess might be of neither sound mind nor judgment; the tests were transparent and responses easily faked. For example, one of the more famous questions from the Woodworth was, "I drink a quart of whiskey each day." From a social desirability perspective, it is even very easy for persons with an addiction to alcohol to see the consequences of such a question. No real procedures were in place for cross-validation of responses, so clinicians frequently made decisions based on untruthful responses, resulting in tremendous criticism of this burgeoning and promising area of assessment.

Test developers again went to work devising "validity scales," subscales that attempt to measure a client's forthrightness when answering questions. A milestone in personality and clinical test construction occurred in 1940, when Starke R. Hathaway and J. Charnley McKinley published the *Minnesota Multiphasic Personality Inventory* (*MMPI*). This test led a resurgence of self-report personality inventories because it addressed the issue of respondent forthrightness and developed several validity scales that helped examiners to identify potentially invalid test protocols. The *MMPI* has become the most commonly used and widely researched structured clinical inventory in the history of assessment. Importantly, the *MMPI* was developed and used to assess the clinical population for mental and emotional disorders, not the personality functioning of nonclinical individuals. However, the success of the *MMPI* in addressing the critics of self-report inventories spurred numerous other clinical inventories (e.g., *Millon Clinical Multiaxial Inventory* (*MCMI*), *Beck Depression Inventory* (*BDI*), *Achenbach System of Empirically Based Assessment* (*ASEBA*) and behavioral inventories (e.g., *Conners' Rating Scales* (*CRS-R*), *Behavior Assessment System for Children* (*BASC*) for clinical purposes, as well as personality inventories used with the general population (e.g., *Myers-Briggs Type Indicator, 16 PF*). The *MMPI* is now in its second edition (*MMPI-2*) (Butcher et al., 1989) and also has an adolescent version, the *Minnesota Multiphasic Personality Inventory—Adolescent* (*MMPI-A*) (Butcher et al., 1992). The *MMPI* is also somewhat different because it was not developed using factor analysis; instead it relies on items that are empirically derived and criterion based. Currently, *trait* perspectives and the *five-factor model* (Costa & McCrae, 1992) dominate the field of structured personality assessment. Traits are enduring characteristics, and the research on personality assessment appears to consistently identify a limited number of traits that underlie personality functioning (e.g., optimism, extroversion, openness to experience). This model and numerous clinical and personality inventories are explored further in Chapter 8.

Another method of personality assessment was conceived at about the same time as Woodworth's self-report measure. In 1921, Swiss psychiatrist Hermann Rorschach created a set of inkblots that aspired to provide examiners an x-ray view of a client's personality. The *Rorschach Inkblot Test* sought to explore individuals' unconscious thoughts and feelings by allowing them to "project" these thoughts, feelings, needs, hopes, fears, and motivations onto ambiguous stimuli in an unstructured task—in this case a blot of ink on a piece of paper that was folded in half to form an otherwise meaningless, bilaterally symmetrical design. The inkblot itself holds no meaning; clients attempt to structure the activity by projecting meaning from the perspective of their own worldviews and particular personalities. Response requirements are purposefully unclear, and the scoring criteria often are very subjective. The technique did not catch on immediately in Europe but became very popular in the United States during the 1930s and 1940s, when it was adopted by many psychoanalysts, who viewed it as consistent with Freud's goal of exploring the unconscious. The technique became even more popular in the 1950s and 1960s as the field of clinical psychology and personality assessment in general grew tremendously.

Numerous other projective tests have been developed, including single-word associations (e.g., "Say the first thing that comes into your mind when I say the word *mother*"); incomplete-sentence blanks (e.g., "Complete this sentence: Friends think I _____"); and drawing and storytelling tasks. In 1935, Henry A. Murray and Christiana D. Morgan published the *Thematic Apperception Test* (*TAT*), which aimed to give clinicians insight into client personality functioning by having the client look at ambiguous pictures and tell a story about each. Ostensibly, clients would project their needs and motivations into the story, yielding valuable clinical insight. Well-known drawing techniques include the *House-Tree-Person* (*H-T-P*) and *Kinetic Family Drawing* (*KFD*) techniques. For example, in the *H-T-P* clients draw pictures of a house, a tree, and a person, and the examiner generally asks a number of follow-up questions about each drawing. Each technique shares a common thread: There are no right or wrong answers, just what is on one's mind and projected into the situation. Projective tests have the advantage of promoting forthrightness in clients because they usually have no idea what is expected, and therefore find it difficult or unnecessary to be deceitful.

> **Think About It 2.1**   What events or issues appear to consistently spark the interest of the government and citizenry in testing?

General Historical Events Affecting Assessment

While the specialized disciplines of assessment (intellectual, achievement, career, personality) each contributed milestones of import, many more general events contributed to the integration and advancement of the field. And while many of the landmark advances in testing stemmed from wartime needs, the successful use of tests in the military led to their widespread use in other avenues of society, including education and industry. Important societal needs during the middle decades of the 20th century drove this utilization, including free public education, substantial population increases, mandatory school attendance, large increases in the number of college-bound youth, civil rights movements for women and minorities, and the rights of handicapped children and adults. Many of these testing initiatives stemmed not only from general societal concerns, but also from specific test-related issues such as sexual bias, cultural bias, and unfairness to certain segments of the population, all leading to improvement in the development of tests.

The rapid advancement of testing in the 1920s and 1930s led to a tremendous need to identify, catalog, and provide critical evaluations of available instruments. To fill this need, in 1938 Oscar K. Buros published the first edition of the *Mental Measurements Yearbook* (*MMY*). A new edition of these test reviews is produced every couple of years and is now available in full text (online or CD-ROM) through most university library systems.

With the proliferation of thousands of tests being published during the first half of the 20th century, test developers and examiners realized that there was a lack of standards governing the development and use of psychological and educational tests. The American Psychological Association published a guidebook of technical recommendations for test use in 1954 and was joined by the American Educational Research Association (AERA) and the National Council for Measurement and Evaluation (NCME) in 1974 to publish the first edition of *Standards for Educational and Psychological Tests.* These standards were revised in 1999 and continue to serve as a resource for the use and evaluation of tests. Likewise, the Association for Assessment in Counseling and Education (AACE) published the *Responsibilities of Users of Standardized Tests* (*RUST-3*) statement, which is now in its third edition (AACE, 2003a).

In one of the first cooperative mergers among test publishers, the American Council on Education (ACE), the Carnegie Corporation, and the College Entrance Examination Board (CEEB) combined forces during the 1950s to establish the Educational Testing Service (ETS). This merger centralized the publication and scoring of some important tests into a profitable and convenient joint endeavor. ETS continues to publish the *Scholastic Assessment Test* (*SAT*) and the *Graduate Record Exam* (*GRE*) to this day.

In education, the pendulum continues to swing. Most notably, the humanistic orientation of the 1970s was replaced by a back-to-basics movement and the current standards-based and high-stakes approaches to assessment. The back-to-basics movement led many states to develop minimum competency examinations that were designed to ensure that students graduating from high school had the minimum essential academic skills to function in a modern society (Lerner, 1981). High-stakes testing (a chapter on this subject is available on the companion website) may result in students not being promoted to the next grade or not graduating from high school unless achieving a certain minimum level of proficiency measured by the test. Similarly, some states have mandated examinations for teachers to demonstrate that they can read, write, and communicate effectively and that they have mastered the content of the subject they were hired to teach.

Several significant pieces of legislation were passed during the 1970s, including the 1974 Family Educational Rights and Privacy Act (FERPA), which mandated the rights of parents and children over the age of 18 years to view school records and required parental consent for assessment conducted around specific topics.

Computers have changed the complexion of assessment and will continue to do so for the foreseeable future. Computers can now be used to administer, score, and interpret numerous psychological and educational tests, greatly aiding the efficiency of the process. Now examiners can receive scoring and interpretive services in the comfort of their own offices for assessment instruments as diverse as career, achievement, and intelligence tests—even the *MMPI-2* and *Rorschach*.

Computer-assisted career guidance programs were devised in the 1960s and continue to grow in strength and purpose even today. High school students regularly cruise the Internet to take online career inventories, find information about career and educational opportunities, and even locate scholarship funds and complete online college and job applications. Accessible, low-cost, and quick, the immediate results and feedback of such innovations are the primary reasons for their continued success (Zunker & Norris, 1998).

Adaptive testing has made administration and scoring of large-scale testing programs even more efficient. College students taking the GREs can now spend less time on the computer-administered version than they would sitting in a classroom with a paper-and-pencil version, and they can even find out their scores at the conclusion of the tests rather than anguishing for weeks. Schools can now receive computer-generated interpretive reports that can be given to parents so that they may understand their children's performances. Clients can take tests online, via the Internet, making assessment incredibly convenient and efficient for everyone. However, with technological innovation come ethical and legal challenges, topics that are addressed later in this chapter.

Issues of diversity in assessment have been addressed by several professional organizations, and the AACE has compiled a list of these standards (http://aace.ncat .edu). During the 1990s, education experienced a shift toward *performance-based, authentic assessment,* which strives to assess students' depth of understanding by having them perform a task rather than take a pencil-and-paper examination. Likewise, an assessment initiative known as *portfolio assessment* became very popular during this time. Used for decades in modeling, art, and architecture, portfolios are a collection of performance products or samples that can be displayed and evaluated according to quality indicators. Breadth and depth of understanding displayed through real-life performance is key to this form of assessment.

In summary, the past century has witnessed the many ups and downs of testing as well as professional and technological innovations. Many criticisms have been proposed, leading to changes in test development procedures and administration practice. The next section explores some of these concerns in more detail.

PUBLIC AND PROFESSIONAL CONCERNS ABOUT ASSESSMENT

Millions of tests are given annually to help make decisions about peoples' lives. The scope of test use in the United States alone is immense. The No Child Left Behind Act of 2001 requires standardized testing of all public school students in grades 3 through 8. Nearly 2 million high school students take a college admissions test such as the *SAT* or *ACT* each year. Almost 75,000 take a special admissions test for business school, and more than 100,000 take one for law school admission.

Tests are important and helpful sources of information that, when used appropriately, help decision makers make better, more accurate decisions than can be made without the use of assessment instruments. However, sometimes the process does not work as planned. Decision makers may sometimes misunderstand the purpose of a test or use tests to make decisions for which the test scores were never validated. Sometimes the actual assessment process or the criteria for success are perceived as unfair by professionals or the public. Finally, the issue of testing has sometimes been viewed as a political tool, and has been used as one by some critics. Testing is big business, meaning big money. Also, allocation of resources for schools and individuals with disabilities or certain economic considerations is frequently tied to test performance. For example, in some states higher-performing schools meeting state goals have been rewarded with monetary compensation (e.g., program funding). In others, lower-performing schools have received increased levels of funding for new academic initiatives to help close the achievement gap. In mental health clinics and practices around the country, third-party reimbursement is achieved through assessment and diagnosis of mental disorders. Eligibility for special education services under IDEA or accommodations under Section 504 of the U.S. Rehabilitation Act of 1973 involve assessment procedures preceded or followed by funding allocations. In many ways, funding and assessment go hand in hand, meaning that politics are inevitably involved.

Ebel (1976) indicated that primary critics of testing include professional educators concerned about the effect standardized testing has on accountability and curriculum in the schools, reformers who view standardized testing as outmoded and counterproductive to quality instruction, and media representatives looking to reveal scandalous proceedings in social institutions. In fairness, the majority of teachers and the vast majority of parents support the use of standardized testing, but a vocal, politically motivated minority keeps the issue at the forefront of national attention.

This is not to say that standardized testing has not been used in ways deserving of criticism. Table 2.2 lists numerous issues creating public concern, even complaints. Throughout this book, best practices meant to mitigate each of these complaints will be addressed in some manner. Here we give a brief treatment of these complaints.

Table 2.2   Some public complaints about tests

- Decisions about children's lives should not be made on the basis of a single high-stakes test score.
- Tests are biased and unfair to minorities and women.
- Tests create anxiety and stress.
- Tests label and categorize.
- Test developers dictate what students must know or learn.
- Teaching to the test inflates scores.
- Multiple-choice questions punish intelligent, creative thinkers; trivialize the complexities of the learning process; and reward good guessers.

Decisions About Peoples' Lives Should Not Be Made on the Basis of a Single High-Stakes Test Score

We couldn't agree more! Professional counselors who make decisions about the lives of others using a single test score are behaving unprofessionally, unethically, and, depending on the location of practice, perhaps illegally. All major national professional organizations agree on this point, as a quick perusal of major national organization position statements on high-stakes testing will support. The same is generally true in education. For the past 30 years and continuing through today, U.S. law has forbidden placement of students in special education classes on the basis of a single test. Today, legal battles have ensued over a state's ability to withhold a diploma from a high school student who met all curricular requirements and passed all academic coursework but failed to obtain a minimum acceptable score on the state's high-stakes test. Numerous universities "require" a certain *SAT* or *ACT* score for admittance but state that the admissions process "takes other factors into consideration." An axiom in assessment by counseling professionals should be that *decisions about peoples' lives should be made using multiple sources of information provided by multiple respondents.* Using a single piece of data or data provided by a single source to make an important decision about a person is just plain wrong.

Tests Are Biased and Unfair to Minorities and Women

This issue receives far greater treatment later in this chapter, but for now it is important to understand that tests are used to predict some performance criterion, and that the concepts of fairness and bias have to do with how effectively tests accomplish this goal for differing groups of individuals (e.g., race, gender). Thus, if an intelligence test differentially holds some groups to an advantage and others at a disadvantage in predicting the performance criterion, it could be biased. In modern practice, test authors regularly go to great lengths to ensure fairness in test content, but because cultures vary, bias of individual items may vary also.

Of course, it is essential that the performance criterion be equally free from bias. An example is the sometimes-reported observation that standardized achievement tests must be biased against girls because boys sometimes outperform girls on multiple-choice tests, but girls get higher grades in school-based classes. It is easy to jump to this conclusion, except for one thing. Consider that the standardized test scores are objectively derived and subjected to bias analyses. Can the same claim be made for school grades? Nearly any school teacher will confirm that, on average, girls turn in homework more frequently, prepare for exams and study more, are better behaved in the classroom, and generally get higher test scores than boys. If this is the case, girls should get higher grades than boys, but higher grades do not necessarily mean that one knows more or has better mastery of the course content. Given this context, it is just as logical to conclude that the criterion (grades) is more biased against boys than standardized tests against girls. The point is, always consider the bias and fairness of both the predictor (i.e., the variable/test score used to predict the criterion) and the criterion.

Tests Create Anxiety and Stress

That tests create anxiety and stress is, of course, true; but not always in the way many fear. Large-scale group-administered testing certainly creates a degree of stress that, hopefully, reaches a moderate level. Remember the Yerkes-Dodson law: Moderate anxiety maximizes performance; low and high anxiety minimize performance. Of greatest concern is a student's phobic or panicked reaction due to a high degree of anxiety, usually with high-stakes tests. While there is certainly anecdotal evidence to support this claim of high degrees of pressure being placed upon students (including physical illness, vomiting, and crying), this claim is not true for the vast majority of students. Professional counselors understand that a small percentage of the population suffers from test phobia and take steps to treat it when appropriate. Professional counselors also understand that a significant proportion of the school-aged population may be diagnosed with an anxiety disorder (see Chapter7), usually Generalized Anxiety Disorder, and take steps to treat these difficulties when appropriate. Anxious people are likely to get upset about tests *and* myriad other life events. Professionals need to predict who will be affected and to take preventive and interventive measures. All told, the vast majority of individuals are not harmed or unduly upset by standardized testing. In fact, most educators are far more concerned about the other end of the spectrum—unmotivated students who care too little and do not get anxious enough about tests.

Tests Label and Categorize

While it is true that tests label and categorize, technically speaking, it is the decision makers (e.g., professional counselors, multidisciplinary team members, or mental health professionals) who label and categorize. Frequently, labeling is a necessary evil in society because labels are used to identify individuals in need of, and entitled to, services. For example, identifying a child with a learning disability is a step toward obtaining the educational services the child may need for academic success. Clinical tests are often used to identify individuals with mental disorders so that third-party (i.e., insurance company) reimbursement can be obtained for counseling services. In this way, tests can be a valuable aid in making more accurate decisions about the categories that clients and students are determined to fit.

While the public holds many concerns about labeling of clients and students, much of the concern about the use of labels lies in two areas: (1) that tests may be used to mislabel an individual, and (2) that labels may be used as an excuse for some remediable (or even nonexistent) condition. Professional counselors must always be aware of the potential for misidentification. Tests are not perfect predictors; nothing is. Tests are instruments that inform the decisions of professional counselors and must be used with other sources and types of information to arrive at accurate decisions. Inaccurate labels tend to have detrimental consequences for clients, sometimes lasting for many years. For example, a 7-year-old boy inaccurately identified as mentally retarded may spend three or more years in an instructional program specially designed for students with mental retardation. A young man inaccurately diagnosed with schizophrenia may not only receive improper treatment, but be followed by an erroneous paper trail and even wrongful discrimination in the workplace.

Others may use a label as an excuse for not trying in school or not pursuing effective treatment strategies. For example, children with Attention-Deficit/ Hyperactivity Disorder (AD/HD) may use the condition as an excuse for not trying hard in math. Worse, teachers and parents may use the diagnosis as an excuse for not encouraging such students to put more effort into their studies. Excuses such as, "He has a poor memory," "She can't write well so shouldn't be expected to," or "He'll always be disorganized" may be true to a certain degree but also may become self-fulfilling prophecies with no effort put forth to ever cope and compensate for difficulties.

Test Developers Dictate What Students Must Know or Learn

Developers of achievement tests select items that measure the domain of knowledge being assessed. They use several methods in this process, including curriculum and textbook reviews, reviews of previously available tests, and consultation and evaluation of experts in the given content area. The goal is to develop a test that faithfully and accurately samples the domain of knowledge. In today's standards-based and large-scale (group) assessment atmosphere, it is common for state departments of education to develop their own learning standards and instructional objectives and to contract with publishers to measure those standards and objectives. Good curriculum evaluation starts with well-defined standards, which are then implemented through an effective curriculum (including benchmarks, instructional objectives, and instructional activities) and appropriately assessed.

The key is for the test or assessment program to align perfectly with the curriculum, and for the curriculum to align perfectly with the standards. In the past, many large-scale achievement tests were "off the shelf" and thus may or may not have aligned with a given school's curriculum. Misalignment can result in lowered test scores. For example, if a curriculum teaches only half of what an achievement test measures (i.e., 50% overlap between test and curriculum), then low scores will result. Unfortunately, it was difficult for educators to determine whether low student scores were due to misalignment (i.e., students were not taught half of what they needed to know to do well on the test) or poor skills (i.e., students did not master the half of the items that they were taught).

Recently, educators and test publishers have worked collaboratively to develop large-scale tests that are tailored to state needs and aligned with state learning standards. Frequently, these tests are composed of "off the shelf" items that do apply to the state standards and are augmented with item pools that measure additional specific state standards. In this way, test items align more precisely with state standards, and the burden is on school systems and individual teachers to develop and implement an effective curriculum. The mechanics of this issue is addressed in the chapter on high-stakes testing, which is available on the companion website for this text.

"Teaching to the Test" Inflates Scores

As a continuation of the previous criticism, teachers are supposed to implement a curriculum that provides the bridge between standards and assessment. "Teaching to the test," a phrased loathed by most educators, means that the focus of instruction becomes so precribed that only content that is sure to appear on an exam is addressed in instruction. Obviously, if this occurs, test scores should rise.

Whether test scores are inflated in this instance is a matter of content mastery. Consider an example from the classroom. Teachers "teach to the test" all the time in the regular curriculum. They have a learning objective—say single-times-single-digit multiplication (e.g., $3 \times 6 = 18$, $7 \times 8 = 56$); instruct students in the process for arriving at correct solutions; assign activities in class and for homework to enhance student mastery; and then, finally, test student knowledge with some kind of teacher-made or textbook examination. If the students are prepared and motivated, and the teacher implements the instruction efficiently, students should receive high scores. Whether the scores are inflated depends on whether the student scores reflect mastery of the domain of behavior—that is, can the students effectively solve nearly all single-by-single-digit multiplication problems. If the answer is yes, great—that was the goal. In contrast, assume the teacher decides ahead of time that the test will be comprised of 10 items and the students are instructed and drilled only on those 10 items. It is quite likely that the students will do very well on the examination but not be very proficient at calculating items from the broader domain. In this example, the test scores do not accurately reflect the level of mastery of the total domain. As a result, it can be said that the scores are inflated.

To solve this dilemma, test publishers, state education departments, and local educators must work collaboratively to develop test items that adequately sample the broad content domain and standards. Equally important, these entities must protect and secure the test content so that teachers do not know which items will appear. This ensures that student test performance reflects content mastery, not the teaching of how to solve specific items. In the end, if teachers understand the standards, are provided with an effective curriculum and material resources, and effectively implement the instructional strategies, then motivated, prepared students will master the domain of knowledge being assessed. (Note that there are a lot of "ifs"!)

Multiple-Choice Questions Punish Intelligent, Creative Thinkers; Trivialize the Complexities of the Learning Process; and Reward Good Guessers

While multiple-choice questions can effectively measure knowledge and skills in diverse areas, it would be absurd to propose that they can effectively measure everything. Sometimes extended-response items (e.g., essays) or performance evaluations are necessary because they allow for the assessment of applied skills and more thorough explanations. For example, in the training of professional counselors, it is a necessary and common occurrence for the trainee to be observed actually counseling clients, either live or on video. No multiple-choice or essay test can substitute for this performance assessment. That is not to say that certain knowledge components of the counseling process cannot be tested—only that the act of counseling is a fluid, applied process that happens with real people. In some instances, indirect measures cannot be substituted for direct measures.

Whether multiple-choice items measure trivial or meaningful information is really in the hands of the test developer. Remember from the discussion above that test items are created to measure some standard or objective so that an inference can be made about the mastery of a domain of behavior. Thus if the standard or objective is trivial, so will be the question. Well-crafted multiple-choice questions can measure advanced, high-level thinking every bit as well as other response formats. It all comes down to the skill of the item writer.

The criticism is often made that students who are "good guessers" or "lucky guessers" can get significantly higher scores on a multiple-choice test. However, the facts simply do not support this assertion. On a typical four-choice, multiple-choice question, the likelihood of getting a question correct just by guessing is 25% (0.25). Now if the test has very few items on it, getting one additional question correct might make a difference, but most large-scale assessments have hundreds of questions, and subtests usually have dozens. Thus to get an appreciably higher score, one would have to guess correctly on several to perhaps dozens of questions. Anyone can beat the odds, of course; but what are the odds of beating the odds? Let's use as an example that students would need to guess correctly on four questions in order to appreciably increase their score. When you know that a student has a 25% (0.25) chance of guessing correctly on each item, the odds are easy to compute: $0.25 \times 0.25 \times 0.25 \times 0.25 = 0.004$—a 0.4% chance of guessing correctly on all four items. This means that 4 out of 1,000 students taking that subtest might get a substantially higher score. Now if one is a die-hard gambler, these odds are about four times higher than hitting the "Pick 3" Lotto—something to get excited about, perhaps. But in the assessment arena, few would bet their college admission prospects, or their grade in an assessment course, on them.

Learning From Past Mistakes and Criticisms

Periodically throughout history, the use of tests has come under attack, and such attacks sometimes limit the widespread application of test use in society. These movements are often double edged; they highlight fair criticisms of the power that tests sometimes wield in decision making but fail to replace the current system with one that is more objective, accurate, and fair. This is the dilemma: Tests have risen to current prominence because they provide more objective, accurate, and fair information on which decisions can be made . . . *but* . . . because no test is perfect, errors can and do occur in the decisions made. What critics often fail to mention is that a systematic decision-making process using standardized tests most often results in fewer poor decisions than a nonsystematic decision-making process based on "judgment," in which the decision maker becomes the instrument (more on this in Chapter 7). Individuals exercising judgment are just as susceptible to threats to reliability and validity as tests.

To prevent biased judgments, professional counselors receive substantial training in assessment. Professional counselors must understand the important concepts that guide the development of assessment instruments in order to become informed consumers. The future of assessment in counseling depends on professional counselors being able to use assessments effectively to benefit students and clients, to base their decisions on objective facts, and to replicate and justify those decisions on the basis of scientific evidence, not subjective "feel." Professional counselors have a professional duty and responsibility to know as much as they can about all facets of counseling in order to best serve and advocate for students and clients.

ETHICS AND ASSESSMENT

Counseling, like many other professions, is guided both by laws and by ethical standards. **Laws** regulate who can perform what type of counseling, in which settings, and with which clients. Additionally, in the area of assessment, myriad policies and procedures regulate who can be or is assessed, under what circumstances, for what reasons, and who is qualified to administer and interpret the assessments. However, despite the controls that exist within the area of assessment, there is still tremendous room for judgment on the part of the professional regarding these issues. Responsibility for final decisions regarding conduct rests with counselors themselves (Wickwire, 2002). In the absence of laws, policies, and procedures, ethical standards are the basis for appropriate and professional behavior. **Codes of ethics** propose guidelines for standards of professional behavior, and it is essential for professional counselors to be familiar with and follow these standards in order to provide high-quality, professional counseling services.

Both laws and ethical standards are based on generally accepted societal norms, beliefs, customs, and values (Fischer & Sorenson, 1997) and exist for the good of society. However, laws are more prescriptive, have been codified, and generally carry penalties for failure to comply. Ethical standards are generally developed by professional associations to guide the behavior of a particular group of professionals. According to Herlihy and Corey (1996), ethical standards serve three purposes: to educate members about sound ethical behavior, to provide a mechanism for accountability, and to serve as a means for improving professional practice. They also serve a fourth purpose—to educate, and therefore protect, the public about the standards of behavior they can expect from a particular group of professionals. Associations periodically update their ethical codes to ensure continuing relevance and applicability and involve stakeholders in the process. The enforcement of ethical standards is the responsibility of the association, which is usually limited in what it can do to members who fail to comply. It is the responsibility of each member to voluntarily comply and behave ethically because it is the right thing to do, although sanctions for noncompliance may occur.

Forester-Miller and Davis (1996) suggested that Kitchener's five moral principles are the cornerstone of the American Counseling Association's ethical standards. The first is *autonomy,* which refers to clients' independence and right to make sound and rational decisions on their own. *Nonmaleficence* is often referred to as "do no harm"; professional counselors must avoid behaviors that place clients at risk or could potentially cause harm. *Beneficence* involves contributing to the positive welfare of clients and their growth. *Justice* means treating each client according to what is best for that client—fair treatment and consideration of each client. The last principle is *fidelity,* which refers to honoring commitments and establishing an accepting relationship in which the client can trust the professional counselor. These moral principles are critically important in the field of assessment to ensure that clients receive professional and appropriate services that are in their best interest.

There are a number of codes of ethical standards, since different associations and divisions within the counseling profession promulgate their own codes. However, since all of the ethical standards are based on either the moral principles previously discussed or similar common values, the similarities among the codes are greater than the differences. These differences usually pertain to workplace setting. The American Counseling Association's *Code of Ethics* (2005a) will be used as the basis for the discussion that follows here. The *Code of Ethics* delineates the responsibilities of professional counselors toward their clients, their colleagues, the workplace, and themselves. It is divided into eight sections: The Counseling Relationship; Confidentiality; Privileged Communication and Privacy; Professional Responsibility; Relationships With Other Professionals; Evaluation, Assessment, and Interpretation; Supervision, Training, and Teaching; Research and Publication; and Resolving Ethical Issues. Section E: Evaluation, Assessment, and Interpretation is reviewed below.

Section E: Evaluation, Assessment, and Interpretation covers standards related to the assessment of clients, the counselor's skills, and appropriateness of assessment, including: general appraisal issues, competence to use and interpret tests, informed consent for appraisal, releasing information, proper diagnosis of mental disorders, test selection, conditions of test administration, diversity in testing, test scoring and interpretation, test security, obsolete tests and outdated test results, and test construction.

Each subsection delineated below in italics is quoted from the *ACA Code of Ethics* (2005a) and accompanied by commentary.

Section E: Evaluation, Assessment, and Interpretation

Introduction. Counselors use assessment instruments as one component of the counseling process, taking into account the client personal and cultural context. Counselors promote the well-being of individual clients or groups of clients by developing and using appropriate educational, psychological, and career assessment instruments.

E.1. General

E.1.a. Assessment. The primary purpose of educational, psychological, and career assessment is to provide measurements that are valid and reliable in either comparative or absolute terms. These include, but are not limited to, measurements of ability, personality, interest, intelligence, achievement, and performance. Counselors recognize the need to interpret the statements in this section as applying to both quantitative and qualitative assessments.

E.1.b. Client Welfare. Counselors do not misuse assessment results and interpretations, and they take reasonable steps to prevent others from misusing the information these techniques provide. They respect the client's right to know the results, the interpretations made, and the bases for counselors' conclusions and recommendations.

It is the responsibility of the professional counselor to use assessment techniques and results appropriately and to ensure that others do as well. As mentioned in the discussion of the moral principles underlying the ethical standards, professional counselors must operate in the best interest of the client. Salvia and Ysseldyke (2004, p. 58) go further and state that "those who assess . . . must accept responsibility for the consequences of their work, and they must make every effort to make certain their services are used appropriately." In so doing, professional counselors use instruments that will yield reliable and valid scores so that decisions made using these instruments will benefit clients.

E.2. Competence to Use and Interpret Assessment Instruments

E.2.a. Limits of Competence. Counselors utilize only those testing and assessment services for which they have been trained and are competent. Counselors using technology-assisted test interpretations are trained in the construct being measured and the specific instrument being used prior to using its technology-based application. Counselors take reasonable measures to ensure the proper use of psychological and career assessment techniques by persons under their supervision. . . .

E.2.b. Appropriate Use. Counselors are responsible for the appropriate application, scoring, interpretation, and use of assessment instruments relevant to the needs of the client, whether they score and interpret such assessments themselves or use technology or other services.

E.2.c. Decisions Based on Results. Counselors responsible for decisions involving individuals or policies that are based on assessment results have a thorough understanding of educational, psychological, and career measurement, including validation criteria, assessment research, and guidelines for assessment development and use.

Professional associations, employers, test publishers, and test users have put safeguards in place to ensure the qualifications of professionals using assessments. A number of guidelines and resources have been developed to assist professional counselors in this area, including the *RUST-3* statement (AACE, 2003a) and the *Standards for Educational and Psychological Testing* (AERA et al., 1999). These guidelines and resources are discussed in other chapters of this book. However, the responsibility for appropriate use and interpretation of assessments lies with the professional counselor. Professional counselors should conduct a thorough search to ensure that the instrument or assessments selected are appropriate for the client, the intended purpose, and the information needed (Wickwire, 2002). Additionally, the professional counselor must be trained in the assessment procedure and qualified to conduct the assessment. Often students take assessment classes in graduate school but gain little additional training during their careers. Thorndike (1997) suggested that the assessor withdraw from the process if insufficiently trained to provide the quality of services and expertise required. Professional counselors have an obligation to maintain or increase their expertise in the area of assessment if they are going to conduct assessment activities.

Standard E.2 mandates that professional counselors receive periodic training and retraining on assessments used. Just as important, simply knowing how to administer and score a test does not satisfy this requirement. Professional counselors endeavor to know as much as possible about the construct or content under study, including the test psychometrics, purposes for which the test has been validated, and other research related to the test's use.

Professional counselors are highly trained and ensure that those under their supervision are trained to use assessments for intended purposes. When supervisees or employees under a counselor's supervision behave unethically, it is the supervising professional counselor who bears responsibility for their misactions.

3. Informed Consent in Assessment

E.3.a. Explanation to Clients. Prior to assessment, counselors explain the nature and purposes of assessment and the specific use of results by potential recipients. The explanation will be given in the language of the client (or other legally authorized person on behalf of the client), unless an explicit exception has been agreed upon in advance. Counselors consider the client's personal or cultural context, the level of the client's understanding of the results, and the impact of the results on the client. . . .

E.3.b. Recipients of Results. Counselors consider the examinee's welfare, explicit understandings, and prior agreements in determining who receives the assessment results. Counselors include accurate and appropriate interpretations with any release of individual or group assessment results. . . .

E.4. Release of Data to Qualified Professionals

Counselors release assessment data in which the client is identified only with the consent of the client or the client's legal representative. Such data are released only to persons recognized by counselors as qualified to interpret the data. . . .

Informed consent implies that the person granting permission understands exactly what assessments will be conducted, why the assessments are being conducted, what will happen to the results, and who will be given the results. **Confidentiality** is the cornerstone of counseling and is critical to the area of assessment, particularly when the assessment concerns very personal questions or asks for sensitive information. Frequently, permission to conduct assessments requires signed, informed consent from either the client or, in the case of a minor child, the parent or legal guardian. The legitimacy of informed consent rests upon three essential facets: capacity, comprehension, and voluntariness. *Capacity* refers to the right one holds to consent. For example, precious few circumstances exist that would allow a 9-year-old boy the right to consent to anything. This is because in the United States, the parent or legal guardian almost always holds this right. Likewise, someone who has mental retardation or is mentally disabled may not have the ability to consent. *Comprehension* means the consenter understands the implications of consent. If the evaluator cannot communicate the purpose of the assessment in a language or terms the client can understand, consent cannot be obtained. *Voluntariness* means the assessment involves no coercion or duress. As with any ethically conducted research study, a client has the right to withdraw from an assessment at any time.

The Family Educational Rights and Privacy Act of 1974 (FERPA) and subsequent amendments govern student records in schools and universities. FERPA mandates that only those persons with a legitimate educational interest have the right to access a student's records, including assessment information, and that psychological evaluations and some other assessments and surveys require signed, informed consent. In school settings, it may be clearer who has a legitimate need to access a student's assessment results, but there may also be more professionals involved due to the number of support staff and teams operating within schools. Professional counselors should ensure that the persons with whom assessment results are shared, whether in the clinic or at school team meetings, have a legitimate need to know the results and are fully capable of understanding the results. Professional counselors must also safeguard the maintenance of assessment protocols and results. Under normal circumstances, protocols and raw interview data are released only with client permission and only to professionals who can understand and use the information to make decisions in the best interest of the client.

The same limits to confidentiality that exist within the counseling relationship also exist within the assessment area unless informed consent is provided. The client (or parent or guardian of a minor) always has the right to request in writing that information be shared. Professional counselors must be aware that assessment information is subject to court orders and subpoenas and duty-to-warn situations. In addition, sharing information with third parties (e.g., insurance companies); allowing clerks, secretaries, and other personnel to handle assessment information; and consultation are all legitimate limitations to confidentiality.

Think About It 2.2   What makes confidentiality and informed consent such important aspects of assessment?

E.5. Diagnosis of Mental Disorders

E.5.a. Proper Diagnosis. Counselors take special care to provide proper diagnosis of mental disorders. Assessment techniques (including personal interview) used to determine client care (e.g., locus of treatment, type of treatment, or recommended follow-up) are carefully selected and appropriately used.

E.5.b. Cultural Sensitivity. Counselors recognize that culture affects the manner in which clients' problems are defined. Clients' socioeconomic and cultural experiences are considered when diagnosing mental disorders. . . .

E.5.c. Historical and Social Prejudices in the Diagnosis of Pathology. Counselors recognize historical and social prejudices in the misdiagnosis and pathologizing of certain individuals and groups and the role of mental health professionals in perpetuating these prejudices through diagnosis and treatment.

E.5.d. Refraining from Diagnosis. Counselors may refrain from making and/or reporting a diagnosis if they believe it would cause harm to the client or others.

Standard 8.8 of the *Standards for Educational and Psychological Testing* (AERA et al., 1999) advises that the least stigmatizing label should always be assigned when reporting test results. This does not mean that a less serious code is used, but rather the diagnosis should be an appropriate one and described precisely. Contextual factors (e.g., the client's cultural or socioeconomic experiences) must be considered when diagnosing clients because of the significant impact diagnostic labels can have on a client's life (Whiston, 2005). In some cases, the diagnostic code drives treatment protocols and/or payment for treatment. This factor presents a serious dilemma for many practitioners, as the specified number of sessions for one diagnostic code may be insufficient to adequately assist the client, while a different code would allow a sufficient number of sessions. Still, the *Code of Ethics* requires that professional counselors use the proper diagnosis. A great deal of research is currently under way exploring the congruence of diagnoses across diverse populations. For example, the context of living in a low-socioeconomic inner-city neighborhood may elevate the number of criteria for Conduct Disorder the average adolescent male may meet. But if these behaviors have become "normative" due to context, is it equitable that the diagnosis of Conduct Disorder is made at a substantially increased rate for these inner-city youth? Or should a more culture-normative, context-sensitive process be pursued? This question is becoming critically important and will likely receive tremendous attention in the coming years.

E.6. Instrument Selection

E.6.a. Appropriateness of Instruments. *Counselors carefully consider the validity, reliability, psychometric limitations, and appropriateness of instruments when selecting assessments.*

E.6.b. Referral Information. *If a client is referred to a third party for assessment, the counselor provides specific referral questions and sufficient objective data about the client to ensure that appropriate assessment instruments are utilized. . . .*

E.6.c. Culturally Diverse Populations. *Counselors are cautious when selecting assessments for culturally diverse populations to avoid the use of instruments that lack appropriate psychometric properties for the client population. . . .*

Professional counselors should choose assessments that are the most appropriate for the targeted purpose of the assessment and for the clients they are assessing (Anastasi & Urbina, 1997). Doing so may involve a thorough search and evaluation of potential assessment instruments. According to Wickwire (2002), this step is essential, as the "professional is seeking an appropriate and workable fit, with the highest quality and greatest benefit" (p. 8). The implication of "fit" for clients from diverse populations is particularly important. Professional counselors must explore each instrument's psychometric properties and ensure its appropriateness and usefulness for clients from diverse cultures.

E.7. Conditions of Assessment Administration . . .

E.7.a. Administration Conditions. *Counselors administer assessments under the same conditions that were established in their standardization. When assessments are not administered under standard conditions, as may be necessary to accommodate* *clients with disabilities, or when unusual behavior or irregularities occur during the administration, those conditions are noted in interpretation, and the results may be designated as invalid or of questionable validity.*

E.7.b. Technological Administration. *Counselors ensure that administration programs function properly and provide clients with accurate results when technological or other electronic methods are used for assessment administration.*

E.7.c. Unsupervised Assessments. *Unless the assessment instrument is designed, intended, and validated for self-administration and/or scoring, counselors do not permit inadequately supervised use.*

E.7.d. Disclosure of Favorable Conditions. *Prior to test administration of assessments, conditions that produce most favorable assessment results are made known to the examinee.*

The previous discussion has concerned the need for care in the selection of assessment tools. Equal care must be taken with the use of these tools and the administration of all assessments in order to achieve the optimal result. Changing the way in which assessments are given or the conditions under which they are given may negate the usefulness and validity of the results. Professional counselors must be sensitive to conditions that may affect assessment performance (Anastasi & Urbina, 1997). This awareness is particularly important when some clients are advantaged by having access to experiences or information about how to perform better on a test—sometimes referred to as *test sophistication.* Certainly an individual who takes a standardized test and has had multiple exposures to sample test questions and the "bubble" response format (i.e., penciling in answers on a machine-scored form) will have advantages over someone who doesn't know what to expect or how to respond appropriately ahead of time. Professional counselors seek to "level the playing field" by ensuring that all students have requisite information and skills.

E.8. Multicultural Issues/Diversity in Assessment

Counselors use with caution assessment techniques that were normed on populations other than that of the client. Counselors recognize the effects of age, color, culture, disability, ethnic group, gender, race, language preference, religion, spirituality, sexual orientation, and socioeconomic status on test administration and interpretation, and place test results in proper perspective with other relevant factors. . . .

According to recent projections, the United States racial population will approach 50% non-White by the year 2050. Communities and schools are becoming increasingly diverse. In some schools, the number of different languages spoken exceeds 150. This increasing diversity poses serious concerns for assessment if professional counselors are to behave ethically. **Diversity** concerns are discussed in depth later in this chapter. For now, it is important to understand that it is the burden of test authors to demonstrate that the test scores are not affected by diverse examinee characteristics. In the absence of a declarative statement by test authors in this regard, the examiner should assume that cultural differences may exist and approach use of the test with culturally diverse clients with caution.

E.9. Scoring and Interpretation of Assessments

E.9.a. Reporting. In reporting assessment results, counselors indicate reservations that exist regarding validity or reliability due to the circumstances of the assessment or the inappropriateness of the norms for the person tested.

E.9.b. Research Instruments. Counselors exercise caution when interpreting the results of research instruments not having sufficient technical data to support respondent results. The specific purposes for the use of such instruments are stated explicitly to the examinee.

E.9.c. Assessment Services. Counselors who provide assessment scoring and interpretation services to support the assessment process confirm the validity of such interpretations. They accurately describe the purpose, norms, validity, reliability, and applications of the procedures and any special qualifications applicable to their use. The public offering of an automated test interpretations service is considered a professional-to-professional consultation. The formal responsibility of the consultant is to the consultee, but the ultimate and overriding responsibility is to the client. . . .

Professional counselors are ultimately responsible for the accuracy of the assessment results and must make every effort to ensure that their services are used appropriately (Salvia & Ysseldyke, 2004) and that the best interest of the client is served. This is equally true when using computerized interpretive programs. While information derived from an interpretive report is often accurate and helpful, professional counselors realize that these interpretations are based on statistical models and that the software author has never met the client. Thus, as is *always* the case, professional counselors validate and supplement all scores and interpretation with additional information from multiple sources before making decisions that affect clients' lives.

Also, while professional counselors strive to administer tests exactly as specified, mistakes and outside interference do occur. Professional counselors document these circumstances and consider them when interpreting test scores. If the circumstances are serious enough to invalidate the test scores, professional counselors state such and then *do not use the invalid scores to describe client performance or make decisions affecting a client's life.* If the professional counselor has any reservations about the assessment results, it is the responsibility of the counselor to communicate those reservations to the client and/or other appropriate parties, such as parents. The professional counselor must ensure that accurate and appropriate interpretations accompany the dissemination of any assessment results so that the recipients of the information are clear as to what the results actually are.

E.10. Assessment Security

Counselors maintain the integrity and security of tests and other assessment techniques consistent with legal and contractual obligations. Counselors do not appropriate, reproduce, or modify published assessments or parts thereof without acknowledgment and permission from the publisher.

E.11. Obsolete Assessments and Outdated Results

Counselors do not use data or results from assessments that are obsolete or outdated for the current purpose. Counselors make every effort to prevent the misuse of obsolete measures and assessment data by others.

E.12. Assessment Construction

Counselors use established scientific procedures, relevant standards, and current professional knowledge for assessment design in the development, publication, and utilization of educational and psychological assessment techniques.

Professional counselors must preserve the integrity of the assessments and the accompanying protocols. Testing materials should be stored in a locked facility to prevent theft or misuse by unauthorized individuals. All published tests are copyright protected and cannot be photocopied for use with clients. Tests are very expensive to develop, norm, and print. Development of these products is done through financial risks by authors and publishers. For those professional counselors who are involved with the development of assessments, it is important to adhere to current scientific standards and methodology. Among numerous sources, the *RUST-3* statement (AACE, 2003a) and the *Standards for Educational and Psychological Testing* (AERA et al., 1999) are important to consult when developing tests.

If the assessment information is outdated, professional counselors must take care with its use, as the validity and usefulness of the information may be questionable. In brief, professional counselors should discontinue use of older versions of tests, and cease using them to make client decisions. However, it is not always easy to make this call. Previous versions of tests often have a rich research base and numerous studies exploring psychometric integrity. Also, it is, unfortunately, not unusual for new norms and new test manuals to have errors. Thus it is often prudent to phase in use of new instruments and to use the new instrument exclusively once its quality has been established.

E.13. Forensic Evaluation: Evaluation for Legal Proceedings

E.13.a. Primary Obligations. When providing forensic evaluations, the primary obligation of counselors is to produce objective findings that can be substantiated based on information and techniques appropriate to the evaluation, which may include examination of the individual and/or review of records. Counselors are entitled to form professional opinions based on their professional knowledge and expertise that can be supported by the data gathered in evaluations. Counselors will define the limits of their reports or testimony, especially when an examination of the individual has not been conducted.

E.13b. Consent for Evaluation. Individuals being evaluated are informed in writing that the relationship is for purposes of an evaluation and is not counseling in nature, and entities or individuals who will receive the evaluation report are identified. Written consent to be evaluated is obtained from those being evaluated unless a court orders evaluations to be conducted without the written consent of individuals being evaluated. When children or vulnerable adults are being evaluated, informed written consent is obtained from a parent or guardian.

E.13.c. Client Evaluation Prohibited. Counselors do not evaluate individuals for forensic purposes they currently counsel or individuals they have counseled in the past. Counselors do not accept as counseling clients individuals they are evaluating or individuals they have evaluated in the past for forensic purposes.

E.13.d. Avoid Potentially Harmful Relationships. Counselors who provide forensic evaluations avoid potentially harmful professional or personal relationships with family members, romantic partners, and close friends of individuals they are evaluating or have evaluated in the past.

Forensic evaluation and court testimony is a burgeoning specialty within counseling, psychology, and psychiatry. The standard regarding avoidance of potentially harmful relationships is a new addition to the 2005 *Code of Ethics* and seeks to make sure that professional counselors understand the importance of making inferences based on firsthand knowledge of the client, rather than speculation or generalities. Professional counselors can expect much more attention to this area of study in the future because of the increasing need of courts, lawyers, and those accused of crimes to have mental health experts provide testimony regarding psychological status. Also, this is another issue that psychological boards across the country are pursuing in order to attempt to limit the scope of professional counselors' practice.

Source: Section E of the *ACA Code of Ethics and Standards of Practice* has been reprinted with permission. No further reproduction is authorized without written permission from the American Counseling Association.

Think About It 2.3   When assessments are conducted with clients and students, it is essential that results be used correctly. What are some consequences of inappropriate use? How could these problems be resolved?

While the *ACA Code of Ethics* is helpful in describing ethical test use, the reader is again referred to the *RUST-3* statement for a comprehensive and explanatory treatise of responsible, professional test use. Assessment information, used in conjunction with other sources of information about the client, can be extremely useful in working with clients. As can be seen from this discussion, it is critically important for professional counselors to practice ethically in order to do no harm. But what should a professional counselor do if unsure of the correct ethical course of action? For answers, we now turn to a brief discussion of ethical decision making as applied to assessment issues.

ETHICAL DECISION MAKING

One of the greatest professional challenges facing most counselors is ethical behavior—that is, determining the ethically appropriate course of action in any situation. Professional counselors must also be acutely aware of the behavior of their colleagues and have a responsibility to act if a colleague is behaving in an unethical manner. To assist professional counselors with these issues, the ACA's Ethics Committee developed the *Practitioner's Guide to Ethical Decision Making* (Forester-Miller & Davis, 1996), which delineates a seven-step model for working through ethical dilemmas:

1. *Identify the problem.* One should gather all relevant information and determine whether the problem is an ethical issue or a legal, practice, or other issue. If it is an ethical issue, continue with the process.
2. *Apply the ACA* Code of Ethics (2005a). Determine which section of the *ACA Code of Ethics* addresses the issue most directly. The relevant section may outline the course of action to follow. If the answer is not indicated, then one should proceed to the next step of the model.
3. *Determine the nature and dimensions of the dilemma.* Forester-Miller and Davis suggested that professional counselors should consider the moral principles that underlie the *Code of Ethics* for direction, current research, and consultation to determine an appropriate course of action.
4. *Generate potential courses of action.* Professional counselors should consult at least one colleague to ensure that all potential courses of action are identified.
5. *Consider the potential consequences of all options and determine a course of action.* The impact of potential consequences on the client, professional counselor, and others should be considered in determining which option is optimal for addressing the dilemma.
6. *Evaluate the selected course of action.* Evaluate the selected course of action to ensure that implementing that choice will not create new or additional ethical dilemmas.
7. *Implement the course of action.* The professional counselor should implement the selected course and follow up to ensure that the selected action had the desired outcome.

The following scenario highlights the use of the ethical decision-making model in practice for an assessment-related issue. The Student Services Team (SST) at Happy Days Middle School meets once a month to discuss students who are experiencing problems that are interfering with their ability to be successful academically or socially in school. Ms. Jones is a licensed professional counselor who works in the school-based mental health center and routinely attends the SST meetings as a team member. A student new to the school who was experiencing both academic and social difficulty was referred for assessment. At the meeting the next month, the results of the student's assessment were presented and discussed. Ms. Jones reviewed the assessment results and had a number of concerns. In particular, she questioned whether the assessments used were appropriate for the student, wanted to know why an older version of the *WISC* had been used, and also questioned whether the person administering the assessments (the learning disabilities teacher) was qualified to do so. When she tried to raise these issues, the SST members ignored her concerns and agreed to change the student's program based on the assessment results and anecdotal information.

Ms. Jones believed that this situation was an ethical dilemma and therefore used the ethical decision-making model. She first identified the problem and then applied the *ACA Code of Ethics.* In this case, she identified three problems and the applicable sections of the *Code of Ethics:* the use of obsolete and inappropriate assessment instruments (E.6.a), the competence of the person administering the assessments (E.2.a), and the use of the assessment results in placement (E.2.b). To determine the nature and dimensions of the issue, she went to her supervisor to discuss her concerns. Since she is not employed by the school system, she wanted to make sure that she was considering all facets of the situation and recognized that perhaps there were processes in the schools she did not understand.

Ms. Jones concluded that the problems she had identified were ethical dilemmas in this case and suspected that they might also exist in other cases as well. She then determined possible courses of action. Ms. Jones's supervisor identified a supervisor in the school system with whom Ms. Jones could discuss her concerns. Ms. Jones also thought about going back to the team and discussing her concerns again, and also talking with the person who performed the assessment to determine why these particular assessments were used and what credentials the assessor held. After considering all options and their potential consequences, Ms. Jones chose to speak to the assessor. She felt this was particularly important since the *Code of Ethics* also indicates that if one is concerned about the ethical behavior of a colleague, the first step is to discuss the concern directly with the colleague, even one who is not a counselor bound to uphold the *ACA Code of Ethics.*

Through Ms. Jones's discussion with the assessor, it became clear to her that the assessor lacked the experience and training to conduct an assessment using current tools and that the school system had not purchased current versions of assessments and had not provided appropriate professional development for the staff. Ms. Jones then went to the school system supervisor to discuss her concerns. As a result of this discussion, the school system recognized the need to change some of its practices, and the assessments for the student in question were redone by a qualified assessor using current tests.

As Ms. Jones discovered, professional counselors must continually review their behavior and that of their colleagues to ensure that the best interests of the client always come first, that their practice reflects current best practices, that they use and/or interpret only those assessments for which they are trained, and that the assessments chosen are appropriate for the client and the intended purpose.

LEGAL ISSUES IN ASSESSMENT

While ethical issues in assessment are important, professional counselors must be even more aware of important legal rulings. Ethical codes represent high standards of professional practice; however, laws must be followed, even if they conflict with ethical standards. Both federal and state legislatures enact legislation that impacts the way professional counselors must practice. Local boards of education, state and local agencies, and other organizations also implement **regulations** and **policies** that impact counseling practice. While not the same as laws, regulations and policies govern the practices of the professionals to whom they pertain. For example, a licensed professional counselor (LPC) who violates a state regulation can be cited or even sanctioned. A professional school counselor who violates a school board policy can be reprimanded or even terminated for cause. These steps can be taken because professionals who are licensed, certified, or employed are frequently required to abide by such regulations as a condition of licensure, certification, or employment.

While the purpose of laws is not specifically to direct or limit assessment, they have been enacted to protect the rights of clients, students, parents, and employees, and therefore influence how assessment may or must be conducted. **Case law** is the result of litigation or court cases and often does direct how professional counselors must practice. Professional counselors need to keep current with legislation and court cases, as this is an ever-changing area. Some of the major legal issues affecting assessment are reviewed in the rest of this section.

The Family Educational Rights and Privacy Act of 1974 (FERPA) and Related Legislation

Prior to the 1970s, educators and researchers frequently conducted assessments without parental consent and often stored these assessments in student files. In addition, access to student files was virtually unlimited; a simple request to the principal was often enough to get access to a student's files by entities, professionals, and employers outside of a school system. The **Family Educational Rights and Privacy Act** of 1974 (FERPA) is the federal law that protects the privacy of all student records in schools and institutions of higher learning. Often referred to as the Buckley Amendment, this law has several provisions and applies to all pre-K-12 and postsecondary institutions that receive federal funding from the U.S. Department of Education for any program. Nonpublic schools that do not accept federal funding are exempt from these regulations.

FERPA defines education records as all information a school collects for attendance, achievement, group and individual testing and assessment, behavior, and school activities. FERPA gives parents specific rights regarding this information. The first provision is that parents have the right to inspect and review their children's records. Each school system must annually send a notice to parents detailing this review process and the procedure for filing a complaint if they disagree with anything in the record. The school system has 45 days in which to comply with the parents' request to review the record and faces penalties, including the loss of all applicable federal funding, for failure to comply. Second, the law limits who may access records. Under FERPA, only those persons with a "legitimate educational interest" can access a student's record. Some personally identifiable information may be released without parental consent. This information is usually referred to as *directory information,* or *public information,* and generally includes such material as the student's name, address, telephone number, date and place of birth, honors and awards, and attendance records. The major exemption to the confidentiality of student records relates to law enforcement issues. The school must comply with a judicial order or lawfully executed subpoena. In cases of emergency, information about the student relevant to the emergency can be released without parental consent (see www.ed.gov/print/policy/gen/guid/fpco/ferpa/index.html for details). All states and local jurisdictions have incorporated FERPA's requirements into state statutes and local policies with some degree of variance among specifics, such as directory information.

The rights of consent transfer to students upon their 18th birthday. The law does not specifically limit the rights of parents whose children are over the age of 18 and continue to attend a secondary school (i.e., high school). The law also does not specifically limit parental rights for a student who attends a postsecondary institution but is older than 18 years, although most institutions of higher learning adhere to a policy of informed consent for a student who is 18 years or older. Noncustodial parents have the same rights as custodial parents, unless a court order has limited or terminated the rights of one or both parents. Stepparents and other family members who do not have legal custody of the child have no rights under FERPA without court-appointed authority.

The **Protection of Pupil Rights Amendment** of 1978 (PPRA), often referred to as the Hatch Amendment or the Grassley Amendment, for the members of Congress who introduced it, gives parents additional rights with regard to surveying minor students. PPRA does not apply to postsecondary schools. If the survey is funded with federal money, informed consent must be obtained for all participating students if students are required to take the survey and if questions about particular personal areas are asked. PPRA also requires informed parent consent for any psychological, psychiatric, or medical examination, testing, or treatment of students or any school program designed to affect the personal values or behavior of students. PPRA also gives parents the right to review instructional materials in experimental programs.

The **No Child Left Behind Act** of 2001 includes several changes to FERPA and PPRA (see www.ed.gov/about/offices/list/index.html for specific details). The changes apply to surveys funded in whole or part by any program administered by the U.S. Department of Education (USDE). PPRA (20 U.S.C. 1232h) requires that schools and contractors make instructional materials available for review by parents of participating students if those materials will be used in any USDE-funded survey, analysis, or evaluation and that schools and contractors obtain written parent consent prior to the participation of minor children in any USDE-funded survey, analysis, or evaluation if information in any of the following areas would be revealed:

- Political affiliations or beliefs of the student or parent
- Mental and psychological problems of the student or family
- Sex behavior or attitudes
- Illegal, antisocial, self-incriminating, or demeaning behavior
- Critical appraisals of other individuals with whom respondents have close family relationships
- Legally recognized privileged or analogous relationships, such as those of lawyers, physicians, and ministers
- Religious practices, affiliations, or beliefs of the student or the student's parent
- Income other than such information required to determine eligibility/participation in a program

These new provisions of PPRA also apply to any survey that is not funded in any way with USDE money. Under these provisions, parents have the right to inspect, upon request, any survey or instructional materials used as part of the curriculum created by a third party if one or more of the eight above-outlined areas are involved. Parents also have the right to inspect any instrument used to collect personal information from students for marketing or selling. Parents may opt their child out of this data collection process or any survey involving one or more of the eight above-delineated areas. PPRA does not apply to any survey that is administered as part of the Individuals with Disabilities Education Improvement Act of 2004 (IDEIA).

As can be ascertained from the explanation of FERPA and PPRA, there are many constraints to assessment, testing, and surveys in public schools. As each school district may further define policies involving this legislation, it is critical for professional counselors to become familiar with what types of assessments fall under these regulations, how the assessment results may be used or disseminated, and to whom. It has become increasingly difficult for professional counselors to give any type of formal or informal assessment to students without informed parent consent. And other school mental health professionals, such as school psychologists, may have even more restrictions placed on their ability to conduct any form of assessment without signed, informed parent consent. One assessment issue that is becoming more problematic in schools concerns the desire of parents to review the actual protocol used after their child has completed the assessment. The problem revolves around the issue of whether the actual assessment forms become part of the educational record or just the results. Most professional associations believe that the actual protocol is not part of the record and that parents usually lack the training to completely understand the assessment tools.

FERPA, PPRA, NCLB, and related legislation all have provisions aimed at protecting the rights of school-aged children and their parents from the collection of information that violates the privacy of all students. Additional provisions have also been put in place to protect the rights of handicapped citizens; these provisions are discussed in the section on IDEIA later in this chapter.

Minimal Competency Assessment and the No Child Left Behind Act of 2001

"High-stakes" testing has been used in education for years, starting with the initial premise that all students should master the basics of a curriculum before being granted a diploma. Such a premise has tremendous support among adults in the United States, but establishing minimal competency for graduation has a controversial sociopolitical dimension.

In the 1970s, many states began to develop minimal competency tests as a requirement for graduation. The *Debra v. Turlington* (1979) case questioned in the Florida state courts the *Florida State Assessment Test*. Lawyers for 10 African American students who had been denied diplomas on the basis of their failure to pass the state assessment examination argued that the test was discriminatory because the students had been educated in a segregated system and had not acquired the skills that would have allowed them to pass the test. The judge ruled that the test was not discriminatory but did suspend its use for four years and directed that the school must show the assessment covered only information taught. While the intent behind minimal competency assessment was noble, educators and legislators soon realized that such a system revolved around low expectations rather than a striving for higher standards.

The discussions of higher-standards-based education led to implementation of the No Child Left Behind Act of 2001 and its requirements for high-stakes testing and accountability. A high-stakes test is any test that results in a decision about a student or school that can change a student's or school's status (e.g., graduation from high school; admittance into a college; and a school that comes under State Department of Education oversight for poor performance). Almost all states now require students to pass tests as part of high school graduation requirements. In addition, students are assessed at identified grade levels from 3rd grade through high school to meet the requirements of the No Child Left Behind Act. Both students and schools are feeling the increased pressure to perform well on the assessments, lest the school fail to meet annual yearly progress for five years in a row and risk being reconstituted (i.e., being put under external control, leading to the possible replacement of administration, staff, curriculum, etc.). Many laud the intent of ensuring that all children learn and achieve to high academic levels. However, many educators are also concerned that the focus on assessment competes with the focus on learning.

Numerous professional organizations have weighed in on the high-stakes testing issue. The American Counseling Association (ACA) appointed a Task Force on High-Stakes Testing in 2003 and some of the areas considered by this task force are particularly noteworthy. In a position statement adopted by the ACA Governing Council (ACA, 2005b), the task force recognized the importance of assessment and accountability and its relationship to high achievement. (This position statement may be found on the companion website for this text, in the chapter on high-stakes testing.) **High-stakes testing** (HST) is one objective means of assessing student performance, and HST assessments are generally well developed. However, the task force specified some important cautions. Using a single test score resulting from a group administration of the test to make decisions about individual students has inherent problems; many students are at a disadvantage on HST, and the results may not accurately reflect their abilities. The task force points out that special education law does not allow decisions to be made about children based on a single test, but the accountability provisions of HST do allow this type of decision making. While accountability remains a major requirement for schools and school systems, it must be balanced with providing assessment tools for students that truly assess what they should know in a way that maximizes student performance and reflects best practices in assessment.

Individuals With Disabilities Education Improvement Act of 2004 (IDEIA) and Related Legislation

The Education for All Handicapped Children Act, also known as PL 94-142, was initially enacted in 1975 after a long struggle to equalize the opportunities for disabled students and to provide opportunities similar to those of their nonhandicapped peers through a free, appropriate education in the least restrictive environment. This special education law has been reauthorized several times since its enactment, renamed the Individuals With Disabilities Education Act (IDEA) in 1990, and most recently signed by President Bush on December 3, 2004 as the **Individuals With Disabilities Education Improvement Act (IDEIA)**. The bill outlines the process for referring, assessing, identifying, placing, and instructing students with handicapping conditions who warrant additional services under the law. The law requires that all decisions are made by a multidisciplinary team that includes the parents, special educator, regular educator, school system representative, and frequently the professional school counselor and school psychologist. Parental consent is required for assessment and placement activities. The multidisciplinary team makes all placement and educational decisions; each eligible child is required to have an **Individual Education Plan (IEP)**, which outlines the goals for the child and the services that will be provided.

Part B, Section 614 (2) (3) of IDEIA outlines the requirements for conducting the evaluation to determine if a child has a handicap. It states that the local education agency (i.e., school system) shall

- use a variety of assessment tools and strategies to gather relevant functional, developmental, and academic information, including information provided by the parent, that may assist in determining if the child is a child with a disability and the content of the IEP;
- not use any single measure or assessment as the sole criterion for determining whether a child is a child with a disability or determining an appropriate educational program for the child;
- use technologically sound instruments that may assess the relative contribution of cognitive and behavioral factors, in addition to physical or developmental factors; and
- ensure that assessments and other evaluation materials used to assess the child
  - are selected and administered so as not to be discriminatory on a racial or cultural basis;
  - are provided and administered in the language and form most likely to yield accurate information;
  - are used for purposes for which the assessments or measures are valid and reliable;
  - are administered by trained and knowledgeable personnel; and
  - are administered in accordance with any instructions provided by the producer of such assessments.

The above language clearly delineates requirements that are actually best practices in assessment and which are discussed earlier in this chapter and in other chapters of this book. This reauthorization of the law strengthened the development of new approaches to determine whether students are learning disabled that are not based solely on the IQ discrepancy model (see Chapter 12, Table 12.1). Additionally, the law focuses on addressing the problem of the over- and misidentification of linguistic and cultural minority students and directs districts with significant over representation of minorities to create and operate programs to reduce this problem (see www.cec.sped.org/law_res/doc/law/index.php or further details).

The Health Insurance Portability and Accountability Act of 1996 (HIPAA)

Privacy issues of the general citizenry regarding medical and mental health fields are of critical importance. The rise of managed care, frequent switching of health insurance plans by employers, and the sensitive nature of questions frequently asked by these entities often lead to privacy concerns. The **Health Insurance Portability and Accountability Act** of 1996 (HIPAA) required that the U.S. Department of Health and Human Services (HHS) adopt national standards for the privacy of individually identifiable health information, outlined patients' rights, and established criteria for access to health records. Included in this law was a provision that HHS must adopt national standards for electronic healthcare transactions. In response to this mandate, regulations named the Privacy Rule were adopted in 2000 and became effective in 2001. This rule set national standards for the protection of health information as it applied to health plans, health clearing houses, and healthcare providers who conduct transactions electronically. All covered entities had until April 14, 2003, to comply with the Privacy Rule (see http://www.hhs.gov/ocr/hipaa for further details).

The HIPAA Privacy Rule has a number of provisions, including giving patients the right to obtain and examine a copy of their health records and request corrections, allowing patients some ability to control the uses and disclosures of their health information, allowing patients to know how their information might be used and if disclosures have been made, setting limits on the use and release of health records, and providing a complaint process. The Privacy Rule also requires that providers give clients a privacy notice and should obtain a signed acknowledgement of this notice.

States and health entities continue to work on the details of the implementation of HIPAA. Clearly, it has implications for professional counselors, particularly those who work in health settings, clinics, agencies, and private practice. Professional counselors must be aware of this law and its requirements and ensure that their practices are in accordance with its provisions. Importantly, the laws apply whether the client is a self-payer or the professional counselor receives payment through insurance companies or health organizations. Professional counselors should also be sure to adhere to HIPAA provisions when client information is shared.

HIPAA protects health information much the same way FERPA protects student records and information. While the USDE has indicated that FERPA will continue to regulate student information in schools, the schools are finding that HIPAA has complicated the process. Schools frequently depend on assessments conducted by nonschool providers, particularly for handicapped students, who are regulated by HIPAA. In past years the assessments and health information would routinely become part of the child's educational record. What schools are now finding is often documents are stamped with "do not redisclose" or other indications that information should not be made a permanent part of the educational record of the child and must be returned to the assessor if the child leaves the school. As healthcare providers and patients become more aware of the requirements of HIPAA, these issues will likely be resolved.

It should be noted that the mandates of HIPAA are consistent with ethical standards and therefore should not be a barrier to sound professional practice. Signed, informed consent; limits to disclosure; and the confidentiality of patient information are all part of the ethical standards and should drive the practice of professional counselors.

Guidelines of the Equal Employment Opportunity Commission (EEOC)

According to Kaplan and Saccuzzo (2001), the government exercises its power to regulate testing largely through interpretations of the 14th Amendment to the Constitution, which guarantees all citizens due process and equal protection under the law. This is evidenced by the government's actions concerning personnel practices, particularly employee testing. Title VII of the Civil Rights Act of 1964 and its subsequent amendments created the Equal Employment Opportunity Commission (EEOC), whose guidelines outlaw discrimination in employment based on race, color, gender, national origin, religion, pregnancy, gender, age 40 and above, or status as a Vietnam veteran.

The EEOC developed guidelines for the use of tests and assessments in employment practices. The commission was particularly interested in any procedures that might have an adverse impact on selection and worked to ensure that tests and assessments were not used to discriminate based on race. It ruled that any assessment used as a basis for employment decisions that adversely affected hiring, promotion, transfer, or any other activity protected by the law constituted discrimination unless the test was validated for the reason it was being used and the person handling the personnel matter could not use other procedures (Drummond, 2000).

Following the Civil Rights Act, a number of U.S. Supreme Court cases challenged the concept of adverse impact and refined employment practices. The first landmark case was *Griggs v. Duke Power Company* (1971). The case involved several African American employees of the power company who sued because they felt the criteria used for promotion (a high school diploma and two tests) were discriminatory. In this case, and in the subsequent cases of *Albemarle Paper Company v. Moody* (1975) and *Washington v. Davis* (1976), the U.S. Supreme Court's decisions placed the burden of proof on the employer. The decisions indicated that employment tests must be valid and reliable, and forced the employers to define how job performance relates to test scores (Kaplan & Saccuzzo, 2001).

A 1988 U.S. Supreme Court's decision in *Watson v. the Fort Worth Bank and Trust Company* involved an African American woman who was passed over for promotion for a supervisory position at the bank. She argued that racial minorities were underrepresented in selections for higher-level jobs. The court ruled that by adding one subjective item to objective tests, employers could protect themselves from discrimination suits as adverse impact does not apply to subjective criteria. This ruling was followed by *Wards Cove Packing Company v. Antonio* in 1989. This case was filed by cannery workers at an Alaskan packing company who claimed that the company was keeping them out of higher-paying and more skilled jobs. The U.S. Supreme Court refused to hear the case and remanded it back to the lower court. In so doing, they noted that the burden of proof should be shifted to the plaintiff to demonstrate that there are problems with selection procedures. This ruling obviously favored employers as few employees have the resources and knowledge necessary to prove bias in personnel practices.

As a result of these cases, Congress passed the Civil Rights Act of 1991, which incorporated many of the principles of the *Griggs v. Duke Power Company* case. The act placed the burden of proof back on the employer and outlawed differential cut-off scores or score adjustments.

The Americans With Disabilities Act of 1991 (ADA)

Just prior to the enactment of PL 94-142 in 1975 to address the needs of school-aged youth with educational handicaps, Congress passed the U.S. Rehabilitation Act of 1973. Section 504 of this act contains important provisions for individuals with medical or mental disorders (see Chapter 12 for a fuller discussion of this act). Some of the implications of the U.S. Rehabilitation Act of 1973 and related legislation involved the requirements for access by handicapped citizens to ramps and elevators in public buildings, as well as handicapped parking spaces and curbs cut to allow wheelchair access. These landmark laws were added to by important new laws in the1990s. The Americans With Disabilities Act (ADA) of 1991 was enacted to remove barriers for persons with physical and mental disabilities to employment, education, and public services. The law requires that reasonable accommodations must be made for persons who are determined to be impaired, including accommodations in testing and assessments. The law does not delineate what accommodations are required, so they must be determined on a case-by-case basis. There are tremendous concerns in the assessment community regarding how to provide accommodations and fairly assess individuals with disabilities without compromising the reliability and validity of the assessment instruments. Murphy and Davidshofer (2001) suggested that this issue will occupy test developers for years to come. Of course, the implications of the ADA go far beyond assessment. But for now, realize that Americans with disabilities are given full protection under the law, and that reasonable accommodations must be offered.

Court Decisions Related to Diversity in Assessment

Tests have long been used to "sort" and "select." When certain groups are over- or underselected for participation in programs, the specters of bias and fairness will certainly arise. There have been a number of court cases involving the use of testing in education, decisions that have shaped amendments to special education law and practice. The first major case that examined the validity of psychological test scores was *Hobson v. Hansen* (1967). Students in the District of Columbia public schools, which were integrated, were placed in classes based on the results of group ability tests, which resulted in establishment of a de facto segregation or tracking system. Hobson, the parent of two children, sued the school system, arguing that African American students were tracked into the basic track while White students were placed in the honors and other tracks. The U.S. Supreme Court found that ability tests that had been developed on White students could not be used to place African American students (Kaplan & Saccuzzo, 2001). Current test development standards specify that students about whom decisions will be made *must* be well represented in a test's standardization sample. The *Hobson v. Hansen* case brought this point home very clearly. In fact, present-day test developers owe much of their "commonsense" procedures to the issues resolved by early pioneers in test development *and* civil rights cases.

The case of *Diana v. State Board of Education* concerned the use of intelligence tests for bilingual Mexican American students. The plaintiffs argued that bilingual Mexican American students were inappropriately placed in classes for the educable mentally retarded (EMR) based on tests that failed to take into account their bilingual status. The students retested in Spanish all scored too high to meet the EMR criteria. An out-of-court agreement established that bilingual students would be tested in both English and their native language; that placement in EMR classes would be based on both test scores and a comprehensive developmental assessment of the child; and that tests that emphasize areas that might be unfair to minority children could not be used for placement. Again, today we see this issue as "common sense," but in the1960s and 1970s, almost all tests were published in English. Today, greater diversity in languages occurs to test clients.

Chapter 10 explores the interaction of race and socioeconomic status on intellectual development, an issue that, however, was not widely studied in the 1960s and 1970s. The placement of African American students in EMR classes based on IQ tests was at the heart of the California case *Larry P. v. Riles* (1979). The plaintiffs contended that use of these intelligence tests was invalid for African American students and that IQ tests should therefore not be employed for placement purposes. Many testing experts testified at the trial, some in support of the validity of IQ tests for African American and other children, others in opposition to the use of such tests. The judge in the case ruled that the "tests are racially and culturally biased, have a discriminatory impact on African American children, and have not been validated for the purpose of (consigning) African American children into educationally dead-end, isolated, and stigmatizing classes" (Kaplan & Saccuzzo, 2001, p. 580). This decision was appealed but upheld in 1984. As a result, intelligence tests could not be used to place African American students in special education classes. This ban was expanded in 1986 to include testing all African American children for special education in California but does not apply to other minority children. Enter the law of unintended consequences. Because qualification for special education services required assessment of ability (i.e., intelligence), these laws virtually eliminated minority students from qualifying for services intended to help them. Some civil rights advocates viewed special education as a way to "segregate" minorities within the educational system, but the alternative of failing children with disabilities was seen as even more egregious. As a result of a subsequent case, *Crawford v. Honig,* the ban on testing African American children was lifted in 1992. Legislation related to test bias and discrimination against clients of diverse backgrounds has become a source of hot debate within the assessment field, so the final pages of this chapter are dedicated to an exploration of this essential foundational issue.

DIVERSITY ISSUES IN ASSESSMENT

For years, U.S. Census data have indicated that the United States is becoming increasingly diverse. The U.S. population is multiracial, multiethnic, and multilingual. Approximately 7% of this population reported in the 2000 Census having a disability, and 18% reported living below the poverty level (U.S. Census Bureau, 2003).

These demographics demand that professional counselors be able to work effectively with clients and students from a multitude of cultures (Constantine, 2001; Lee, 2001). Professional counselors are involved in numerous ways in administering and ensuring that clients receive appropriate assessment. This section discusses some of the basic aspects of diversity in assessment and provides professional counselors with practical steps to approaching fairness in assessment in the clinical and school settings.

Understanding Diversity

Conversations of diversity often focus on race and ethnicity. *Race* is an anthropological construct based on the classification of physiological characteristics (Gladding, 2001) and includes a political and socioeconomic dimension related to differences in physical appearance (Brace, 1995; Yee, Fairchild, Weizmann, & Wyatt, 1993). *Ethnicity* is the "group classification in which members believe they share a common origin and a unique social and cultural heritage such as language or religious belief" (Gladding, 2001, p. 45). While important, these two factors alone do not describe the extent of diversity that professional counselors face.

Culture is another important diversity issue. Culture is both complex and multidimensional. Professional counselors may recognize several cultures and subcultures within a population. Although this adds to the complexity of the construct, understanding and appreciating culture and its multidimensionality gives professional counselors valuable insight into their clients' sense of self, language and communication patterns, dress, values, beliefs, use of time and space, relationships with family and significant others, food, play, work, and use of knowledge (Whitefield, McGrath, & Coleman, 1992). Succinctly, *culture* can be described as the set of "values, beliefs, expectations, worldviews, symbols, and appropriate behaviors of a group that provide its members with norms, plans, and rules for social living" (Gladding, 2001, p. 34).

Diversity also encompasses gender, sexual orientation, language, socioeconomic status, ability, and disability. *Diversity* simply means difference: difference in the many aspects and dimensions used to help understand student development and behavior. The professional counselor must therefore appreciate and understand diversity in all of its manifestations and its implications for assessment.

For well over 40 years, the counseling profession has been deeply concerned about appropriate assessment for clients and students of diverse populations (Anastasi & Urbina, 1997; Sattler, 2001; Whiston, 2005). Some of this discussion has resulted from legislation and legal proceedings regarding the specific areas of multidisciplinary assessment, assessment in a client's native language, assessment used for selection purposes, assessment procedures, informed consent, and due rights notification (Rogers, 1998; Sattler 2001). Ethical guidelines also address appropriate assessment. Beyond global charges to respect diversity and work in the best interest of students and clients, Section E of the *ACA Code of Ethics* (2005a) specifically addresses diversity in testing. Further direction regarding diversity in assessment, however, is delineated in the Association for Assessment in Counseling and Education's *Standards for Multicultural Assessment* (AACE, 2003b).

Standards for Multicultural Assessment

Recognizing the importance of **multicultural assessment**, the Association for Assessment in Counseling and Education (AACE) studied and compiled standards of many professional organizations. The result was a document outlining 68 competencies specific to the assessment and counseling of diverse populations (see http://aace.ncat.edu). The competencies cover assessment content and purpose; norming, reliability, and validity beyond general standards issues; administration and scoring; and interpretation and application of assessment results. Many of the competencies have significant consequences for professional counselors, psychologists, and other diagnosticians involved in psychological assessment and placement processes. In addition, professional counselors should be aware of the competencies because of their relationship to culturally appropriate counseling and assessment services (AACE, 2003b).

Diversity Factors Involved in Assessment

Thus far we have outlined the mandate for professional counselors to be aware of legal and ethical responsibilities regarding multicultural assessment. Following is a more specific discussion of the ways in which diversity factors affect assessment.

Difference

Inherent in the concept of diversity is an understanding of difference. Difference does not imply better than or worse than. Difference may, however, become advantage or disadvantage in the realm of assessment. Imagine that all mental health professionals are asked to take an assessment on providing services to clients. Professional counselors, psychologists, psychiatrists, family therapists, and social workers (among others) gather to take the test. Clearly, each of these groups of professionals differs in training, credentials, experience, and perhaps views of clients. No group is better than the other. The groups are different. If the assessment is based largely on the Council for Accreditation of Counseling and Related Educational Programs (CACREP) (2001) curricular standards using the language and orientations of professional counselors, professional school counselors may have an advantage on the test. Their scores may be somewhat higher than those of psychologists, psychiatrists, family therapists, or social workers. This simplistic example demonstrates how cultural difference and test content can interplay. In more subtle ways (e.g., test words, pictures, format), test content must be examined to ensure that information specific to certain cultures is controlled in assessment (Rogers, 1998).

Worldview

Worldview is a second factor involved in assessment. Every aspect of counseling occurs in a cultural context. This includes assessment. As a result of cultural context, assessment can be undergirded by cultural worldviews that are unique to a specific culture and unfamiliar or offensive to another. Worldview includes beliefs, values, perspectives, and perceptions (Whiston, 2005). The rather common practice of timed assessment deserves consideration in respect to worldview. In America, speed is often valued. Think of Americans' fascination with fast food, microwaveable products, instant messaging, and turbo-charged cars. In many other cultures, however, speed is not valued. Reflection is considered sacred. Given this difference in worldview, it is not hard to see why a 4th-grade student new to this country may not score well on a timed multiplication test, even though the student may have mastered multiplication facts.

Acculturation and Language

Acculturation and language are additional diversity factors involved in assessment. Acculturation is a change process that occurs when an individual of one culture comes in contact with an individual or individuals of another culture. As a result of this process, individuals may take on different values, beliefs, and behaviors (Drummond, 2004; Fouad & Chan, 1999). The degree and rate of change depend on a number of factors, including power dynamics, issues of immersion, and individual personality characteristics (e.g., cultural identity development status, generational status). Professional counselors often have the opportunity to work with clients, students, and families dealing with various stages of acculturation. It is not unusual for a professional school counselor to work with a student who, due to the school setting and peer interactions, is bicultural yet lives in a family setting that largely maintains the traditions and practices of the student's native culture. A culturally competent counselor is prepared to recognize and effectively handle the counseling implications these issues of acculturation may have for students and clients.

A growing number of Americans have the ability to communicate in more than one language, but proficiency in the languages they speak may vary considerably (Rogers, 1998). This growing phenomenon affects assessment in many interesting and diverse ways. Language is more than words and pronunciation. Language includes structure, nuance, denotation, and connotation. These components preclude the simple use of translations or unstandardized forms of a test (Fouad & Chan, 1999; Whiston, 2005). For example, it is inappropriate to have a staff member simply translate a test for Spanish-speaking clients. The process of ensuring that the "translation" is equivalent to the original test involves sophisticated statistical and content analyses that extend beyond the scope of this chapter. It is important to note that it is equally inappropriate to assume that a Caribbean student who has just moved to this country must take a test with no accommodation simply because the child has always been educated in "English." Differences in sentence structure, word meaning, idioms, and nuance may affect the student's ability to perform on the test. Of course, there are times when mastery of the English language is the objective of the test. In these cases, students and clients should be given the opportunity to demonstrate their understanding of the language by being tested in the given language. When English competence is not the issue, however, the language considerations discussed must be examined. Although professional counselors are not often involved in developing assessments, in their role as advocates, they must ensure that issues of language are fully explored when assessing students and clients with limited English proficiency, bilingual abilities, or multilingual capabilities.

Socioeconomic Status

Research suggested that **socioeconomic status** is a significant factor in assessment (Flanagan, 1993). Herring (1997) suggested that social class is the most important factor affecting the counseling process. Furthermore, there is a line of research describing the confounding issues of race, ethnicity, and social class (Fouad & Chan, 1999). Although social class cuts across all races and ethnicities, poverty disproportionately affects clients and families of color. When these findings are merged with census data regarding poverty rates, it becomes evident that professional counselors must be aware of issues of socioeconomic status and assessment. Socioeconomic status is about much more than money. Social class may affect students' values, worldviews, emotional resources, and support systems (Payne, 2003).

Student and Client Factors

A host of student and client factors, including test-taking attitudes, experience and capabilities, motivation, and social desirability, can affect assessment (Cohen & Swerdlik, 1999; Drummond, 2000; Fouad & Chan, 1999). These factors, discussed in much greater detail in Chapter 8, are unique to the individual and may change from test situation to test situation. For example, it is conceivable that a teenager may perform better on a multiple-choice test on social studies vocabulary than a true-false test on the same vocabulary. The difference in performance may be due only to the student's familiarity with the test format. Or clients with a visual impairment may have their test performance greatly diminished by their Braille and keyboarding skills rather than their knowledge of the material. Additionally, it is not difficult to imagine a situation in which clients give the answer they feel the professional counselor wants, or the answer that is the most socially desirable. There is a strong literature base that suggests social desirability is a significant issue in assessment for many groups of clients (Marin & Marin, 1991). This factor may differentially affect cultural groups.

Traditionally, professional counselors work with clients and students individually and in small groups on decreasing test anxiety and strengthening test-taking strategies. Professional counselors should also provide direct student and client service and work as advocates to address these and other factors affecting assessment.

Counselor and Examiner Factors

Counselor and examiner factors comprise a final category of diversity issues that must be considered in assessment. Counselor and examiner factors include professional competence; comfort with the assessment process; perceptions and worldview; race, ethnicity, and culture; and social influence. These important issues are addressed in the *Standards for Multicultural Assessment* (AACE, 2003b):

> *Culturally competent counselors have training and expertise in the use of traditional assessment and testing instruments. They not only understand the technical aspects of the instruments but also are aware of the cultural limitations. This allows them to use test instruments for the welfare of clients from diverse cultural, racial, and ethnic groups.*
>
> Selection of Assessment Instruments: Content and Purpose

> *Culturally competent counselors have knowledge about their social impact on others.*
>
> Interpretation and Application of Assessment Results

BIAS IN ASSESSMENT

Some or all of the factors discussed in the preceding section can result in assessment bias. Standardization samples may also affect bias (Reynolds & Brown, 1984). According to Whiston (2005, p. 211), **bias** "refers to the degree that construct-irrelevant factors systematically affect a group's performance." Construct-irrelevant factors are those facets not related to the idea being assessed. An assessment or test item is said to be biased when "empirical evidence shows that it is more difficult for one group member than another, the general ability level of the two groups is held constant, and no reasonable rationale exists to explain the group difference on the same items" (Drummond, 2000, p. 356). Three types of bias—content bias, internal structure bias, and predictive bias—have particular implications for diverse populations.

Content Bias

Content bias refers to test material being more familiar to one group than another. Our earlier example involving professional counselors, psychologists, psychiatrists, family therapists, and social workers provides a simplistic illustration of content bias. Content bias is often less obvious when affecting multicultural populations, however. Content bias may involve hidden messages or values of a culture that are not readily visible due to cultural encapsulation. Consider two well-documented items from the *Wechsler Intelligence Scale for Children—Revised* (*WISC-R*) (Kaplan & Saccuzzo, 2001; Sattler, 2001). One question asks, "What would you do if you were sent to buy a loaf of bread, and the grocer said he did not have any more?" Another question, which has been subject to much controversial investigation, asks, "What should you do if a child smaller than you begins to fight with you?" Although research findings differ, these questions appear to contain embedded cultural values, behaviors, and norms that may not hold consistent over all multicultural groups

(Hardy, Welcher, Mellitis, & Kagan, 1976; Koh, Abbatiello, & McLoughlin, 1984; Sandoval, Zimmerman, & Woo-Sam, 1983). Student responses to these questions may not be a measure of intelligence, but rather a measure of cultural values, behaviors, and norms.

Internal Structure Bias

Scores on an assessment may be reliable for one group, but not reliable for another. Or scores on an instrument may be more reliable for one group than another. This phenomenon is called **internal structure bias.** Internal structure bias can be due to norming factors or the underlying factor structure of an instrument. In light of this, some assessment instruments report differences between groups of test takers. For example, an assessment instrument may report differential reliability data based on gender, age, or ethnicity.

Predictive Bias

A test can also be biased if it systematically over- or underpredicts a group's performance. This type of bias is called **predictive bias.** Many professional counselors are familiar with debate about the ability of standardized assessments like the Scholastic Assessment Test-I *(SAT-I)* to predict students' performance in college (McCornack & McLeod, 1988). "Gifted and talented" testing and success in special accelerated educational programming embody another common area of concern regarding predictive bias. Generally, predictive bias is investigated along the lines of gender, race, and ethnicity.

Interpreting Test Scores With Caution

Some test manuals and texts, including this one, use the phrase "interpret with caution" to warn readers about possible problems with the interpretations of scores. So what does the warning actually mean? In the context of this discussion on diversity, it usually means that we don't know the consequences of interpreting the score for a given individual with diverse characteristics. For example, some tests have norms that undersampled participants from various cultural backgrounds. If test norms undersampled African Americans, for instance, interpretations of an African American client's score may result in some inaccuracies. Unfortunately, without extensive empirical study, it is often extremely difficult to determine what the possible effects of undersampling may be. Empirical studies often explore differences between participants with diverse characteristics and provide helpful conclusions about whether scores generated by the test yield appropriate inferences about the examinee. While it is best practice to use tests that will yield reliable and valid scores for the individual being tested, often such tests either do not exist or are suspect for individuals with certain characteristics. So when you encounter the phrase "interpret with caution," it may have several different potential meanings, but the phrase always should be taken into account when making decisions about the client's life.

Ensuring Fairness in Assessment

Test bias is a critical and alarming issue. Nonetheless, tests and other forms of assessment do have an important role in educational and clinical settings. Sattler (2001) suggested that good assessment offers an objective standard, reveals disparity, appraises functioning, obtains appropriate programming, and evaluates programs. All of these functions of assessment are significant to the professional counselor's work with clients and students. How, then, can the professional counselor work to ensure fairness in testing? The question is complex and multifaceted. The following suggestions offer some initial strategies, interventions, and recommendations:

- Remember that the professional counselor's primary responsibility is the welfare of all clients. Ensure that the focus of any and all assessment is to benefit the client.
- Engage in professional development opportunities (e.g., continuing education and training) to continue to learn about self, multicultural counseling, and diversity in educational and clinical issues and settings.
- Continually monitor and challenge personal belief systems and attitudes regarding all aspects of diversity.
- Demonstrate competence in multicultural counseling knowledge, skills, and beliefs. Employ culturally sensitive approaches when working with clients and families.
- Abide by the *ACA Code of Ethics* (2005a) and other pertinent standards, including the *Standards for Multicultural Assessment* (AACE, 2003b) and the *Multicultural Counseling Competencies and Standards* (Sue, Arredondo, & McDavis, 1992).
- Become familiar with assessment instruments and procedures for the given population. As appropriate, become fully competent in all aspects of administration, interpretation, and application of assessment results.
- Do not attempt to use assessment procedures outside of your scope of experience.
- Refer students and clients for assessment as warranted.
- Consult with other mental health professionals, including clinical psychologists, school psychologists, and social workers, to become familiar with the ways they use assessment to serve clients.
- Test clients and students in the appropriate language. Use only translations with established validity.
- Use only valid and appropriate test adaptations and modifications. Do not assume that counselor- or teacher-made changes are appropriate without first consulting the test manual.
- Consult with special educators, school psychologists, and other specialists to ensure that students receive appropriate test accommodations. Accommodations may include changes in setting, scheduling, timing, presentation, or response format (Spinelli, 2002).
- Use multiple assessment methods to gain a more complete picture of a client or student.

- Clarify test purpose, procedure, and expectations to clients and students.
- Provide individual and group counseling support for stress and anxiety related to assessment as needed.
- Provide individual and group counseling support for motivation and test preparation as needed.
- Actively advocate for continued research on culturally appropriate assessment and counseling intervention for all clients and students.

SUMMARY/CONCLUSION

This chapter has discussed various historical, ethical, legal, and diversity issues in assessment, and provided resources for understanding how best to use assessment results in clinical practice. However, because legislation and litigation are an ongoing process, professional counselors must stay updated on current issues in assessment and must also continuously assess their behavior to ensure that it meets the highest ethical standards. Best practices in assessment are really ethical and legal practices.

This chapter has also highlighted and summarized key events in the evolution of assessment, from its historic roots to its current ethical concerns. Knowledge of such events and issues helps present-day professional counselors to understand the context for today's concerns, both within the profession and in society at large. Today, professional counselors are involved in a variety of ways in ensuring that clients and students receive quality assessment. Legal and ethical standards mandate that all clients receive assessment that is appropriate, unbiased, and meaningful. This mandate challenges professional counselors to understand the implications of diversity and assessment, and all that is involved in administering culturally competent assessment and in interpreting results. With this charge in mind, assessment can offer useful and important information for diverse client populations.

KEY TERMS

acculturation
achievement
aptitude
bias
career assessment
case law
clinical assessment
code of ethics
confidentiality
content bias
culture
diversity
Family Educational Rights and
 Privacy Act (FERPA)

Health Insurance Portability and
 Accountability Act (HIPAA)
high-stakes testing (HST)
Individual Education Plan (IEP)
Individuals With Disabilities
 Education Improvement Act
 (IDEIA)
informed consent
intelligence
internal structure bias
laws
multicultural assessment
No Child Left Behind Act (NCLB)
personality assessment

policy   regulation
predictive bias   socioeconomic status
Protection of Pupil Rights   vocational development
  Amendment (PPRA)   worldview

CHAPTER 3

Reliability

by Dimiter Dimitrov

Reliability of scores is a critical issue in measurement. This chapter reviews basic principles in reliability, such as classical test theory and standard error of measurement in classical test theory. It also discusses the types of reliability commonly used by test developers, including internal consistency, test-retest, alternate form, criterion-referenced, and interscorer reliability. Finally, the concepts of attenuation and reliability of composite scores are discussed. Advanced concepts of dependability and generalizability of scores are included on the companion website for this text.

WHAT IS RELIABILITY?

Reliability means consistency. Measurements in the physical sciences can often be conducted with great precision (e.g., millimeters, grams). However, measurements in counseling, education, and related fields are not completely accurate and consistent—and are sometimes far from it. There is always some error involved, usually due to a person's conditions (e.g., mood, fatigue, momentary distraction) and/or external conditions (e.g., noise, temperature, light), that may randomly occur during the measurement process. The way instruments of measurement (e.g., tests, inventories, or raters) are designed or the way questions or items are phrased may also affect the accuracy of the scores (observations).

For example, it is unlikely that the scores of a person on two different forms of an anxiety test would be equal, because differently worded items often yield varying results. Also, different scores are likely to be assigned to a person when different professional counselors evaluate a specific attribute of the person (e.g., introversion, sociability, self-esteem). In another scenario, if a group of people takes the same test twice within a short period of time, one can expect the rank order of their scores on the two test administrations to be somewhat similar, but not exactly the same. In other words, one can expect a relatively high, yet not perfect, positive correlation of test-retest scores for this group of examinees. As still another example, when it comes to making placement decisions about clients, inconsistency may occur in different criterion-referenced classifications (e.g., pass-fail group labels or mastery-nonmastery group labels) based on measurements obtained through testing or subjective judgments of raters (e.g., teachers, parents).

In measurement parlance, the higher the accuracy and consistency of measurement scores, the higher the reliability. The **reliability** of scores indicates the degree to which they are *accurate*, *consistent*, and *repeatable* when (a) different people conduct the measurement, (b) different instruments are used that purport to measure the same trait (e.g., proficiency, ability, attitude, anxiety), and (c) there is incidental variation in measurement conditions (e.g., lighting, seating, temperature). In other words, reliable scores are produced by tests that are free from errors of measurement. Reliability is a key indicator of quality measurements with tests, surveys, inventories, or individuals (e.g., raters, judges, observers). Most important, reliability is a necessary (albeit not sufficient) condition for the validity of measurements. *Validity* refers to the meaningfulness, accuracy, and appropriateness of interpretations and decisions based on measurement data. Thus if professional counselors cannot measure a client characteristic consistently (reliability), they cannot make accurate interpretations (validity).

It is important to note that reliability refers to the scores obtained with a test and not to the instrument itself. Previous studies and recent editorial policies of professional journals (e.g., Dimitrov, 2002; Sax, 1980; Thompson & Vacha-Haase, 2000) emphasize that it is more accurate to refer to "reliability of measurement data" than to "reliability of tests" (e.g., items, questions, tasks). Tests cannot be accurate, stable, or unstable, but observations (scores) can be (i.e., tests are neither reliable or valid, but scores on tests can be). Therefore, any reference to reliability of a test should be interpreted to mean the reliability of scores derived from the test.

As is discussed in Chapter 4, the most important characteristic of any measurement is its validity—that is, the degree to which scores lead to meaningful and appropriate interpretations. To allow for such interpretations, however, the scores should be accurate and consistent (i.e., reliable). The criterion-related validity of an entrance examination, for example, is assessed by the correlation between the examinees' scores on this test and their scores on a criterion (e.g., grade point average at the end of the first academic year). However, under the classical model of reliability, *a criterion-related validity coefficient of test scores cannot exceed the square root of their reliability.* More simply put, the reliability of scores predetermines a "ceiling" for the validity of a test's scores. How closely this ceiling will be approached depends on other factors as well. But at this point it is essential to understand that reliability is a necessary, but not sufficient, condition for validity. That is, high validity *can* occur if test scores are highly reliable but *cannot* occur if test scores have low levels of reliability. On the other hand, just because test scores are highly reliable does not mean they will have high validity. For example, just because you can measure your height consistently (high reliability) does not mean that height indicates intelligence (low validity).

THE CLASSICAL MODEL OF RELIABILITY

True Score

Scores on performance tests, personality inventories, expert evaluations, and even physical measurements are not completely accurate, consistent, and repeatable. For example, although the height of a person (i.e., one's "true height") remains constant throughout repeated measurements within a short period of time (say, 15 minutes) using the same scale, the observed values would be scattered around this "true height" due to the equipment being used or imperfection in the visual acuity of the measurer (whether the same examiner or somebody else). Thus, if T denotes the person's constant true height, then the observed height (X) in any of the repeated measurements will deviate from T with an *error of measurement* (E). That is,

$$X = T + E \qquad\qquad (3.1)$$

In classical test theory, one often refers to a client's **observed score** (X, the score the client received on a test) and the client's **true score** (T, the score the client would have received if the test and testing conditions were free of error [E]). Thus, if $E = 0$ (i.e., there is no error), the observed score *is* the true score (i.e., if $E = 0$, then $X = T$).

To grasp what is meant by true score in classical test theory, imagine that a person takes a standardized intelligence test each day for 100 days in a row. The person would likely obtain a number of different observed scores over these occasions. The mean of all observed scores would represent an approximation of the person's true score (T) on the standardized intelligence test. In general, the true score is the average of the (theoretical) distribution of scores that would be observed in repeated independent measurements of a person with the same test. Importantly, the true score (T) is a hypothetical concept, for it is not practically possible to test the same person infinity times in independent repeated measurements because each testing could influence the subsequent testing (i.e., practice effects, memory effects).

It is important to note that the error in Equation 3.1 is assumed to be random in nature. Possible sources of **random error** are (1) fluctuations in the mood or alertness of persons taking the test due to fatigue, illness, or other recent experiences; (2) incidental variation in the measurement conditions due, for example, to outside noise or inconsistency in the administration of the instrument; (3) differences in scoring due to factors such as scoring errors, subjectivity, or clerical errors; and (4) random guessing on response alternatives in tests or questionnaire items. Conversely, **systematic errors** that remain constant from one measurement to another do not lead to inconsistency and therefore do not affect the reliability of the scores. Systematic errors will occur, for example, when one professional counselor assigns 2 points lower than another professional counselor to each person in a group of examinees. So, again, *the reliability of any measurement is the extent to which the measurement results are free of random errors.* Random error affects reliability; systematic error does not.

Classical Definition of Reliability

Equation 3.1 represents the classical assumption that any *observed score* (*X*) consists of two parts: *true score* (*T*) and *error of measurement* (*E*). Because errors are random, it is assumed that they do not correlate with the true scores (i.e., $r_{TE} = 0$). Indeed, there is no reason to expect that persons with higher true scores would have systematically larger (or smaller) measurement errors than persons with lower true scores. Under this assumption, Equation 3.2 is true for the *variances* (σ^2) of observed scores, true scores, and errors for a population of test takers:

$$\sigma_X^2 = \sigma_T^2 + \sigma_E^2 \qquad (3.2)$$

that is, the observed score variance (σ_X^2) is the sum of true score variance (σ_T^2) and error variance (σ_E^2). Given this, *the reliability of measurements, r_{XX}, indicates what proportion of the observed score variance is true score variance.* The analytic translation of this definition is

$$r_{XX} = \frac{\sigma_T^2}{\sigma_X^2} = \frac{\sigma_T^2}{\sigma_T^2 + \sigma_E^2} \qquad (3.3)$$

The definition of reliability implies that the reliability takes values from 0.00 to 1.00. The closer r_{XX} is to 1.00, the higher the reliability, and, conversely, the closer r_{XX} is to zero, the lower the reliability. *Perfect reliability* ($r_{XX} = 1.00$) can theoretically occur when the total observed score variance is true score variance ($\sigma_X^2 = \sigma_T^2$) or, equivalently, when the error variance is zero ($\sigma_E^2 = 0$).

In general, reliability coefficients in the 0.80s are desirable for screening tests, 0.90s for diagnostic decisions (Salvia & Ysseldyke, 2004). Reliabilities of less than 0.80 indicate substantial error variance and subsequent inconsistent conclusions. This is not to say that scores based on $r_{XX} < 0.80$ cannot be helpful for hypothesis generation (exploring problems or strengths in areas of client functioning); for hypothesis validation (confirming suspected problems or strengths in areas of client functioning); or for instruments used in research studies for the purpose of defining a construct (e.g., self-efficacy, anxiety). However, important decisions about a client's life should be based on more consistently derived information.

Standard Error of Measurement (SEM)

Classical test theory also proposes two additional assumptions: (a) that the distribution of observed scores that a person may obtain under repeated independent testings with the same test is normal, and (b) that the standard deviation of this **normal distribution,** referred to as the **standard error of measurement** (*SEM*), is the same for all persons taking the test. Figure 3.1 represents a hypothetical normal distribution of observed scores for a person with a true score of 20 for a specific test. The

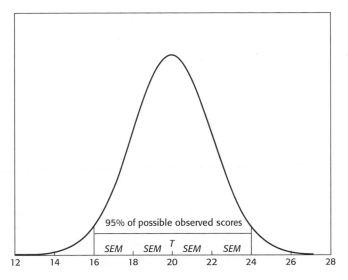

95% of possible observed scores

SEM | SEM | T | SEM | SEM

12   14   16   18   20   22   24   26   28

Figure 3.1   Theoretical distribution of observed scores for
repeated independent testings of one person with the
same test

mean of the distribution is the person's true score (T = 20), and the standard deviation is the standard error of measurement (SEM = 2).

Based on the statistical properties for normal distributions, about 95% of the scores fall in the interval from 2 standard deviations below the mean to 2 standard deviations above the mean. In Figure 3.1, this is the interval from $T - 2(SEM)$ to $T + 2(SEM)$, which in this case is from 16 to 24 [i.e., 20 − 2(2) to 20 + 2(2)]. This property can be used to construct (approximately) a 95% confidence interval of a person's true score (T) falling within the given observed score (X) range based on the person's performance in a single testing:

$$X - 2(SEM) < T < X + 2(SEM) \tag{3.4}$$

For example, if 23 is the person's observed score in a single real testing (X = 23), then the true score of this person is expected (with about 95% confidence) to fall in the interval from 23 − 2(SEM) to 23 + 2(SEM). This range of scores within which the true score probably lies is called a **confidence interval** because it gives the degree of confidence an examiner can expect regarding whether the client's true score lies within the given interval. In this example, with SEM = 2, the 95% confidence interval for the person's true score is from 23 − 2(2) to 23 + 2(2), or from 19 to 27.

When it comes to understanding and using confidence intervals, it is useful to know that (a) about 68% of all possible observed scores in Figure 3.1 fall in the interval from $T - 1(SEM)$ to $T + 1(SEM)$—i.e., from 18 to 22 in this case; (b) about 95% of all possible observed scores in Figure 3.1 fall in the interval from $T - 2(SEM)$ to $T + 2(SEM)$—i.e., from 16 to 24 in this case; and (c) almost all (99.7%) of the observed scores in Figure 3.1 are in the interval from $T - 3(SEM)$ to $T + 3(SEM)$, which in this case is from 14 to 26. You may have noticed that these percentages (i.e., 68%, 95%, 99.7%) are the same percentages under the normal curve used in the discussion of standard deviation. This is because the *SEM* is, in effect, the standard deviation for the individual, with the individual's true test score standing at the center and the *SEM* serving as the "personal standard deviation," based on the test score reliability coefficient.

A smaller *SEM* will produce smaller confidence intervals for the person's true score, thus improving the accuracy of measurement. Also, because the *SEM* is inversely related to reliability, high reliability indicates high accuracy of measurements (lower *SEM*). *SEM*s are much more helpful than reliability coefficients when reporting client test scores. The reliability coefficient is a unitless number between 0 and 1 conveniently used to report reliability in empirical studies. But the *SEM* relates directly to the meaning of the test's scale of measurement (e.g., raw number–right score, deviation IQ score, T score, z-score) and is therefore more useful for score interpretations (e.g., Feldt & Brennan, 1989; Thissen, 1990). The *SEM* is related to the reliability, r_{XX}, and the standard deviation of the observed scores, as follows:

$$SEM = \sigma_X \sqrt{1 - r_{XX}}. \qquad (3.5)$$

To compute the *SEM*, one needs to know the reliability and standard deviation of the client's test score. For example, if the reliability is 0.90 and the standard deviation of the client's observed scores is 15 (such as is the case for the deviation IQ, a standard score scale with an $M = 100$ and $SD = 15$—a scale commonly used in intelligence and achievement tests), then the standard error of measurement is

$$SEM = 15\sqrt{1 - 0.9} = 15(0.3162) = 4.743.$$

Some test manuals leave it to the test user to compute the client's confidence interval, sometimes providing only reliability coefficients; others provide confidence intervals in norm conversion tables. Professional counselors understand that even though it is often necessary to make decisions about clients based on an observed or obtained score, it is not appropriate to interpret a single observed score to a client. Instead, it is appropriate to report and interpret the *range* of scores within which the true score probably lies.

Furthermore, it is most appropriate to interpret these scores at the 95% level of confidence (± 2 *SEM*). Some test manuals and computer scoring programs recommend interpretation at the 68% level of confidence, which means that the client's true score will fall outside the suggested range in 1 out of every 3 reports (i.e., the 68% level results in an average "mistake rate" of 32%!). Most clinicians (and clients) find it unacceptable to be wrong in one 1 of every 3 decisions—especially decisions related to diagnosis and treatment. Using the 95% level of confidence (± 2 *SEM*) means that the true score falls in the reported range 95 out of 100 administrations. A 5% error rate is much more acceptable in clinical practice, especially when making decisions about peoples' lives that may influence treatment for months or years into the future.

Consider the following examples of how to apply *SEM* to score interpretation. If a client's full-scale IQ (FSIQ) score on the *WAIS-III* is 110, and the *SEM* is equal to 4 standard score points, the client's IQ could be interpreted at the 95% level of confidence (± 2 *SEM*) as 110 ± 8 (e.g., 2 × 4). Thus, on 100 alternative-form administrations of the *WAIS-III,* the client's FSIQ would probably fall within the FSIQ range of 102–118 about 95 times. This means that the professional counselor may have 95% confidence that the client's true IQ score falls between 102 and 118 (also referred to as the Average to High Average range). Likewise, the client's *Conners' Adult ADHD Rating Scales* (*CAARS*) (Conners, Erhardt, & Sparrow, 1999) *DSM-IV* inattention scale T score of 71, with an *SEM* = 3 points (T score units), would be interpreted at the 95% level of confidence (±2 *SEM*) as 71 ± (2 × 3) = 71 ± 6. Thus, on 100 alternate form administrations of the *CAARS DSM-IV* inattention scale, the client's T score would probably fall within the T score range of 65–77 about 95 times.

Think About It 3.1   If a client's observed score on the *MMPI-2* Depression scale is a T score ($M = 50$, $SD = 10$) of 67, and the scale's reliability is 0.82, what is the client's likely range of scores at the 95% level of confidence? Given this information, would you be inclined to support a diagnosis of depression for this client? Explain.

TYPES OF RELIABILITY

The reliability of test scores for a population of examinees is defined as the ratio of their true score variance (*T*) *to* observed score variance (see Equation 3.3). Equivalently, the reliability can also be represented as the squared correlation between true and observed scores (i.e., $r_{XX} = r_{XT}^2$). Unfortunately, in empirical research, true scores cannot be directly determined. Thus the reliability is typically estimated by coefficients of internal consistency, test-retest, alternate forms, and other types of reliability estimates adopted in the measurement literature. It is important to emphasize that different types of reliability relate to different sources of measurement error and, contrary to common misconceptions, are generally not interchangeable.

Internal Consistency

Internal consistency estimates of reliability are based on the average correlation among items within a test or scale. A huge advantage of internal consistency is that participants need to receive only one administration of a single test on a single occasion. A widely known method for determining internal consistency of test scores is **split-half reliability**. Using the split-half method, the researcher literally divides the questions into two halves, either by an odd-even method or by some other strategy. Each half of the items is treated as a separate test, and the total scores of these two half-tests for each participant are correlated together. With this method, the two halves are assumed to be parallel (i.e., the two halves have equal true scores and equal error variances).

However, because halving the number of items on a test substantially lowers the correlation (i.e., all other things being equal, the greater the number of items, the higher the correlation—thus halving the number of items lowers the correlation), an estimation formula is required to predict what the internal consistency of the items would be if returned to the size of the original complement of items. The score reliability of the whole test is estimated using the *Spearman-Brown Prophecy formula:*

$$r_{XX} = \frac{2r_{12}}{1 + r_{12}} \qquad (3.6)$$

where r_{12} is the Pearson correlation between the scores on the two halves of the test. For example, if the correlation between the two test halves is 0.6, then the split-half reliability estimate is: $r_{XX} = 2(0.6)/(1 + 0.6) = 0.75$.

The Spearman-Brown Prophecy formula can also be used to determine the likely result of adding more items to a given scale. Following on the example above, if the number of test items yielding the internal consistency coefficient of 0.75 were doubled yet again (this is what the value *2* in the numerator designates), the resulting reliability coefficient would be $r_{XX} = 2(0.75)/(1 + 0.75) = 1.50/1.75 = 0.83$.

How one splits the items into two equivalent halves when computing internal consistency is very important. One commonly used approach to forming test halves, called the *odd-even method,* is to assign the odd-numbered test items to one half and the even-numbered test items to the other half of the test. This method is particularly appropriate when the items are presented in order of increasing difficulty, such as on an achievement or intelligence test. Perhaps an even more appropriate method would be to stagger the assignments to even out the item difficulty levels (i.e., sum items 1, 4, 5, 8, 9 versus items 2, 3, 6, 7, 10).

A more recommended approach, called *matched random subsets*, involves three steps. First, two statistics are calculated for each item: the proportion of individuals who answered the item correctly (i.e., the item difficulty) and the point-biserial correlation between the item and the total test score. Second, each item is plotted on a graph using these two statistics as coordinates of a dot representing the item. Third, items that are close together on the graph are paired, and one item from each pair is randomly assigned to each half of the test.

Computer programs, such as *SPSS,* are frequently used to compute internal consistency estimates. Researchers and test users should use caution to ensure that proper item matching procedures were used, lest the computer default to a procedure that will overestimate a scale's internal consistency, leading to undue confidence in score reliability. Importantly, if the instrument consists of different scales yielding interpreted scores, internal consistency should be estimated for each scale. For example, the *Disruptive Behavior Rating Scale (DBRS)* (Erford, 1993) is composed of four subscales: Distractible, Oppositional, Impulsive-Hyperactive, and Antisocial Conduct. There is no interpretable total score, and each subscale score is interpreted as a separate subscale. Thus internal consistency coefficients for the observed scores on each scale are of interest.

The Spearman-Brown Prophecy formula is not appropriate when there are indications that the test halves are not parallel (e.g., when the two test halves do not have equal variances). In such cases, the internal consistency of the scores for the whole test can be estimated with the Cronbach's *coefficient* α (Greek letter *alpha*) using the formula (Cronbach, 1951):

$$\alpha = \frac{2[\text{VAR}(X) - \text{VAR}(X_1) - \text{VAR}(X_2)]}{\text{VAR}(X)}, \tag{3.7}$$

where $\text{VAR}(X)$, $\text{VAR}(X_1)$, and $\text{VAR}(X_2)$ represent the sample variance of the whole test, its first half, and its second half, respectively. For example, if the observed score variance for the whole test is 40 and the observed variances for the two test halves are 12 and 11, respectively, then coefficient *alpha* (α) = 2(40 − 12 − 11)/40 = 0.85.

The coefficient *alpha* is usually calculated for more than two components of the test, and when item response formats are multiscaled (e.g., Very Dissatisfied, Dissatisfied, Satisfied, Very Satisfied; or Almost Never, Sometimes, Frequently, Almost Always). Each test component is an item or a set of items. Sometimes it is helpful to see the mathematical formulas to understand what comprises α. But if you find this confusing, don't worry. Computers do all of these computations nowadays in a split second, using programs such as *SPSS*.

The general formula for *alpha* (see Equation 3.8) is simply an extension of Equation 3.7 for more than two test components:

$$\alpha = \frac{n}{n-1}\left[1 - \frac{\sum \text{VAR}(X_i)}{\text{VAR}(X)}\right], \tag{3.8}$$

where n is the number of test components (usually the number of items), X_i is the observed score on the ith test component, $\text{VAR}(X_i)$ is the variance of X_i, X is the observed score for the whole test (i.e., X = X_1 + X_2 + . . . + X_n), $\text{VAR}(X)$ is the variance of X, and Σ (Greek capital letter *sigma*) is the summation symbol.

When each test component is a dichotomously scored item (1 = correct [or true], 0 = incorrect [or false]), the coefficient α can be calculated by an equivalent formula, called *Kuder-Richardson formula 20* (see Equation 3.9), with the notation KR-20 (or α-20) for the coefficient of internal consistency:

$$\text{KR-20} = \frac{n}{n-1}\left[1 - \frac{\sum p_i(1 - p_i)}{\text{VAR}(X)}\right], \tag{3.9}$$

where n is the number of test items, X is the observed score for the whole test, $\text{VAR}(X)$ is the variance of X, p_i is the proportion of persons who answered correctly item i, and $p_i(1 - p_i)$ is the variance of the observed binary scores on item i (X_i = 1 or 0)—that is, $\text{VAR}(X_i) = p_i(1 - p_i)$.

Again, high-speed computer programs, such as *SPSS*, make the computation of coefficient α, or KR-20, rather simple.

Recall from Chapter 1 that speeded tests are those on which few clients miss any items, but the score is determined by how many items a client finishes in a given period of time. With a **speed test**, the split-half correlation coefficient ordinarily would be close to zero if the test were split into the first half of items versus the second half of items, since most examinees would correctly answer almost all items in the first half and (running out of time) would miss most items in the second half of the test. Likewise, if the odd-even splitting method is used for a speeded test, the resulting correlation would be artificially high because clients usually would get all items correct up until the point at which time ran out, and all subsequent items would be marked incorrect. Thus the score for odd items would almost always be within 1 point of the even-item total. When determining the internal consistency of speeded tests, it is generally appropriate to split the test by time intervals, rather than items, and to combine the raw scores for these intervals into the two test halves. For example, on the *WISC-IV*'s Coding subtest, one could observe how many items were responded to correctly during each of the eight 15-second intervals that comprise the 2-minute subtest. Then the number of items correctly responded to during the odd (1st, 3rd, 5th, and 7th) 15-second intervals could be summed and correlated with the sums of the even (2nd, 4th, 6th, and 8th) 15-second intervals for each participant in the study.

Test-Retest Reliability

The extent to which the same persons consistently respond to the same test, inventory, or questionnaire administered on different occasions is known as the **test-retest reliability** of test scores. Sometimes test-retest reliability is also called *temporal stability,* meaning stability over time. Test-retest reliability is estimated by the correlation between the observed scores of the same people taking the same test twice; that is, the same participants take the same test on two separate occasions. The resulting correlation coefficient is also referred to as the *coefficient of stability,* because the primary source of measurement error is stability over time. Because tests are frequently used to track therapeutic progress or the effects of medication, test-retest reliability can provide helpful insights into how client scores are likely to vary simply due to a readministration of the same test on a second occasion.

The major problem with test-retest reliability estimates is the potential for carryover effects between the two test administrations. Readministration of the test within a short period of time (e.g., a few days or weeks) may produce carryover effects due to memory and/or practice. For example, students who take a math or vocabulary test may look up some answers they were unsure of after the first administration of the test, thereby changing their true knowledge on the content measured by the test. Likewise, the process of completing an anxiety inventory could trigger an increase in the anxiety level of some people, thus causing their true anxiety scores to change from one administration of the inventory to the next. This happens if the client is more or less anxious on a second administration of the anxiety inventory.

If the construct (attribute) being measured varies over time (e.g., cognitive skills, depression), a long period of time between the two administrations of the instrument may produce carryover effects due to biological maturation, cognitive development, or changes in information, experience, and/or moods. For example, if a student learns a lot about math between the first and second administration of a math achievement test, the student's score may increase substantially. Likewise, a client with depression who is administered the *Beck Depression Inventory—Second Edition* (*BDI-II*) (Beck, Steer, & Brown, 1996) may receive a lower score on the second administration of the *BDI-II* six months later, regardless of whether treatment was successful.

Thus, test-retest reliability estimates are most appropriate for measurements of traits that are stable across the time period between the two test administrations (e.g., visual or auditory acuity, personality, work values). In addition to problems with carryover effect, there is also a practical limitation to retesting, because it is usually time consuming and/or expensive. For many tests, retesting solely for the purpose of estimating score stability may be impractical, although it is frequently of interest to clinicians using tests as an outcome measure to know what degree of consistency to expect on test readministration.

On a final note, researchers should always report the time interval between the first and second administrations of the test. This is because, normally, the longer the period of time between the two administrations, the lower the reliability (e.g., the greater the chances that some external factor or developmental change will occur).

Alternate Forms Reliability (Equivalent Forms Reliability)

One way of counteracting the practice effects that occur in test-retest reliability is to design two equivalent versions of a test. If two versions of an instrument (test, inventory, or questionnaire) have very similar observed score means, variances, and correlations with other measures, they are called alternate forms or equivalent forms of the instrument. In fact, any decent attempt to construct parallel tests is expected to result in alternate test forms, as it is practically impossible to obtain perfectly parallel tests (i.e., equal true scores and equal error variances). Alternate forms usually are easier to develop for instruments that measure, for example, abilities and aptitudes or specific academic abilities because of the larger potential item pools (i.e., domains of knowledge) than those that measure constructs that are more difficult to represent with measurable variables (e.g., personality, motivation, temperament, anxiety). Thus professional counselors will frequently see alternate forms of achievement tests (i.e., Forms A and B of the *WJ-III ACH* [Woodcock, Mather, & McGrew, 2001] and the Blue and Tan forms of the *WRAT-III* [Wilkinson, 1993]), but they only rarely see alternate forms purposefully designed by a test author in the intellectual, behavioral, or personality domains.

Alternate form reliability is a measure of the consistency of scores on alternate test forms administered to the same group of individuals—that is, two equivalent tests administered to the same participants on two separate occasions. The correlation between observed scores on two alternate test forms, referred to as the *coefficient of equivalence,* provides an estimate of the reliability of each of the alternate forms based on item content, scorer, *and* temporal stability. Just as with the test-retest reliability coefficients, the estimates of alternate form reliability are subject to carryover (practice) effects, but to a lesser degree, as the persons are not tested twice with the same items. To minimize carryover effects, a recommended rule of thumb is to have a 2-week time period between administrations of alternate test forms.

Whenever possible, it is important to obtain both internal consistency coefficients and alternate forms correlations for a test. If the correlation between alternate forms is much lower than the internal consistency coefficient (e.g., a difference of 0.20 or more), this might be due to (a) differences in content, (b) subjectivity of scoring, and (c) changes in the trait being measured over time between the administrations of alternate forms. To determine the relative contribution of these sources of error, it is usually recommended to administer the two alternate forms on the same day for half a sample of respondents, and then after a 2-week time interval for the other half of the sample (so long as the number of participants in each group is at least 10 or more for empirical purposes). If the correlation between the scores on the alternate forms for the same-day administration is much higher than the correlation for the 2-week time interval, then variation in the trait being measured is a major source of error (i.e., temporal instability). For example, it is likely that measures of mood will change over a 2-week time interval, and thus the 2-week correlation will be lower than the same-day correlation between the alternate forms of the instrument. However, if the two correlations are both low, the persons' scores may be stable over the 2-week time interval, but the alternate forms probably differ in content.

Likewise, when scores on alternate forms of an instrument are assigned by raters (e.g., counselors, parents, teachers), one may check for scoring subjectivity by using a three-step procedure: (1) randomly split a large sample of persons; (2) administer the alternate forms on the same day for one group of people; and (3) administer the alternate forms after a 2-week time interval for the other group of people. If the correlations between raters are high for both groups, there is probably little scoring error due to subjectivity. If the correlation over the 2-week time interval and the same-day correlation are both consistently low across different raters, it is difficult to determine the major sources of scoring errors. Such errors can be reduced by training the raters in using the instrument and by providing clear guidelines for scoring behaviors or traits being measured.

Reliability of Criterion-Referenced Tests

Criterion-referenced measurements show how the examinees stand with respect to an external criterion. The criterion is usually some specific educational or performance objective, such as "can apply basic algebra rules," "is able to recognize patterns," or even "is at risk for depression."

Most teacher-made tests are criterion referenced because the teacher is more interested in how well students master coursework (criterion referenced) rather than how students did when compared with other students (norm referenced). Likewise, professional counselors frequently want to know whether a client has "enough" of a mental disorder (depression, anxiety, oppositional behavior) to warrant a diagnosis. This is also a situation calling for criterion-referenced measurement. Because a criterion-referenced test may cover numerous specific objectives (criteria), each

Table 3.1   Contingency table for mastery-nonmastery classifications

		Form B		
		Master	*Nonmaster*	
Form A	*Master*	p_{11}	p_{12}	P_{A1}
	Nonmaster	p_{21}	p_{22}	P_{A2}
		P_{B1}	P_{B2}	

objective should be measured as accurately as possible. When the results of criterion-referenced measurements are used for classifications related to mastery or nonmastery of the criterion, the reliability of such classifications is often referred to as *classification consistency*. This type of reliability shows the consistency with which classifications are made, either by the same test administered on two occasions or by alternate test forms.

Two classical indices of classification consistency are (a) P_o = the observed proportion of persons consistently classified as mastery versus nonmastery and (b) Cohen's κ (Greek letter *kappa*) = the proportion of nonrandom consistent classifications. Their calculation is illustrated for the two-way data layout in Table 3.1, where the entries are proportions of persons classified as masters or nonmasters by two alternate test forms of a criterion-referenced test (Form A and Form B). Specifically, p_{11} is the proportion of persons classified as "mastery" (those who mastered the content to the specified level) by both test forms; p_{12} is the proportion of persons classified as "mastery" by Form A and "nonmastery" by Form B; p_{21} for "nonmastery" of Form A and "mastery" on Form B; and p_{22} as "nonmastery" on both forms of the test. Also, P_{A1}, P_{A2}, P_{B1}, and P_{B2} are notations for marginal proportions—that is: $P_{A1} = p_{11} + p_{12}$; $P_{B1} = p_{11} + p_{21}$; $P_{A2} = p_{21} + p_{22}$; and $P_{B2} = p_{12} + p_{22}$. The observed proportion of consistent classifications (mastery/nonmastery) is

$$P_o = p_{11} + p_{22} \tag{3.10}$$

However, P_o can be a misleading indicator of classification consistency, because part of it may occur by chance. Cohen's *kappa* (see Equation 3.11) takes into account the proportion of consistent classification that is theoretically expected to occur by chance, P_e, and provides a ratio of nonrandom consistent classifications

$$\kappa = \frac{P_o - P_e}{1 - P_e}, \tag{3.11}$$

where P_e is obtained by summing the cross-products of marginal proportions in Table 3.1: $P_e = P_{A1}P_{B1} + P_{A2}P_{B2}$. In Equation 3.11, the numerator $(P_o - P_e)$ is the proportion of nonrandom consistent classification being detected, whereas the denominator $(1 - P_e)$ is the maximum proportion of nonrandom consistent classification that may occur. Cohen's *kappa* indicates, then, what proportion of the maximum possible nonrandom consistent classifications is found with the data.

Think About It 3.2   Administering a substance abuse screening test along with a *DSM-IV-TR* diagnostic process, let us assign specific values to the proportions in Table 3.1 (see Table 3.2): $p_{11} = 0.3$, $p_{12} = 0.2$, $p_{21} = 0.1$, and $p_{22} = 0.4$. These are nice even numbers, meaning that 30%, 20%, 10%, and 40% of the cases (decisions) fell into each category, respectively. The marginal proportions are: $P_{A1} = 0.3 + 0.2 = 0.5$, $P_{A2} = 0.1 + 0.4 = 0.5$, $P_{B1} = 0.3 + 0.1 = 0.4$, and $P_{B2} = 0.2 + 0.4 = 0.6$.

Table 3.2   Contingency table for mastery-nonmastery classifications for identifying individuals with substance abuse

		Form B—*DSM*-diagnosis		
		Diagnosed	*Not diagnosed*	
Form A Substance Abuse Test	*Diagnosed*	0.3	0.2	0.3 + 0.2 = 0.5
	Not diagnosed	0.1	0.4	0.1 + 0.4 = 0.5
		0.3 + 0.1 = 0.4	0.2 + 0.4 = 0.6	

With these data, calculate the observed proportion of consistent classification P_o. You should have gotten $P_o = 0.3 + 0.4 = 0.7$ by using Equation 3.10.

Next, calculate κ using Equation 3.11. The proportion of consistent classifications that may occur by chance in this hypothetical example is: $P_e = (0.5)(0.4) + (0.5)(0.6) = 0.5$. Using Equation 3.11, the Cohen's *kappa* ratio is: $κ = (0.7 - 0.5)/(1 - 0.5) = 0.2/0.5 = 0.4$.

Finally, interpret these results. For this example of using a substance abuse test, the initially obtained 70% of observed consistent classifications ($P_o = 0.7$) is reduced to 40% consistent classifications after taking into account consistent classifications that may occur by chance. Because *kappa* provides "conservative" estimations of consistency, it is reasonable to report in this case that the classification consistency is between 0.40 and 0.70 (i.e., between κ and P_o). *Note:* For practical purposes, it is recommended to report both P_o and Cohen's *kappa,* as the latter is very conservative, thus underestimating the actual rate of consistent classifications. Previous research [e.g., Chase, 1996; Subkoviak, 1988] provides some additional procedures for estimating classification consistency, including scenarios with a single test administration or prior to the initial application of the test.)

Interscorer and Interrater Reliability

The chances of measurement error usually increase when the scores are based on subjective judgments of the person(s) doing the scoring. In general, the less objective the scoring procedures, the lower the **interscorer reliability**. Such situations occur, for example, with classroom assessment of essays or portfolios where the teacher is, in fact, the "judge" of performance. In another scenario, involving some projective tests of personality, the scorer (e.g., professional counselor, psychotherapist) should decide if the person's responses suggest normal functioning or some form of psychopathology. Subjective judgments of raters (experts, judges) are also used for classification purposes (e.g., to determine a "minimum level of competency" in pass/fail decisions). In all scenarios of rater-based scoring, it is important to estimate the degree to which the scores are unduly affected by the subjective judgments of the raters. Such estimation is provided by coefficients of **interrater reliability** (also called coefficients of interrater agreement).

Depending on the context of measurement, there are different methods of estimating interrater reliability. Frequently used classical measures of interrater reliability are the Pearson correlation coefficients, observed proportion of consistent classification (P_o) and Cohen's *kappa* coefficient. The Pearson r is by far the most commonly used measure of interscorer reliability when scores are interval, as most test scores (e.g., standard scores) are, or ratio. Otherwise, the two indices of classification (P_o and Cohen's *kappa*) can be used as estimates of interrater reliability when two raters (instead of two test forms) classify persons as mastery or nonmastery. When more than two categories are used by two raters to classify persons (or their products), one can still use Equation 3.11 for Cohen's *kappa*, but P_o and P_e should be calculated with a contingency table for the respective number of categories. For example, with three classification categories (e.g., low, medium, and high performance), P_o and P_e are calculated as follows: $P_o = p_{11} + p_{22} + p_{33}$ and $P_e = P_{A1}P_{B1} + P_{A2}P_{B2} + P_{A3}P_{B3}$.

Interrater reliability is also sometimes used to refer to two independent observers who rate another individual, such as when sets of mothers and teachers rate children on a behavior rating scale and the results are correlated. This type of relationship is better described as a type of criterion-related validity (see Chapter 4). In this instance, one set of scores (e.g., teachers) serves as the criterion for the other set of scores (e.g., mothers). If two raters independently assign scores (say, to portfolios) of students, then the Pearson correlation coefficient for the two sets of scores can be used as an estimate of interrater agreement. The higher the correlation coefficient, the lower the error variance due to scorer differences, and the higher the interrater agreement.

When scoring of alternate forms of a measurement instrument is done by two or more raters, one can check for measurement error due to subjectivity of scoring by administering the alternate forms (a) on the same day for one group of subjects and (b) with a 2-week delay for another group of subjects. If the correlations between raters are high for both groups, there is probably little error due to subjectivity of scoring. If, however, the correlation over the 2-week time interval and the same-day correlation are both consistently low across different raters, it is difficult to determine the major source of unreliability (subjectivity of scoring or, say, differences in content for the two alternate forms of the instrument). The interrater reliability can be improved by training the raters in the use of the instrument and providing clear guidelines for scoring (e.g., a more specific rubric or more specific criteria).

Overall, researchers and test users can reduce measurement error and improve reliability by (1) writing items clearly, (2) providing complete and understandable test instructions, (3) administering the instrument under prescribed conditions, (4) reducing subjectivity in scoring, (5) training raters and providing them with clear scoring instructions, (6) using heterogeneous respondent samples to increase the variance of observed scores, and (7) increasing the length of the test by adding items that are (ideally) parallel to those that are already in the test. The general principle behind improving reliability is *to maximize the variance of relevant individual differences and minimize the error variance.*

THE IMPORTANCE OF RELIABILITY

Reliability in Validation

The most important characteristic of any measurement is its *validity*—a concept referring to the meaningfulness, appropriateness, and usefulness of the inferences made from the measurement scores. Validation is an ongoing process of gathering evidence to support such inferences. It is essential to understand that it is the inferences made from measurement scores that are being validated, not the instrument (e.g., test, survey, or questionnaire) being used to obtain such scores.

The score reliability is an important (necessary, but not sufficient) condition in the validation process. For example, as noted earlier in this chapter, the reliability of scores predetermines a "ceiling" for their criterion-related validity, but how closely this ceiling will be approached depends on other factors as well. The validation of measurements in counseling usually deals with constructs (e.g., proficiency, motivation, anxiety, empathy, and beliefs) and involves different types of evidence. The quality of such evidence depends, among other things, on the reliability of the data collected from different sources. The reliability also affects the results from correlational analyses and other statistical procedures used in the validation process. The term *attenuation* is used to indicate the reduction of the magnitude of such results due to unreliability of scores.

ATTENUATION

If the reliability of the scores on two variables X and Y is not perfect (i.e., $r_{XX} \neq 1$ and/or $r_{YY} \neq 1$), the observed correlation between X and Y, r_{XY}, is attenuated (i.e., lower than the "actual" correlation between the person's true scores on the two variables: T_X and T_Y). One can estimate the correlation between the true scores T_X and

T_Y by using Equation 3.12, referred to as the *correction for attenuation formula* (Spearman, 1904):

$$r_{T_X T_Y} = \frac{r_{XY}}{\sqrt{r_{XX} r_{YY}}}$$

(3.12)

Think About It 3.3   The correlation between two variables, Self-esteem (X) and Persistence decisions (Y), in a study on academic persistence for college undergraduates was found to be $r_{XY} = 0.35$. Professional counselors involved in this study found also that the reliability of the two measures, X and Y, for the study data was relatively low: $r_{XY} = 0.68$ and $r_{YY} = 0.71$, respectively. To estimate what would be the correlation between the two variables if their measurements were perfectly reliable, the professional counselors used Equation 3.12, thus obtaining much higher correlation (0.50) between the students' true scores (i.e., no error involved) on Self-esteem and Persistence decisions:

$$r_{T_X T_Y} = \frac{0.35}{\sqrt{(0.68)(0.71)}} = 0.50$$

Importantly, because perfect reliability is generally not obtainable, one cannot observe the corrected-for-attenuation correlation values. Such values indicate the highest correlation coefficients for perfectly reliable scores. Important conditions for using Equation 3.12 are (1) The reliability estimates, r_{XX} and r_{YY}, should also be accurate and (2) The components in the right-hand side of Equation 3.12 (r_{XY}, r_{XX}, and r_{YY}) should be affected by the same measurement error—for example, if r_{XY} is estimated when X and Y are measured during one testing session and their internal consistency estimates are used for r_{XY} and r_{XX} in Equation 3.12. However, if r_{XX} and r_{YY} are alternate form reliabilities, error of measurement involved in their estimation (due to time lapse and change of test form) would not be involved in the estimation of the correlation between X and Y (r_{XY}). Then Equation 3.12 will produce an overestimated true score correlation between X and Y $\left(r_{T_X T_Y}\right)$.

Attenuation effects due to unreliability of data occur also in hypothesis testing with statistical methods. It should be noted, for example, that although the Pearson correlation coefficient between an independent variable X and a dependent variable (criterion) Y is attenuated by error of measurement, the regression coefficient (slope) in the regression of Y on X is attenuated by measurement errors in X but not in Y (Bohrnstedt, 1983). Therefore, particular attention should be paid to the reliability of the pretest scores when they are used as a covariate (X), say, in the comparison of treatment groups, using the statistical method analysis of covariance (ANCOVA). The power of statistical tests is also attenuated by unreliability of the measurement data (to remind: the power of a statistical test of a null hypothesis is the probability that this test will lead to the rejection of the null hypothesis when it is false indeed). Specifically, the unreliability shrinks the observed effect size (e.g., produced by a specific treatment), thus reducing the power of the statistical test (for more details, see, e.g., Cohen, 1988; Maxwell, 1980; Zimmerman & Williams, 1982).

RELIABILITY OF COMPOSITE SCORES

In many situations, scores from two or more scales are combined into *composite scores* to measure and interpret a more general dimension (trait, ability, or proficiency) related to these scales. Composite scores are often used with test batteries for achievement, aptitude, intelligence, depression, or eating disorders, as well as with local school measurements such as performance and portfolio assessments. One frequently reported composite score, for example, is the sum of verbal and quantitative scores of the *Graduate Record Examination* (*GRE*). Another example is the *WISC-IV*'s 10 core subtests, which yield four index scores (i.e., Verbal Comprehension Index [VCI], Perceptual Reasoning Index [PRI], Working Memory Index [WMI] and Processing Speed Index [PSI]), which are subsequently combined to yield the full-scale IQ (FSIQ). The scores on nine scales of the *Symptom Checklist-90-Revised* (*SCL-90-R*) (Derogatis, 1990) are combined into three "global" (composite) scores in measuring current psychological symptom status. A Total Aggressive Expression score with the Driving Anger Expression Inventory (DAX) (Deffenbacher, Lynch, Oetting, & Swaim, 2002) is also obtained as a sum of three scales: Verbal Aggressive Expression, Personal Physical Aggressive Expression, and Using the Vehicle to Express Anger. Thus, composite scores are frequently encountered in psychological and educational testing.

Although the composite score may be simply the sum of several scale scores, its reliability is usually not just the mean of the reliabilities for the scales being combined. The issue of reliability estimation for composite scores is addressed in this section when the composite score is (a) the sum of two scale scores (e.g., *GRE*s, *SAT*s); (b) the difference score (e.g., *gain* score for pretest to posttest measurements or the difference between two independent scorers of a single set of portfolios); and (c) the sum of three or more scale scores (e.g., *WISC-IV, SCL-90-R*).

Reliability of Sum of Scores

Let the composite score Y be the sum of two scale scores, X_1 and X_2: $Y = X_1 + X_2$. With the *GRE* scoring, for example, the composite score is the sum of the verbal and quantitative scores. The *reliability of the sum of two scores*, r_{YY}, can be estimated as

$$r_{YY} = 1 - \frac{\sigma_1^2(1 - r_{11}) + \sigma_2^2(1 - r_{22})}{\sigma_Y^2}, \qquad (3.13)$$

where σ_1^2 is the variance of X_1, that is: $\sigma_1^2 = \text{VAR}(X_1)$, σ_2^2 is the variance of X_2, that is: $\sigma_2^2 = \text{VAR}(X_2)$, σ_Y^2 is the variance of the composite score Y, that is: $\sigma_Y^2 = \text{VAR}(Y)$, r_{11} is the reliability of X_1, and r_{22} is the reliability of X_2.

Think About It 3.4   The estimation of the reliability for a composite score, $Y = X_1 + X_2$, is illustrated in this example with data from a study on attitudes and behaviors of students related to their sexual activities. Specifically, X_1 is the score on a scale labeled "Love as Justification for Sexual Involvement," and X_2 is the score on a scale labeled "Sex for Approbation." With the notations adopted in Equation 3.13, the following results were obtained from the study data for (a) the variances of X_1, X_2, and Y: $\sigma_1^2 = 13.750$, $\sigma_2^2 = 10.433$, $\sigma_Y^2 = 38.5992$; and (b) the reliabilities of X_1 and X_2: $r_{11} = 0.8334$, $r_{22} = 0.8217$.

Replacing these components for their values in Equation 3.13, we obtain:

$$r_{YY} = 1 - \frac{13.750(1-0.8334)+10.433(1-0.8217)}{38.592} = 0.892.$$

Thus, the reliability estimate of the composite score Y (0.892) in this example is higher than the reliability estimates of its components, X_1 (0.8334) and X_2 (0.8217). While this frequently occurs, it is not always the case. In reality, the larger the difference between r_{11} and r_{22}, and the lower the correlation between the two components (r_{12}), the less likely that r_{YY} will exceed each individual component's reliability.

Although not explicitly present, the correlation between X_1 and X_2, denoted r_{12}, affects the reliability of the composite score. When X_1 and X_2 do not correlate ($r_{12} = 0$), the reliability of their sum ($Y = X_1 + X_2$) is simply the average of their reliabilities: $r_{YY} = (r_{11} + r_{22})/2$.

In many cases, the scores that are combined into a composite score come from scales with different units of measurement (e.g., 3-point and 5-point survey scales). Therefore, to present the measurements on a common scale (and for some technical reasons), the raw scores are often converted into standard scores (z-scores) before being summed (this is done, for example, with the raw scores of the primary psychological symptoms measured with the self-report symptom inventory *SCL-90-R*). For the special case of standard (z-) scores, Equation 3.13 is converted into a simpler form (Equation 3.14):

$$r_{YY} = 1 - \frac{2-\left(r_{11}+r_{22}\right)}{\sigma_{YZ}^2}, \tag{3.14}$$

where σ_{YZ}^2 is the variance of the sum of the z-scores for X_1 and X_2 (i.e., $Y_z = z_1 + z_2$), r_{11} is the reliability of X_1, and r_{22} is the reliability of X_2. Assume that $\sigma_{YZ}^2 = 3.203$ and that $r_{11} = 0.8334$ and $r_{22} = 0.8217$. With this, using Equation 3.14, we obtain the value for the reliability of the composite score $Y = X_1$ and X_2 (or, equivalently, for $Y_Z = z_1 + z_2$):

$$r_{YY} = 1 - \frac{2-(0.8334+0.8217)}{3.203} = 0.892.$$

Note that Equation 3.14 follows directly from Equation 3.13, taking into account that the variance of the standard (z-) scores for any variable is 1 and, thus, $\sigma^2(z_1) + \sigma^2(z_2) = 2$.

Equations 3.13 and 3.14 can be readily extended for cases where the composite score is a sum of more than two scale scores (e.g., Nunnally & Bernstein, 1994). For the sum of three scores, for example, the reliability of the composite score $Y = X_1 + X_2 + X_3$ can be estimated by extending Equation 3.14 to form Equation 3.15 as follows:

$$r_{YY} = 1 - \frac{3 - (r_{11} + r_{22} + r_{33})}{\sigma_{YZ}^2},\tag{3.15}$$

where σ_{YZ}^2 is the variance of the sum of the standard (z-) scores for X_1, X_2, and X_3; that is, $Y_Z = z_1 + z_2 + z_3$ (r_{11}, r_{22}, and r_{33} are the reliabilities for X_1, X_2, and X_3, respectively).

Reliability of Difference Scores

The difference between two observers' scores for the same person, called *difference score,* is widely used in behavioral research primarily (a) to measure the person's growth across time points and (b) to compare the person's scores on academic, psychological, or personality variables. For example, measurement of *change* using the person's difference (or *gain*) score from pretest to posttest is used to assess the effect of specific educational programs, counseling treatments, and rehabilitation services or allied health interventions, all important facets of outcomes research in the mental health field. Clearly, the quality of the results and the validity of interpretations in studies on change and profile analysis depend, among other things, on the reliability of difference scores.

Think About It 3.5 The data in this example also come from the study on attitudes and behaviors of students related to their sexual activities. However, instead of summing the scores on two scales, the composite score is now the difference (gain) from pretreatment to posttreatment measurements on a scale labeled "Self-affirmation"; that is, $Y = X_2 - X_1$, where X_1 is the pretreatment score and X_2 the posttreatment score on this scale. With the study data, the variance of the difference $Y_z = z_2 - z_1$ (where z_1 and z_2 are the standard score values for X_1 and X_2) was found to be $\sigma_{YZ}^2 = 0.786$.

The reliability coefficients (*alpha* coefficients) for X_1 and X_2 were $r_{11} = 0.8282$ and $r_{22} = 0.8374$, respectively. Using Equation 3.14, the reliability of the difference scores is

$$r_{YY} = 1 - \frac{2 - (0.8282 + 0.8374)}{0.786} = 0.575$$

Evidently, the reliability of the difference score (0.575) is smaller than the reliability of the scores entering the difference (0.8282 and 0.8374). As noted earlier, the reliability of the difference score, r_{YY}, is (implicitly) influenced by the correlation between X_1 and X_2 (in this case, $r_{12} = 0.606$), because this correlation affects the value of σ_{Yz}^2 in Equation 3.15.

The use of difference (gain) scores in measurement of change has been criticized because of the (generally false) assertion that the difference between scores is less reliable than the scores themselves (e.g., Cronbach & Furby, 1970; Linn & Slindle, 1977; Lord, 1956). This assertion is true, however, if the pretest scores and the posttest scores have equal variances and equal reliability. When this is not the case, which may happen in many measurement situations, the reliability of the gain score is reasonably high (e.g., Overall & Woodward, 1975; Zimmerman & Williams, 1982). The relatively low reliability of gain scores does not preclude valid testing of the null hypothesis of zero mean gain score in a population of examinees, but it is not appropriate to correlate the gain score with other variables for these examinees. An important practical implication is that, without ignoring the caution urged by some authors, researchers should not always discard gain score and should be aware when gain scores are useful.

Reliability of Weighted Sums

When different components are of varying importance, but need to be combined into a composite score, the components must first be "weighted" before being combined. Let the scores from two tests, X_1 and X_2, have different "weights" (w_1 and w_2, respectively) in a composite score, $Y = w_1X_1 + w_2X_2$. To estimate the reliability of the composite score, Y, given the reliabilities of X_1 and X_2, one can (for simplicity) use the weighted composite score, Yz, of the standardized variables Z_1 and Z_2, which are obtained by transforming the raw scores of X_1 and X_2 into z-scores. That is,

$$Y_Z = w_1X_1 + w_2X_2.$$

With this, the reliability of the composite score, Y (or Y_Z), is given by Equation 3.16:

$$r_{YY} = 1 - \frac{(1-r_{11})w_1^2 + (1-r_{22})w_2^2}{\sigma_{YZ}^2}, \qquad (3.16)$$

where r_{YY} is the reliability of the composite score Y (or Yz), r_{11} is the reliability of X_1, r_{22} is the reliability of X_2, and σ_{YZ}^2 is the variance of the composite score Yz (the weighed sum of Z_1 and Z_2).

Think About It 3.6   The examination score of counseling students in a lifespan development course is obtained as a composite score of midterm and final examinations, with 40% importance assigned to the midterm and 60% importance to the final examination. The task is to estimate the reliability of the composite score.

The reliability estimates (Cronbach's *alpha* coefficients) for the scores on the first test, X_1 (midterm), and the second test, X_2 (final), are $r_{11} = 0.72$ and $r_{22} = 0.80$, respectively. Given that the weight for X_1 is $w_1 = 0.4$ (40% importance) and the weight for X_2 is $w_2 = 0.6$ (60% importance), the composite score is: $Y = (0.4)X_1 + (0.6)X_2$. After transforming the scores on X_1 and X_2 into z-scores to obtain the standardized variables Z_1 and Z_2, respectively, the variance of $Y_Z = (0.4)Z_1 + (0.6)Z_2$ is found to be $\sigma_{YZ}^2 = 1.27$. Using Equation 3.16, the reliability of the composite score Y is then

$$r_{YY} = 1 - \frac{2 - (1-0.72)(0.4)^2 + (1-0.80)(0.6)^2}{1.27} = 0.908.$$

Equation 3.16 can be easily extended to estimate the reliability of a weighted sum of the scores on more than two tests. In the case of three tests, for example, the reliability of the composite score $Y = w_1X_1 + w_2X_2 + w_3X_3$ can be obtained by extending Equation 3.16 to Equation 3.17:

$$r_{YY} = 1 - \frac{\left(1 - r_{11}\right)w_1^2 + \left(1 - r_{22}\right)w_2^2 + (1 - r_{33})w_3^2}{\sigma_{YZ}^2}, \tag{3.17}$$

where σ_{YZ}^2 is the variance of $Yz = w_1Z_1 + w_2Z_2 + w_3Z_3$. Equations 3.16 and 3.17 (as well as their extensions for more than three tests) apply equally well when some of the weights are negative numbers.

SUMMARY/CONCLUSION

This chapter has introduced the concept of reliability, types of reliability, different methods of estimating reliability, and principles in interpreting and comparing reliability coefficients. Generally, reliability of measurements (e.g., test scores and survey ratings) indicates their accuracy and consistency under random variations in measurement conditions, such as a person's conditions (e.g., fatigue or mood) and/or external sources (e.g., noise, temperature, different raters, and different test forms).

In classical test theory, the *true score* of a person is defined as the theoretical mean of the observed scores that this person may have under numerous independent testings with the same test. A basic assumption is that the examinee's observed score is a sum of the person's true score and an error ($X = T + E$). Tests with equal true scores and equal error variances, for any population of examinees, are referred to as *parallel tests*. The *reliability* of test scores is equivalently defined as (a) the correlation between observed scores on parallel tests, (b) the ratio of true score variance to observed score variance for the same test, or (c) the squared correlation between observed and true scores. *Standard error of measurement* (*SEM*) is the standard deviation of the (assumed normal) distribution of the difference between examinees' observed scores and their true scores.

Five types of classical reliability were discussed in this chapter: internal consistency, test-retest reliability, alternate form reliability, classification consistency, and interrater reliability.

Internal consistency estimates of reliability are based on the average correlation among items within an instrument. If the instrument consists of different scales, internal consistency should be estimated for each scale. Widely used estimates of internal consistency are the *split-half* reliability coefficient and Cronbach's coefficient *alpha* (or its equivalent version, KR-20, for dichotomously scored items). It is always useful to report the internal consistency of test scores even when other types of reliability are of primary interest. With *speed* tests, however, it would be misleading to report estimates of internal consistency.

Test-retest reliability indicates the extent to which persons consistently respond to the same test, inventory, or questionnaire administered on more than one occasion. It is estimated by the correlation between the observed scores of the same people taking the same test twice (*coefficient of stability*). The major problem with test-retest reliability estimates is the potential for carryover effects between the two test administrations (e.g., due to biological maturation, cognitive development, changes in information, experience, and/or moods). Thus, test-retest reliability estimates are most appropriate for measurements of traits that are stable across the time period between the two test administrations (e.g., personality or work values).

Alternate form reliability relates to the consistency of scores on two alternate test forms administered to the same group of individuals. It is estimated by the correlation between observed scores on two alternate test forms, referred to also as *coefficient of equivalence.* Estimates of alternate form reliability are also subject to carryover effects. A recommended rule of thumb is to have a 2-week time period between administrations of alternate test forms.

Criterion-referenced reliability shows the consistency with which decisions about mastery-nonmastery of a specific objective (criterion) are made, using either the same test administered on two occasions or alternate test forms. Widely used classical indices of classification consistency are the observed proportion of consistent classifications, P_o, and Cohen's *kappa* coefficient, which takes into account consistent classifications that may occur by chance.

Interrater (or interscorer) reliability refers to the consistency (agreement) in subjective judgments of raters (experts, judges) used for classification purposes (e.g., to determine a "minimum level of competency" in pass-fail decisions) or scoring rubrics in alternative assessments (e.g., portfolios, projects, and products). Depending on the measurement case, frequently used estimates of interrater reliability are correlation coefficients, P_o, and Cohen's *kappa* coefficient (or *kappa*-like coefficients).

Often the person's scores from two or more scales of some instruments are combined into *composite scores* to measure and interpret a more general dimension (trait or proficiency) related to these scales (i.e., achievement, intelligence, aptitude, depression). Although the composite score may be simply the sum of several scale scores, its reliability is usually not just the mean of the reliabilities for the scales being combined. In this chapter, the reliability for composite scores is addressed for cases when the composite score is a sum (or difference) of scale scores or a weighted sum of scores.

KEY TERMS

alternate form reliability
confidence interval
internal consistency
interrater reliability

interscorer reliability
normal distribution
observed score
random error

reliability   systematic error
speed test   test-retest reliability
split-half reliability   true score
standard error of measurement

CHAPTER 4

Validity

by Alan Basham and Bradley T. Erford

This chapter focuses on the concept of validity of scores in testing and assessment. It examines how reliability and validity are related and distinct, the different methods by which evidence for validity can be established, and key principles professional counselors should apply in determining whether a test is appropriate for use with a client or group. Methods for making accurate decisions using a single test or multiple tests are also discussed.

VALIDITY DEFINED

While reliability indicates the degree to which scores on an instrument are measured consistently, **validity** considers the degree to which test scores measure what the test claims to measure. In both cases, test developers attempt to amass evidence that indicates, either logically or through probability, that test scores are trustworthy. In reliability, test scores are trustworthy to the degree that they reflect an accurate assessment of some trait or ability, minimizing randomly occurring testing error. Evidence for validity, however, is concerned with verifying exactly what the test is measuring. Test results can be trusted, not just because they can be measured consistently, but because they measured what they were supposed to measure.

Suppose you and a group of friends had an opportunity to demonstrate your skills at an archery range. Supplied with a bow and several arrows, you each fired at targets the same distance away. Some people's arrows hit the target, others careened off nearby trees and rocks, and one person nearly skewered the instructor with a singularly wild shot. Only you hit the bulls-eye five shots in a row. The instructor, thinking you might have been just lucky, gives you five more arrows, all of which you calmly sink into the center of the target. Clearly, you are the most reliable archer in the group, because you keep getting the same result over and over. That's reliability, of course. However, if the amazed instructor asks you how you came to be so academically gifted, you might be well advised to question the instructor's judgment. Why? Because your demonstrated consistency at archery has little or nothing to do with the concept of academic giftedness. Imagine a scholarship program that awarded grants for tuition in counselor education based on consistency and proficiency of archery scores. Your archery score may be consistent (and therefore reliable) but is probably not a reasonable measure of academic potential. The meaning of the consistent, repetitive bulls-eyes, then, has become a question of validity.

So, the validity of test scores is about two things: (1) what the test actually measures and (2) how well the test scores measure it (Anastasi & Urbina, 1997). Some common methods for establishing evidence for validity are described in the *Standards for Educational and Psychological Testing* (AERA/APA/NCME, 1999). The *Standards* identified three major types of evidence for validity: content-related, criterion-related, and construct-related. While each of these types is distinct in its approach to demonstrating score validity, it is important not to assume that they are unrelated to each other. In fact, many test authors use more than one of these techniques to support the validity of test scores. Much of this chapter is devoted to outlining these techniques and providing examples. Although face validity is no longer generally accepted as a legitimate form of validity assessment, a brief discussion of this type of validity follows.

FACE VALIDITY

Face validity is derived from the obvious appearance of the measure itself and its test items. Items in instruments marked by face validity ask directly for information that is expected and wanted by the test user. Face validity is quite appropriate for survey instruments in which the person being queried is responding to questions such as "What is your age?" or "What is the highest level of education you completed?"

A major problem with self-report tests with high face validity is that when the trait or behavior in question is one that many people will not want to reveal about themselves, the likelihood of a truthful (and therefore valid) answer is minimal. A well-known example of the problem with face validity is that of the *Woodworth Personal Data Sheet* (Woodworth, 1920). This first structured personality test was developed during World War I for use in screening applicants for the military. Designed to standardize the psychiatric interview, it was based on the incorrect assumption that the content of an item and people's truthful response to it could be taken at face value. The assessment device included questions such as "I wet the bed" and "I drink a quart of whiskey every day," to which the person was asked to respond yes or no. The false assumption that people would answer such questions truthfully and that they interpreted the questions the same as everyone else essentially made the test results untrustworthy (Kaplan & Saccuzzo, 2001). Because of these limitations, the *Standards* (AERA et al., 1999) does not include face validity as a legitimate type of validity in psychological assessment. However, the above information is noteworthy because professional counselors may see the term in other documents. Even so, for tests in certain domains (e.g., achievement, intelligence), face validity can add credibility or acceptance to the assessment process.

CONTENT-RELATED VALIDITY

Content-related validity is widely used in educational testing (Kaplan & Saccuzzo, 2001) and in tests of aptitude or achievement. It is used in achievement tests to determine how well an individual has mastered a skill or the content of a course of study (Anastasi & Urbina, 1997). The main focus in content-related validity is on how the instrument was constructed and how the content of the test was determined (Whiston, 2005). The focus on content reflects the examiner's concern with how well the test items reflect the domain of the material being tested. The term **domain** refers to the total informational field from which the items are drawn.

For example, a teacher of U.S. history could write an exam to assess students' knowledge of the Civil War. The domain of information from which test items would be drawn is composed of the dates, battles, important persons, sociopolitical and economic factors, and causes of the war itself. The test would have validity to the effect that its content reflected all the important aspects of the domain of Civil War knowledge. A test that asked only about specific battles but ignored persons, causes, and political outcomes would hardly yield valid test scores of one's comprehensive knowledge of the U.S. Civil War.

Determining the content validity of a test requires a systematic evaluation of the test items to determine whether adequate coverage of a representative sample of the content domain was measured (Anastasi & Urbina, 1997). Obviously, the test cannot ask questions about all the information in the domain, but it should contain some items that assess knowledge of each of the domain's areas or categories. The domain itself should be examined to make sure that all major aspects are covered by the test, and the test should be constructed so that the number of items from each category within the domain is consistent with the size and importance of that category. Demonstrating how the test is constructed to represent the content of the domain provides evidence of content-related validity. The following is another example illustrating the concept.

Most professional counselors have taken a graduate course in counseling theories. Imagine an exam (much like one you have probably come across yourself in your academic journey) that covered the counseling theories of Freud, Adler, Jung, Ellis, and Rogers. (Please note that the number of theorists is limited here for the sake of a manageable example). To create a test that assessed knowledge of these progenitors and their contributions to the field, the professor would first analyze the important content areas of the domain. Let's assume the professor divided the overall domain of each of these five therapeutic pioneers into five subcategories identifying the salient content of each, including theoretical underpinnings of the model, therapeutic techniques, history of the founder, differences between each model and the others, and important terms and concepts unique to the model. The professor's organized analysis of the domain would look something like that contained in Table 4.1.

Table 4.1   Content analysis of important information regarding five counseling theorists

Freud	Adler	Jung	Ellis	Rogers
Theory	Theory	Theory	Theory	Theory
Techniques	Techniques	Techniques	Techniques	Techniques
History	History	History	History	History
Differences	Differences	Differences	Differences	Differences
Terms, i.e.,	Terms, i.e.,	Terms, i.e.,	Terms, i.e.,	Terms, i.e.,
Id, ego, superego	*inferiority complex*	*archetypes, shadow*	*catastrophizing, A-B-C-D-E*	*unconditional positive regard*

The professor would then write items reflecting each of the 25 categories listed above and select items from each category. If the items of the test adequately assessed some knowledge of each area of the domain, the test would have content-related validity. However, if the professor asked questions only about the terms of Jungian psychology, the history of Sigmund Freud's life, and the techniques of Rationale-Emotive Behavior Therapy (REBT) (Ellis), the test items probably would not be valid measures of the content under study because the questions did not adequately reflect knowledge of the domain being considered.

CRITERION-RELATED VALIDITY

Criterion-related validity is derived from comparing scores on the test to scores on a selected criterion. What is a **criterion**? It is a person's performance score on activities the test is designed to predict. Specifically, a sample of participants in the validation study has two scores that may be correlated with each other. One is the person's score on the test being studied, and the other is a score indicating the person's actual level of ability in the skill or behavior under question as measured by some criterion. The Scholastic Assessment Test (*SAT*) and Graduate Record Exam (*GRE*), for example, are used to predict performance in college and graduate school, respectively. The criterion measure for each of these tests is actual academic performance as measured by grade point average at some point later in the students' academic career. Similarly, the *Armed Services Vocational Aptitude Battery* (*ASVAB*) (USMEPCOM, 2005) is designed to identify the occupational specialties in which military personnel will be most skilled, given the proper level of training. Job performance in the military is the criterion measure for the *ASVAB*.

Anastasi and Urbina (1997) delineate several sources of criterion scores:

- *Academic achievement*, such as school grades and achievement test scores.
- The *amount of education* a person has.
- *Performance in specialized training*, such as music, accounting, or flying airplanes.
- *Job performance*, including in business, industry, and the military.
- *Psychiatric diagnosis*, which is used especially in development of tests measuring personality and psychopathology.

- *Ratings by job supervisors,* teachers, and others in a position to evaluate the performance effectiveness of subordinates.
- *Correlations with a previously available test,* especially when the new test is a simpler form of the original test.

There are two forms of criterion-related validity, **predictive criterion-related validity** and **concurrent criterion-related validity**. The main difference between the two is *when* the criterion measure is taken. In predictive criterion-related validity, the test is administered first, and scores on the criterion measure are collected on the same sample of persons at a later date (i.e., some time in the future). In concurrent criterion-related validity, the scores on the test and criterion measure are collected at the same point in time. Let's consider examples of each form of criterion-related validity.

Suppose that a professional counselor has been asked by a local business owner, Ms. Schmidlapp, to help her make more accurate hiring decisions at her factory, the Schmidlapp Widget Company. Ms. Schmidlapp wants the professional counselor to construct a test that will enable her to select those job applicants who will be most effective at widget assembly. The professional counselor develops a test believed to help her make the right choices and conducts the necessary studies to determine that, in fact, the test scores are quite reliable. However, the professional counselor does not yet know whether the test scores are valid measures of one's potential as a widget assembler. The professional counselor gives the next 100 job applicants the test, Ms. Schmidlapp hires them all on a three-month probationary status, and three months later each new employee is observed to identify the number of flawless widgets assembled in one week. Each employee's score on the test (predictor) is correlated with the employee's (score on) widget assembly proficiency (criterion). The direction and magnitude of the correlation between predictor and criterion variables tells the professional counselor the degree to which the test is associated with assembly skill. Because the criterion measure was collected some time later than the predictor, this study measured the test's *predictive* criterion-related validity.

Of course, there are some problems with using this form of validity assessment. First, the employer has to hire all the applicants in the pool of 100, regardless of ability or test scores, so that the predictor test accuracy will not be compromised by **restricted range**. If Ms. Schmidlapp hires only "qualified applicants," she will have criterion scores only on qualified applicants. How will she know if the test will identify unqualified applicants if the sample will contain no unqualified applicants? However, hiring everyone can create some major costs in terms of lost productivity and dissatisfied customers who receive faulty widgets. Thus, the delay between collection of predictor and criterion measures means that the problem the test was designed to resolve continues for that length of time. Second, conducting a time-delayed study creates the risk of *attrition,* in which one may lose some of the original sample (and their criterion scores) because they quit the job, go on sick leave, or are rapidly promoted to management.

Concurrent criterion-related validity solves some of these problems but creates others. In this scenario, the professional counselor creates the test and conducts reliability studies, just as explained above. Then the professional counselor administers the test to all current employees who assemble widgets and assesses their level of productivity at the same time. Finally, the professional counselor correlates the scores to determine the relationship between scores on the test and concurrent efficiency of widget assembly. As before, if high scores on the test are associated with high efficiency at widget assembly and low scores with low proficiency, the professional counselor has established criterion-related evidence for validity, and Ms. Schmidlapp will probably give the professional counselor a bonus. However, the major problem with the test scores is that they are likely afflicted with a restricted range in the sample of current employees. If the test is supposed to identify which job applicants have an aptitude for widget assembly and which do not, how do we know it will do so when the criterion measure is derived only from those who *can* assemble widgets, as evidenced by their employment? That is, Ms. Schmidlapp has probably already rid her employee production line of inefficient widget assemblers, some, no doubt, reassigned to management. The advantage of the concurrent method, though, is that there is no long delay in the construction of the test, with all its real-world adverse effects, and no risk of attrition.

Perhaps you can readily see how this same scenario would apply to the construction of aptitude and achievement tests as predictors of future performance. With the *SAT,* for example, one could give the test to a group of high school students and later correlate each student's score to the student's college grade point average. To be most accurate, though, all the high school students should be admitted to college, preferably the same college. This presents obvious problems. One could also give the test to a group of current college students and compare their test scores to their college grade point averages. The problem, of course, is that of restricted range, again; only college students are in the sample, but the test is intended to be used with those who are still in high school. The above examples are of predictive and concurrent criterion-related validity, respectively.

To determine with even greater certainty how valid test scores are and how accurately each predicts future behavior, one can develop a *prediction equation* representing the relationship between the predictor and criterion measures and then calculate the *standard error of estimate* in one's predictions.

Standard Error of Estimate

A correlation coefficient represents the relationship between two variables (X and Y). A correlation of 0.87 means the same thing, no matter what variables X and Y are. Their relationship in this case is a positive one; as X increases, Y increases. High scores on X are associated with high scores on Y; low scores on X are associated with low scores on Y. Squaring the correlation coefficient produces the *coefficient of determination* (r^2), the amount of variability in X that is accounted for by the variability in Y.

Recall also that the relationship between X and Y can be represented by a regression equation:

$$Y = a + bX \tag{4.1}$$

This equation is the algebraic formula that indicates both the **slope** and **intercept** of the line that is closest to all the data points in a scatter diagram or bivariate data plot. The intercept (a) is the point at which the line crosses the vertical y axis. The intercept may also be defined as the value of Y when $X = 0$. The slope (b) is the amount Y increases when X increases by 1.0. Like the correlation coefficient, the slope and intercept are calculated using the scores in the X and Y distributions. Once these statistical values are determined, the equation for the regression line can be used to predict the value of Y when we have a value of X for a given person.

For example, consider a prediction equation derived from two variables, the predictor (X) and criterion (Y): $Y' = 5.0 + 0.7X$. We can use this quantified relationship between X and Y to predict a person's eventual performance on Y (Y') using their score on our test, X. A person whose score on $X = 30$ would have a predicted value of 26 on Y. [$Y' = 5.0 + (0.7 \times 30) = 26$].

This process of prediction is widely used in education, business, and industry. Standards called **cutoff scores** are often set by those making decisions about hiring, promotion, and admission to educational and occupational training opportunities. Those whose predicted performance on the criterion variable is below the cutoff score are not likely to be selected, while those attaining the highest scores are. Because decisions affecting people's lives are made using their scores on predictor variables, it is imperative to have the most accurate tests we can and to know just how accurate a given test is. The method used to determine the accuracy of prediction is the standard error of estimate.

The **standard error of estimate** (SE_{est}) is derived from examining the difference between our predicted value of the criterion (Y') and the person's actual score on the criterion (Y). This difference is known as prediction error or *residual*. Recall that all test scores contain some degree of random error, and that a reliable test is one that produces scores that are mostly truth with little error. However, there is no such thing as a perfectly reliable test. Further, both our predictor and criterion measures are imperfect, despite our best efforts. Knowing this, it is certain that, even with the best of criterion and predictor measures, we are destined to be inaccurate to some degree when estimating future scores using a prediction equation. Fortunately, SE_{est} enables us to determine how accurate test scores are likely to be.

The easiest way to understand SE_{est} is to reflect on the concept of the standard deviation of a sample of scores. The standard deviation is the average amount of distance between a given score and the sample mean in a distribution of scores. Using the standard deviation, we can determine how far away from the mean the scores tend to be, and thus how accurately the mean represents the sample scores as a measure of central tendency. A large standard deviation indicates that the scores are spread widely around the mean; a small standard deviation indicates less variability because the scores tend to be clustered around the mean.

The standard error of estimate operates in a similar fashion, quantifying the average distance between predicted scores and persons' actual scores on the criterion. A large SE_{est} indicates that we are typically not very accurate in our predictions of a person's eventual performance on the criterion measure. This means that, however noble our intentions, our test is not a very good one, at least for this purpose.

However, if the SE_{est} is small, our predictions, though not perfect, on average are coming close to the person's eventual performance on the criterion measure. The formulas for the standard error of estimate are

$$SE_{est} = \sqrt{\frac{\sum(Y-Y')^2}{N-2}} \quad \text{or} \quad (4.2)$$

$$SE_{est} = S_Y\sqrt{1-r_{XY}^2} \quad (4.3)$$

In Equation 4.2, each person's predicted score (Y') is subtracted from the person's criterion score (Y). This residual is then squared for each person, and all the squared residuals are added up. This numerator is divided by a denominator, the value of which is the number of persons in the sample minus two (N – 2). Take the square root to attain SE_{est}. Equation 4.3 multiplies the square root of 1 minus the square of the validity coefficient (r_{XY}^2) times the standard deviation of the criterion scores (s_Y) in the validity study.

The SE_{est} can be used to identify the overall level of accuracy of predictions by referring to a table of areas under the normal curve. For example, the area of the normal curve that lies between a z-score of 1.96 and –1.96 is 0.95, or 95% of the area. In a normal distribution of scores, 95% of the scores fall between these points. Similarly, because errors of prediction are random, 95% of criterion scores lie within 1.96 standard scores (1.96 × SE_{est}) of their predicted value. Consider a distribution of predicted scores with a SE_{est} of 2.0. If a person's predicted score (Y') on the criterion measure was 30, simple arithmetic would indicate a 95% probability that the person's actual eventual criterion score would be somewhere between 33.92 [30 + (1.96 × 2.0) = 30 + 3.92 = 33.92] and 26.08 [30 – (1.96 × 2.0) = 30 – 3.92 = 26.08]. Whether this is accurate enough is a judgment call embedded with ethical ramifications made by those using the test against cutoff scores.

To conclude this section, let's return to the Schmidlapp Widget Company with the prediction equation (Y' = 5.0 + 0.7X) and standard error of estimate (SE_{est} = 2.0). Ms. Schmidlapp has informed you that, on average, her employees must be able to assemble 40 widgets per week to keep the company solvent. To be on the safe side, Ms. Schmidlapp determines that no applicants should be hired whose predicted score on the criterion (Y') is less than 40. What cutoff score on the test should the professional counselor recommend? Substituting the available values into the prediction equation, 40 = 5.0 + 0.7X, and using simple algebra procedures, it is determined that X = 50. Thus, the professional counselor recommends that Ms. Schmidlapp hire only those applicants who score 50 or higher on the test, understanding that some will produce fewer than 40 widgets and some will produce more than 40. In fact, Ms. Schmidlapp can be 95% certain that all applicants with a test score of 50 will produce somewhere between 36.08 and 43.92 widgets each week. Of course, because the test is imperfect (as all tests are), Ms. Schmidlapp will hire a few applicants who will not perform adequately and will not hire others who could have made numerous magnificent widgets. Also, if Ms. Schmidlapp needs to boost profits at some point, she always can raise the present minimum acceptable score of 50 to a higher score.

> **Think About It 4.1**   As an example of how to calculate the Standard Error of Estimate (SEE), assume that for the T score scale ($M = 50$ and $SD = 10$) of the *Conners' Adult ADHD Rating Scales* (*CAARS*) *Diagnostic and Statistical Manual of Mental Disorders—Fourth Edition* (*DSM-IV*) Inattention subscale, the score reliability for a sample of clients is 0.91. Using Equation 3.5 for the SEM and Equation 4.3 for the SEE, we obtain:
> $$\text{SEM} = 10\sqrt{1-0.91} = 3.00 \quad \text{and} \quad \text{SEE} = 10\sqrt{(0.91)(1-0.91)} = 2.86.$$

CONSTRUCT VALIDITY

Evidence for **construct validity** is established by defining the construct being measured and by gradually collecting information over time to demonstrate or confirm the meaning of what the test measures (Kaplan & Saccuzzo, 2001). Construct validity is widely used in assessment of theoretically defined domains, such as personality traits, psychological disorders, and intelligence. In each case, the test author carefully defines the construct under consideration, then designs a test to measure it, and collects evidence supporting the validity of the test as a measure of the construct. The principal means by which construct validity is established include convergent evidence, discriminant evidence, factor analysis, meta-analysis, developmental changes, and distinct groups (Whiston, 2005).

Convergent validity evidence is gathered by correlating the scores on a test with scores on other tests believed to measure the same or very similar constructs. High positive correlations are evidence of convergent validity, in that scores on the two tests converge on each other, pointing toward the same psychological characteristic. For example, both the *Minnesota Multiphasic Personality Inventory—Second Edition* (*MMPI-2*) (Butcher et al., 2001) and the *California Psychological Inventory* (*CPI*) (Gough & Bradley, 1996) have scales that measure the construct "Dominance." High scores on both scales would be convergent validity evidence. A strong negative correlation with a scale that measures the same trait using a reversed scaling method or measures an opposite trait would also indicate convergence. For example, valid scores on a scale on dominance should be expected to correlate negatively with a scale that measures passivity.

Discriminant validity evidence is derived by demonstrating that test scores are not highly correlated with measures of other, unrelated constructs. A personality scale that accurately measures self-esteem should not correlate highly with a measure of extraversion, though high levels of self-esteem may be associated with social participation in some people. Introverts with high self-esteem, however, will not be as likely to engage in social activity with people they do not know well. To be a distinct measure of self-esteem, scores on the instrument in question should not be impacted by the introversion or extraversion of the test taker, theoretically speaking. Low correlations between measures of these unrelated constructs provide evidence of discriminant validity. Discriminant and convergent techniques are especially important in the validation of personality tests (Anastasi & Urbina, 1997).

> **Think About It 4.2**   How is a combination of evidence of convergent and discriminant validity useful in determining the overall validity of test scores?

Factor analysis conducts a complex statistical evaluation to determine the degree to which the items contained in two separate instruments tend to group together along factors that mathematically indicate similarity, and thus a common meaning. In addition, factor analysis can determine to what degree the subscales of two tests are similar to each other, as indicated by their lining up together on factorial vectors (Whiston, 2005). For example, subscales measuring dominance, sensitivity, or tolerance should line up with similar scales on another test if the evaluated scores are valid.

Meta-analysis considers the results of a number of validation studies, combining the results to identify an overall effect, if one exists. Synthesizing the results of numerous validity studies can demonstrate strong evidence for the validity of a given test.

Developmental changes indicate support for the construct validity of a test when the test measures changes that are expected to occur over time. For example, we may be interested in measuring the thinking processes of children in light of Piaget's model of cognitive development. A valid test would discriminate between concrete operations and formal operations and would show increased levels of formal operations thought among young people as they moved from childhood to adolescence, as is expected developmentally. More generally, older children would be expected to obtain higher raw scores on intelligence or achievement tests than younger children. Note that developmental age or grade changes are necessary but not sufficient conditions for establishing construct validity; that is, achievement test scores had better become higher as children get older, or the test developer has some real explaining to do.

Distinct groups can provide evidence of construct validity if their scores are different in an expected direction from scores of people in other groups or the general population. If we had a test designed to measure leadership, we would expect a group of military officers to score higher, on average, than the general population. Because the identified distinct group is logically assumed to possess the characteristic in question, one expects them to score high on the test. The degree to which they do indicates the extent to which the test measures leadership.

In conclusion, it is important to remember the crucial step of defining the construct carefully before attempting to demonstrate the validity of an assessment instrument. There are many tests that measure intelligence, self-esteem, depression, and marital compatibility, to name just a few constructs. No two tests are necessarily measuring the same construct just because they use the same name for that construct. Referring back to an earlier example, both the *MMPI-2* and *CPI* have scales measuring the personality trait of "Dominance" (Duckworth & Anderson, 1995; Gough & Bradley, 1996). The *CPI*'s scale defines a dominant person as "being strong in face-to-face situations and as being able to influence others, to gain their automatic respect, and, if necessary, to control them" (Gough

& Bradley, 1996, p. 76). The *MMPI-2* identifies its Dominance scale as "a fairly simple measure of a person's ability to take charge of his/her own life" (Duckworth & Anderson, 1995, p. 340) and as measuring "poise, self-assurance, resourcefulness, efficiency, and perseverance" (p. 341). Note that the *MMPI-2* Dominance scale has no indication of a desire to influence or control others, while the *CPI's* scale does. In fact, the *MMPI-2* scale indicates the desire to influence others only when other scales are elevated. Both scales carry the name "Dominance," but they do not measure identical constructs.

Finally, keep in mind that the definitions of various **constructs** change as society evolves and knowledge changes over time. Consider the emergence of emotional intelligence (Goleman, 1995), a construct derived from research in behavior and the processes of the brain, but not specifically measured by any of the major intelligence tests currently in use.

THE INTERACTION OF RELIABILITY AND VALIDITY

Quite simply, a test can never be more valid than it is reliable. Recall that a reliable test score is a mostly true estimate of a person's actual ability or characteristic, with only a little error contained in the test. If a test score is mostly composed of testing error, it cannot possibly be mostly composed of accurate assessment of the construct or ability in question. Stated another way, because unreliable test scores do not measure accurately and/or consistently, it is difficult to demonstrate that they measure any particular construct or ability accurately and consistently. It is possible to have a reliable test without knowing exactly what it measures. Whatever it measures, a reliable test does so consistently. Logically, though, it is not possible to have valid test scores that are unreliable.

The reliability of predictor and criterion measures in criterion-related assessment is also an important factor in determining test score validity. Equally important is the reliability of comparison instruments used in convergent and discriminant construct-related validity and in factor analysis. Using instruments with low reliability in an effort to compile validity data on a test of interest inevitably introduces error into the resultant validity coefficients.

VALIDITY AND TESTING PRACTICE

Test validity is important because decisions about which test to use and conclusions as to what scores indicate about clients are derived from our understanding of what the test measures. Following are some important considerations when using a particular test with clients:

- Because a test cannot be more valid than it is reliable, always become familiar with the reliability of test scores, including the methods by which evidence for reliability was established.
- Consider the size and makeup of the samples used in reliability and validity studies. As in other forms of research, smaller samples make it less reasonable to generalize results of the study to the population (Harris, 1998). If at all possible, the

norming samples should be representative of the client(s) with whom you plan to use the test. If it is not, use caution in interpretation, taking into consideration the reality that factors other than those the test is designed to measure may be affecting your client's score.

- Examine any test you use for biased items. Items may be more familiar to some identifiable groups of people than others. For example, a test item picturing a winter snow scene may be perceived differently by those who grew up in tropical climates than by those whose winters were routinely snowy.

- Language is a significant contributor to potential bias, especially if the test is written in a language in which the test taker is not proficient. Use caution in applying scores from tests that place the client at a disadvantage due to linguistic differences.

- Ethnicity can be a source of response variation in testing. Cultural differences can lead to different outcomes on a personality test, for example, even when language difference is not an issue. One culture's definition of appropriate behavior can be very different from another's, leading to erroneous assumptions about an individual's personality that actually emerge from cultural norms.

- Do not assume that the name of a test or scale accurately reflects the actual meaning of the test score. Always read the test manual to determine the exact definition of the skill or construct being measured.

- Where possible, use more than one test or scale to increase the accuracy of assessment. Using more than one predictor increases the likelihood of correctly predicting a client's outcome score. Using more than one personality assessment provides more complete information about the trait under consideration, especially if the tests purport to measure the same construct.

- Tests are not *proven* to be valid. The validity of a particular test score for use with a particular client under the circumstances at hand is a judgment call made by the professional counselor based on the amassed evidence supporting the test's validity and defining its meaning. Because professional counselors should use tests only with the intent of being helpful to the client, ask if this is the right test for the right client for the right reasons.

THE APPLICATION OF VALIDITY: DECISION MAKING USING TEST SCORES

The primary purpose behind administering psychological and educational tests is to help make accurate decisions that will benefit clients and students. Psychometricians and statisticians have developed a number of procedures for making decisions using a single test and multiple tests.

Decision Making Using a Single Score

By definition, decision making using a single test is relegated to the realm of a screening procedure. There are three popular procedures for single-score decisions: decision theory, linear regression, and setting a cutoff score.

Decision theory

Decision theory (Anastasi & Urbina, 1997) involves the collection of a screening test score and a criterion score, either at the same point in time (i.e., concurrent decision) or at some point in the future (i.e., predictive decision). Some common examples of concurrent decisions would be virtually any clinical or diagnostic study in which a screening test for a mental or emotional disorder (i.e., depression, anxiety, Attention-Deficit/Hyperactivity Disorder [AD/HD], dementia) would be administered concurrently with a clinical diagnosis from a qualified mental health professional (sometimes called *diagnostic validity*), or the administration of an academic achievement test to a group of children and concurrent identification of low-performing students or students "at risk" for academic failure by a teacher or diagnostician (sometimes called *decision reliability*). Examples of predictive decisions would involve any of these previous examples, but with the criterion of diagnosis or determination of "at risk" status being collected months or years after the screening test was administered. In this way, the screening test would be used to predict future problems, usually allowing professional counselors and educators to put prevention or early intervention programs in play to lower the incidence of future problems. Whether used for concurrent or predictive purposes, the goal of the procedure is to maximize the likelihood of accurate decisions (sometimes called *hits*) while minimizing inaccurate decisions (sometimes called *misses* or *errors*). Remember, the ultimate purpose of a screening procedure is to identify clients or students in need of deeper-level diagnostic assessment.

As an example of applying decision theory, assume that a professional counselor has been asked to develop an accurate screening procedure to identify adults at risk for depression. The professional counselor first explores the literature and selects a published, efficient screening device for depression whose scores have previously demonstrated sufficient reliability and validity for screening-level purposes. To determine the adequacy of the depression inventory for the requested service, the professional counselor arranges for each new adult referral to several area clinics to complete the depression inventory and undergo a diagnostic evaluation with a qualified mental health professional. Selection of the criterion is critical. It is often viewed as the "gold standard" and should have the qualities of excellent score reliability and validity. This diagnostic evaluation would normally serve to identify mental and emotional disorders related to the clients' presenting problems and to aid in establishing goals for counseling but because of the study's focus will also result in a clinical determination regarding the degree of clinical depression in the clients on a 5-point scale (e.g., 1 = Absence of Depressive Symptoms, 2 = Slightly Depressed, 3 = Mildly Depressed, 4 = Moderately Depressed, 5 = Severely Depressed). (*Note:* Admittedly, the diagnosis of depressive disorders is complex; for the sake of this example, the process has been simplified). The professional counselor then collects two pieces of data for each of the next 50 adult clients to the area clinics: (1) the screening test score and (2) the clinical decision of the presence of clinical depression on the 5-point scale. The results of these 50 participants are presented in Figure 4.1.

As can be seen in Figure 4.1, the distribution of scores is somewhat broad, ranging from 0 to 50 on the depression screening test (0 indicates the Absence of

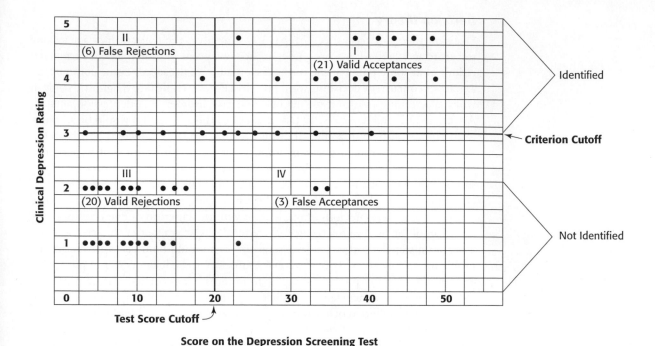

Figure 4.1   An application of decision theory using a criterion cutoff score of 3

Depression; 50 is the highest score possible and indicates Severe Depression), and from 1 to 5 on the clinical diagnostic rating (1 indicates the Absence of Depressive Symptoms; 5 indicates Severe Depression). The professional counselor now needs to use judgment in applying the decision-making model. How this judgment is applied may vary and, as will be seen below, has implications for the accuracy of decisions (i.e., the hit rate). One can see from Figure 4.1 that a criterion score cutoff line has been placed at scores of 3 or higher, and a test score cutoff line at scores of 20 or higher. The criterion cutoff was established at 3 or higher because, in the professional counselor's judgment, people who are Mildly Depressed qualify for mental health services with a diagnosis of depression and should receive treatment. The test score cutoff was established at 20 or higher because, in the professional counselor's judgment (and based on the test manual), people scoring 20 or higher are likely Mildly Depressed and should receive further diagnostic assessment to determine the nature and extent of any problems related to depression.

These two cutoff lines divide the participants' scores into four quadrants, each of which has implications for decision accuracy. Quadrant I is referred to as **valid acceptances** (VAs) (or *true positives*) because clients in this quadrant were identified as having elevated scores on both the screening test and clinician rating. Thus these were accurate decisions, or "hits." Note that 21 of the 50 participants fell into this category (42%). Quadrant II is referred to as **false rejections** (FRs) (or *false negatives*) because clients in this quadrant were not identified as having an elevated score on the screening test but were elevated on the clinician rating. Thus these were inaccurate decisions, or "misses." Note that 6 of the 50 participants fell into this category (12%). Quadrant III is referred to as **valid rejections** (VRs) (or *true negatives*) because clients in this quadrant were not identified as having elevated scores on the screening test or clinician rating. Thus these were accurate decisions, or "hits." Note that 20 of the 50 participants fell into this category (40%). Finally, quadrant IV is referred to as **false acceptances** (FAs) (or *false positives*) because clients in this quadrant were identified as having elevated scores on the screening test, but not on clinician ratings. Thus these were inaccurate decisions, or "misses." Note that 3 of the 50 participants fell into this category (6%).

Overall, the screening test's **total predictive value** (TPV) was 0.82, or 82% accurate decisions and 18% inaccurate decisions. TPV is computed using Equation 4.4:

$$\text{TPV} = \frac{VAs + VRs}{VAs + VRs + FAs + FRs} \text{ or } \frac{hits}{hits + misses}. \tag{4.4}$$

Whether this result (82%) is accurate enough is again left to the judgment of the professional counselor conducting the study. One way of determining the sufficiency of the total predictive value is to consider the impact of not using the screening test. In this instance, it could be reasoned that without any preliminary information, the likelihood of an accurate decision on this population of clients just by chance guessing would be about 50%. Of course, this likelihood of accuracy is far more complicated in most clinical situations and has to do with the base rate of the diagnosis in the population under study. That is, if the population under study was the general adult population rather than those who turn up at clinics for counseling, the base rate would probably be much closer to 5–15% of a sample. The "gain" in accuracy by using the screening test rather than chance guessing is called *incremental validity.* The reader is referred to Anastasi and Urbina (1997) for a more in-depth discussion of base rates and incremental validity and their application to decision making.

Another way of determining whether an accuracy rate is sufficient is to examine the potential downside of using the screening test. While it would be wonderful to have 100% accuracy, such accuracy is seldom the case. But a primary goal of screening is to ensure that all potential clients get the help they need. Two quadrants of particular interest are quadrants II and IV, because they represent erroneous decisions. But in a screening procedure, errors in quadrant IV (false acceptances) are of little concern because these clients have been identified by the screening test and will receive further diagnostic assessment, even though they will not be diagnosed as having a depressive disorder. Yes, it is somewhat more expensive to provide the "unnecessary" service to these three clients, but in the final analysis, they are evaluated and determined to not need further treatment. Their needs have been addressed. However, professional counselors must be very concerned with the errors present in quadrant II (false rejections). Because these clients' screening test scores are below the criterion score of 20, they will not receive follow-up diagnostic services and may not receive the counseling services required. In this example, quadrant II housed 12% of the sample—clients who have the problem, but who will not receive the help they need. The goal of decision theory is to minimize occurrence within this group while not sacrificing efficiency.

Knowing the constitution of each of the four quadrants allows researchers to compute several helpful indexes: sensitivity, specificity, positive predictive power (PPP), and negative predictive power (NPP) (Erford, 2004; Erford & Stephens, 2005; Widiger, Hurt, Frances, Clarkin, & Gilmore, 1984).

A screening test's **sensitivity** is the proportion of the test's valid acceptances out of all those identified by the criterion (i.e., diagnosed with depression, learning problems). This is the test's "hit rate" out of only those who are diagnosed with the disorder (i.e., the proportion of people with depression the test would identify). The formula for sensitivity is Equation 4.5:

$$\frac{VAs}{VAs + FRs}, \tag{4.5}$$

and thus the sensitivity of the screening test in Figure 4.1 is $\frac{21}{21+6} = 0.78$.

A screening test's **specificity** is the proportion of the test's valid rejections out of all those *not* identified by the criterion (i.e., not diagnosed with depression, learning problems). This is the test's "hit rate" out of only those who are not diagnosed with the disorder (i.e., the proportion of people without depression the test would identify as not having depression). The formula for specificity is Equation 4.6:

$$\frac{VRs}{VRs + FAs}, \tag{4.6}$$

and thus the specificity of the screening test in Figure 4.1 is $\frac{20}{20+3} = 0.87$.

A screening test's **positive predictive power** (PPP) is the proportion of the test's valid acceptances out of all those identified by the screening test (i.e., elevated scores on the screening test). This is the criterion's "hit rate" out of only those whom the test identifies with the disorder. The formula for PPP is Equation 4.7:

$$\frac{VAs}{VAs + FAs}, \tag{4.7}$$

and thus the positive predictive power of the screening test in Figure 4.1 is $\frac{21}{21+3} = 0.88$.

A screening test's **negative predictive power** (NPP) is the proportion of the test's valid rejections out of all those not identified by the screening test (i.e., no elevated scores on the screening test). This is the criterion's "hit rate" out of only those who are not identified with the disorder by the test. The formula for NPP is Equation 4.8:

$$\frac{VRs}{VRs + FRs}, \tag{4.8}$$

and thus the negative predictive power of the screening test in Figure 4.1 is $\frac{20}{20+6} = 0.77$.

Now let's explore the implications of altering judgments in the decision model. Figure 4.2 presents the same client depression study scenario and data, but this time the decision parameters have been slightly altered so that the criterion cutoff line has been moved to ratings of 4 or higher (i.e., Moderate Depression); the test score cutoff remains at 20. It is determined that quadrant I (VAs) has 14 partici-

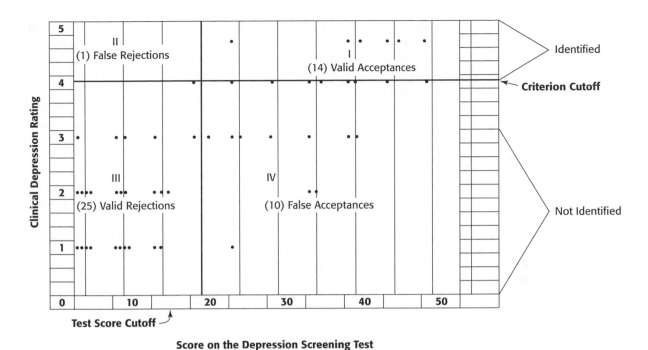

Figure 4.2   An application of decision theory using a criterion cutoff score of 4

pants, quadrant II (FRs) has 1 participant, quadrant III (VRs) has 25 participants, and quadrant IV (FAs) has 10 participants. Using the formulaic information presented above, TPV = 0.78; Equation 4.5 = 0.93; Equation 4.6 = 0.71; PPP = 0.58; and NPP = 0.96. Changing the criterion to a higher criterion score lowered the total accuracy slightly (TPV went from 0.82 to 0.78) while substantially diminishing the number of false rejections (FRs went from 6 to 1) and substantially increasing the number of false acceptances (FAs went from 3 to 10). The implication of this second model is that nearly everyone (except one client) with moderate to severe depression will be referred for further evaluation, but now only 58% of those who receive further assessment will actually qualify for the diagnosis—a more inclusive, but less efficient process. The point is, different judgments will lead to different results. Perhaps most importantly, *the higher the validity (correlation) coefficient between the selection test and criterion, the fewer errors there will be.*

Linear regression

Linear regression was discussed earlier in this chapter (remember Ms. Schmidlapp?). Suffice it to say that if a professional counselor has a large sample of scores on both the screening test and criterion and can accurately determine the critical criterion score upon which a decision will hinge, the counselor has everything needed to use a linear regression decision-making system for a screening-level decision. For example, if the regression equation for the depression screening example was $Y' = 0.40 + 0.10X$, then a score of 20 on the screening test (X) would lead to a predicted score on the criterion of 3.0, meaning mild depression. Likewise, a minimum possible score of 0 on the screening test would lead to a predicted criterion score of 0.40 (little to no depression), and a maximum possible score of 50 on the screening test would lead to a predicted criterion score of 6.9 (an impossible score given the scale, but nonetheless indicating severe depression). Again, *the higher the validity (correlation) coefficient between the selection test and criterion, the fewer errors there will be.*

Setting a cutoff score

When a screening decision is made using a single score, professional counselors will sometimes designate a single cutoff score upon which to make a decision. This is frequently the case with criterion-referenced assessments in which some rationally derived determination of mastery is made. For instance, in the internship for a graduate counseling program, the instructor for the course may decide that a passing grade on the internship is a B– or higher, so any intern achieving this level of proficiency or higher can graduate; any intern who doesn't, won't. Sometimes a single test score may be (mis)used to determine a student's eligibility for a remedial education program. If the test score is criterion referenced, the standard may be a certain cutoff score, say, 70% correct. If a norm-referenced score, educators will sometimes choose a percentile rank of ≤ 25. This method differs from the decision theory discussion above primarily because little, if any, consideration is given to a criterion score, or the negative or unintended complications of adverse (or even undue favorable) decisions.

Regardless of the test or cutoff score selected, the critical issue becomes the standard-setting process. A standard set too high will deny access to needy clients or students; a standard set too low will allow unqualified individuals to access sometimes limited services. The American Psychiatric Association constantly struggles with this issue when producing diagnostic criteria settings for mental disorders in the *DSM*. For example, the behaviors associated with Conduct Disorder have remained more or less the same over the past three editions of the *DSM*, but how the disorder is conceptualized and categorized has changed somewhat. In the *DSM-III-R* (APA, 1987) the disorder was subclassified as "group" and "solitary" subtypes, while the current *Diagnostic and Statistical Manual of Mental Disorders—Fourth Edition—Text Revision* (*DSM-IV-TR*) (APA, 2000) uses the subclassifications of "adolescent-onset" and "childhood-onset." Perhaps more importantly, much concern has been raised that the current criteria overidentify children and adolescents from certain racial, cultural, and socioeconomic categories while underidentifying others. Indeed, there are substantial cautions in the *DSM-IV-TR* warning clinicians to take culture and other background factors into consideration; some researchers even suggest raising the number of diagnostic criteria necessary for diagnosis in some cases. These concerns over misclassification point to the great care required of professional counselors when establishing criteria and setting a cutoff score. All other things considered, the higher the stakes and implications of the decision to be made, the less appropriate any single cutoff score method becomes.

Decision Making Using Multiple Tests

Although multiple tests can be used to make screening-level decisions, this category of decision making also allows for diagnostic or placement decisions. Several decision-making strategies are commonly used with multiple tests. In this chapter, three will be reviewed: (1) multiple regression, (2) multiple cutoff, and (3) clinical judgment.

Multiple regression

Multiple regression allows for several variables to be weighted in order to predict some criterion score. The formula was $Y' = a + b_1X_1 + b_2X_2 + b_3X_3 + b_iX_i$. By simply knowing the client's scores on the several predictor tests, this formula allows computation of a predicted criterion score.

As an example of the application of multiple regression, suppose that a professional counselor needs to develop an efficient decision-making model for the screening or diagnosis of students with Attention-Deficit/Hyperactivity Disorder—Predominantly Inattentive Type (AD/HD-PIT). The professional counselor searches the literature, evaluates a number of tests appropriate for the intended purpose and chooses the *Disruptive Behavior Rating Scale* (*DBRS*) (Erford, 1993). The professional counselor selects as the criterion score the number of diagnostic criteria determined to exist through a structured clinical interview. The *DSM-IV-TR* (APA, 2000) specifies nine AD/HD-PIT criteria, and the client must have at least six of the nine to qualify for a diagnosis.

To derive the regression equation, the professional counselor would need to administer the *DBRS* to the parents and teachers of many students and to subject each client or case to the structured clinical interview. Thus the professional counselor administers the *DBRS-T* (teacher version) to the students' primary teachers (X_1), and the *DBRS-P* (parent version) to students' mothers and fathers (designated X_2 and X_3, respectively). Importantly, the criterion score is collected as the number of AD/HD-PIT criteria (ranging from 0 to 9), and the *DBRS* scores are reported as T scores ($M = 50$; $SD = 10$). When the data have been collected, the professional counselor then subjects the data to statistical analysis using *SPSS* and derives the following regression equation: $Y' = a + b_1X_1 + b_2X_2 + b_3X_3 = 1.21 + 0.031X_1 + 0.024X_2 + 0.017X_3$ (that is, $a = 1.21$, $b_1 = 0.031$, $b_2 = 0.024$, and $b_3 = 0.017$). Having now derived the formula, the professional counselor is ready to evaluate new cases, and will identify students with $Y' \geq 6.0$ and will not identify students with $Y' < 6.0$ (or more likely will conduct additional assessment with borderline cases).

Then, for the next student that presents for evaluation, Juanita, the professional counselor will have the teacher, mother, and father complete the respective versions of the *DBRS*, then plug their scores into the regression formula. For Juanita, assuming $X_1 = 73$, $X_2 = 67$, and $X_3 = 55$, the prediction formula would be: $Y' = 1.21 + (0.031)(73) + (0.024)(67) + (0.017)(55) = 1.21 + 2.263 + 1.608 + 0.935 = 6.016$. Thus Juanita would be identified as having fulfilled the diagnostic criteria for AD/HD-PIT. For another, more distractible child, Nakita, presenting with scores of

Table 4.2   T Scores on the *DBRS* Distractible Subscale for Three Students and Criterion Cutoff Scores

Student name	Teacher score (X_1)	Mother score (X_2)	Father score (X_3)	Decision
Juanita	70	67	55	No
Nakita	78	88	90	Yes
Susanna	37*	49*	40*	No
Cutoff score required	65	65	65	

Note: * designates a score falling below the required cutoff score of T = 65.

X_1 = 78, X_2 = 88, and X_3 = 90, the prediction formula would be: Y' = 1.21 + (0.031)(78) + (0.024)(88) + (0.017)(90) = 1.21 + 2.418 + 2.112 + 1.530 = 7.270. Thus, Nakita would be identified as having fulfilled the diagnostic criteria for AD/HD-PIT. For a third, less distractible child, Susanna, presenting with scores of X_1 = 37, X_2 = 49, and X_3 = 40, the prediction formula would be: Y' = 1.21 + (0.031)(37) + (0.024)(49) + (0.017)(40) = 1.21 + 1.147 + 1.176 + 0.68 = 4.213. Thus, Susanna would not be identified as having fulfilled the diagnostic criteria for AD/HD-PIT.

The primary advantage of the multiple regression technique is that it allows some scores to compensate for other scores. For instance, while the results were not in doubt in either Nakita's or Susanna's case, in Juanita's case, her father viewed her level of distractibility to be more or less normal (T = 55), while her teacher's and mother's scores were elevated (T = 73 and 67, respectively). These scores compensated for the low score of the father and put Juanita in the "diagnose" category. A primary disadvantage of the multiple regression technique is the necessity of labor-intensive preliminary data collection, data analysis, and standard setting. It is a lot of work to collect the several hundred protocols necessary to yield a reliable multiple regression equation.

Multiple cutoff method

The **multiple cutoff method** is far simpler to set up and implement than the multiple regression procedure. Basically, *multiple cutoff* means that the professional counselor must establish a minimally acceptable score on each measure under consideration, then analyze the scores of a given client or student and determine whether each of the scores meets the given criterion. Importantly, failure to meet even one of the cutoff scores will eliminate an examinee from consideration. As an example, consider the scores on the *DBRS* for the three girls, which are now presented in Table 4.2 for ease of comparison.

The criterion score standard-setting decision is of critical importance in the multiple cutoff technique because criterion scores set too low will overidentify individuals who do not have the condition, and criterion scores set too high will underidentify individuals who do have the condition. In the context of this multiple cutoff technique example, Nakita would be identified with AD/HD-PIT because each of her T scores on the *DBRS* exceeded the minimum criterion T score of 65. Likewise, Susanna would not be identified because none of her T scores on the

DBRS was high enough to warrant diagnosis. Interestingly, Juanita, who did qualify under the multiple regression procedures explained in the preceding section, would not be identified with AD/HD-PIT using these criterion scores because her father's rating of her did not meet the specified criterion (i.e., his rating of Juanita was a T score of 55, and a minimum score of 65 was required).

It is important to understand that multiple cutoff techniques use hard-and-fast criteria, and violations are not allowed. Thus a low score on one test can effectively eliminate someone from consideration; other scores are not allowed to compensate for deficient scores, such as was the case in the multiple regression model. Therefore, a less than optimal administration for any reason (i.e., low motivation, response bias, faking bad or good) could result in a selection error. Because the multiple cutoff method is easier to set up and manage than the multiple regression method, it is more widely used. However, most clinicians use a third method, clinical judgment and diagnosis using a test battery.

Think About It 4.3   How could you apply the multiple regression or multiple cutoff models to a decision-making problem in your area of counseling specialty?

Clinical judgment and diagnosis using a test battery

Clinical judgment relies on the experiences, information processing capability, theoretical frameworks, and reasoning ability of the professional counselor to make sense out of sometimes-conflicting information, to arrive at a rational decision about the disposition of a client or student. Clinical judgment is not a statistics-driven decision-making method per se. Test results, interview information, behavioral observations, and other data are interpreted and integrated, leading to a reasoned judgment or decision. Clinical decision making using a test battery can be a very complex undertaking, depending on the presenting problem(s), and requires a good deal of education, supervised training and experience, and analytical capabilities. It is also subject to theoretical differences and examiner bias; that is, the same information often leads to different conclusions based on a professional counselor's theoretical orientation(s) and personal or professional biases. A clinical case of a young girl evaluated for problems with distractibility is presented in Box 4.1 to demonstrate how data can be interpreted and integrated so that a clinical decision can be made.

Box 4.1   Clinical Judgment Using a Battery of Tests: Case Study of Nakita

Identifying Information

Name: Nakita
Chronological Age: 12 years, 2 months
Grade Placement: 6.6

continued

Box 4.1 continued

Reason for Referral and Initial Case Conceptualization

Nakita was referred for psychoeducational evaluation by her mother. The primary referral concerns were distractibility, difficulty understanding and/or following directions, and poor school performance in the academic areas of reading, science, and written expression. No significant emotional issues were reported by the parents or school. Initially, this evaluator sought to explore the existence of a significant learning disorder in reading and writing and significant degrees of inattention commonly associated with AD/HD. A general emotional and behavioral screening was also undertaken to rule in or rule out conditions that mask and mimic the symptoms of inattention, as well as determine Nakita's general level of emotional adjustment.

Assessment Techniques

Because the referral concern was both behavior (inattention) and academic (language arts, science), the examiner chose instruments that would be useful in the identification of potential learning problems and behavior disorders, such as AD/HD, and would also screen for emotional adjustment. The following assessments were intentionally selected at the outset of the evaluation:

- *Wechsler Intelligence Scale for Children—Fourth Edition* (*WISC-IV*) (as an intellectual assessment to establish an anchor score for expected achievement levels and to determine learning strengths and weaknesses)
- *Beery's Developmental Test of Visual-Motor Integration* (*VMI-3, Motor, and Visual*) (as a gross screen for visual perception, fine-motor coordination, and visual-motor integration)
- *Woodcock-Johnson Tests of Achievement—Third Edition* (*WJ-III ACH*) (to establish achievement levels in the major academic subject areas and determine whether a learning disorder is evident)
- *Conners' Parent and Teacher Rating Scale—Revised: Long Versions* (*CPRS-R:L* and *CTRS-R:L*) (to screen for inattention and other behavioral/emotional concerns)
- Clinical interview (exploration of developmental history and clinical conditions using structured protocols found in Appendixes A and C of Erford, 2006).

The following tests were also administered as a result of additional questions and hypotheses that came up during the evaluation:

- *Test of Auditory Perceptual Skills-Revised* (*TAPS-R*)—Word Discrimination and Auditory Processing subtests (to rule out auditory perceptual and processing deficiencies)
- *Jebsen Writing Speed* subtest (to assess for handwriting speed, sometimes deficient in clients with fine-motor coordination and processing speed difficulties)
- *Stanford-Binet Intelligence Scale—Fourth Edition: Memory for Sentences* subtest (to assess for language-loaded short-term auditory memory skills)

- *Wide Range Achievement Test—Third Revision* (*WRAT-3*): *Spelling* subtest (as a validating spelling test)
- *Slosson Written Expression Test* (*SWET*) (for further exploration of writing mechanics)
- *Visual Aural Digit Span Test* (*VADS*) (for further exploration of short-term auditory and visual memory difficulties)

Background Information

Clinical interviewing using a structured protocol and reports from the teachers provided a wealth of helpful background information. Nakita is a 12-year, 2-month-old African American girl currently attending grade 6 at XYZ Middle School. Her mother reports the primary concerns to be age-inappropriate inattention and difficulty in the academic areas of language arts and sciences. Nakita is reported to be easily distracted by the slightest sound and easily frustrated. She is very artistic and enjoys drawing. She has struggled with reading since the first grade. Currently, reading comprehension appears to be problematic, as well as understanding word problems in math. Recently, Nakita has begun to struggle in science, and this difficulty appears to result from a complex interaction of reading comprehension, conceptual difficulties, and teaching style. Nakita also reportedly has difficulty following multistep directions, although it is unclear whether this difficulty is due to a lack of understanding or to a lack of motivation. She has a wonderful sense of humor, but is becoming more temperamental when it comes to academic tasks.

Previous group-administered testing indicated Average to High Average school ability on the *Otis-Lennon School Ability Test* (*OLSAT*). Her 5th-grade achievement testing indicated Average math achievement (46th percentile), reading comprehension (58th percentile), and writing mechanics (30th percentile). Mr. Trig, Nakita's math and social studies teacher, is concerned about Nakita's weak skill retention in math. Nakita reportedly needs a lot of practice and relearning to keep her grades in the passing range. He also reports that Nakita is very distractible and impulsive. Socially and emotionally, Mr. Trig describes Nakita as a very pleasant and kind student who is always smiling. Mrs. Bookworm, Nakita's language arts teacher, reports that Nakita often becomes talkative and "clowns around" during inappropriate moments in class—often when answering questions or presenting in front of the class. Because of being behaviorally off-task, Nakita often misses important information and displays inconsistent comprehension. Mrs. Bookworm also reports that Nakita has a wonderful zeal for learning and a sense of humor that often energizes classroom activities. She is a hard worker and frequently participates in classroom discussions. She is also very loyal and supportive of friends. Although Nakita struggles with higher-order thinking skills, comprehension, and writing mechanics, Mrs. Bookworm believes that she is a bright, tenacious, and capable student.

continued

Box 4.1 continued

Nakita attended XYZ Elementary from kindergarten through grade 5. Reading has always been an area of academic difficulty. She has traditionally displayed a poor sight-word vocabulary and reading comprehension. She has not displayed letter-number reversals since grade 1. Nakita is currently placed in the "low" math group, according to her mother. Her math calculation skills appear satisfactory, but Nakita is struggling with the story problems. Nakita's short-term memory (both auditory and visual) is reportedly poor. Written language has also been an area of consistent difficulty. Her spelling, capitalization, and punctuation skills are reportedly deficient. She has excellent penmanship, and is a fast keyboarder. Nakita taught herself to keyboard and is very proud of her ability in this regard.

Nakita's parents divorced five years ago. Nakita has an older sister who is a very strong student. Nakita does engage in periodic day visits with her father, but no overnight stays. Nakita's birth and developmental history was normal, and she met all developmental milestones either on time or ahead of time. Her medical history is unremarkable. Nakita is reportedly a happy, sociable child. She is very outgoing and popular with peers. Her mother and teachers report that Nakita's social and emotional development is within normal limits and not of primary concern at this time.

Maternal family history reportedly is negative for learning and emotional problems. Her mother reports she was a straight-A student and not at all distractible. She completed one year of college and is currently employed in real estate management. Nakita's birth father was not available for interview. Nakita's mother reports seeing many similarities in learning styles between Nakita and her father. She indicated that Nakita's father was a strong math student, but struggled academically—although no specific details were provided. He did not finish high school and is currently a construction worker. She indicated that Nakita's father enjoyed reading and was very artistic but had poor writing skills. He reportedly had great difficulty focusing his attention on task and was easily distracted. A paternal grandmother reported that, as a child, Nakita's father was very overactive. A paternal brother has been diagnosed with depression and, reportedly, is aggressive and possesses a temper. Nakita's father also reportedly has difficulty controlling his temper.

The formal evaluation was conducted over two mornings in consecutive weeks. Formalized evaluation centered on the areas of intellectual, perceptual, achievement, behavioral, and emotional development. Nakita was a well-mannered child and was very cooperative during the evaluation. Rapport was easily established, and she attempted all items presented to her. Nakita displayed a quite high interest level throughout the evaluation. She displayed no obvious physical or sensory deficits, nor did she appear anxious. Therefore, the obtained results are considered to be an accurate representation of Nakita's current level of functioning. Her test results, briefly interpreted. are given in Tables 4.3 through 4.6.

Nakita was administered the *Wechsler Intelligence Scale for Children—Fourth Edition* (*WISC-IV*) to establish a level of expectation for scholastic

Table 4.3   What Nakita's scores mean

Standard score	Scale score	T score	Interpretive range meaning
130+	16+	70+	Very Superior
120–129	14–15	63–69	Superior
110–119	12–13	57–62	High Average
90–109	9–11	43–56	Average
80–89	6–8	37–42	Low Average
70–79	4–5	30–36	Borderline
55–69	3	20–29	Mildly Deficient
40–54	2	10–19	Moderately Deficient
<40	0–1	<10	Severe and Profoundly Deficient

Wechsler Intelligence Scale for Children—Fourth Edition (WISC-IV)

	IQ; Range	Percentile rank; Range	Interpretive range
Verbal Comprehension Index	119; 111–125	90; 77–95	High Average to Superior
Perceptual Reasoning Index	117; 108–123	87; 70–94	Average to Superior
Working Memory Index	74; 68–84	4; 2–14	Mildly Deficient to Low Average
Processing Speed Index	75; 69– 87	5; 2–19	Mildly Deficient to Low Average
Full Scale IQ	100; 95–105	50; 37–63	Average

Verbal Comprehension Index subtests		Perceptual Reasoning Index subtests	
Similarities	14 S*	Block Design	11
Vocabulary	12	Picture Concepts	13
Comprehension	14 S	Matrix Reasoning	14 S

Working memory index subtests		Processing speed index subtests	
Digit Span	5 W*	Coding	5 W
Letter-Number Sequencing	5 W	Symbol Search	6 W

Note: * S = Intrapersonal strength; W = Intrapersonal weakness.

achievement and identify her learning strengths and weaknesses. Nakita's Verbal Comprehension Index (VCI) score was measured to lie in the High Average to Superior range (percentile rank = 90; percentile rank range = 77–95), commensurate with her Perceptual Reasoning Index (PRI) score, which fell in the Average to Superior range (percentile rank = 87; percentile rank range = 70–94). While Nakita currently performs in the Average range of general cognitive ability (Full Scale percentile rank = 50; percentile rank range = 37–63), her true educational potential is probably much closer to her VCI and PRI capabilities (standard score of approximately 118; High Average to Superior capabilities), and it is this score that will serve as the anchor score for determining intrapersonal weaknesses and achievement areas in need of improvement. Nakita's Working Memory Index (WMI) score fell

continued

Box 4.1 continued

in the Mildly Deficient to Low Average range (percentile rank = 4; percentile rank range = 2–14), as did her Processing Speed Index (percentile rank = 5; percentile rank range = 2–19). Both the WMI and PSI were significantly below current ability estimates and are considered significant intrapersonal weaknesses. Subtest analysis indicates that Nakita displayed intrapersonal strengths on tasks requiring verbal abstract reasoning (Similarities subtest percentile rank = 90); social comprehension (Comprehension subtest percentile rank = 90); and visual analogical reasoning (Matrix Reasoning subtest percentile rank = 90). Significant intrapersonal weaknesses were noted on tasks requiring short-term auditory recall (Digit Span subtest percentile rank = 5); recall and organization of auditory stimuli (Letter-Number Sequencing percentile rank = 10); short-term visual recall and psychomotor speed (Coding subtest percentile rank = 5); and speed in processing visual information (Symbol Search subtest percentile rank = 10). Thus Nakita presents as a bright child with potential weaknesses in processing speed and in short-term auditory and visual memory.

Stanford-Binet Intelligence Scale—Fifth Edition: Sentence Memory subtest
                    Standard Score = 92   Percentile Rank = 29

Test of Auditory Perceptual Skills-Revised (TAPS-R)
Auditory Word
    Discrimination subtest   Scaled Score = 11   Percentile Rank = 63
Auditory Processing
    subtest   Scaled Score = 12   Percentile Rank = 75

Because a presenting concern had to do with Nakita's ability to understand directions, it was important to explore the possible existence of a language processing disorder and central auditory processing disorder. The above-mentioned *WISC-IV* VCI subtest results do not support the existence of a language processing disorder because they all fell in the above-average ranges. To rule out the existence of a central auditory processing disorder, two subtests from the *Test of Auditory Perceptual Skills-R* were administered. Nakita performed in an Average to High Average capacity on each subtest. She scored at the 63rd percentile rank on a task requiring auditory word discrimination and the 75th percentile rank on a task purporting to measure auditory processing. Thus little support was garnered for the existence of a central auditory processing disorder.

To further assess Nakita's short-term auditory recall, the Memory for Sentences subtest of the *Stanford-Binet Intelligence Scale—Fourth Edition* was administered. Nakita performed at the 29th percentile on this task, commensurate with WMI estimates and significantly below intellectual estimates.

Visual Aural Digit Span Test (VADS)   Visual Memory   10th percentile
                                               Auditory Memory   25th percentile

Next, the *VADS* was administered to validate weaknesses in short-term auditory and visual memory observed during administration of the *WISC-*

IV. On this administration of the *VADS,* Nakita scored at the 10th and 25th percentiles on the visual and auditory memory components, respectively. Both performances were significantly below expected levels and validate the weaknesses observed during administration of the *WISC-IV.* Thus the existence of significant distractibility in the auditory and visual channels remains as a primary explanation for Nakita's difficulty in successfully performing in class and carrying out multistep directions.

Notice that each "hypothesis" generated from the presenting problem is being systematically explored through clinical interviewing and results from selected tests.

| *Jebsen Writing Speed* Subtest | Trial 1 = 22 seconds | (approximately the 15th percentile) |
| | Trial 2 = 23 seconds | (approximately the 15th percentile) |

To validate the apparent weakness in processing speed, the *Jebsen Writing Speed* subtest was administered and resulted in deficient writing speed performances. The 15th percentile is one standard deviation below the mean, indicating that about 85 percent of same-aged girls can write faster than Nakita. This slow motor speed was commensurate with the deficient Processing Speed Index scores reported above. These results are extraordinarily important when trying to understand the academic difficulties that Nakita is currently facing. These results indicate that Nakita's processing and writing speed are substantially slower than expected for a child of her ability. This is likely to be evidenced in the classroom through slower writing, note-taking, and task completion speeds.

Test of Visual Motor Integration	VMI Standard Score = 120	Percentile Rank of 91
	Visual Standard Score = 122	Percentile Rank of 93
	Motor Standard Score = 90	Percentile Rank of 25

Nakita's performance on *Beery's Developmental Test of Visual-Motor Integration—Third Edition* (*VMI-3*) exceeded that of 91% of other children her age, falling in the High Average to Superior range of performance. This edition of the Beery also allows exploration of visual-perceptual and motor capabilities. Nakita's fine-motor coordination performance exceeded only 25% of age-mates (Low Average to Average), while her performance on the visual-perceptual task of the *VMI-3* was High Average to Superior (93rd percentile rank). Altogether, Nakita's visual-motor and visual discrimination capabilities appear well developed at this time, actually exceeding current intellectual ability estimates. However, her fine-motor coordination is poorly developed.

In an effort to explore Nakita's current educational achievement and determine whether significant learning problems are occurring in the areas of reading and writing, selected subtests of the *Woodcock-Johnson: Tests of Achievement—Third Edition* (*WJ-III*), the *Wide-Range Achievement Test—Third Edition* (*WRAT-3*), and the *Slosson Written Expression Test* (*SWET*) were administered.

continued

Table 4.4   *Woodcock-Johnson Tests of Achievement—Third Edition (WJ-III)* (Conversions based on age norms)

Subtest	Standard score	Percentile rank	Range
Word identification	105; 97–113	64; 41–80	Average to High Average
Passage comprehension	114; 102–126	83; 56–96	Average to Superior
Reading fluency	90; 85– 95	25;16–37	Low Average to Average
Math calculation	103; 93–113	59; 32–80	Average to High Average
Applied problems	96; 84–108	39; 15–70	Low Average to Average
Math fluency	78; 74– 82	8; 4–12	Borderline to Low Average
Spelling	86; 76– 96	18; 6–39	Borderline to Average
Writing samples	111; 97–125	77; 43–95	Average to Superior
Writing fluency	88; 83–93	21;17–32	Low Average to Average

Table 4.5   *Slosson Written Expression Test (SWET)*

Subscale/Scale	Scaled/Standard score	Percentile rank	Interpretive range
Writing maturity	100; 90–110	50; 25–75	Average
Type-token Ratio	11; 9–13	63; 37–84	Average to Above Average
Av. Sentence Length	9; 6–12	37; 10–75	Below Average to Average
Writing mechanics	81; 76– 90	10; 5–25	Deficient to Average
Spelling	7; 5– 9	16; 5–37	Deficient to Average
Capitalization	6; 4– 8	10; 1–25	Very Deficient to Average
Punctuation	8; 6–10	25; 10–50	Below Average to Average
Written expression total SS*	89; 83– 97	23; 13–42	Below Average to Average

Note: * SS = Standard Score (*M = 100; SD = 15*)

Box 4.1 continued

Wide-Range Achievement Test—Third Revision
        Spelling Subtest Standard Score = 88   Percentile Rank = 21

Nakita was administered the *Woodcock-Johnson Tests of Achievement— Third Edition* (*WJ-III*) to explore reported weaknesses in language arts content areas. On the tests of reading, some task variability was noted as her passage comprehension skills (*percentile* rank range = 56–96; Average to Superior) were slightly better developed than her sight-word vocabulary (*percentile* rank range = 41–80; Average to High Average). Both of these areas were commensurate with current ability estimates. However, her reading fluency was significantly below expected levels given current ability estimates (*percentile* rank range = 16–37; Low Average to Average). Reading fluency is a function of processing speed, reading speed, and attentional control, and this performance represented a 28-point discrepancy below ability.

In mathematics, Nakita's calculation skills were Average to High Average, exceeding approximately 59% of age-mates (*percentile* rank range = 32–80), while her problem-solving capabilities were Low Average to Average, exceeding approximately 39% of age-mates (*percentile* rank range = 15–70). Her math problem-solving skills were slightly to significantly below current ability estimates (a 22-standard-score-point discrepancy). However, her math fluency score was very significantly below expected levels given current ability estimates (*percentile* rank range = 4–12; Borderline to Low Average). Math fluency is a function of processing speed, computational speed, and attentional control, and this performance represented a 40-standard-score-point discrepancy below ability.

Nakita's written expression in context (Writing Samples subtest) was significantly better developed (*percentile* rank range = 45–95; Average to Superior) than her spelling skills in isolation (Spelling subtest *percentile* rank range = 6–39; Borderline to Average). Her written expression was commensurate with ability estimates, while her spelling skills were significantly deficient. The *WRAT-3* Spelling subtest was administered to further explore Nakita's spelling skills and she performed at the 21st percentile (Low Average to Average), confirming deficient spelling skills. She appears to struggle substantially with nonconventional spelling patterns. Interestingly, her Writing Samples responses were frequently inappropriately punctuated and capitalized and were comprised of simple vocabulary and sentence structure. To further explore the nature of suggested writing difficulties, the *Slosson Written Expression Test* (*SWET*) (Hofler, Erford, & Amoriell, 2001) was administered. The *SWET* requires the student to compose a story about a picture cue, and the product is scored for writing maturity and mechanics. On this administration of the *SWET*, Nakita's Writing Maturity Index was slightly below expected levels, but her Writing Mechanics Index was 37 standard-score points below current ability estimates. Importantly, her capitalization, punctuation, and spelling were consistently poorly developed. Thus, a Disorder of Written Expression (mechanics) is evident to a significant degree. In addition, Nakita's Writing Fluency subtest score was very significantly deficient in comparison with current ability estimates (percentile rank range = 17–32; Low Average to Average). Writing fluency is a function of processing speed and attentional control, and this performance represented a 30-point discrepancy below ability.

Because a referral question was whether Nakita possessed significant problems with inattention, clinical and behavioral assessments focused on the presence of age- and ability-inappropriate levels of distractibility, primary symptoms of an Attention-Deficit/Hyperactivity Disorder (AD/HD).

Mr. Trig and Mrs. Bookworm, teachers who have instructed Nakita and who are well acquainted with her academic and behavioral performance, completed the *Conners' Teacher Rating Scale—Revised, Long Version* (*CTRS-R:L*). Nakita's mother completed the *Conners' Parent Rating Scale—Revised, Long Version* (*CPRS-R:L*). All respondents indicated substantial concerns regarding Nakita's inattentive behaviors, indicating that Nakita frequently

continued

Table 4.6   [Nakita's results from the Conners' Rating Scales—Revised]

Conners' Parent Rating Scale Revised: Long Version (CPRS-R:L)		Conners' Teacher Rating Scale Revised: Long Version (CTRS-R:L)		Conners' Teacher Rating Scale Revised: Long Version (CTRS-R:L)	
Respondent: Nakita's mother		Respondent: Mr. Trig		Respondent: Mrs. Bookworm	
Scale	T Score	Scale	T Score	Scale	T score
A. Oppositional	61	A. Oppositional	46	A. Oppositional	50
B. Cognitive Problems	67*	B. Cognitive Problems	76*	B. Cognitive Problems	74*
C. Hyperactivity	49	C. Hyperactivity	54	C. Hyperactivity	48
D. Anxious/shy	49	D. Anxious/shy	46	D. Anxious/shy	46
E. Perfectionism	42	E. Perfectionism	41	E. Perfectionism	49
F. Social Problems	45	F. Social Problems	46	F. Social Problems	46
G. Psychosomatic	51				
L. *DSM-IV:* Inattentive	67*	L. *DSM-IV:* Inattentive	76*	L. *DSM-IV:* Inattentive	68*
M. *DSM-IV:* Hyper-Impulsive	47	M. *DSM-IV:* Hyper-Impulsive	55	M. *DSM-IV:* Hyper-Impulsive	46

Note: * designates a score falling above the required cutoff score of T = 65.

Box 4.1 continued

avoids engaging in tasks requiring sustained mental effort; fails to give close attention to details; has difficulty sustaining attention on tasks; is easily distracted by sights and sounds; loses things needed for tasks; and has difficulty concentrating. Each of these items loads heavily on inattention, a core component of AD/HD—Predominantly Inattentive Type. All other personality and behavioral functioning was reported to be well within normal limits.

A clinical interview involving both Nakita and her mother confirmed much of the evidence substantiating a mild to moderate attentional deficiency without the associated hyperactive features. However, because it has been well documented in research literature that myriad conditions exist that mask and/or mimic the symptoms associated with AD/HD, an exhaustive interview was conducted to rule out more than two dozen clinical and cognitive disorders that often lead to misdiagnosis (see Appendix C of Erford, 2006). Upon concluding this interview, Nakita was determined to not display substantial symptoms associated with disruptive behavior, anxiety, or depressive disorders. No medical history of lead poisoning, hyperthyroidism, or allergies in Nakita or family members was reported. Nakita does not exhibit a visual or auditory processing disorder, and her history is reportedly negative for physical or sexual abuse and abuse of alcohol or other drugs. No tic or seizure disorders, hallucinations, or delusions were reported or evidenced, and Nakita displayed a history of positive social relationships and interactions. Thus myriad conditions shown to mask and/or mimic AD/HD were ruled out.

In conclusion, behavior rating scales, cognitive-perceptual information, and clinical interview confirm that Nakita fulfills the diagnostic criteria for

Table 4.7 *DSM-IV-TR* diagnostic summary for Nakita

Axis I—314.00 AD/HD—Predominantly Inattentive Type
      314.5—Developmental Coordination Disorder (fine-motor)
      315.2—Disorder of Written Expression (mechanics, spelling)
      315.9—Learning Disorder—NOS (processing speed)
Axis II—None
Axis III—None
Axis IV—Academic/testing problems
Axis V—Global Assessment of Functioning (GAF) (current) = 69

AD/HD—Predominantly Inattentive Type, Developmental Coordination Disorder, and Disorder of Written Expression. These conditions are presently mild to moderate in severity and are affecting her schoolwork production and performance. Also of concern is a deficiency in processing speed [Learning Disorder—Not Otherwise Specified (NOS)] that adversely impacts her motivation to engage in written expression and other academic activities and affects the quality of written expression and other academic output.

Final Conceptualization and Recommendations

Nakita is a 12-year-old girl currently attending grade 6 at XYZ Middle School. She currently performs in the Average range of general intellectual ability, but her VCI and PRI index scores indicate her intellectual capabilities are much higher (deviation IQ estimate = 118). Deficiencies in processing speed and short-term auditory and visual recall were noted. A significant achievement deficiency was noted in written expression and spelling (Disorder of Written Expression). This inconsistency is often apparent in children with deficient processing speed because the speed of their written expression cannot keep up with the flow of ideas they are trying to communicate. Frequently inattentive and disorganized, Nakita fulfills the diagnostic criteria for Attention-Deficit/Hyperactivity Disorder—Predominantly Inattentive Type. In addition, Nakita displays a Developmental Coordination Disorder (fine motor). At this time, the extent of these disorders appears mild to moderate in severity and affects Nakita's schoolwork production and performance.

The following recommendations are offered:

1. Nakita's mother is encouraged to share the results of this evaluation with Nakita's physician and to seek the physician's guidance in developing a treatment plan that addresses Nakita's inattentiveness and disorganization.
2. Nakita may benefit from short-term remedial tutoring in written expression and mechanics. In particular, this course of action should address a review of written-language mechanics rules (punctuation, capitalization, and

continued

Box 4.1 continued

grammar in context), as well as composition construction strategies and skills.

3. Nakita can be helped to better understand task directions when she and her teachers and parents break down multistep directions into a sequence of ordered steps. It will help to:

- *Write them down* and number the steps so Nakita can complete the steps one at a time.
- Have Nakita check with an adult after completing each step and before moving on to the next step. She currently is experiencing a good deal of frustration by making mistakes and misunderstanding directions in the early steps of a multistep task. Having an adult check her progress at each step before moving on will help eliminate some of this frustration.
- Be sure Nakita is on the right track when beginning the assignment.
- Give an example of what she is to do.
- Check her progress frequently.
- Have Nakita rephrase directions in her own words to be sure she understands them.
- Have a well-organized student help Nakita transition from step to step.
- Have Nakita do two or three examples under the supervision of a teacher, parent, or student helper to be sure she understands the process before beginning to complete items independently.
- Make sure multistep directions are *written down,* whether on the paper, a chalkboard, or an index card.

4. Classroom and home-study modifications that may facilitate Nakita's academic performance include:

- Consider creating compositions with a written outline and verbally constructing the composition on audiotape. A transcription of the audiotape can then be made, embellished on, and proofread. This procedure will capitalize on Nakita's verbal strengths and minimize the frustration that ensues by her forgetting good ideas when trying to construct compositions from memory.
- Encourage Nakita to further develop keyboarding skills to facilitate her typing. She should strive to type at a rate of greater than 40 words per minute by the beginning of her 9th-grade year.
- Allow Nakita to compose compositions and other written work on a word processor. She should immediately begin to type and edit her written work using the word processor.
- Cut back repetitive homework assignments beyond the point of mastery.
- Give Nakita preferential seating near the primary area of instruction, with her back facing any distracting students or stimuli.
- Surround her with focused role models who will not distract her and who will not allow Nakita to distract them.

5. Classroom and home-study modifications that may facilitate Nakita's behavioral and work habit adjustments include:
    - A daily assignment notebook that allows daily or at least weekly communication between the parents and teachers.
    - Praise and encouragement that emphasize Nakita's accomplishments and successes (no matter how small).
    - Brief verbal reprimands addressing behaviors, not perceived motivations, followed by praise and encouragement for successes.
    - Behavioral contracts that identify specific academic and behavioral goals.
    - The use of a timer to break assignments into smaller time units of more intense focus. For a preteenager with a short attention span, timed units should not generally exceed 15 to 30 minutes. After a short break with plenty of performance feedback and encouragement, as well as some physical movement or exercise, the next timed task can ensue.
    - Appropriate home and school study spaces, with set times, no distractions, and a recognized routine.
6. Treatment of AD/HD can be addressed best through a combination of:
    - Parent, teacher, and student education on the nature and treatment of AD/HD.
    - Behavior modification to address educational and behavioral issues.
    - Educational modifications to make Nakita more successful in the classroom.
    - Medical intervention as determined by Nakita's attending physician.
7. Because of Nakita's slow processing speed, she will benefit from extra time given to complete standardized tests, particularly timed, group-administered tests of achievement. Extra time should also be given, as needed, on in-school tests so that Nakita's grades will reflect mastery of content, rather than suppression due to time constraints.

A primary strength of using clinical judgment is the flexibility it affords the decision maker. A seasoned examiner will be quick to admit that the various data accumulated during an evaluation do not always agree. There are times when two tests purporting to measure a similar construct may yield dissimilar results. There are times when teachers, spouses, mothers, and fathers who are asked the same set of questions about the same client will vary widely in their responses, sometimes due to varying perceptions, response bias, or the intent to deceive. In fact, it is more often the case that some data do conflict, thus requiring great skill and judgment on the part of the examiner to realize what to focus on and what not to focus on. In these instances, clinical judgment is indispensable as a tool for reckoning divergent information from diverse data sources. However, this same flexibility can also lead to examiner bias and a decision-making process that lacks reliability (i.e., consistency) and usefulness. Indeed, some have demonstrated that statistical models, compared to clinical judgment models, lead to more reliable and valid decisions.

Table 4.8 Example of a multiple regression/multiple cutoff hybrid decision-making model

In the following scenario, a decision must be made to select the three most qualified applicants. X_1, X_2, and X_3 are the scores on the selection tests. Y' is the predicted criterion score based on the multiple regression equation: $Y' = a + b_1 X_1 + b_2 X_2 + b_3 X_3$. The minimum cutoff scores for each selection variable are $X_1 = 20$, $X_2 = 15$, and $X_3 = 25$. The "All met" column indicates whether the client's scores on each of the selection tests (X_1, X_2, and X_3) met or exceeded the minimum cut score and, therefore, can be considered for final selection. "Final Rank" indicates the final ranked position of the "surviving" candidates. The top three ranked candidates (marked by an asterisk) will be deemed most qualified and offered the positions. (Note that Candidate H was selected even though Candidate J had a higher Y', because X_2 for Candidate J was below the minimum criterion, effectively eliminating Candidate J from consideration.)

Participant	X_1	X_2	X_3	Y'	All met	Final rank
A	22	20	20	22.65	Yes	5
B	18	19	25	23.17	No	X
C	14	12	21	18.74	No	X
D	20	15	25	22.99	Yes	4
E	24	19	30	27.20	Yes	1*
F	17	16	25	22.21	No	X
G	22	19	28	25.72	Yes	2*
H	21	18	25	23.95	Yes	3*
I	11	11	12	13.85	No	X
J	23	14	28	25.00	No	X

Note: * = the top three ranked candidates.

Combining decision-making models

Sometimes a combination of these three methods can lead to greater accuracy. For example, strict adherence to a multiple cutoff method may at times be softened by clinical judgment that takes into account a client's or student's extenuating circumstances—circumstances not accounted for by the multiple cutoff method, but nonetheless important. This happens frequently with educational decisions (i.e., grade retentions, exceptions to course requirements, college admission and scholarship applications) and clinical decisions (i.e., use of the designation "Not Otherwise Specified"). Alternatively, multiple regression and multiple cutoff methods can be used in conjunction to select the "cream of the crop" in a two-stage process. Stage 1 involves applying the multiple regression equation to client scores and rank ordering the client's scores according to the magnitude of the client's predicted criterion score (Y'). Stage 2 involves standard setting to determine the minimal cutoff for each selection test score and then applying these multiple cutoff criteria to the same scores analyzed in stage one. This process, an example of which is provided in Table 4.8, may eliminate some of the individuals who benefited from the multiple regression process, which allowed a compensation for low scores, and may eliminate them from final selection. Such a procedure is particularly helpful when the cost of selecting an unqualified person may be too prohibitive or the risk of failure too detrimental. Of course, any decision-making method has strengths and weaknesses, and will virtually never be foolproof. Selection of an appropriate decision-making model must be undertaken with great care to ensure the rights and protection of clients and students.

SUMMARY/CONCLUSION

Test validity is about whether or not (and to what degree) a test score measures what it claims to measure. Validity is closely related to, and dependent on, test reliability. Evidence for test score validity is determined in several ways. Content validity considers the degree to which a test adequately represents the breadth of content of the domain being examined. Criterion-related validity correlates scores on the predictor variable (test score) with those on the criterion or outcome measure. Criterion-related validity may be predictive, in which the predictor and criterion measures are gathered at different times, or concurrent, in which both are gathered at the same time. A prediction equation can be used to predict a person's score on the outcome measure from the individual's score on the predictor variable. The standard error of estimate indicates the degree of accuracy of predictions. Construct validity uses convergent and discriminant forms of validity assessment. Convergent construct validity is established by showing high correlations between the new test and other established measures of the same or similar constructs. Discriminant construct validity is evidenced by low correlations between the new test and measures of unrelated constructs. It is important to establish a clear definition of the construct in order to know what the test score means. Finally, the use of a given test is a based on informed judgment to be made by a competent counselor for the benefit of the client.

Decision making using a single test score is generally done through one of three processes: setting a cutoff score, linear regression, and application of decision theory. Decision making using multiple tests frequently makes use of clinical judgment, multiple cutoff, or multiple regression methods. Each of these methods has strengths and weaknesses, and each requires varying degrees of expertise and sophistication. Most professional counselors use clinical judgment methods based on a theoretical framework and previous experience.

KEY TERMS

clinical judgment	decision theory
concurrent criterion-related validity	discriminant validity
construct	domain
construct validity	face validity
content-related validity	false acceptance
convergent validity	false rejection
criterion	intercept
criterion-related validity	linear regression
cutoff scores	multiple cutoff method

multiple regression
negative predictive power
positive predictive power
predictive criterion-related validity
restricted range
sensitivity
slope

specificity
standard error of estimate
total predictive value
valid acceptance
valid rejection
validity

CHAPTER 5

Selecting, Administering, Scoring, and Interpreting Assessment Instruments and Techniques

by R. Anthony Doggett, Carl J. Sheperis, Susan Eaves, Michael D. Mong, and Bradley T. Erford

This chapter begins with issues related to proper test selection, administration, and scoring, followed by discussion of proper interpretation of test scores from both norm-referenced and criterion-referenced tests. A section regarding the appropriate sources for obtaining information about assessment instruments has been included to assist the reader in proper test selection. Finally, common errors committed during the assessment process are discussed, along with recommendations for addressing these issues.

TEST SELECTION

Appropriate test selection is crucial in the assessment process. Before selecting instruments, the professional counselor must first determine the purpose for engaging in assessment activities. As discussed in Chapter 1, sometimes clinicians administer different tests to determine if the individual meets criteria for a particular diagnosis, to develop interventions or treatments for clients, to evaluate the integrity of services, or to evaluate the outcome of receiving treatment. In any of these cases, the professional counselor must ensure that the instrument being used is adequate for the stated purpose of the assessment. As such, the instrument must be normed (or criterion-referenced) on a representative population, contain items that are appropriate for evaluating the current referral concern, have adequate psychometric properties, and provide scores that lend themselves to appropriate outcome comparisons. Choosing instruments that are not linked to the original purpose of the assessment, lack technical adequacy, or are not appropriate for the referred problem or individual will reduce the professional counselor's ability to meet the client's needs and could potentially expose the client to harmful and unwarranted experiences. Table 5.1 offers summary suggestions that professional counselors should consider when selecting an instrument.

TEST ADMINISTRATION

After determining the purpose of the assessment, the professional counselor must determine the best way to obtain the information needed from the client. While assessments are designed to yield meaningful information about a client, the quality of the information obtained is closely linked to the skills and abilities of the clinician administering the test.

Administrator Requirements

It is important to mention that each assessment instrument requires a certain level of training and/or education by the administrator. In other words, legally and ethically, professional counselors can select instruments only from the category of instruments available for use according to their level of training. In clinical practice, these requirements are often determined by state licensure laws. In schools and agency work, state certifications or exemptions often exist that allow examiners to administer tests they would otherwise be unable to use in the private sector. For example, unlicensed professional counselors working in a correctional institution or for a nonprofit agency may be allowed to administer clinical or intelligence tests as a condition of employment. But, because they not licensed by a state counseling board, they may not be able to administer those same tests to the public for a fee in a private practice. The same is often true for professional school counselors and school psychologists. They may be able to administer the *Wechsler Intelligence Scale for Children—Fourth Edition* (*WISC-IV*) or *Woodcock-Johnson Tests of Achievement—Third Edition* (*WJ-III ACH*) during school hours to students as a condition of employment, but be prohibited from administering these same tests in private practice for a fee. While some instruments can be used with knowledge gained from the manual, others require in-depth supervised training. To assist in the process of delineating which instruments require which level of training, a majority of publishers use a level system similar (albeit not identical) to that described below.

Level A

Level A instruments can be administered, scored, and interpreted after studying the manual, with no additional training or education required. However, employment

Table 5.1   Guide to proper test selection

Test information
- What is the name of the test?
- Who are the test authors?
- What company published the test?
- When was the test published?
- Are alternative forms of the test available?
- How much does the test cost?
- How long does it take to administer the test?
- Is the test manual comprehensive (i.e., includes information on psychometrics, norms, item development, etc.)?
- Does the test have current norms and items?
- Who is included in the standardization sample?

Test interpretation aids
- Does the manual provide clear descriptions of the purposes and applications of the test?
- Does the manual provide clear information regarding the training and qualifications needed to administer the test?
- Does the manual include example cases to aid in interpretation of the results?

Examinee considerations
- What skills are needed by the examinee to take the test?
- In what language are the test items written?
- What is the reading/vocabulary level of the test items?
- How are the test items presented?
- How is the examinee expected to respond to the test items?
- What adaptations can be made to the test items or test presentation to accommodate any examinee disabilities?
- Is the test free from bias?
- Is the test administered to individuals or groups?

Technical adequacy
- What types of reliability studies have been performed on the test scores?
- What types of validity studies have been performed on the test scores?
- Are the reliability and validity estimates adequate for the intended purpose?

Administration and scoring
- Are the directions for administering the test appropriate and clear?
- Are the directions for scoring the test appropriate and clear?
- What options are available for scoring the test?

Interpretive scores and norms
- Are the scales used for reporting test scores adequately presented and described?
- Are the normative scores presented in an appropriate format (e.g., standard scores, percentile ranks)?
- Is the standardization sample appropriate and clearly described?
- If more than one form of the test is available, are equivalent scores on the different forms provided?
- Does the test manual provide guidance on establishing local norms?

---

or affiliation with an institution or organization is sometimes required before the publisher will agree to send the instrument. The *Self-Directed Search* (Holland, Fritzche, & Powell, 1994) is a Level A test.

Level B

Level B instruments require specialized knowledge of psychometric issues and test score properties, usually obtained by taking a graduate-level course in assessment. To qualify for this level's criteria, the professional counselor administering the test must have a master's degree in counseling, psychology, or a related field. In addition, the professional counselor must have specific training and/or licensure or certification recognized by the test publisher. The *Reynolds Adolescent Depression Scale—Second Edition RADS-2*, *(WJ-III ACH)*, and *Slosson Intelligence Test—Revision 3 SIT-R3* are examples of Level B tests.

Level C

Level C instruments require substantial knowledge about the construct being measured and about the instrument being used. Often, a doctorate in counseling, psychology, or a related field and/or appropriate licensure or certification is required. In addition, the professional counselor should have specific coursework or training related to assessment (generally) and to the instrument (specifically) or class of instruments (e.g., intelligence, personality, projectives). Test publishers commonly use the general levels described, although the designations sometimes vary. In addition, there are often exceptions and variations due to state laws or regulations that the professional counselor should check prior to selecting an instrument. The *Rorschach Inkblot Test*, the *Wechsler Adult Intelligence Scale—Third Edition* (*WAIS-III*), and the *Minnesota Multiphasic Personality Inventory—Second Edition* (*MMPI-2*) are examples of Level C tests.

Finally, it is a magnificent practice to administer, score, and interpret a test under the supervision of a highly trained practitioner a number of times and on volunteer participants prior to using the test for decision-making purposes with clients. How many "practice administrations" depends largely on the complexities of the test. Practice administrations allow professional counselors to hone their skills on a new instrument under competent supervision and in no-risk situations to enhance the ultimate competence of the examiner.

Examinee Preparation

The first step in any assessment is to prepare the test takers for the test they are about to take. Because many standardized tests are administered in school settings or to school-aged youth in agency or private settings, professional counselors who work with children and adolescents must be able to adapt their assessment skills and knowledge toward younger age groups.

The professional counselor's job is to familiarize clients and students with the type of assessment they will be taking. This may seem like common sense, but many professional counselors fail to take into account the client's familiarity with the test and the testing procedure. People should be informed of the type of test (e.g., math achievement, career interest inventory, personality inventory), whether the test is timed, and what the test is designed to measure. Professional counselors should approach the assessment positively while helping clients and students to ease and manage their test anxiety.

Environmental Concerns

Another important aspect of preparing students for assessments is preparing and maintaining the proper testing environment. The proper assessment environment is one that is distraction-free, provides proper space for working, and discourages cheating. While the ideal assessment environment can be difficult to provide, test administrators should strive to ensure there are relatively few distractions during the testing process. Minimizing distractions can be accomplished by not allowing examinees to wander around the room, make unnecessary noise, or have materials unrelated to the test with them in the testing session. Likewise, the examiner should ensure the testing environment provides sufficient lighting, temperature, and work space for the task at hand.

Testing Procedures

The actual process of test administration is often very straightforward. Standardized test administration is a very rigid and scripted process. The primary requirement for administering a published test is that the examiner strictly follows testing procedures described in the test's manual. Due to the many variations in testing procedures found in different published tests, it is critically important that the test administrator be familiar with the specific test procedures and materials used. Testing procedures can include, but are not limited to, test directions, time limits, and registration and identification procedures.

The majority of test manuals stress the importance of the manner in which test directions are given. In most cases, test directions are to be read word for word following a script that is laid out in the manual. Any deviation from the protocol may result in invalid test results. The primary function of verbatim instructions is to ensure that uniform testing conditions are present for all test takers. Whenever possible, professional counselors should memorize directions for administering and scoring test items. Even though the test manual is still referred to, memorization tends to help the administration flow more seamlessly, significantly reducing pauses by the administrator to locate a needed passage or judge the accuracy of a client response. Thus the professional counselor's demonstrated knowledge of and comfort with the test helps to establish a relational rapport and projects administrator competence and confidence.

While not all tests employ time limits, time limits are frequently a vital part of the testing procedure. Test administrators should be familiar with the time limits for different items or subtests. Administrators should also carry some sort of timing device (i.e., stopwatch, wristwatch, clock, egg timer) with them so that they are aware of the time limits at all times. Ending a testing session too early or ending late may result in invalid test results.

Many published tests also have specific procedures for examinee registration and identification, particularly high-stakes aptitude or achievement tests (e.g., *SATs*, graduate record examinations, advanced placement examinations). Sometimes examinees must identify themselves through means such as their names or Social Security numbers. In an attempt to discourage cheating, some tests also require examinees to present one or more forms of identification, both before and after a testing session. Professional counselors conducting assessments for employers, government program eligibility, or even community mental health services must be equally vigilant to ensure that client results are accurate and legitimate.

Despite the test publisher's vigorous attempts to provide a uniform testing experience for all examinees, there are sometimes deviations. According to the *Responsibilities of Users of Standardized Tests* (*RUST-3*) statement (AACE, 2003a) and *Standards for Educational and Psychological Testing* (AERA/APA/NCME, 1999), any deviations from the test procedure should be documented by the test administrator. Many test protocols contain a section in which the examiner may record and describe problems or unusual circumstances that may occur during the testing session. The professional counselor should take any irregularities under consideration when interpreting test results.

While deviations from standardized testing procedures are not required for the average examinee, test administrators should be aware of the special considerations given to examinees with disabilities or to very young examinees. The majority of published group-administered tests (particularly those administered by schools, institutions of higher education, or licensure or other professional boards) require that an examinee show proof of a disability before being given special accommodations under the Individuals with Disabilities Education Improvement Act of 2004 (IDEIA), the Americans With Disabilities Act of 1991 (ADA), or Section 504 of the U.S. Rehabilitation Act of 1973. While there is no set standard on the requirement of proof of disability, many institutions or test publishers require that the examinee in question have a written report on file that documents the disability. The reports must come from a legitimate source, usually a licensed specialist, and must be current (usually less than three years, depending on the test). Common considerations for individuals with disabilities include extended time on tests, longer breaks, Braille tests, oral instructions, dictated responses, and computer-assisted technology.

Factors Affecting Test Scores

During the process of test administration, the test administrator should be aware of the many factors that can affect test scores. While the administrator should strive to maintain these variables at a minimum level, not all variables can be controlled. Table 7.1 (see Chapter 7) contains a summary of important test-related factors. A comprehensive treatise of these factors affecting client and student responses is provided by Erford (2006).

TEST SCORING

By definition, **test scores** are simply the numerical result of testing. Test scores summarize the information obtained through the testing process by using numbers that the test administrator may interpret. The use of numbers allows test administrators to describe and quantify examinee performance in a standardized manner.

Assessment instruments may be scored by a wide array of people. For example, some instruments are designed to be self-scored (i.e., Level A tests). This type of scoring usually consists of adding columns of scores or counting the number of items responded to. Some tests can also be scored by persons other than the client or examiner (e.g., clerical staff, interns). While having others score assessments may save the test administrator time on the front end, the test administrator should always recheck the test scores to minimize the chance of error. Under most circumstances in clinical practice, the professional counselor will score the protocols for Level B and Level C tests. As stated above, the reason for this practice is because use of Level B and C tests requires advanced education and training.

While most assessment instruments may be scored by hand, computer-assisted scoring programs are becoming increasingly common. Some tests may also provide templates to aid the examiner in scoring the test by hand. Despite the aid offered by test templates, hand scoring for many tests is tedious to even the most experienced examiner. Due to the increased time consumption necessary for hand scoring, many examiners prefer to use computerized scoring programs and services for the longer or more complicated tests. For example, for the *MMPI-2,* computer scoring time is virtually instantaneous after the items are entered into the scoring program (which usually requires 5 to 10 minutes). Depending on the scoring program used, many to most of the *MMPI-2* scales listed in Table 7.10 (see Chapter 7) can be obtained in a matter of seconds. In contrast, using the scoring stencils may require well more than an hour to obtain the same set of scores. Of course, both methods have risks of inaccuracies due to human error. Thus, when using computerized scoring programs, it is essential to double-check all score entries; when using scoring forms or stencils, it is equally important to double-check the derived scores.

Wise and Plake (1990) conducted a study in which computer scoring was compared to hand scoring. The researchers concluded that computer scoring is more accurate, faster, and more thorough than hand scoring. An added advantage of computer scoring is the fact that computers are completely unbiased. Unless modified by the examiner, computers will not discriminate against examinees on the basis of individual differences such as sex, religion, race, sexual preference, or socioeconomic status. Computers can also aid examiners in complex test interpretations that can take human interpreters days. Of course, this does not mean that the interpretations derived by the computer are more accurate than those of a skilled clinician.

While computerized scoring procedures are a useful aid to clinicians, they are not infallible due to their reliance on human programmers. In an attempt to minimize computer scoring errors, the *Standards for Educational and Psychological Testing* (AERA et al., 1999) requires test scoring services to provide documentation of their programming procedures.

Despite the increasing availability of computer scoring programs, some types of tests require human interpretation. For example, projective personality tests usually require a professional counselor to interpret information that computers are unable to perform, although recent efforts have resulted in attempts to standardize scoring and interpretations of some techniques (Exner, 2002; McArthur & Roberts, 2005). Professional judgment may also be required for some individually administered intelligence, aptitude, achievement, personality, and clinical tests.

It is always important for the professional counselor to remember that test scores serve a wide variety of functions in a variety of different settings. School personnel can use test scores to determine student placement. Teachers use test scores to analyze their lesson plans and teaching methods. Professional counselors can use test scores to communicate examinee performance to clients, parents, or other stakeholders. The common link among all the above examples is that professionals use test scores to guide them in their decision-making responsibilities.

Professional Standards in Testing

Although each test publisher generally includes a set of minimum standards for the examiner to follow, several professional organizations provide additional ethical guidelines or standards for proper test administration and scoring. For example, the American Counseling Association's *Code of Ethics* (ACA, 2005a), the *RUST-3* statement (AACE, 2003a), the *Standards for Educational and Psychological Testing* (AERA et al., 1999), and the National Board of Certified Counselors' *Code of Ethics* (1989) all encourage professional counselors administering tests to use appropriate procedures, techniques, and strategies related to the consideration of individual differences in sex, gender, ethnicity, and socioeconomic status of the examinee. Table 5.2 is offered as an amalgamated guide for the proper administration and scoring of tests.

Table 5.2   Summary guidelines for administering and scoring tests

Examiner preparation
1. Administer only tests for which you have been thoroughly trained.
2. Read and learn all instructions.
3. Adhere to standardization procedures.
   a. Cite instructions to examinees exactly as the test manual prescribes.
   b. Present test items according to prescribed time limits.
   c. Follow scoring guidelines rigidly.
   d. Document any deviations from standardized procedures or testing irregularities.
4. Administer the test in an objective manner.
   a. Reinforce participation but give no indication of accuracy or inaccuracy of examinee's responses (e.g., "You're doing fine. Keep trying your best.").
   b. Remember that you are testing, not teaching. Pay close attention to verbal (e.g., intonation of voice) and nonverbal cues (e.g., eye glances, head nods).
5. Administer the test in a natural manner.
   c. Achieve rapport with the examinee before administering any test items.
   d. Use standardized wording in a normal and nonthreatening manner.
6. Prepare the testing environment by removing distractions and avoiding clutter.
   a. Have the examinee face away from doors, windows, or other areas that may distract attention from the test.

    b. Have the examinee complete the test in a quiet area.

    c. When possible, avoid testing the examinee when he or she presents as hurried, worried, or ill (unless these are the conditions that prompted the evaluation or the client's normal state).

7. Provide optimum testing conditions.

    a. Provide the examinee with comfortable seating and make sure he or she can see the test materials clearly.

    b. Provide a well-lit room with a comfortable temperature.

    c. Provide instructions in a clear, audible voice at a moderate rate of speed.

    d. Help the examinee maintain interest through enthusiastic presentation of the items and attention for effort.

    e. Provide social attention and encouragement for general performance, not for specific items.

    f. For maximum performance tests, let the examinee know that you want to see how well he or she can do on this test administration.

Test administration

1. Administer the test in an efficient manner. Have an efficient system for

    a. Recording answers.

    b. Viewing the manual without distracting the examinee.

    c. Bringing out test materials and storing them away after use.

    d. Avoiding delays.

2. Make smooth transitions from (sub)test to (sub)test.

3. Know test administration guidelines and test materials well enough to avoid overextending the test experience for the examinee.

    a. Always begin at designated starting points.

    b. Score each item correctly and efficiently.

4. Learn how to appropriately handle distractions from the examinee.

    a. Avoid attending to inappropriate remarks.

    b. Ignore inappropriate movements if they are not distracting to the examinee's test performance.

    c. Redirect the examinee to the task at hand if remarks or movements become too distracting.

Scoring the test items

1. Know the scoring standards well, so you thoroughly understand the intent behind each item.

2. Remember that scoring standards provide guidelines for scoring items. When in doubt, score examinee answers in relation to the intent behind the item.

3. Review the guidelines in the manual to verify any unclear answers provided by the examinee.

4. Check and recheck every step of the scoring procedure.

5. Check and recheck all figures and calculations.

Test storage and care of materials

1. Place all examinee protocols and other information in client folders in a proper storage (i.e., locked) cabinet to protect the confidentiality of the responses and personal information.

2. Store all materials in a safe, secure place to prevent unwarranted wear and exposure to untrained personnel.

3. Replace any materials that are worn so that these materials do not become distracting to the examinee.

4. Point to pictures with a finger or eraser of the pencil to avoid placing marks on the page.

5. Replace any materials that are lost or damaged with objects identical to the original from the testing company.

NORM-REFERENCED INTERPRETATION

Tests are usually administered to assess important domains in the examinee's life. For example, intelligence tests evaluate cognitive functioning; achievement tests evaluate academic functioning; adaptive behavior measures evaluate important daily living skills (e.g., communication, motor skills, social functioning); career inventories measure interests, skills, and values; and clinical or personality measures evaluate inter- and intrapersonal functioning. When these large domains of functioning are assessed, the examinee's **raw score** is usually transformed and then compared to the performance of other individuals with similar characteristics (e.g., age, gender, ethnicity). For a norm-referenced test, this population of individuals is referred to as the **standardization sample**, normative sample, or the norm group. The comparison scores are called derived scores and are placed into two groups: *developmental scores* and *scores of relative standing* (Salvia & Ysseldyke, 2004).

Developmental Equivalents

One type of transformed or derived score is called a **developmental equivalent**. The two most common types of developmental equivalents are *age equivalents* and *grade equivalents*. Both of these equivalent scores are obtained by determining the average score obtained on a test by different groups of examinees who vary in age or grade placement. Specifically, an age equivalent means that the examinee's raw score is the average (mean or median) performance for a particular age group. For example, if the average raw score for 11-year-old children (11 years, 0 months) on a particular test is 15 items correct out of a 30-item test, then any examinee obtaining a score of 15 would receive an age-equivalent score of 11-0 (11 years, 0 months). Therefore, the age-equivalent score is obtained by computing the mean or median raw score on a test for a group of children of a specific age. It is also important to note that age-equivalent scores are expressed in years and months with a hyphen between the year and the month (i.e., 11 years, 2 months is expressed as 11-2).

A grade-equivalent score is obtained by computing the average (mean or median) raw score on a test obtained by examinees in a specified grade. For example, if the average score of 6th-graders on a mathematics test is 25, then any examinee obtaining a score of 25 is reported to have math knowledge at the 6th-grade level. Grade-equivalent scores are expressed in grades and tenths with a decimal between the two numbers (i.e., 6.5 refers to the average performance of children at the middle of the 6th grade; 2.1 refers to the average performance of children during the first month of the 2nd grade)

Salvia and Ysseldyke (2004, pp. 92–93) appropriately pointed out five concerns when using age- and grade-equivalent scores. These are:

1. *Systematic misinterpretation.* Examinees who earn an age-equivalent score of 11-0 have answered as many questions correctly as the average for examinees that are 11 years of age. Obtaining this score does not mean that the examinee performed on the test in the same manner that an 11-year-old student would have performed. In a similar fashion, a 2nd-grader and a 6th-grader may have both

earned a grade equivalent of 3.0; however, it is very probable that they did not attack the items on the test in the same manner. Developmentally, their thought processes may be quite different. In other words, it is essential to communicate to clients, teachers, and parents that just because a 4th-grader receives a grade equivalent (GE) of 8.5, this does not mean the student is as "smart" as an 8th-grader.

2. *Interpolation and extrapolation.* It is important to remember that average age- and grade-equivalent scores are only estimates of functioning and represent groups of examinees that were not actually tested. Loosely defined, *interpolation* means guessing within the bounds of what is known. Thus, if one knows that a raw score (RS) of 25 yields a grade equivalent of 2.5 (GE = 2.5) and a raw score of 35 (RS = 35) yields a grade equivalent of 3.5 (GE = 3.5), it is reasonable to conclude that each raw score point between 25 and 35 raises the grade equivalent by 0.1. Thus, a RS of 27 would be a GE = 2.7, and a RS = 33 would be a GE = 3.3. Whether this has been demonstrated empirically or not, such interpolations make sense because some empirical results do exist upon which to base a conclusion. Interpolation, while often somewhat inaccurate, is quite benign in comparison to extrapolation. *Extrapolation* involves guessing *outside* the bounds of what is known. Following with the example above, what grade equivalents might one assign to raw scores of less than 25, particularly if no one younger than a grade level of mid-2nd grade actually made up the norm group? Extrapolation provides these estimations. A test developer may extrapolate that the linear relationship noted between GEs of 2.5 and 3.5 continues in the downward direction. Thus the author assumes that a RS = 15 would yield a GE =1.5, and a RS = 19 would yield a GE = 1.9, etc. Of course, such guesswork without the benefit of empirical support is shoddy at best, dangerous at worst. This is just one reason why developmental equivalents should be avoided.

3. *Typological thinking.* Examinees are always being compared to an average that does not actually exist. For example, the average American family may be reported to have 1.7 cars, with a 2.5-bedroom house, and 2.4 children. However, it is simply impossible to have 0.4 of a child. Therefore, the average score simply represents a statistical abstraction.

4. *False standards of performance.* Students are expected to perform at their age and grade levels. Eleven-year-olds are expected to perform at the 11-0 level on a test, and 6th-graders are expected to perform at the 6.0 level. However, equivalent scores are constructed in such a manner that at least half (50%) of any age group or grade group will perform at or below the age or grade level, because half of the group always earns scores at or below the median. This means that a principal who insists that all 2nd-graders complete the year reading at a GE = 2.9 or higher is being statistically naïve. The professional counselor should explain that in the average classroom, only 50% of 2nd-graders can be expected to be at GE = 2.9 or higher.

5. *Scales are ordinal, not equal-interval.* The scales often used to obtain age and grade equivalents are ordinal; therefore, the intervals are not equal. As a result, the scores on these scales cannot be added, subtracted, or multiplied. Thus

school systems that determine student eligibility for remedial services by requiring the student's reading or math achievement to be "two grade levels below current grade placement" are being statistically inappropriate. A two-grade-level difference yields very different results at different grade levels.

It is essential to note that developmental equivalents are frequently misunderstood, miscommunicated, and misused. While professional counselors should be aware of the existence of developmental equivalents and be prepared to explain them, professional counselors should avoid using developmental quotients when explaining client or student scores.

Scores of Relative Standing

Unlike developmental scores, **scores of relative standing** have equal units of measurement. As such, scores on the same test for several different examinees of different ages can be compared. Additionally, different scores on several different instruments can be compared for the same person. The major types of scores of relative standing used in norm-referenced measurement include standard scores and percentile ranks. Figure 5.1 demonstrates the relationship between these scores.

Standard scores

Standard scores are raw scores that have been mathematically transformed to have a designated mean and standard deviation. A standard score expresses how far an examinee's score lies in relation to the standard deviation of the norm group. Five commonly used standard-score distributions include: z-scores, T scores, deviation IQs, normal-curve equivalents, and stanines.

Z-scores

A **z-score** has a mean of 0 and a standard deviation of 1. As such, a z-score simply indicates how many standard deviations above or below the mean a given score falls. A z-score is obtained by subtracting the mean of the norm group (M_x) from the examinee's raw score (X) and then dividing by the standard deviation (SD_x) of the norm group $\left(z = \dfrac{X - M_x}{SD_x}\right)$. Almost all z-scores (99.7%) lie between −3.0 and +3.0.

If an examinee obtains a z-score of 2.0, the examinee has performed 2.0 standard deviations *above* the mean of the group. A z-score of −1.5 is 1.5 standard deviations *below* the mean of the group. A z-score of 0 is at the mean performance of the group. Z-scores are commonly used in empirical research studies.

T scores

In order to remove the − and + signs, z-scores are often transformed into other scores, such as T scores. A **T score** has a mean of 50 and a standard deviation of 10. Many test manuals transform raw scores directly into T scores, but a z-score can be transformed into a T score using the following formula: T = 10(z) + 50. Using the examples above, a z-score of 2.0 would be transformed into a T score of

Number of scores

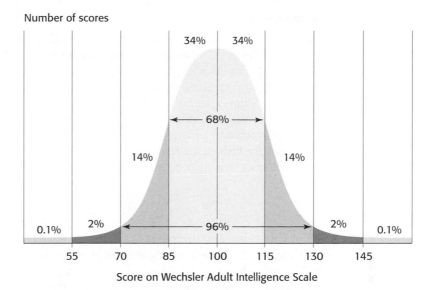

Score on Wechsler Adult Intelligence Scale

Figure 5.1   The normal curve and related standardized scores

70 (T = 10(2.0) + 50 = 70). A z-score of –1.5 would be transformed into a T score of 35 (T = 10(–1.5) + 50 = 35). A z-score of 0 would be transformed into a T score of 50 (T = 10(0) + 50 = 50). T scores are commonly reported in behavioral, personality, and clinical inventories.

Deviation IQs

Deviation IQs have a mean of 100 and a standard deviation of 15 or 16, depending on the instrument used (nearly all currently use *SD = 15*). All of the *Wechsler Scales* have a standard deviation of 15; however, the *Slosson Intelligence Test—Revised* (*SIT-R3*) (Nicholson & Hipshman, 1990) uses a standard deviation of 16. While most test manuals transform raw scores directly into deviation IQs (*M* = 100, *SD* = 15), a z-score can be transformed into a deviation IQ score using the following formula: Dev. IQ = 15(z) + 100. Therefore, an examinee with a z-score of 2.0 would have a deviation IQ of 130 (Dev. IQ = 15(2.0) + 100 = 130). A z-score of –1.5 would be transformed into a deviation IQ of 78 (Dev. IQ = 15(–1.5) + 100 = 78). A z-score of 0 would be transformed into a deviation IQ of 100 (15(0) + 100 = 100). It is important to note that the formula would change if the instrument has a standard deviation of 16. For example, a z-score of 2.0 would be transformed into a deviation IQ of 132 (16(2.0) + 100 = 132). Deviation IQ scores are frequently reported for tests of intelligence, achievement, and perceptual skills.

Normal-curve equivalents

Normal-curve equivalents (NCEs) are standard scores with a mean of 50 and a standard deviation of 21.06. The standard deviation is set at 21.06 because this transformation divides the normal curve into 100 equal units or intervals.

Stanines

Stanines is shortened from the term "standard nines." Stanines are standard-score bands that divide a distribution into nine parts with a mean of 5 and a standard deviation of 2. These scores are expressed as whole numbers from 1 to 9. When scores are converted to stanines, the shape of the original distribution changes into a normal curve. Stanines are frequently provided by publishers of large-scale testing programs. Their use should be limited, and caution in interpretation is warranted because educators and parents often express concern that a client's score has dropped from, say, the fifth to the fourth stanine. In actuality, this "drop" could be a difference of a single raw score point.

Percentile Ranks

Percentile ranks, also referred to as *percentiles,* are derived scores indicating the percentage of individuals whose scores fall at or below a given raw score. It is important to note that the terms *percentile rank* and *percentage correct* are not the same. For example, a **percentage** score of 50 means 50% of the items were correct (a proportion of correct to total points), while an examinee who obtains a percentile rank of 50 on a standardized test has scored the same or better than 50% of the examinees in the norm group. Percentiles allow comparison of a client's score with other scores. Percentages only allow comparisons with some standards. Although percentile ranks are fairly easy to understand, their psychometric properties limit their usefulness. Still, percentile ranks are essential staples in test interpretation because of their ease of understanding. Unlike z-scores or T scores, percentile ranks are not evenly distributed across the normal curve. In fact, raw score differences between percentile ranks are smaller near the mean of the distribution and larger at the extremes of the distribution.

It is also essential to understand that small differences in a client's raw score around the mean can lead to large changes in percentile rank. It is often helpful to explain percentile ranks using a visualization of a line of 100 individuals of the same age (or grade), with the 1st individual in the line being the lowest performer (e.g., poorest math student, least depressed, least hyperactive) and the 100th person in the line being the highest performer (e.g., best math student, most depressed, most hyperactive). Thus an individual scoring at the 95th percentile rank exceeded the performance of 95% of same-aged peers. A person scoring at the 5th percentile rank outperformed only 5% of same-aged peers. Importantly, because the normal curve theoretically runs in each direction to infinity, it is theoretically impossible to achieve the percentile rank end points of 0 or 100.

> **Think About It 5.1**   How would you interpret a percentile rank score of 84 to a client being assessed for depression? Be sure to include a good explanation of what percentile ranks are.

Table 5.3 *SEM* at a given age level

Age (yr-mth)	Reliability	68% LOC (± 1 *SEM*)	95% LOC (± 2 *SEM*)	99% LOC (± 2.58 *SEM*)
12-0–12-11	0.80	±6.7	±13.4	±17.3
13-0–13-11	0.83	±6.2	±12.4	±16.0
14-0–14-11	0.86	±5.6	±11.2	±14.5
15-0–15-11	0.90	±4.7	±9.5	±12.2
16-0–16-11	0.93	±4.0	±7.9	±10.2
17-0–17-11	0.96	±3.0	±6.0	±7.7

Note: Ages presented in years and months. Confidence intervals are reported in standard scores (M = 100; SD =15).

Quartiles

Percentile ranks that divide a distribution into four equal parts are called *quartiles*. With quartiles, each part contains 25% of the norm group. The first quartile (Q1) contains percentile ranks of ≤25; Q2 contains percentile ranks of 26–50; Q3 contains percentile ranks of 51–75; and Q4 contains percentile ranks of >75.

Applying Standard Error of Measurement (SEM) to Test Scores

The score that a client or student obtains on a given test is called the observed score. Recall from the discussion of reliability and standard error of measurement (*SEM*) in Chapter 3 that all test scores have some measurement error, and this score error can be expressed using a band of confidence around the observed score to indicate the likely presence of the true score (i.e., the client's actual score if no measurement error was present). This confidence band reflects the test's standard error of measurement, which is influenced by a test's reliability (see Chapter 3 for an explanation of how *SEM* is computed). *SEM* is essential to test score interpretation because it is misleading to report a score as if it is "the truth, the whole truth, and nothing but the truth." Realistically, the score a client receives on a test may vary up or down on readministration of that test—and this is normal. The more reliable a test score is, the less variability will be expected upon retest; conversely, the lower the reliability, the greater the variability.

Most test manuals and computer scoring programs provide *SEM* for standard scores (SS) obtained by students and clients. Sometimes this information is included in a table that indicates the *SEM* at a given age level and for a certain level of confidence, such as provided in Table 5.3. In these cases, the confidence interval (CI) is computed as CI = SS ± *SEM*. For example, if the observed score is a standard score of 105 and the *SEM* equals 5 standard-score points, then the confidence interval is 105 ± 5 or a range of 100–110. However, an important consideration in determining confidence intervals is the level of confidence to display. Recall from Chapter 3 that ± 1 *SEM* is the 68% level of confidence, ± 2 *SEM* is the 95% level of confidence, and ± 2.58 *SEM* is the 99% level of confidence. Under normal circumstances,

Table 5.4   Observed scores with ranges of standard scores

Test	Standard scores; range	Percentile rank; range	Interpretive range
WISC-IV—IQ	111; 101–121	77; 53–92	Average–Superior
WJ-III—Math Calculation	92; 82–102	29;12–55	Low Average–Average
WJ-III—Applied Problems	77; 67–87	6;1–19	Deficient–Low Average
VMI-4	95; 85–105	37; 16–63	Low Average–Average

Note: For the purpose of this example, it is assumed that 1 *SEM* = 5 standard score points for all four measures. Note that this is *not* usually the case. All scores are interpreted at the 95% level of confidence (i.e., ±10 standard score points).

professional counselors should interpret scores at the 95% level of confidence (± 2 *SEM*), meaning the client's true score will probably lie within the given range 95 times out of 100 (alternate-form administrations of the test).

Table 5.4 presents an example of several observed scores with ranges of standard scores determined at the 95% level of confidence. Note that these scores have also been converted into percentile ranks and interpretive ranges.

Notice that the observed *WISC-IV* IQ score is 111. Interpreting this score at the 95% LOC (level of confidence) with 1 *SEM* equal to 5 standard score points means the range of scores surrounding the score is 111 ± 10, or 101–121 (i.e., if 1 *SEM* = 5 SS points, then 2 *SEM* = (2 × 5) = 10 SS points; thus 111−10 = 101 and 111 + 10 = 121). Next, these standard scores should be converted to percentile ranks to make them easier to explain to clients, students, parents, teachers, or other stakeholders. This can be easily accomplished by using Table 5.5. In this case, a deviation IQ of 111 converts to a percentile rank of 77. Also, a SS of 101 is a percentile rank of 53, and SS or 121 is a percentile rank of 92. Finally, the standard score range of 101–121 is converted to the appropriate interpretive ranges (i.e., brief verbal descriptors), which can also be found in Table 5.5. In this case, a SS of 101 is in the Average range, and a SS of 121 is in the Superior range. Thus the interpretive range is Average to Superior.

A professional counselor's interpretation of the scores in Table 5.4 when presenting them to clients, teachers, parents, guardians or other stakeholders might go like this:

> Juan's performance on the *WISC-IV* exceeded that of 77% of other children his age. His true score probably falls in the percentile rank range of 53 to 92. This performance is Average to Superior. His score on the *WJ-III ACH* Math Calculation subtest exceeded the performance of 29% of other children his age. His true score probably falls in the percentile rank range of 12 to 55. This performance is Low Average to Average. Juan's performance on the *WJ-III ACH* Applied Problems subtest, a measure of math problem-solving abilities, exceeded that of only 6% of other children his age. His true score probably falls in the percentile rank range of 1 to 19. This performance is Deficient to Low Average. Finally, his score on the Developmental Test of Visual-Motor Integration *(VMI-4)* exceeded the performance of 37% of other children his

Table 5.5   Score conversion table

IQ	Percentile rank	Scaled score	Stanine	Z-score	T score	NCE	Interpretive range
155	99.99	19	9	+3.67	87	99	Very Superior
154	99.98	19	9	+3.60	86	99	Very Superior
153	99.98	19	9	+3.53	85	99	Very Superior
152	99.97	19	9	+3.47	85	99	Very Superior
151	99.97	19	9	+3.40	84	99	Very Superior
150	99.96	19	9	+3.33	83	99	Very Superior
149	99.95	19	9	+3.27	83	99	Very Superior
148	99.93	19	9	+3.20	82	99	Very Superior
147	99.91	19	9	+3.13	81	99	Very Superior
146	99.89	19	9	+3.07	81	99	Very Superior
145	99.87	19	9	+3.00	80	99	Very Superior
144	99.83	19	9	+2.93	79	99	Very Superior
143	99.79	19	9	+2.87	79	99	Very Superior
142	99.74	18	9	+2.80	78	99	Very Superior
141	99.69	18	9	+2.73	77	99	Very Superior
140	99.62	18	9	+2.67	77	99	Very Superior
139	99.53	18	9	+2.60	76	99	Very Superior
138	99	17	9	+2.53	75	99	Very Superior
137	99	17	9	+2.47	75	99	Very Superior
136	99	17	9	+2.40	74	99	Very Superior
135	99	17	9	+2.33	73	99	Very Superior
134	99	17	9	+2.27	73	99	Very Superior
133	99	17	9	+2.20	72	99	Very Superior
132	98	16	9	+2.13	71	93	Very Superior
131	98	16	9	+2.07	71	93	Very Superior
130	98	16	9	+2.00	70	93	Very Superior
129	97	16	9	+1.93	69	90	Superior
128	97	16	9	+1.87	69	90	Superior
127	96	15	9	+1.80	68	87	Superior
126	96	15	9	+1.73	67	87	Superior
125	95	15	8	+1.67	67	85	Superior
124	95	15	8	+1.60	66	85	Superior
123	94	15	8	+1.53	65	83	Superior
122	93	14	8	+1.47	65	81	Superior
121	92	14	8	+1.40	64	80	Superior
120	91	14	8	+1.33	63	78	Superior
119	90	14	8	+1.27	63	77	High Average
118	88	14	8	+1.20	62	75	High Average
117	87	13	7	+1.13	61	74	High Average
116	86	13	7	+1.07	61	73	High Average
115	84	13	7	+1.00	60	71	High Average
114	82	13	7	+0.93	59	59	High Average
113	81	13	7	+0.87	59	68	High Average
112	79	12	7	+0.80	58	67	High Average
111	77	12	7	+0.73	57	66	High Average
110	75	12	6	+0.67	57	64	High Average

continued

Table 5.5   continued

IQ	Percentile rank	Scaled score	Stanine	Z-score	T score	NCE	Interpretive range
109	73	12	6	+0.60	56	63	Average
108	70	12	6	+0.53	55	61	Average
107	68	11	6	+0.47	55	60	Average
106	66	11	6	+0.40	54	59	Average
105	63	11	6	+0.33	53	57	Average
104	61	11	6	+0.27	53	56	Average
103	58	11	5	+0.20	52	54	Average
102	55	10	5	+0.13	51	53	Average
101	53	10	5	+0.07	51	52	Average
100	50	10	5	0.00	50	50	Average
99	47	10	5	−0.07	49	48	Average
98	45	10	5	−0.13	49	47	Average
97	42	9	5	−0.20	48	46	Average
96	39	9	5	−0.27	47	44	Average
95	37	9	4	−0.33	47	43	Average
94	34	9	4	−0.40	46	41	Average
93	32	9	4	−0.47	45	40	Average
92	30	8	4	−0.53	45	39	Average
91	27	8	4	−0.60	44	37	Average
90	25	8	4	−0.67	43	36	Average
89	23	8	4	−0.73	43	34	Low Average
88	21	8	3	−0.80	42	33	Low Average
87	19	7	3	−0.87	41	32	Low Average
86	18	7	3	−0.93	41	31	Low Average
85	16	7	3	−1.00	40	29	Low Average
84	14	7	3	−1.07	39	27	Low Average
83	13	7	3	−1.13	39	26	Low Average
82	12	6	3	−1.20	38	25	Low Average
81	10	6	2	−1.27	37	23	Low Average
80	9	6	2	−1.33	37	22	Low Average
79	8	6	2	−1.40	36	20	Borderline
78	7	6	2	−1.47	35	19	Borderline
77	6	5	2	−1.53	35	17	Borderline
76	5	5	2	−1.60	34	15	Borderline
75	5	5	2	−1.67	33	15	Borderline
74	4	5	2	−1.73	33	13	Borderline
73	4	5	2	−1.80	32	13	Borderline
72	3	4	1	−1.87	31	10	Borderline
71	3	4	1	−1.93	31	10	Borderline
70	2	4	1	−2.00	30	7	Borderline
69	2	4	1	−2.07	29	7	Very Deficient
68	2	4	1	−2.13	29	7	Very Deficient
67	1	3	1	−2.20	28	1	Very Deficient
66	1	3	1	−2.27	27	1	Very Deficient
65	1	3	1	−2.33	27	1	Very Deficient
64	1	3	1	−2.40	26	1	Very Deficient
63	1	3	1	−2.47	25	1	Very Deficient
62	1	2	1	−2.53	25	1	Very Deficient

Table 5.5   continued

IQ	Percentile rank	Scaled score	Stanine	Z-score	T score	NCE	Interpretive range
61	0.47	2	1	−2.60	24	1	Very Deficient
60	0.38	2	1	−2.67	23	1	Very Deficient
59	0.31	2	1	−2.73	23	1	Very Deficient
58	0.26	2	1	−2.80	22	1	Very Deficient
57	0.21	1	1	−2.87	21	1	Very Deficient
56	0.17	1	1	−2.93	21	1	Very Deficient
55	0.13	1	1	−3.00	20	1	Very Deficient
54	0.11	1	1	−3.07	19	1	Very Deficient
53	0.09	1	1	−3.13	19	1	Very Deficient
52	0.07	1	1	−3.20	18	1	Very Deficient
51	0.05	1	1	−3.27	17	1	Very Deficient
50	0.04	1	1	−3.33	17	1	Very Deficient
49	0.03	1	1	−3.40	16	1	Very Deficient
48	0.03	1	1	−3.47	15	1	Very Deficient
47	0.02	1	1	−3.53	15	1	Very Deficient
46	0.02	1	1	−3.60	14	1	Very Deficient
45	0.01	1	1	−3.67	13	1	Very Deficient

Note: IQ means deviation IQ, or standard score (SS) (M = 100; SD = 15); %ile rank is a Percentile Rank (P); scaled score means (M = 10; SD = 3); stanine means (M = 5; SD = 2); z-score means (M = 0; SD = 1); T score means (M = 50; SD = 10); NCE means normal-curve equivalent (M = 50; SD = 21.06).

age. His true score probably falls in the percentile rank range of 16 to 63. This performance is Low Average to Average.

It is important to note that the interpretations offered above are *statistical interpretations*. Statistical interpretation gives meaning and context to quantitative scores. Another type of interpretation that is equally valuable is called *qualitative or contextual interpretation*. In this type of interpretation, the professional counselor describes what tasks the client can and cannot do, or provides rich content descriptions to help the reader understand the nature of client developmental and clinical issues. The quality of contextual interpretations is determined primarily by the level of expertise and the theoretical or practical orientations of the professional counselor. For example, professional counselors who are expert in describing the characteristics of personality disorders and the behaviors observed in a client with such a condition may be able to provide a rich contextual description of the client's current circumstances and how the personality disorder is expressed and affects the client.

Often statistical and contextual interpretations are combined in evaluation reports. For example, when interpreting the results of a *WAIS-III* protocol, a more statistically oriented interpretation may be appropriate, supplemented by contextual comments, as in the following example:

Intellectually, Jaime currently performs in the Average to High Average range of general cognitive ability (Full Scale percentile rank = 82; percentile rank range = 75–89), as measured on the *Wechsler Adult Intelligence Scale–Third Edition*

(*WAIS-III*). Her Verbal Comprehension skills were measured to lie in the Average to High Average range (percentile rank = 82; percentile rank range = 70–90), commensurate with her Perceptual Organizational skills, which also fell in the Average to High Average range (percentile rank = 73; percentile rank range = 53–86). Because of these results, Jaime's Full Scale IQ is the best choice of anchor scores to represent her educational and intellectual potential and to determine strengths and weaknesses.

On the Verbal Comprehension subtests from the *WAIS-III,* Jaime displayed an intrapersonal strength on a task requiring social comprehension and problem solving (Comprehension subtest percentile rank = 99; Very Superior). No intrapersonal weaknesses were noted as her profile of verbal cognitive performance was well balanced. She performed in an Average to High Average capacity on tasks requiring verbal abstract reasoning (Similarities subtest percentile rank = 75), and general information (Information subtest percentile rank = 63). Her word knowledge and facility performance (Vocabulary subtest) exceeded 95% of age-mates, falling in the Superior range of performance.

On the Perceptual-Organizational subtests of the *WAIS-III,* Jaime displayed no significant strengths, but did display a significant intrapersonal weakness on a task requiring nonverbal spatial reasoning (Block Design subtest percentile rank = 25; Low Average to Average). Nonverbal spatial reasoning is usually associated with math problem solving and advanced mathematical reasoning, an area that Jaime has claimed as a challenging academic subject since her elementary years. Jaime's performance on a task of logical reasoning (Matrix Reasoning subtest percentile rank = 95) fell into the High Average to Very Superior range, while her ability to sequence socially meaningful stimuli (Picture Arrangement percentile rank = 75) and to attend to visually detailed missing elements (Picture Completion percentile rank = 75) both revealed an Average to High Average capacity.

Jaime's Working Memory Index score from the *WAIS-III* fell into the Average to High Average range (percentile rank = 73; percentile rank range = 55–84), commensurate with current ability estimates. Her performance on the Letter-Number Sequencing subtest (percentile rank = 63; Average to High Average range) was slightly less developed than her performance on the Digit Span subtest, which fell in the High Average to Very Superior range (percentile rank = 95). Both areas were better developed than her Arithmetic subtest (percentile rank = 37; Average), a traditionally poor area of achievement for Jaime. Overall, little distractibility in the auditory channel appears to exist.

Jaime's Processing Speed Index score from the *WAIS-III* fell in the Borderline to Average range (percentile rank = 18, percentile rank range = 8–42), very significantly below current ability estimates, given Jaime's Average to High Average intellectual capabilities—a 32-point discrepancy. Jaime's psychomotor speed and short-term visual memory (Coding subtest) and her speed in processing visual information (Symbol Search subtest, which does not have a memory component) both fell into the Borderline to Average range. These results are important, because distractibility frequently shows up in a client's cognitive profile as a short-term memory deficiency. As will be seen in the *WJ-III* fluency testing that follows below, Jaime displays a processing speed deficiency. In addition, these and previous assessment results documented an intra-personal weakness in short-term visual memory.

As a second example, a more contextual description can sometimes help those who will work with the client better understand the client's current situation:

Because a question arose regarding whether Ben possessed significant problems with inattention, clinical and behavioral assessments focused on the presence of age- and ability-inappropriate levels of distractibility, a primary symptom of an Attention-Deficit/Hyperactivity Disorder (AD/HD). Miss Wallace (2nd-grade teacher), and Mrs. Davis (reading teacher), educators who have instructed Ben and who are well acquainted with his academic and behavioral performance, completed the *Conners' Teacher Rating Scale—Revised, Long Version* (*CTRS-R:L*). Miss Wallace also completed the *Achenbach System of Empirically Based Assessment* (*ASEBA*) *Teacher Rating Form* (*TRF*). Mr. and Mrs. Smith completed the *Conners' Parent Rating Scale—Revised, Long Version* (*CPRS-R:L*). Mr. and Mrs. Smith and Mrs. Davis reported substantial concerns related to inattention and disorganization; Miss Wallace did not. All were in agreement that Ben displayed the following behaviors associated with inattention to a significant degree: forgets things he has already learned and has difficulty engaging in tasks requiring sustained mental effort. In addition, Mr. and Mrs. Smith and Mrs. Davis agreed that Ben frequently fails to give close attention to details and makes careless mistakes, has difficulty organizing tasks and activities, and is easily distracted by extraneous stimuli. Mrs. Smith and Mrs. Davis also agreed that Benjamin frequently does not seem to listen to what is said and has difficulty sustaining attention on tasks. Finally, Mr. and Mrs. Smith agreed that Ben does not follow through on instructions, fails to finish assigned work, and loses things necessary for tasks and activities. Each of these behaviors is a criterion for diagnosis of AD/HD—Predominantly Inattentive Type, and Ben fulfills the diagnostic criteria for this condition. All other behavioral and personality characteristics were reported to be within normal limits, although some concern over social relationships and development was expressed by Miss Wallace.

Such descriptions not only provide contextual understanding, but can aid treatment planning and outcomes evaluation.

Think About It 5.2   Why is it important to demonstrate a client's scores as a range instead of as an individual score? How would you explain this process to a client?

CRITERION-REFERENCED INTERPRETATION

As mentioned previously, norm-referenced scores compare an examinee's performance to other individuals in the norm group who share similar characteristics. *Criterion-referenced scores,* on the other hand, compare the examinee's scores against an absolute standard (i.e., criterion) of performance. In other words, this form of testing measures *levels of mastery.* As such, performance on criterion-referenced testing is often helpful in making important instructional decisions regarding the mastery of specified curriculum goals and objectives or diagnostic decisions when a certain number of criteria or level of severity is required. Criterion-referenced interpretation is often divided into two categories: *single-skill scores* and *multiple-skill scores.*

Single-Skill Scores

Single-skill scores can be obtained for almost any target measured against an established criterion. However, most single-skill targets are related to academic, occupational, or social domains. For example, an educator may score a math problem worked by a student. A vocational rehabilitation counselor may evaluate the feeding ability of an individual who recently experienced a stroke. An observer may note the number of adult instructions with which a referred child complies. Scoring can be *dichotomous* (e.g., pass-fail, right-wrong) or *continuous* (i.e., allowing partial credit for the item). In this case, each point on the continuum (e.g., never, seldom, often, always) would have to be carefully defined. In single-skill probes, raw scores are often transferred into a ratio. For example, an examinee may correctly complete 40 of 50 items on a test. Therefore, the score would be represented as 40/50.

Multiple-Skill Scores

Many activities are not comprised on single-skill units but contain multiple skills. For example, measures of oral reading involve decoding of words, fluency, knowledge of grammatical rules, and, often, comprehension of material read. Additionally, educators often obtain answers to several questions on a mathematics exam composed of varying calculations (e.g., addition, subtraction, multiplication, division) rather than an answer to one problem. Multiple-skill scores are often divided into three areas of reporting: *accuracy, retention,* and *verbal labels for percentages* (Salvia & Ysseldyke, 2004).

Accuracy

An *accuracy percentage* is obtained by dividing the number of correct responses provided by the examinee by the total number of items and then multiplying by 100. For example, a student who correctly responded to 9 out of 10 items on a test would receive a percent correct score of 90 ($9/10 \times 100 = 90\%$). Although educators often convert raw scores into this format to report student outcomes, remember that such scores are not equivalent in the same way as standard scores. A score of 90% on a mathematics test is not the same as a score of 90% on a spelling test, because the subject content is completely different and the items are presented in different formats as well. Note that the score of 90% does not allow for comparison of scores. The 90% could be the highest or lowest score in a distribution, and without access to the distribution of scores, further comparative analysis is hindered.

Retention

Retention refers to the percentage of information previously learned that is remembered at a later date. It also has been referred to as *recall, memory,* or *maintenance.* Retention is calculated by dividing the initial number of items remembered by the total number of items initially learned and then multiplying by 100. For example, an examinee may have learned 50 new words and recalled 40 of them two weeks later. This examinee's retention would be 80% ($40/50 \times 100 = 80\%$).

Percentages expressed as verbal labels

Sometimes percentages are expressed as labels. Two methods in which percentages are expressed as labels include level of performance and grades. Level of performance is often divided into two levels: *mastery level* and *instructional level* (Salvia & Ysseldyke, 2004). In many educational contexts, mastery is set at 90% or above, and nonmastery is set at any percentage below 90%.

Instructional level is further divided into *frustrational, instructional,* and *independent* levels of performance. Frustrational-level performance is usually defined as less than 85% correct. Instructional-level performance is defined as 85–95% correct. Independent-level performance is defined as above 95% correct.

Grades have also been used as verbal labels for percentages. For example, many college professors use a grading scale in which any one scoring 90–100% correct would receive a grade of an "A," anyone scoring 80–89% correct would receive a grade of a "B," and anyone scoring 59% or below would receive a grade of "F."

SOURCES OF INFORMATION ABOUT TESTS

Selection of an assessment tool is an important clinical decision and a vital part of the counseling process. The information gained from the assessment itself often serves as the foundation of counseling as it gives the professional counselor much necessary information that will aid in determining therapeutic goals and interventions and which will be a great asset in measuring progress and outcomes.

Professional counselors must carefully choose instruments that are designed to address the referral questions and which are appropriate to their levels of education and training. However, the amount of assessments available today can prove overwhelming, and many professional counselors find themselves relying on less than appropriate tools simply out of habit or lack of information. This kind of choice is not necessary given the resources available to help make an informed decision regarding assessment selection. Although there is no one source that contains every assessment tool developed, there are a variety of sources that professional counselors should

Table 5.6 Evaluation of sources of information about tests

Source type	Advantages	Disadvantages
Test manuals	Usually contain much information about theoretical basis, item development, reliability, validity, standardization, and norms. Are often the best single source.	Test authors vary in comprehensiveness and psychometric sophistication. External empirical validation of results is not available for years after publication of the manual.
Publisher catalogs	Provide current information on tests, even on new tests not found elsewhere. Give costs and ordering information.	Information may be biased. Necessary basic information is often lacking.
Test review volumes	Offer critical reviews by experts, with evaluation of weaknesses and strengths of each test.	Information is often dated. Reviews often do not include a thorough discussion of purposes of test.
Journals	Give research on issues in testing. Often show application of test. Contain validity and reliability studies.	Information is often theoretical and technical and may be dated due to publication backlog.
Textbooks	Give in-depth information on certain tests. Provide an overview of tests in general.	Information may be biased, dated, oversimplified, or technical.
Electronic sources	Give easy access to current information. Are easy to search by subject matter. Provide links to other sources.	Information may be biased or incongruent in presentation. Access to information may be difficult for some.

search on a regular basis. To help in this process, several sources are listed below (and in Table 5.6) that provide assistance in selecting and evaluating tests most suitable and technically sound.

> **Think About It 5.3**   When deciding which test to administer to a client, why would it be important to thoroughly research the test using several of the resources described in Table 5.6?

Published Resources

One of the most basic and essential assessment resources is the *Mental Measurements Yearbook* (*MMY*). First published in 1938 by Oscar K. Buros, this series of yearbooks is currently published by the Buros Institute of Mental Measurements of the University of Nebraska—Lincoln. This series of yearbooks contains thorough critiques of many commercially available instruments. Each *MMY* includes descriptive information about each test, including the purpose of the instrument, for whom the instrument is appropriate, cost, and the publisher. Additionally, the yearbooks contain critical reviews of each instrument, written by knowledgeable professionals. These reviews contain the strengths and weaknesses of the instrument.

Another resource published by the Buros Institute is *Tests in Print*, which is especially useful for quickly identifying which instruments are most appropriate for a

Table 5.7 What to include in a test critique

1. Exact name of the instrument (or technique)
2. Author (person, organization, or company)
3. Publisher
4. Copyright date(s)
    a. Date first published
    b. Date(s) of revision(s)
    c. Date of version being reviewed
5. Purpose and recommended use
6. Appropriate respondent characteristics (e.g., age, grade, reading level, mental abilities, physical characteristics)
7. Available forms
8. Current cost information
9. Content
    a. Categories assessed or measured
    b. Types of items used
    c. Type(s) of responses required
10. Administration procedures and requirements
11. Time factors and considerations
12. Administrator qualifications
13. Interpreter or user qualifications
14. Scoring options and procedures
15. Type(s) of scores derived or reported
16. Normative data
17. Validity information
18. Reliability information
19. Statistical information other than validity or reliability
20. Multicultural issues
21. Evaluation
    a. Limitations for use in counseling or student development
    b. Advantages for use in counseling or student development

particular content area or for a particular use. Once a test is located, the professional counselor can then cross-reference it with the more thorough descriptions found in the *MMY.* For information relevant to critiquing tests, see Table 5.7.

PRO-ED

While the Buros Institute has several prominent resources, PRO-ED, Inc., has useful sources for locating and evaluating tests. One, *Tests: A Comprehensive Reference for Assessments in Psychology, Education, and Business* (PRO-ED, 2003), contains more than 3,000 published tests. Each test listed includes a brief description, a statement of its purpose, and information regarding cost, scoring, and the publisher. Tests, though not reviewed, are easily accessed through the classifications and categories used to organize the resource.

For reviews and evaluations of tests, PRO-ED provides *Test Critiques,* a series of volumes containing test critiques written by measurement and assessment experts.

Each critique includes emphasis on information that will aid the professional counselor using the test, such as guidelines for administration, scoring, and interpretation. Especially helpful are the explanations of technical terms that will make the information more understandable, even to those with little testing experience.

Publisher Catalogs

Some test publishers will send catalogs upon request; others are available online. Catalogs can be especially useful for locating new tests and recent editions of previously published tests—information that sometimes cannot be found in the sources discussed above. These catalogs provide information regarding uses of the test, cost, administration time, and other brief descriptions.

Professional Journals and Textbooks

Other sources of information include professional journals and some textbooks. Journal articles often contain test reviews and may discuss the nature and use of particular tests. These articles can be most easily located through electronic databases. The professional counselor will find many journals very helpful in finding current extant research on commonly used assessments, including *Measurement and Evaluation in Counseling and Development, Educational and Psychological Measurement, Psychological Reports, Psychological Assessment,* and *Assessment for Effective Intervention.* Recently, desk references of different types of tests (e.g., *Achievement Test Desk Reference* [Flanagan, Ortiz, Alfonso, & Mascolo, 2002], *Intelligence Test Desk Reference* [McGrew & Flanagan, 1998]) have been published to assist examiners in selecting appropriate instruments. In addition, some textbooks contain appendices with lists of widely used testing instruments. However, texts such as this one mainly supply a brief overview of available instruments.

Several resources exist to help the professional counselor identify and locate appropriate assessments in an efficient manner. When searching for an instrument that will test a specific content area, *Tests* or *Tests in Print* will provide quick information that can then be further explored in the *Mental Measurements Yearbook.* When additional information is needed to help in understanding the specific mechanics of a test, *Test Critiques* may prove beneficial. Both of the latter resources provide sufficient information to weed out tests that are inappropriate or which have obvious weaknesses. Although all of the above publications provide comprehensive coverage of available tests, catalogs, journals, and textbooks can also prove useful.

Electronic Resources

Changes in technology have greatly improved access to possible assessment instruments. The Buros Institute of Mental Measurements provides test information through an electronic source, in addition to its printed version. Various search engines are available that allow viewing of a large amount of information on tests and testing. "Test Reviews Online" is a web-based service of the Buros Institute of Mental Measurements, available at www.unl.edu/buros, and makes test reviews available to individual users exactly as they appear in the *Ninth* through *Fifteenth Mental Measurements Yearbook* series. In addition, monthly updates are provided from the institute's latest test review database. For a small fee, users may download reviews for over 2,000 tests that include specifics on test purpose, population, publication date, administration time, and descriptive test evaluations.

Another service of the Buros Institute is *Tests in Print. Tests in Print (TIP)* can be accessed through the above website and serves as a comprehensive bibliography to all known commercially available tests that are currently in print in the English language. Now in its sixth edition, *TIP* provides vital information to users, including test purpose, test publisher, in-print status, price, test acronym, intended test population, administration times, publication date(s), and test author(s). *TIP* also guides readers to critical, candid test reviews published in the *Mental Measurements Yearbook* series.

The Educational Testing Service (ETS) offers an electronic source for its test collection as well. The ETS Test Collection includes an extensive library of 20,000 tests and other measurement devices from the early 1900s to the present. The collection is advertised as the largest in the world and was established to make information on standardized tests and research instruments available to researchers, graduate students, and teachers. The ETS database can be accessed at www.ets.org/testcoll. From there, one can search by topic for instruments with each result providing descriptive information. Orders can also be placed at this site.

PRO-ED has a useful source for locating and evaluating tests at www.proedinc.com/store/index.php. Through PRO-ED's online catalog products, available assessments can be located by a topic, title, or author name search. This search will give results with brief descriptions of each test, including price of test, materials included in each testing kit, and an option to place an order.

Finally, another valuable electronic source can be found at http://aace.ncat.edu. This website is the home page of the Association for Assessment in Counseling and Education, a division of the American Counseling Association. Through AACE's "resources" option, professional counselors can find invaluable links to the ERIC test locator, some test reviews, assessment journals, and key documents such as *Ethics in Assessment, Standards for Qualifications of Test Users,* and *Rights and Responsibilities of Test Takers: Guidelines and Expectations.*

COMMON ERRORS

Regardless of level of training or expertise, professional counselors are human and are therefore susceptible to committing errors during the testing process. In interpreting assessment instruments, professional counselors sometimes may commit inference and attribution errors. Although the assessments provide basic information about the client, the professional counselor must then sort the information and formulate overall conclusions and implications. While much is known about how to develop and evaluate psychological tests, much less is known about how to use the information generated. By familiarizing the professional counselor with common errors, it is hoped that these errors will be minimized in test interpretation and decision making.

The tendency to seek *confirmatory evidence* (confirmatory bias) is one of the most common mistakes in test interpretation. Humans are prone to self-confirmation and often search for confirmatory information. In other words, one often believes what one wants to believe. Research supports this claim and shows that the human tendency is to search out and attend only to evidence that conforms to one's hypothesis. Though professional counselors have been trained to attend to all information in clinical decision making, they are just as prone to attend to narrow paths of evidence. Because of this tendency, professional counselors often conclude what they already suspect. This process of searching for confirmation can lead to inaccurate conclusions and may lead to an increased confidence in one's conclusions and abilities. Some evidence suggests that beginning counselors are particularly subject to confirmatory bias, thinking they understand the problem before they really do and, thus, working on the wrong problem.

A second error commonly made is the *tendency to see patterns* where no patterns actually exist. Because humans strive for predictability in life, we are prone to attribute order to ambiguous information. This tendency can have implications in test interpretation, as themes and patterns may be said to exist where none have actually emerged.

Finally, the use of *preconceived biases* is a form of error commonly found in test interpretation. Primarily, there is a tendency to *overpathologize* clients. Professional counselors are prone to search for information indicative of pathology and then interpret this information in a way that indicates more pathology than may actually exist. This tendency is exaggerated when the client is from a lower social class, nonwhite, disabled, or female.

Professional counselors must be aware of these common errors throughout the assessment process, as inaccurate decisions regarding clients can be easily made. The use of quality information provided in psychological assessments is not enough to remedy the errors involved in the interpretation process. Given these concerns, the following recommendations are provided:

- Do not confuse the ability to explain current data with the ability to predict future performance.
- Continue to assess skills over time instead of relying on one evaluation of the examinee's performance.
- Collect data from multiple sources. Do not rely solely on self-report or observation of one informant.
- Consider all other possibilities, and rule out alternative hypotheses.
- Choose the highest quality and most appropriate assessment instruments.
- Recognize personal biases, especially those pertaining to age, gender, class, and ethnicity.
- Be aware of the norms used during test construction, as well as the differences between the client and the norm group used.

As humans, professional counselors must continually strive to overcome any potential biases or attribution errors that may affect their decisions regarding client performance. While psychological tests improve the accuracy of decision making, care must still be taken in their interpretation and application.

SUMMARY/CONCLUSION

Testing involves administering questions to an individual or individuals in order to obtain a score. Assessment differs from testing in that it includes such processes as interviewing, records review, observations, rating scales, standardized testing, and many other provisions that create a larger process. When administering tests, take into account the test qualifications specified by the test's manual. Also, professional counselors should ensure that examinees are prepared and familiar with the procedures and process of testing before beginning testing.

The testing environment is a very important aspect to consider when one wishes to obtain accurate results. One should always try to strictly follow time specifications, directions, registration and identification procedures, and any other procedural guidelines laid out by the test's manual. If any deviation from the specified procedures occurs during testing, it should be thoroughly documented by the examiner.

Many factors can affect test scores. First, the examiner-examinee relationship should be one that is neutral. Reinforcement or negativity during testing can greatly affect scores. Professional counselors should always take into account individual differences when administering tests and interpreting scores. Furthermore, expectancy of the examiner can affect test scores.

Scoring a test can allow quantification of scores and aid in interpretation. Several formats for scoring tests exist. Tests can be self-scored, scored by others, or scored by computers. While computer scoring is the most accurate form of scoring, computers are often incapable of making the judgments required for test interpretation.

Norm-referenced interpretation involves comparing the obtained score of the examinee to the norm group. These scores can be expressed in developmental equivalents such as age equivalents, which compare the examinee to others of the same age, and grade equivalents, which compare the examinee to others of the same grade level. There are many problems with making comparisons like those made in developmental equivalents, and interpretation should be done with care. In order to interpret developmental equivalents, the test interpreter compares the examinee's chronological and mental age to obtain a developmental quotient.

Scores on the same test for several different examinees of different ages can be compared by using scores of relative standing. Common types of scores of relative standing are standard scores, which have a designated mean and standard deviation. T scores, z-scores, deviation IQs, normal-curve equivalents, and stanines are common types of standard scores.

Criterion-referenced scores compare the examinee's scores against an absolute standard (i.e., criterion) of performance. Types of criterion-referenced scores include single-skill scores, which assess a solitary academic, occupational, or social domain, and multiple-skill scores, which measure any area that is compowsed of several skills. Multiple-skill scores can be reported by expressing accuracy, retention, verbal labels for percentages, and instructional-level scores.

There are many available sources of information on tests, test administration, test scoring, and psychometric properties of tests. The chapter covers in detail the many published sources of this information and electronic information.

Lastly, professional counselors should take into account sources of error in testing and assessment. First, although professional counselors are trained to take all sources of information into account, they often make mistakes. Such mistakes include overpathologizing clients, seeking to confirm their hypotheses with more evidence, and recognizing patterns that may not actually be present. The chapter includes a series of steps and precautions to avoid this type and other types of error.

KEY TERMS

developmental equivalent
deviation IQ
normal-curve equivalent
percentage
percentile rank
raw score
scores of relative standing

standardization sample
standard score
stanine
test score
T score
z-score

CHAPTER 6

How Tests Are Constructed

by Carl J. Sheperis, Carey Davis, and R. Anthony Doggett

his chapter provides readers with preliminary information related to the construction and evaluation of psychological and educational tests, including: the purposes of tests; observables; item generation (multiple-choice, essay, true-false); technical analysis (item difficulty, item discrimination); and norms. The chapter also addresses the process of building quality tests that are aimed toward promoting valid score interpretation, and how to evaluate the use of a specific test for a specific purpose. Finally, the chapter reviews the fundamentals of test development, how to choose among already existing tests for a specific purpose, how to use the results of standardized tests to help make decisions about individuals, and how to identify flaws in assessment instruments and procedures.

Many of you reading this book may be highlighting or underlining certain words or phrases to help yourself remember key information you might encounter on the next exam. As you study for that exam, you might also want to ask the instructor some questions to help yourself prepare. First, you might ask the purpose of the test (e.g., the objectives of the test, the way it will be scored, and how the results will affect your final grade). Next, you might ask what content the test will cover (e.g., the chapters to be covered on the test and whether the questions will require memorization of facts or application of knowledge). Finally, you might ask what the format of the test items will be (e.g., multiple-choice, short-answer, essay).

When instructors are constructing a test, they, consciously or unconsciously, will be asking and answering similar questions: "What is the purpose of the test?" "How do I assess the content to be covered by the test?" and "How should I write the items on the test?" Similarly, identifying the *purpose of a test, observables related to the test, item generation procedures,* and *test format* are critical components of any test construction process, whether the test is a simple one to be used in an elementary school classroom, an examination for a graduate-level course, or a published psychological assessment instrument. However, appropriate test construction does not stop when items are developed. Development of a quality test requires appropriate statistical analyses to determine *item difficulty* and *item discrimination*. Some tests, such as published psychological instruments, also use *norms* to help test users interpret test results. Each of the above concepts related to test development is discussed throughout this chapter. The brief introduction to this material given in this chapter, however, will not provide adequate guidance to become a seasoned test developer; those interested in learning more about test construction should see Crocker and Algina (1986).

PURPOSE OF THE TEST

The first step in test construction is to define the general **purpose** of the test. The instructor probably defined the general purpose of your next test on your syllabus (e.g., the test may assess class members' knowledge of the information from Chapters 1 through 6 of this textbook and be worth 40% of your final grade in the course). Although the general purpose of a published test must be more formally defined than that of your next classroom exam, the basic principles are the same. Test development addresses the **population** taking the instrument (i.e., the members of the class) and the **content** of the test (i.e., knowledge of Chapters 1 through 6).

Although course-related tests provide a very basic example of test construction, for a standardized test, the content of the test and the theory on which the test is based may be considerably more complex. There are many questions related to test purpose that the instructor does not necessarily need to consider when writing a course-related test—questions that are, however, crucial in constructing many other types of standardized tests. Test developers must consider such issues as whether a test will be norm referenced or criterion referenced, what objectives will be measured, how items and scores will be scaled, and what approach to test construction will be used. Cohen and Swerdlik (1999, pp. 216–218) suggested that test developers need to consider at least the following 14 questions prior to developing a test:

1. What is the test designed to measure?
2. What is the objective of the test?
3. Is there a need for this test?
4. Who will use this test?
5. Who will take this test?
6. What content will the test cover?
7. How will the test be administered?
8. What is the ideal format of the test?
9. Should more than one form of the test be developed?
10. What special training will be required of test users for administering or interpreting the test?
11. What types of responses will be required by test takers?
12. Who benefits from the results of this test?

13. Is there any potential for harm from administration of this test?
14. How will meaning be attributed to scores on this test?

In addition, the question "How does the test address multicultural/diverse populations?" must be asked.

Examinees

For several reasons, it is important to define who will be in the normative sample when constructing a test. First, the **age range** of the test takers will be a factor in determining the content and how that content will be assessed. Also, the **reading ability** of the test takers will affect the way the items are written and whether the test will be presented in written or oral form. Additionally, the cultural backgrounds of examinees may influence the items that are included on the test and the way items are presented. Finally, it is important to identify who needs to take the test and/or who would want to take it (Cohen & Swerdlik, 1999).

Goals and Theory

The goals of any test are inherently based on a **theory**. For example, a typical classroom test is probably based on the theory that if the examinee is able to answer a certain percentage of questions correctly, the examinee is competent in knowledge of the course content. In this case, knowledge of course content is theoretically related to test performance. Standardized tests are often more complex, because test developers writing an intelligence test would first have to choose a theory of intelligence on which to base the instrument. Likewise, test developers writing a personality test would have to define the aspects of personality the test would purport to measure. The theory on which a test is based links the content of the test to the constructs, characteristics, or attributes that the test is designed to measure.

Norm Referenced or Criterion Referenced

Once the theory that underlies the purpose of the test has been clarified, the next step in the test construction process is to decide whether a test should be **norm referenced** or **criterion referenced**. A *norm-referenced test* is one in which an individual's score is interpreted by comparing it with other individuals' scores (i.e., a normative sample); a *criterion-referenced test* is one in which an individual's score is interpreted in terms of a predetermined criterion of demonstrated skills (i.e., objectives) (Mehrens & Lehmann, 1991). A test developer's decision about whether a test should be norm referenced or criterion referenced must be based on the purpose or goal of the test (Hopkins, 1996). For example, if a test is designed to assist employers in choosing from a large pool of potential employees, its goal should be to make comparisons among the candidates; therefore, a norm-referenced test would be appropriate. On the other hand, if the purpose of a test is to help a teacher determine whether individual students have mastered certain instructional objectives in order to identify the ones who need additional tutoring in specific areas, a criterion-referenced test would be beneficial because it would yield information about the areas in which the students needed help instead of just comparing the students to each another (as a norm-referenced test would do). There are times when a test may be both norm referenced and criterion referenced. When you take your next test, your instructor will probably give you a grade based on a predetermined criterion, such as the number of questions you must answer correctly in order to pass the test. Such a grade would indicate that the test is to be criterion referenced. However, if your instructor gives you information about the class average on the test, enabling you to compare your score to the scores of your classmates, the test could become not only a criterion-referenced test but also a very simple norm-referenced test.

Objectives

Test developers who write criterion-referenced tests must carefully consider **objectives** when writing their tests. The terms *objectives* and *goals* may easily be confused, but in this discussion, the *objectives* refer specifically to instructional objectives measured by criterion-referenced tests, whereas *goals* have a broader reference, applying to many types of tests. For example, when instructors write a class test (which is very likely to be an informal criterion-referenced test), they look at the objectives listed on the syllabus and write the test so that it measures those objectives; the goals of the test are much broader—primarily to determine whether students have mastered course content well enough to pass the course. When considering the objectives to be tested, test developers must take several factors into account. First, the specificity of the objectives will affect the way the test items are written (Hopkins, 1996). Also, Hopkins contended that tests that measure educational objectives must define these objectives in terms of "Bloom's taxonomy," which categorizes objectives into six hierarchical levels: knowledge, comprehension, application, analysis, synthesis, and evaluation. Objectives are important to consider in criterion-referenced tests, but not all tests measure objectives. For example, a personality test does not measure whether an individual has attained mastery of a certain personality type; instead, it measures a person's personality type. Many norm-referenced tests do not measure whether individuals meet certain objectives.

Scaling

Another issue that test developers must consider is **scaling**, which is "the process by which a measuring device is designed and calibrated, and the way numbers (or other indices)—scale values—are assigned to different amounts of the trait, attribute, or characteristic being measured" (Cohen & Swerdlik, 1999, p. 219). In other words, scaling is basically attaching numbers to the construct that the test is theorized to measure. There are cases in which scaling is fairly simple. On your next test, each question will probably be assigned a point value, and your score will reflect the number of questions you answer correctly. The example of your next test represents a **summative scale**, in which correct responses are added together (summed) to calculate the final score.

The example of the scaling for your next test is fairly straightforward; however, scaling can be an extremely complicated process. Scales may be defined in several different ways. For example, scales may be defined by whether they are *nominal, ordinal, interval,* or *ratio.* Scales may also be defined by whether they are *rating scales* or *comparative scales* or by whether they are *unidimensional* or *multidimensional.* For example, some tests use rating scales, which require examinees to rate test items (i.e., "On a scale of 1 to 10, with 1 being poor and 10 being excellent, rate the service you received from your waiter"). On some tests that use such rating scales, the ratings are summed for the final score; therefore, they are summative tests (Cohen & Swerdlik, 1999). Rating scales may take many forms. In some instances, true-false tests may be considered rating scales (i.e., "I felt depressed this morning. Circle one: True/False), or rating scales may be written as a series of faces—such as a sad face, a medium face, and a happy face—that examinees should circle. A very popular type of rating scale is the *Likert scale,* which allows examinees to choose from a continuum of five responses, usually with Agree or Approve on one end of the continuum and Disagree or Disapprove on the other end. *Comparative scales* are somewhat similar to rating scales. When comparative scales are used, an examinee might be given items to sort or rank in a certain order (i.e., from most to least appealing, or from worst to best).

Another way of defining a scale is whether it is unidimensional or multidimensional. *Unidimensional scales* are those in which numbers are assigned only to one dimension; *multidimensional scales* are those in which several different dimensions may underlie the examinee's responses (Cohen & Swerdlik, 1999). For example, if a response to a test item may be interpreted in many different ways, it is likely that the item is part of a multidimensional scale. All of the scales mentioned to this point yield ordinal scores.

Two other types of scales are the Guttman scale and the Thurstone scale. The *Guttman scale* is an ordinal scaling method in which items are arranged to form a hierarchy, so that an examinee who agrees with or confirms one item on the hierarchy also agrees with or confirms the items lower than that item on the hierarchy but disagrees with or disconfirms the items higher than that item on the hierarchy. The Guttman scale is also called the *deterministic* or *monotone model.* Thorndike (2005, p. 393) gave the following example of a Guttman scale:

1. Abortion should be available to any woman who wishes one.
2. Abortion should be legal if a doctor recommends it.
3. Abortions should be legal whenever the pregnancy is the result of rape or incest.
4. Abortion should be legal whenever the health or well-being of the mother is endangered.
5. Abortion should be legal only when the life of the mother is endangered.

Such a graduated scale presumes that a respondent selecting response choice 1 also agrees with the conditions listed in choices 2 through 5. Conversely, an individual selecting choice 5 would be presumed to not agree with choices 1 through 4.

The *Thurstone scale* is a scaling method that yields interval data (Cohen & Swerdlik, 1999). In this method, items are rated by a group of judges, and means and standard deviations of the judges' ratings are calculated for all of the items.

Then, items on which most judges agreed (or items with low standard deviations) are included in the test. Finally, the examinee rates the items, and the examinee's score is determined by the judges' ratings of the items the individual selects. The Thurstone scale is also called the *probability* or *nonmonotone model* or the *equal-appearing interval model*. The type of scale that is used in a test should be selected according to the variables being measured and the examinees for whom the test is intended.

Approaches to Test Construction

After a test developer has defined the general purpose of the test, identified the examinees who are to take the test, described the theory on which the test is based, decided whether the test will be norm referenced or criterion referenced, outlined the objectives that will be measured, and selected a scaling method, the developer must choose an approach to test construction. Approaches to test construction can be divided into three basic categories: the rational approach, the empirical approach, and the bootstrap approach (Janda, 1998).

Test developers who choose the **rational approach** rely on reason and logic to create items instead of relying on collecting data for statistical analysis when constructing items (Janda, 1998). The rational approach is also called the *theoretical approach* because the test developers are theorizing that the items are related to the constructs they are attempting to measure (Hansen, 1999). Your instructor will probably use the rational approach when constructing your next test. In contrast, test developers who choose the **empirical approach** rely on data collection to identify items that relate to the construct they are attempting to measure. In this approach, items are developed randomly, and whether items are used is based on the data gathered when the items are administered to a pool of examinees participating in the test construction process (Janda, 1998). Two different methods used in the empirical approach are the *method of contrast groups* (in which items are examined based on the different responses of two or more groups of people who are selected because of certain characteristics that each group has in common) and the *method of item clustering* (in which factor analysis is used to identify which items correlate with one another) (Lichtenberg, 1999). The **bootstrap approach** is a combination of the rational approach and the empirical approach in that items are written based on a theory (instead of randomly), and then empirical procedures are used to verify that the items actually measure the construct they are theorized to measure (Janda, 1998). Another name for the bootstrap approach is the *sequential method* (Lichtenberg, 1999).

A Test Development Example

The reader now has a basic understanding of many of the decisions that a test developer must consider in order to thoroughly delineate the purpose of the test. General examples of the concepts have been provided, but a more specific example may give a clearer picture of this crucial step in the test construction process. The *Black Adolescent Racial Identity Scale* (*BARIS*) (see Figure 6.1) constructed by Sheperis (2001) serves as an example demonstrating the development of a test purpose.

BARIS

Instructions: Each item may or may not be true for you. To the right of each item is a set of choices that describes how you think about the item. Select one of the choices by circling the number below it:

Strongly Agree	Agree	Disagree	Strongly Disagree
4	3	2	1

Please answer every item, and make only one choice per item. There are no right or wrong answers. If a question does not seem to apply to you, imagine a time that it might and answer the question based on your thought.

Sample Question:	Strongly Agree	Agree	Disagree	Strongly Disagree
A. I like pizza.	4	3	2	1

Queston:	Strongly Agree	Agree	Disagree	Strongly Disagree
1. It is important to take part in Black activities.	4	3	2	1
2. Whites get more chances in life.	4	3	2	1
3. It is good to be around Blacks and other races.	4	3	2	1
4. Whites are more trustworthy than Blacks.	4	3	2	1
5. It is easier to get along with Black people.	4	3	2	1
6. People should be proud of their race.	4	3	2	1
7. Teenagers should only date people from the same race.	4	3	2	1
8. People from all races have good things about them.	4	3	2	1
9. It is good to get along with all kinds of people.	4	3	2	1
10. Children should know what it means to be Black.	4	3	2	1
11. White counselors are better than Black counselors.	4	3	2	1
12. It is good to do things with people from all types of backgrounds.	4	3	2	1
13. It is OK to date somebody from another race.	4	3	2	1
14. White friends are better than Black friends.	4	3	2	1
15. People from all races should get along.	4	3	2	1
16. It's OK for Whites and Blacks to mix.	4	3	2	1
17. Black counselors understand kids better than White counselors.	4	3	2	1
18. It is better to have lighter skin.	4	3	2	1
19. Whites have nicer hair than Blacks.	4	3	2	1
20. It is important to belong to a Black church.	4	3	2	1
21. It is good to learn about the race and background of others.	4	3	2	1
22. It is better to be more like Whites.	4	3	2	1

Figure 6.1   *The Black Adolescent Racial Identity Scale (BARIS)*

Sheperis (2001) created the *BARIS* "to measure racial identity development (RID) in Black adolescent males" (p. vii). This statement outlines the general purpose of the test, including the theory basis for the goals of the test and the examinees for whom the test is designed. Rather than simply creating a test to measure racial identity development, Sheperis constructed the test for the ultimate goal of using the information from the test to provide effective counseling programs for Black adolescent males who are involved in the juvenile justice system. The implicit theory that the test is based upon is twofold. First, the theory is that racial identity development occurs in measurable statuses (defined by Sheperis) for the purposes of the test as assimilation, self-segregation, and universal acceptance. Additionally, the theory is that knowledge of the racial identity development of Black adolescent males would lead to more effective counseling programs. As noted previously, the examinees are identified as Black adolescent males.

The next step that Sheperis (2001) had to consider when constructing the *BARIS* was whether the test would be criterion referenced or norm referenced. Because the purpose of the test is to compare characteristics of individuals (characteristics indicating individuals' status of racial identity development) within a specified group (Black adolescent males), a norm-referenced test was an appropriate choice for the *BARIS*. As such, Sheperis did not need to consider specific criteria or objectives that the test would measure. However, he did need to consider the way he would go about measuring the different statuses of racial identity development, but this is somewhat different from defining objectives and is discussed in the next section.

The next question that Sheperis (2001) had to consider was the question of the scaling method he would use for the *BARIS*. He selected a 4-point scale. Individual items were designed to reflect the different statuses of racial identity, and response scores were summed to yield raw scores for each of the three statuses. Thus the scaling method was a summative rating scale.

The final consideration that Sheperis (2001) had to take into account when defining the purpose of the *BARIS* was the approach to test construction that he would use. He used the bootstrap approach, or sequential model, which is a combination of the rational approach and the empirical approach. He wrote items based on the theory of racial identity development after careful study of other measures of racial identity development and then identified the items to include in the test through empirical methods. An overview of the *BARIS* is provided in Box 6.1.

OBSERVABLES

Now that the purpose of the next course exam is known (including more information than you ever expected to be related to the purpose of any test), you may wonder what content the test will cover. Of course, you know the goals of the test and the instructional objectives that need to be mastered, but to really prepare for the test, you need to know exactly how the instructor is going to go about measuring whether students have met the objectives—for example, whether the test questions will require application of knowledge through scenarios or simply straightforward answers directly from this textbook.

The instructor's decision about how to assess the content to be covered by the course exam is a question of observables. **Observables** are the specific variables and behaviors that are observable aspects of the construct stemming from the implicit theory. In terms of the course exam, the implicit theory is that test performance is

Box 6.1   Overview of the BARIS

The *Black Adolescent Racial Identity Scale* (*BARIS*) was developed in several phases. Initial items for the *BARIS* were generated through a review of existing racial identity development (RID) scales and with attention to the tri-status model of racial identity development. The initial version of the *BARIS,* which was subjected to expert review, contained 59 items related to three RID statuses: assimilation, self-segregation, and universal acceptance. In the initial phase of this study, 327 participants from Mississippi school districts completed the *BARIS* and a feedback form. A factor analysis was used to identify the initial factor structure of the initial *BARIS* version. Based on the respective factor loadings on the three *BARIS* factors (i.e., assimilation, self-segregation, and universal acceptance), 37 items were eliminated from the initial instrument, leaving the 22 items comprising the final version of the *BARIS.*

In an attempt to establish the concurrent and divergent validity (discussed in Chapter 4) of the *BARIS,* a second phase of the study was conducted in which the *BARIS* was administered to 126 Black adolescent males from juvenile offender programs in Mississippi, Florida, and Pennsylvania. One of three additional RID instruments was administered to subgroups of 25 participants along with the *BARIS.* The instruments included in this phase of the study were the *Racial Identity Attitude Scale,* the *Multigroup Ethnic Identity Measure* (*MEIM),* and the *Adolescent Survey of Black Life.*

In order to establish a reliability estimate, Cronbach's *alpha* (discussed in Chapter 3) was computed for *BARIS* scores from the second phase of the study. Demographic information related to age, racial designation, socioeconomic status (SES), arrests, and involvement in the juvenile justice system was collected from participants in the second phase of the study. The results of this study showed statistically significant differences in scores based on demographic characteristics. With regard to concurrent validity, two statistically significant correlations emerged from the analysis. Evidence of divergent validity was demonstrated by the lack of statistically significant correlations between the *BARIS* Assimilation and Universal factor scores and all scales of the *MEIM.*

related to knowledge of course content. The answers given to the questions that the instructor chooses to ask on the test are the specific behaviors the instructor will observe to determine whether students have mastered the course content.

Defining Observables

Test developers should use several steps to specify observables. First, they must *define the content and skills to be measured* by the test. This step is similar to defining objectives for a criterion-referenced test; however, it applies to other types of tests as well. In a criterion-referenced test, the objectives may also serve as the content of the test.

In other types of tests, the content or skills to be measured are more difficult to define and are usually guided by the theory on which the test is based. Next, test developers must *describe traits or characteristics* related to the content domain in behavioral terms. That is, they must decide what behaviors indicate that a person has certain traits or characteristics and describe the way in which they will measure those behaviors. For example, when constructing a course exam, the instructor will probably identify the behavior of answering questions as an indicator that students have the trait of being knowledgeable of the course content; however, answering questions is only one example of a behavior that a test developer can choose to measure. A physical education instructor would probably not choose answering questions as the behavior to measure whether the students were physically fit. Instead, the instructor might choose and describe several physical tasks for the students to perform to indicate their level of physical fitness. Finally, the test developer may need to *perform a job analysis,* breaking the behavior chosen for observation into its smaller required tasks and skills. For example, the instructor should recognize the tasks students must complete to answer the questions on the next course exam (i.e., comprehending each question, recalling the information gained in class and from the textbook, synthesizing that information to decide on a response, planning the response, and writing a response using correct grammar and readable handwriting). By breaking the job of answering the questions into its smaller parts, the instructor can better understand student responses and how they reflect knowledge of the course content.

An Example of Observables

Using the *BARIS* as an example, Sheperis (2001) defined the observables of the test through the following steps: First, he identified the content domain through consideration of the theory of racial identity development and a thorough review of other tests that have purported to measure racial identity development. The content areas he chose to measure were assimilation, self-segregation, and universal acceptance. Next, he defined the traits associated with the identified content areas in behavioral terms. In this step, Sheperis (2001) classified statements of beliefs about race into the different categories that were defined by the content areas. He identified examinee behaviors as agreeing or disagreeing with the belief statements through their responses on a Likert scale. Thus, responding to the test items became the observable behavior Sheperis used to measure examinees' status in racial identity development. Because of the nature of the *BARIS,* Sheperis did not conduct a job analysis of the test items but did conduct a factor analysis.

ITEM GENERATION

Now you know that the questions your instructor is going to ask you on your next test are essentially observables. So, if the test items themselves are really small observable behaviors that the instructor is choosing to determine whether students have adequate knowledge of the course content, it follows that the instructor will probably give a great deal of attention to writing the **items** themselves. Likewise, students will have many questions about the test items when preparing to study for the test.

Students will probably ask how many items will be on the test and what percentages of the test will cover the different content areas included on the test. Students may also ask what the item format will be. These are questions that all test developers must answer when generating test items. They must give special consideration to the number of items to devote to certain topics or areas and the format of the test items.

Allocating Proportionate Numbers of Items

As you know, answers to test items are samples of behavior. It is important to keep the word *samples* in mind. In most instances, it would be virtually impossible for a test to thoroughly measure all aspects of a content area or construct for the simple reason that it would be far too time consuming. Therefore, items must be chosen to provide a representative sample of the behaviors that are included in the content area or construct that the test purports to measure (Hopkins, 1996). Furthermore, it is crucial that the proportion of test items devoted to each topic or area covered by the test reflects the importance of each of the individual areas being measured.

Selecting an Item Format

After test developers have decided what proportions of the test will be devoted to different topics or areas, they must select the format of the items. There are many **item formats** from which to choose, including the free-response format, the multiple-choice format, the true-false format, the Likert scale format, and many others. The format selected depends on what the examiner wants to know and provides a useful method for getting that information. If the test itself is well constructed, there is no technical advantage in using any one particular format for the items; however, test developers should choose an item format based on their own preferences, the setting in which the test will be used (Janda, 1998), and the type of information needed. Additionally, when choosing a format, test developers should be aware of the advantages and disadvantages associated with different item formats. For example, although in some instances multiple-choice formats may not be well suited to measure a broad cognitive range, multiple-choice tests are easy to score and quick to administer. Free-response formats may provide test administrators with more information about the examinees' thought processes, but tests using this format are more difficult to score and more expensive to administer (Martinez, 1999).

Descriptions of Item Formats

Item formats may be very simple, or they may be quite complex. The simplest format is the **dichotomous format**, in which examinees are given two alternatives they must choose between in order to respond to each item. (Note: A true-false item is a dichotomous test item because the examinee must choose from two possible responses—true or false.) Dichotomous formats are used not only for achievement tests but also for personality tests (Whiston, 2005). Some advantages of the dichotomous format are the ease with which tests in this format can be administered and scored and the fact that the examinees must use absolute judgment or decisiveness in choosing between the responses rather than being uncertain or vague. A major disadvantage of the dichotomous format when applied to an educational achievement test is that examinees have a 50% chance of getting an item correct, and it may be difficult to determine whether examinees are merely guessing.

Another relatively simple item format is the **polytomous format**. The polytomous format is much like the dichotomous format except that the examinee is given more than two response choices. (Multiple-choice items and matching items are items written in a polytomous format.) Advantages of tests that use the polytomous format include ease of administering and scoring. Also, compared with the dichotomous format, it is less likely that an examinee will get a correct answer by guessing on an item written in the polytomous format. The polytomous and dichotomous formats are used for all types of tests and are sometimes referred to collectively as the *selected-response format* (Cohen & Swerdlik, 1999).

Both the dichotomous format and the polytomous format are item formats that an instructor may use on your next test because they are well suited to achievement tests. An item format that the instructor is not likely to use is the *Likert format*, described earlier in this chapter, because it also represents a scaling method. As you remember, the Likert format requires examinees to indicate whether or not they agree with a statement or question by selecting from five choices that represent a continuum from Agree to Disagree. The Likert format is often used for personality, attitude, career, and aptitude tests (Whiston, 2005).

Another item format available to test developers is the *category format*. This format is very similar to the Likert format in that examinees are asked to rate items; however, examinees are given more choices for an item written in the category format than they are given for an item written in the Likert format. For example, instead of having 5 choices representing the continuum, examinees may have 10 choices (give or take a few). Giving examinees more choices along a continuum allows them to make finer distinctions in their ratings of the items (Whiston, 2005).

Two other item formats that are sometimes used in personality tests are the checklist format and the Q-sort format. The *checklist format* requires examinees to read through a list of words or statements and check the ones that describe themselves or their opinions, beliefs, or attitudes. Effectively, there are two possible responses an examinee may choose for each item: checked (applies to examinee) or not-checked (does not apply) (Whiston, 2005). The *Q-sort format* allows examinees to describe themselves or others. Examinees are given statements and asked to sort them into a specified number of piles (e.g., nine) to indicate the degree to which they apply to the person they are describing. Examinees would place statements that did not apply in pile 1 and statements that definitely applied in pile 9.

A final item format test developers may choose to use is the *constructed-response format* (also called the *free-response format*) (Janda, 1998), which requires examinees to construct their own responses instead of choosing from a selection of responses. There are three types of constructed-response items: the completion item, the short-answer question, and the essay question (Cohen & Swerdlik, 1999). The *completion item* requires an examinee to respond by supplying a word or phrase to complete a sentence. You may know completion items as fill-in-the-blank items. The *short-answer question* requires examinees to respond by writing a short answer to a question (probably no longer than a paragraph and possibly as short as a single word). The *essay question* also requires an examinee to write an answer to a question; however, in most cases, the answer should be longer than a paragraph (Cohen & Swerdlik, 1999). The constructed-response format is often used for items on tests like a course exam. The advantages of using this type of format include the possibility of assessing examinees' understanding of course content on a deeper level than the level that may be assessed by other item formats. Disadvantages include difficulty in scoring and the length of time examinees may take to answer short-answer and essay questions.

> **Think About It 6.1**   What type of test item format would be the most effective to measure your ability to understand the information in this chapter. What types of item formats do you prefer? What types do you dislike? Why?

An Example of Item Generation

When Sheperis (2001) was generating the items for the *BARIS,* he first had to determine how many items to devote to each of the three statuses of racial identity development that the test was intended to measure (assimilation, self-segregation, and universal acceptance). He chose the proportion of items that would apply to each status. The number of items applying to each status is roughly equivalent, and any differences in proportion are accounted for in the scoring procedures.

The next decision Sheperis (2001) had to make was which item format he would use. Although the dichotomous format is often used in personality and attitude assessments, Sheperis chose the Likert format, which gave examinees more latitude to describe their beliefs than the dichotomous format would have. The dichotomous format would have allowed examinees only to agree or disagree.

TECHNICAL ANALYSES

Many counseling students will take a comprehensive exam prior to graduation. Today many counseling programs use a standardized exam developed by the Center for Credentialing and Education (CCE; www.cce-global.org), called the *Counselor Preparation Comprehension Examination (CPCE)*. Part of the reason for adopting a standardized exam is the difficulty involved in developing appropriate items from semester to semester. It is much easier and less expensive for university counseling program faculty to use a published instrument than to develop a quality comprehensive exam on their own. Developing good items for a test requires the test author to evaluate each item in a number of ways. This process of evaluation is typically referred to as **item analysis** and involves an examination of item difficulty and item discrimination. Item analysis involves a variety of statistical techniques, and the process can be quite complex. Only a cursory overview of the process is presented here. Readers interested in a more in-depth discussion of item analysis are referred to Anastasi & Urbina (1997).

Item Difficulty

When preparing for a "comprehensive exam," it is important to recognize that students probably won't answer all of the items correctly. These types of exams are usually criterion exams and are based on an examination of minimal competency in relation to a criterion rather than on competition among examinees. Some of the items will be difficult for most examinees to answer. So why not make the questions easier? Let's assume that all examinees pass the comprehensive exam with flying colors. This would indicate that each student has met the minimum criterion for knowledge of practice in counseling. However, because the test items did not discriminate among examinees, it would be difficult, if not impossible, to make this assertion. Thus some students who did not possess adequate knowledge of the profession would be granted degrees. Because a main ethical principal is to "do no harm," creating a test that everyone could pass would be highly unethical. Conversely, if one created a comprehensive exam that no one could pass, then it would still fail to discriminate among students. Professors would also have a large number of disgruntled students to manage. Thus the task of item development is complex.

Item difficulty is a central issue in the technical analysis of a test; especially measures of achievement or ability. **Item difficulty** is defined in terms of the number of examinees who answer an item correctly. Thus, if 50% of the participants answer a particular item correctly, that item has an item difficulty index of 0.50. Would this be a good item? Is it difficult enough? The essence of item difficulty analysis is to determine the degree to which an examinee could correctly answer an item by chance alone. If the item with a 0.50 difficulty index is a true-false question, the examinee would have a 50% likelihood of getting the right answer by chance. Although as a student you might like these odds, the truth is that the item would not discriminate adequately between those who truly knew the answer and those who did not.

So how does one set an appropriate discrimination index and make sure that each item meets this index? The first step is to determine the percentage of correct responses related to chance. To illustrate, let's continue with the true-false item and the 50% rate due to chance. To establish the usefulness of this true-false item, we must seek a discrimination index that is higher than 50%. Based on best practices in the field, we usually set the difficulty level halfway between a difficulty level of 100% (i.e., everyone getting the item right) and the rate of chance (i.e., 50%). To calculate the optimum difficulty level for our sample item, we subtract the chance level (50%) from the 100% success level and then divide the result by 2. The last step is to add the result of our division to the chance rate, thus providing an optimum difficulty level. In this case,

$$\frac{100 - 0.50}{2} = \frac{0.50}{2} = 0.25 \qquad 0.25 + 0.50 = 0.75 \text{ (optimal item difficulty level)}$$

Thus it would be expected that 75% of individuals attempting this item would answer it correctly. Considering the purpose of comprehensive exams (i.e., minimum competency), this might be an appropriate difficulty level. However, it is important to vary the difficulty level of items throughout the exam. Most people have taken a test in which the first item completely stumped them and the resulting performance suffered whether one knew the remaining answers or not. For this reason, a good approach to test construction is to place easier items at the beginning of a test and to increase item difficulty as the test progresses. This allows examinees a chance to build confidence in their performance and may reduce anxiety surrounding the test situation. In some cases, test authors may even provide items at the beginning of a test that have a 1.0 item difficulty index to increase the positive psychological state of examinees. However, it should be noted that items that approach 1.0 or 0 are typically discarded because of their inability to discriminate among respondents. The typical item difficulty index ranges between 0.30 and 0.70 for most tests in which responses are marked right or wrong. However, some test authors seeking greater scrutiny of test-taker knowledge may employ a sample of more difficult items. For example, some states are now employing a clinical exam for licensure as a professional counselor. This type of exam is usually related to practice knowledge as opposed to the theory knowledge inherent in the "comprehensive exam" example. Because the public welfare is at stake with regard to a licensure exam, it would make sense to have greater scrutiny of applicants through the use of more difficult items.

Item Discrimination

In theory, the purpose of an item discrimination index is to help assess the quality of a particular item. This task is achieved by examining the relationship between total test performance and performance on each individual item. By determining this relationship, we can decide if an item discriminates positively, discriminates negatively, or does not discriminate at all. A *positively discriminating item* is one that is answered correctly more often by those who perform well on the test. In contrast, a *negatively discriminating item* is one that is answered correctly by those who perform poorly on the test. A *nondiscriminating item* fails to indicate a relationship between correct response and test performance. There are numerous statistically derived, computer-generated, item discrimination indices, and the reader is referred to an *SPSS* manual or statistics text for in-depth study.

Some professional counselors may find the discussion of psychometric evaluation, such as item discrimination, tedious and may even wonder how these types of analyses will apply to work in the field. Although few students will likely pursue a career in test construction, it is important to be a qualified user of psychological instruments in order to function in future work settings. Part of being a qualified user means understanding how to evaluate the usefulness of an instrument as well as understanding the usefulness of items within the instrument. The item discrimination index functions as an indicator of the quality of an item. If one is attempting to interpret the results of a test by comparing an individual's responses to a norm group, the item discrimination index tells the degree of confidence one can have in making an interpretation based on a response to a particular item.

Think About It 6.2   Consider such exams as the *Scholastic Assessment Test* (*SAT*) and the *Graduate Record Exam* (*GRE*). Why would assessing item difficulty and item discrimination for these tests be especially important?

Norms

In order to make individual raw scores or individual scale scores meaningful, test authors often administer the instrument to a large comparison sample, or **norm group**. The examinee's raw score is usually transformed to a standard score (e.g., z-score, T score, percentile rank, deviation IQ, or stanine) and then compared to the performance of other individuals with similar characteristics (e.g., age, grade, gender, ethnicity, etc.). This population of individuals is referred to as the *standardization sample, normative sample,* or the *norm group.* The comparison scores are called *derived scores* and are placed into two groups: *developmental scores* and *scores of relative standing* (Salvia & Ysseldyke, 2004).

Many tests use a procedure called **stratified sampling**, which seeks to sample the general population by replicating the percentage of participants according to demographic characteristics. Some important demographic characteristics commonly used include sex (i.e. male, female); age (in years); grade (for achievement tests); race (e.g. White, African American, Asian American, Hispanic American, Native American); region of (U.S.) residence (e.g., south, west, northeast, north central); socioeconomic level (e.g., parent educational attainment, family income, parent occupational status); and area of residence (e.g., urban, suburban, rural). In America, the U.S. Census is consulted, and participants are sampled according to their occurrence in the general population (e.g., 50% male, 50% female).

An additional consideration is the number of participants to include in a norm group. According to Salvia and Ysseldyke (2004), a general rule of thumb is 100 participants per age category for screening tests, and 200 participants per age category for diagnostic tests. Sampling is an absolutely critical consideration in test development, and particular attention should be paid to multicultural and diversity considerations. If a norm sample underrepresents key groups (e.g., racial, socioeconomic, sex), it becomes difficult to support the accuracy of interpretations for those individuals examined using the test.

As an example, the *BARIS* was normed on a group of Black adolescent males in the southern United States. Thus scores for an individual test taker can be compared to average scores of other Black adolescent males in the same geographic region. However, the development of norm-referenced scores is not as simple a task as is indicated by this example. The nature of this chapter does not allow for extensive discussion of the development of norm-referenced scoring procedures. For further information on this topic, readers are referred to the *Standards for Educational and Psychological Testing* (AERA, APA, & NCME, 1999). Readers should also refer to Chapter 5 in this text for more in-depth discussion on this topic.

SUMMARY/CONCLUSION

The development of psychological tests is an intricate process that often takes several years to complete effectively. In order to select quality tests, professional counselors should develop a basic understanding of the test construction process. In general, test construction occurs in distinct phases:

1. *Needs analysis.* Because the development of quality tests is such a time-consuming process, test authors often establish a need for a certain test before beginning the construction process. Needs analysis can be conducted through formal surveys or through an analysis of current instruments available (Drummond, 2004).

2. *Test purpose.* Once a need for a test is established, it is then important to develop clear, behavioral objectives for the development of the proposed instrument. One of the objectives should be related to the construct or content domain to be measured (AERA et al., 1999). For example, the *BARIS* was designed to measure the racial or ethnic identity of Black adolescent males.

3. *Item format.* Prior to beginning the development of specific items for an instrument, it is important to determine the appropriate format for meeting the stated test purpose. Item formats include multiple-choice, forced-choice, open-response, true-false, essay, or Likert scale (Janda, 1998). In order to provide respondents with a limited range of choices, a forced-choice response format was employed for the *BARIS,* with the choices being (a) Strongly Agree, (b) Agree, (c) Disagree, and (d) Strongly Disagree.

4. *Choosing an approach to test construction.* Several approaches to test construction are available (e.g., rational approach, empirical approach, and bootstrap approach). The bootstrap approach was used to develop the *BARIS.* The bootstrap approach is a combination of the rational approach and the empirical approach. The item pool for the *BARIS* was derived from racial identity development theories. Empirical methods of analyses were used to maintain or discard items from the initial pool.

5. *Item development.* Writing effective test items is a difficult process. Test items should be reviewed by a panel of experts to ensure that the items cover the domain being measured and to determine the degree to which the items match the purpose of the test. Previously exiting theories and item pools should also be explored to ensure the items included on a test represent the domain of content being assessed. Items in the *BARIS* were reviewed by experts in the field of multicultural counseling.

6. *Pilot test.* Prior to administering the instrument to a large sample, a pilot test should be conducted to determine item difficulty, discrimination, and comprehension. Test authors often ask pilot test participants to complete feedback sheets that ask about the participants' (a) perception of the test, (b) particularly easy or difficult items, (c) confusing terms, (d) clarity of directions, and (e) general concerns. Test authors conduct in-depth item analysis studies to be sure items "behave" as expected. This process was completed in the initial pilot test for the *BARIS.*

7. *Item review.* After the initial pilot test, it is important to review findings about item difficulty and discrimination in order to determine items that should be removed from the item pool. Test authors should also examine items for bias (i.e., cultural, gender, socio-economic, ability, and sexuality). According to the *Standards for Educational and Psychological Testing* (AERA et al., 1999, p. 82), "Test developers should strive to identify and eliminate language, symbols,

words, phrases, and content that are generally regarded as offensive by members of racial, ethnic, gender, or other groups, except when judged to be necessary for adequate representation of the domain."

8. *Preparing the test for operational use.* Once the pilot test has been completed and the remaining items are reviewed for bias, it is important to prepare the test for operational use. This means that the author should review the objectives and purpose of the test to ensure that the resulting instrument still meets the original intent of the author; scoring procedures should be independently verified; and the instrument should be reviewed by various committees.

9. *Establishing the psychometric properties of the test.* One of the last steps in test development is to establish the technical properties. The test author must determine an appropriate sample size for the statistical analyses to be performed on the instrument. Sample size can vary greatly depending on the analyses employed. Once sample size is determined, the test author administers the instrument, scores it, and computes reliability and validity coefficients (Drummond, 2004). This process can occur in several phases and several individual research endeavors. Finally, the author develops norms for the test.

10. *Ensuring the appropriateness of the norm or criterion group.* Test authors provide norms derived from appropriate sampling procedures (e.g., stratified or selective samples) that account for multicultural and diversity considerations. Test users must ensure that the test is used to make decisions only about clients for whom the test was designed and validated for use.

> **Think About It 6.3**   Why would it be important to carry out all of these steps when developing a test? What would happen if a step were skipped? Would the test still be an effective measure of the desired construct? Explain.

KEY TERMS

age range
bootstrap approach
content
criterion referenced
dichotomous format
empirical approach
items
item analysis
item difficulty
item format
norm group
norm referenced

objectives
observables
polytomous format
population
purpose
rational approach
reading ability
scaling
stratified sampling
summative scale
theory

CHAPTER **7**

Clinical Assessment

by Bradley T. Erford, Carol Salisbury, Kathleen McNinch,
Carl Sheperis, R. Anthony Doggett, and Ota Masanori

O verall, professional counselors in clinical practice engage in clinical and personality assessment more frequently than any other type of assessment.
Knowing the characteristics and conditions of clients is important regardless of counseling specialty. Clinical and personality assessment is defined and explored in detail in this chapter, and numerous inventories commonly used by professional counselors are presented and reviewed. In addition, the basic process of
clinical interviewing is introduced, both for general and for more specific purposes,
such as when conducting a mental status exam. Personality assessment is viewed
from both the psychoanalytic and the "big-five model" perspectives, thus allowing a
basic introduction to projective and objective personality assessment.

WHAT IS CLINICAL ASSESSMENT?

To some, clinical assessment and personality assessment are one and the same. They
are ways of understanding the dispositions, characteristics, strengths, and limitations of the internal world of a client and how that client interacts and functions
within the client's external world. Some even view personality as a global, holistic,
all-encompassing construct that subsumes all the other facets of life and especially
the facets of assessment covered in this book. In other words, in the broadest sense
of the word, intelligence, aptitude, achievement, career, normal and abnormal behavior and emotions, personal adjustment, family, and everything else are subsumed under the category of personality. Unfortunately, while well intentioned,

such a perspective or approach broadens the study of personality far beyond a manageable degree. The perspective taken throughout this chapter is far more proscribed. Here, **clinical assessment** is defined as the measurement of clinical symptoms and pathology in the human condition—in other words, assessment for the purpose of clinical diagnosis. Personality assessment, on the other hand, is the measurement of client traits, needs, motivations, attitudes, or other facets that describe how the client interacts with the external environment, others within that environment, and within the client's internal world. While some may view some of these intrapersonal or interpersonal interactions to be normal or abnormal, the purpose of personality assessment is more appropriately conceived as describing the personal functioning of an individual globally or within some context.

While some may view this distinction as artificial, the implications are not. Professional counselors are often required to diagnose and treat clients with mental and emotional disorders. A client may present with symptoms of depression, anxiety, disruptive behavior, substance use, and so forth. To diagnose and treat the client in an ethical and professional manner, professional counselors will rely on tests and techniques that facilitate the diagnostic and treatment process, and determine the outcomes of treatment—three primary purposes of clinical assessment. While it may be helpful to understand the personality characteristics of a client, it is not always essential for effective treatment, particularly when using brief treatment approaches. When diagnosing and treating clients, professional counselors often use assessment procedures such as clinical interviewing, structured clinical tests—e.g., the *Minnesota Multiphasic Personality Inventory—Second Edition* (*MMPI-2*), the *Millon Clinical Multiaxial Inventory—III* (*MCMI-III*)—and a mental status exam to facilitate efficient and accurate diagnosis and treatment.

When a client seeks counseling for self-growth or a personal or interpersonal problem not amenable to clinical diagnosis, clinical assessment is probably not warranted. However, personality tests can be helpful in deepening both the professional counselor's and the client's understanding of the client's personality and coping mechanisms when under normal and stressful circumstances. Developing such an understanding of thoughts, feelings, and behaviors provides a basis for clients to understand why they think, feel, and behave the way that they do. To facilitate this understanding, professional counselors often use assessment procedures such as developmental interviewing, structured personality tests—e.g., the Myers-Briggs Type Indicator (*MBTI*), the (*16PF*), the (*NEO-PI-R*)—or unstructured, projective tests and techniques—e.g., *House-Tree-Person, Incomplete Sentences, Thematic Apperception Test*. These instruments and the general topic of personality assessment are addressed in more detail in Chapter 8.

Importantly, many psychological instruments can provide helpful information to understand a client's clinical issues and personality functioning. So, while these categories may seem mutually exclusive, tests and test items can be designed to provide information about both. For simplicity's sake, the authors of this chapter have chosen to present these tests in the domain in which they are most commonly used in clinical practice.

CAUTIONS WITHIN CLINICAL ASSESSMENT

In Chapter 1, the general purposes of assessment were outlined. The three purposes most relevant to clinical assessment are diagnosis, treatment planning, and outcomes assessment. Cohen and Swerdlik (1999, p. 482) indicated three primary questions addressed by clinical assessment: (1) Does this person have a mental disorder, and if so, what is the diagnosis? (2) What is the person's current level of functioning? (3) What type of treatment shall this patient be offered? Erford (2006, p. 9) added another: How effective were the implemented interventions?

Many professional counselors find it most efficient to use a combination of interviewing and structured test administration to quickly and accurately diagnose client concerns. That said, if all clients were totally self-aware, open, and forthright in their responses, clinical assessment would be simple, and the text of this chapter could move immediately to the sections on interviewing and structured inventories. Unfortunately, clients present with varying levels of self-awareness, openness, and forthrightness, and professional counselors must take great care to ensure that the diagnostic and treatment decisions made about a client are based on accurate information. Thus, professional counselors must be well aware of important bias issues in both assessment and decision making (i.e., judgment).

Bias in clinical interviewing has been studied for years. Darley and Fazio (1980) coined the term **hypothesis confirmation bias** to explain the observed phenomenon in which interviewers develop hypotheses to explain the concerns being presented by a client and then proceed to ask questions and elicit responses that confirm those hypotheses. While on the surface this may sound like good, sound practice, Darley and Fazio found that clinicians frequently confirmed incorrect hypotheses by interpreting ambiguous information as supportive of the hypothesis and discounting evidence that did not support the hypothesis. Likewise, the term **self-fulfilling prophecy** (Dipboye, 1982) has been used to describe the client's propensity to change responses and behavior to conform to the expectations of the examiner. Often, the client will actually change thoughts, feelings, or actions to align with the perceived expectations of the interviewer. For example, assume a client with low anxiety responds that he or she feels anxious from time to time to a mild degree. If the professional counselor pursues this issue with a line of questioning aimed at understanding the degree of anxiety involved, especially in the context of situations the client may find otherwise troublesome (e.g., interpersonal or workplace relationships), then the client may perceive and "admit" the anxiety to be more problematic than first suspected. Thus, the client fulfills the perceived prophecy, even though it may not be true. With these possible threats to the validity of interview results, professional counselors in training may wonder why interviewing is so popular among clinicians. Again, bias provides the answers. Arvy and Campion (1982) suggested three reasons: (1) Interviews provide a depth of information and perspective that is difficult to obtain using tests alone, (2) clinicians believe themselves to be unbiased, ostensibly because they are good, helpful people, and (3) clinicians believe they are objective and unbiased because they are highly trained and skilled. Note that the final two reasons involve beliefs on the part of the clinician. No matter how well intentioned, any belief can be biased. After all, that is why it is called a belief and not a truism, fact, or law. Every professional counselor must guard against interview response bias. No one is immune.

Equally important, test results can also be biased and inaccurate. It is not hard to understand that results will be inaccurate if someone responds dishonestly to questions. But in actuality, many factors influence student and client responses to items or questions and their subsequent scores on tests. Sometimes these factors may be related to the test itself, while at other times to examiner or examinee variables. Some clients or students may present themselves dishonestly, or lack self-awareness to respond appropriately. Others may not trust the professional counselor for a variety of reasons, some of which have more to do with the client than the counselor. Still others may respond inaccurately because of the way a question is phrased, or the type of response choices required. Regardless of the cause, the result is problematic. Inaccurate client responses lead to inaccurate scores, inferences, and interpretations (i.e., errors). Table 7.1 provides brief descriptions of a number of factors influencing client responses and performances commonly encountered by professional counselors in clinical practice. A more in-depth discussion of these issues can be found in Erford (2006).

In the context of this discussion of clinical response accuracy, further expansion of this list becomes necessary. In the early years of psychological testing (i.e., 1920s–1930s), little concern was given to the accuracy of client responses to personality or clinical questions. Many assumed that clients would respond honestly, and while many clients did respond honestly, examiners quickly learned that not everyone did. While honesty is a good thing, the present-day field of assessment has evolved in such a way that many clients seek the services of professional counselors for help with issues of great importance: child custody, criminal actions, disability documentation, infidelity, and divorce, to name but a few. Likewise, client self-awareness and the relationship between client and counselor can significantly influence the accuracy of client responses. Thus, to assume that all clients always respond accurately is naïve and dangerous. A professional counselor's judgment frequently has personal, financial, and legal implications in such high-stakes decisions.

During the 1940s and through present day, developers of clinical, personality, and behavioral inventories have expended a great deal of effort to construct validity scales that can help identify client response styles. Identification of these response modes can help professional counselors identify clients whose test protocols may be invalid or should be interpreted with caution. Many tests provide validity scales, and the names and functions of these scales vary widely. A good example of a present-day clinical instrument with helpful validity scales is the 567-item, true-false *Minnesota Multiphasic Personality Inventory—Second Edition* (*MMPI-2*). The *MMPI-2* offers a number of helpful scales, including Cannot Say (?), VRIN, TRIN, F, L, K, and S (Butcher et al., 2001).

While clients are encouraged to answer every one of the *MMPI-2*'s 567 questions, many do not. Because raw scores are summed and used to determine a client's norm-referenced score, a client who does not complete a significant number of questions may have deflated scores. This is because failing to answer a question is scored in the nonkeyed (i.e., not clinically relevant) direction, as if to indicate that the client

Table 7.1   Factors that influence student and client test performance and item responses

Factor	Description
Motivation	Motivated clients provide accurate responses; unmotivated clients provide subpar performance, inaccurate, and/or dishonest responses. Client motivation is the most important performance factor.
Anxiety	High and low levels of anxiety lead to low levels of performance. Moderate levels of anxiety maximize performance. This is referred to as the Yerkes-Dodson law.
Coaching	Coaching is any procedure that gives a respondent an advantage. Coaching can involve anything from a simple review of the domain of information being assessed to instructions on giving specific responses to specific questions that will appear on a test. Suspicions of coaching should be followed up on by the examiner.
Test Sophistication	Test sophistication refers to procedural advantages enjoyed by some test takers, but not others (e.g., experience filling in bubble response forms).
Acquiescence	The tendency to answer yes to yes/no questions and true to true/false questions when an examinee is unsure of the correct answer.
Response format	Clients with reading problems, writing problems, poor vision, or disabilities that make sitting difficult may become frustrated with a test requiring reading or constructed written responses. Allowances should be made for audio-taped administration and oral response procedures when possible.
Reactive effects	Clients may alter response styles and patterns in response to the interview or evaluation process (i.e., a series of questions about depressive symptoms could lead clients to perceive in themselves a greater degree of depression than previously considered).
Response bias	A client's response to a question influences responses to future questions (i.e., students who select "False" three times in a row may be more likely to select "False" on the next item, even though they would have otherwise selected "True").
Physical or psychological condition	Clients sometimes present with visual or auditory acuity problems or psychological processing deficiencies (e.g., central auditory processing disorder). In addition, mental disorders can cause psychological conditions that detrimentally affect test performance, such as moderate to severe depression or anxiety, or other disorders that exacerbate mood or distractibility.
Social desirability	Some clients, consciously or unconsciously, may respond in a way that portrays themselves in a more favorable manner (i.e., faking good) and appear less significantly impaired than they really are. Others may portray themselves in a less favorable light (i.e., faking bad) and appear more severely impaired than they really are.
Environmental variables	Some common individual-specific environmental effects include time of day, testing room, lighting, seating arrangements/comfort, noise, and interruptions. Each could affect a client's or student's motivation and performance, but the effects are so individualized that scientific generalizations are normally lacking. Following standardized procedures and minimizing environmental influences are primarily examiner responsibilities.
Cultural bias	Impressions, interpretations, and diagnoses can be influenced by the culture of the examinee and examiner. The professional counselor strives for multicultural competence to minimize biased conclusions.
Examiner-Examinee variables	Some clients and professional counselors just seem to hit it off; others don't. Race, sex, culture, attractiveness, personality, and other variables *may* influence a client's performance, but scientific study indicates they seldom do.
Previous testing experiences	Positive or negative previous assessment experiences may lead to higher experiences or lower self-confidence, thus influencing motivation and performance. Also, some clients may remember content from a previous administration of a test and may have a "memory" advantage on intelligence and achievement tests.

Source: The Counselor's Guide to Clinical, Personality, and Behavioral Assessment by B. T.Erford, (2006), (ed.). Boston: Lahaska Press/Houghton Mifflin.

does not have a problem. The Cannot Say (?) scale is simply a count of the items to which no response was made. Generally, if clients fail to respond to 30 or more items (about 5%), the protocol may be judged invalid; if 11–29 questions are not answered, caution is warranted because some subscales may be invalid. Several helpful scales are termed "content-free," because the content of the scale is not important in determining score validity. VRIN is the acronym for the **Variable Response Inconsistency scale,** which measures a client's pattern of inconsistent responding to pairs of items nearly identical in content. The VRIN raw score indicates the number of inconsistent client responses. Inconsistent responding may mean the client is not paying attention, not taking the task seriously, or doesn't comprehend the item meanings. TRIN is the acronym for the **True Response Inconsistency scale,** which measures a client's pattern of inconsistent responding to pairs of items of opposite content. The TRIN raw score indicates the degree of client response inconsistency due to "yea-saying" (acquiescence) or "nay-saying" (nonacquiescence). T scores of 80+ on the VRIN or TRIN scales indicate the protocol is invalid.

Other validity scales are content-specific. The Infrequency scale (F) is a measure alerting clinicians to unusual patterns of answers. These 60 items were selected because they were infrequently endorsed by members of the original *MMPI* norm sample. Clients with a high score on the F scale (T = 100+) generally are random responders (i.e., paying no attention to items and just coloring in bubbles) or fixed responders (i.e., mostly all true or mostly all false), or are "faking bad" by deliberately trying to portray themselves in a negative light. Of course, the professional counselor must rule out whether the client may also be accurately portraying severe pathology. The *MMPI-2* also has F_B (Back F) and F_P (Infrequency-Psychopathology) scales. The F_B scale is an infrequency-of-response scale for the latter part of the test and, when compared to the total F score, helps determine whether clients changed their response approach during the administration (e.g., the client got bored and began to respond randomly, or to overreport symptoms). The F_P scale is interpreted in conjunction with VRIN and TRIN scales to determine whether a client may be responding randomly, "faking bad," or exaggerating pathological symptoms.

The L scale was originally developed to assess the existence of a defensive mindset by allowing clients to deny the existence of minor faults and flaws that most others readily admitted. While it may indicate deceit in test taking, the L scale is frequently used in conjunction with TRIN to determine the presence of "faking good" and nonacquiescence (i.e., nea-saying) when responding. The K scale was originally developed to measure client response defensiveness so as to correct for this response style on the clinical scales. It was believed that if a clinician knew that a client was responding in such a way that would invalidate the protocol, corrections could be made to the clinical scales so as to still derive meaningful results from them. Interestingly, some researchers (McCrae & Costa, 1989) have shown that uncorrected scale scores have higher validity than K-corrected scores. On other tests, researchers have also demonstrated this to be the case (Hsu, 1986; Kozma & Stones, 1987; McCrae & Costa, 1983). The S scale (Superlative Self-Presentation) was empirically derived by Butcher & Han (1995) by identifying items that were helpful in discriminating between defensive and normal job applicants and norm sample participants. Similar to the K scale, the S scale may also be helpful in determining whether clients are presenting themselves in a socially desirable or nonacquiescent manner.

Other clinical and personality tests have various validity scales under different names designed to assess client response patterns for varying purposes. And the use of validity scales is on the rise, no doubt due to clinician desire to more accurately identify invalid response protocols and better technology for developing such scales. Professional counselors are advised to seek specialized training and to read the manuals of instruments using these scales in order to fully understand how this technology can be harnessed to enhance scale interpretation, and to understand the implications of elevated scores.

CLINICAL JUDGMENT VERSUS STATISTICAL MODELS

Professional counselors must be wary of bias not only from clients and other information sources, but also from within themselves. Most professional counselors have great faith in their own clinical judgment; after all, professional counselors spend years in education and clinical preparation to practice their craft. They have successes and setbacks but are constantly improving and honing their skills to the point of competent practice. It is easy to assume that such a rigorous program of study and practice under supervision will remove bias and sharpen the professional counselor's clinical objectivity. Unfortunately, such is not always the case. Regardless of how well educated, well trained, and well practiced one becomes, a professional counselor is only as perfect as the information obtained and interpreted and the decision-making model employed. Hopefully, the information presented in the preceding chapters has given readers an appreciation for the imperfection of the information they will encounter, the interpretive strategies they will employ, and the accuracy rates of various decision-making models. Errors will always be with us. However, there are ways that a professional counselor can increase the likelihood of more accurate decision making.

Much has been written about the efficacy of decision-making models employing clinical judgment versus statistical models—and the evidence is that the statistical models are at least as accurate as, and usually superior to, clinical judgment (Dawes, 1971; Dawes & Corrigan, 1974; Goldberg, 1970; Meehl, 1954, 1957, 1965). Intuitively, this makes sense, because statistical models are based on probabilities that can be empirically replicated, studied, and often improved on. **Clinical judgment** is individual-specific, so what makes sense to one professional counselor, may not only *not* make sense to another professional counselor, but also may not be easily replicated by another professional counselor. As with all things related to measurement, reliability (i.e., replicability) sets the upward boundary for validity. So if clinicians cannot replicate a decision model efficiently, the validity of results will be lowered. Such is the advantage of a **statistical decision-making model**; it is easily understood and replicable, therefore *may* produce more accurate decisions, although it may not always be presumed to do so. Betting against a statistical model is similar to betting against the house in a game of chance. Sometimes you will win, but the odds are *always* against you; skill and knowledge helps sometimes, but not *most* of the time.

Statistical models in clinical decision making often rely on the use of cutoff scores that are empirically validated. Professional counselors are wise to consider the implications of "betting against" the statistical model. Experienced clinicians know the value of multiple sources of information from multiple respondents. When clinical judgment disagrees with the statistical model, the experienced clinician usually realizes that it is best to collect more information to arrive at a more reasoned decision that one can endorse with greater confidence.

Think About It 7.1   In your practice as a professional counselor, you will encounter situations in which a decision using your "statistical model" does not agree with your "clinical judgment." How will you reconcile this conflict to arrive at the best decision for your client?

CLINICAL INTERVIEWING

There are several essential components to an effective interview. First, establishing rapport is crucial. A professional counselor must relate a sense of mutual understanding, confidence, respect, and acceptance in order to facilitate effective rapport (Sattler, 2002). Establishing rapport is especially important in the initial interview to help clients feel comfortable enough to openly discuss their reasons for coming to counseling. Second, an interviewer needs to have effective facilitative skills. Effective interviews (a) identify client problems clearly; (b) obtain necessary information related to the problems (e.g., antecedent, consequence); (c) assess client functioning, intellectual level, and psychosocial development; and (d) examine the effects of an intervention during and after the intervention. As Kratochwill, Sheridan, Carlson, and Lasecki (1999) posited, eliciting useful information largely depends on the interviewer's ability to strategically use questions and statements.

Three Types of Interviews:
Unstructured, Semi-Structured, and Structured

Depending on the purpose of the interview, a professional counselor should choose an appropriate interview level from among the following: (1) structured, (2) semi-structured, and (3) unstructured. The **structured interview** has established question formats and is often used to assess or diagnose disorders. Generally, structured interviews are shown to yield more reliable results because they are able to be more accurately replicated by others and are less subject to a clinician's biases. It is unclear whether structured interviews yield more valid results (McReynolds, 1989). In a structured interview, every professional counselor asks the same set of questions in the same order, regardless of the examinee. Some structured interview formats are purposely broad in scope and function, others narrow. Erford provided an example of a structured clinical interview of a narrow focus (see Erford, 2006, Appendix C: *Attention-Deficit/Hyperactivity Disorder [AD/HD] Brief Clinical Parent Interview*

Table 7.2   Published structured interviews

CIDI-Core	Composite International Diagnostic Interview: Authorized Core Version 1.0 (*World Health Organization, 1993*)
DIS	Diagnostic Interview Schedule (*National Institute of Mental Health, 1990*)
DICA-R	*Diagnostic Interview for Children and Adolescents* 8.0 (Reich, 1996)
DISC-IV	*Diagnostic Interview Schedule for Children* (Shaffer, 1996)
CAPA	*Child and Adolescent Psychiatric Assessment* Version 4.2—Child Version (Angold, Cox, Pendergast, Rutter, & Simonoff, 1996)
CAS	*Child Adolescent Schedule* (Hodges, 1997)
K-SADS-IVR	*Schedule for Affective Disorders & Schizophrenia for School-Age Children* (Ambrosini & Dixon, 1996)
K-SADS-PL	*Revised Schedule for Affective Disorders & Schizophrenia for School-Age Children: Present and Lifetime Version* (Kaufman, Birmaher, Brent, Rao, & Ryan, 1996)
K-SADS-E5	*Schedule for Affective Disorders & Schizophrenia for School-Age Children, Epidemiological Version 5* (Orvaschel, 1995)

[*ABCPI*]). Examples of published broad-spectrum structured interviews are provided in Table 7.2.

The **semi-structured interview** may also have a specific question format that is used to assess specific mental health issues or psychological disorders. However, in contrast to the structured interview, a professional counselor can modify questions or change the order in which the questions are asked depending on a client's level of functioning (e.g., verbal or intellectual level) or other situational requirements (Sattler, 2002). Erford provided a good example of a semi-structured interview (see Erford, 2006; Appendix D: *Semi-Structured Mental Status Examination Interview Protocol*). Some other published semi-structured interviews are provided in Table 7.3.

Finally, the **unstructured interview** has no standardized question format. An interviewer chooses questions depending on the client and situation. In order to conduct an effective unstructured interview for clinical diagnostic purposes, a professional counselor should have advanced assessment training and be able to elicit the client's concerns through appropriate questions. The skilled professional counselor can use the unstructured interview as an effective tool to establish rapport and to elicit concerns freely during an intake interview. Regardless of the type of interview

Table 7.3   Published semi-structured interviews

SCID-CV	*Structured Clinical Interview for Axis I DSM-IV Disorders* (First, Spitzer, et al., 1997).
SCID-II	*Structured Clinical Interview for Axis II DSM-IV Disorders* (First, Gibbon, et al., 1997).
PRISM	*Psychiatric Research Interview for Substance and Mental Disorders* (Hassin et al., 1996).
SCICA	*Structured Clinical Interview for Children and Adolescents* (McConaughy & Achenbach, 1994).

employed, it is crucial to establish rapport and to elicit necessary information through effective verbal communication. Like any other facet of effective counseling, facilitative skills are an essential component.

The Intake Interview

The purpose of the **intake interview** is to collect relevant information about a client's history and background in order to quickly ascertain the effects past events may have on the client's current situation. Previous history often helps professional counselors to provide a context for current struggles, determine the longevity of symptoms, and tailor treatment interventions to the client's specific context. For example, a client presenting with a five-year history of substantial symptoms of anxiety likely will require a different diagnostic and treatment approach than someone who has developed substantial symptoms only during the past month.

The major advantage of a structured intake interview is that it can be completed by a client prior to the first session. Then the professional counselor can peruse the client's responses and follow up with any details or questions concerning original client responses. This saves a great deal of time. Of course, the professional counselor should verify client responses and expand on them as necessary, because clients sometimes misunderstand the intent of a given question, or are hesitant to provide full disclosure; that is, some clients understandably reveal more in a person-to-person interview than on a piece of paper. Erford (2006) developed a comprehensive eight-page structured *Client History and Background* intake form that professional counselors will find useful. Erford (p. 8) also specified the eight key areas that make up a comprehensive intake interview:

1. *Demographic information:* name, age, sex, marital status, race or ethnicity, religion, socioeconomic status, occupation, and languages spoken.
2. *Referral reasons:* symptoms or complaints, including whether the complaint is likely to end up as a legal issue.
3. *Current situation:* severity of the referral complaints' resiliency factors, such as client strengths and important support figures. This area also includes changes in functioning as a result of the referral concern.
4. *Previous assessments and counseling experiences:* what led to initiation of previous services, what interventions were attempted, and any outcomes of such interventions. It is also important to determine previously offered diagnoses and medications taken to address mental and emotional issues.
5. *Birth and developmental history:* circumstances of birth and delivery, timing of early developmental milestones, or difficulties encountered during development.
6. *Family history:* composition of family of origin and current family; any educational, medical, or psychological difficulties family members may display or have displayed in the past.
7. *Medical history:* major injuries, surgeries, conditions or illnesses, and medications currently taken. This area also includes the client's current medical status.

8. *Educational and work background:* highest education completed, learning difficulties encountered, special services received, work history, and current work setting and satisfaction.

Think About It 7.2   Describe the importance of a thorough intake interview. How could your ability to establish rapport and use facilitative skills influence the intake interview, the initial session, and future counseling sessions?

Mental Status Exam

A special application of clinical interviewing that professional counselors should become proficient in is called the *mental status exam* (MSE). The MSE is to mental health practitioners what the general physical examination is to medical practitioners. The MSE is a quick screening of a client's intellectual, emotional, and neurological functioning. In general, the MSE is a brief summary narrative of client general mental function and is usually conducted during the first interview. MSEs are frequently required by third-party payers (i.e., insurance companies), and the level of detail required varies substantially. Erford (2006), in a detailed discussion that included a sample *Semi-Structured MSE Interview Protocol*, reported that a comprehensive MSE should assess the following six areas:

1. *Appearance, attitude, and behavior:* manner of dress, cleanliness, appearance, demographic information, occupation, physical characteristics, health, size, hearing, vision, eye contact, attitude toward examiner, attitude toward interview, motor functioning, behavior exhibited.
2. *Cognitive capabilities:* knowledge of name, location, time, day, date; long- and short-term memory; serial 7s; spelling a word backwards; math problem solving; digit span; sentence memory; level of consciousness; concentration; capacity for abstract reasoning; demonstration of reading, math and writing tasks; cognitive functioning.
3. *Speech and language:* description of speech capability; description of language capability; repetition of phrases; read a short passage; write a short passage.
4. *Thought content and process:* description of thought processes; description of thought content; fears or phobias.
5. *Emotional status:* presenting mood, intensity, duration, fluctuations; description of affect, intensity, range, variability; modulation and appropriateness of affect; personality characteristics; emotional, physical, or behavioral problems.
6. *Insight and judgment:* description of insight and judgment; responses to judgment questions; decision making regarding presenting problem, past and future events; defense mechanisms.

Erford (2006, pp. 172–173) provided an example mental status exam:

Matthew was appropriately dressed in jeans and a T-shirt. He appeared clean, well-groomed, and relaxed. He is a 15-year-old, English-speaking, White,

9th-grade male with normal physical features and no sign of handicaps, scars, or other signs of self-mutilation. He is approximately 5' 8", 150 pounds, and his hearing and vision are normal. Matthew maintained appropriate eye contact and was cooperative and open throughout the evaluation. His motor functioning was basically normal, although he did frequently "bounce his knee" and adjust his posture indicating signs of overactivity. He demonstrated poor fine-motor coordination during writing tasks and finger-touching activities. He did not display aggressive, irritable, anxious, or otherwise abnormal behavior throughout the evaluation.

Cognitively, Matthew was oriented × 5 and was able to answer basic information questions, including the current and former president, capital of Maryland, serial 7s, and simple math problems. His short-term memory and delayed recall was appropriate for three objects, as was his dichotic and verbal retention. His consciousness was normal. Dysgraphia was evident and should be ruled out through diagnostic evaluation. He was somewhat distractible in the one-to-one situation, but his cognitive functioning was otherwise normal.

Matthew's speech and language capabilities were normal in all regards. His thought processes were clear, appropriate, and logical, and his thought content was normal—devoid of phobic, obsessive, or psychotic process. Matthew's mood was observed to be friendly, pleasant, and calm, with normal intensity and little fluctuation. His affect was appropriate as he was able to modulate an appropriate affective range and intensity, even when discussing emotional content. He admitted being oppositional and appeared ambiverted. Matthew did not report significant emotional, physical, or behavioral problems.

Finally, Matthew's insight and judgment appeared normal, appropriate, and realistic. He was able to clearly describe his decision-making processes and answer questions requiring judgment. Matthew acknowledged the problems reported by parents and teachers, willingly consented to this evaluation, and was willing to "do whatever it takes" to address the issues.

The mental status exam can be administered either through an unstructured, semi-structured, or structured interview format and, of course, relies heavily on observation of attitudes, behaviors, and appearance. Use of an unstructured format requires a great deal of experience with the content and format of the mental status exam and basically involves asking pertinent questions from the categories specified above. As with any unstructured interview, the questions will vary from client to client and occur in no particular order, maximizing the clinician's flexibility and adaptability to the conditions and client responses.

An example of a comprehensive semi-structured presentation of a mental status examination has been mentioned earlier and can be found in Erford (2006). An example of a quicker, far less comprehensive mental status exam in popular use is the *Mini–Mental State Examination* (*MMSE*). The *MMSE* is a brief, structured interview used to assess only the cognitive mental state (Folstein, Folstein, McHugh, & Fanjiang, 2001). The *MMSE* has 11 categories and takes 5 to 10 minutes to administer. An examiner asks questions or gives instructions, and an examinee responds one by one. For example, an examinee needs to (a) answer questions regarding time and place; (b) repeat, memorize, or recall some words; (c) briefly calculate simple math problems; (d) manipulate a piece of paper according to directions; and (e) copy a design. Summing each score (0 or 1) yields a total score, whose maximum is 30. Though the authors of the *MMSE* recommend using a total score of 26 as a cutoff score, a frequently used cutoff score is 23. A total score of 23 or below indicates the likelihood of cognitive impairment and the necessity of further evaluation (Folstein et al., 2001). The *MMSE* has been shown to produce reliable and valid scores when screening for cognitive impairment. An example of a structured mental status exam in common use is the *Standardized Mini–Mental States Exam* (*SMMSE*) (Molloy, Alemayehu, & Roberts, 1991) (see Figure 7.1).Essentially, Malloy et al. took the *MMSE* and structured its administration to increase the administrative efficiency and enhance the interrater and internal consistency reliability of scores.

Strengths and Limitations of Interviewing

A clinical or behavioral interview allows the professional counselor great latitude in how to collect important information from clients and other stakeholders (e.g., parents, teachers, spouses). A lot of important information can be collected quickly and efficiently. However, it is good practice to validate this information and client perceptions against other information sources. Aside from the important demographic and historical information derived from an interview, the important point of conducting the interview is to generate and validate hypotheses, arrive at an understanding or diagnosis of the client's presenting concerns, and develop a plan of treatment or intervention to help ameliorate the client's concerns. The interview allows for in-depth analysis of issues, flexibility in how the information is garnered, and instantaneous clarification of ambiguous information. The interview also provides the professional counselor with valuable insight into what has been tried previously to ameliorate the client's condition, how motivated the client is to enact proposed treatment strategies, and resources that the client can draw upon to effect necessary changes (Erford, 2006).

But interviewing is not without limitations. Interview responses frequently possess lower levels of reliability and validity than more standardized inventories, although structured interviews frequently rival their counterpart inventories. Unstructured interviews are particularly problematic in this regard because of very low interrater reliability. Professional counselors using unstructured clinical interviews frequently derive very different information from the interview and arrive at very different conclusions. More specifically, clinician bias often determines which questions are asked, what client responses are clarified and explored in depth, and what diagnosis or conclusion is arrived at.

The clinical or behavioral interview can be an important aspect of assessing client problems and needs. Professional counselors must use caution when interpreting interview data, just as when interpreting the results of objective tests or projective measures. The key to competent assessment and diagnosis is using multiple measures from multiple respondents, resulting in convergence of information. When unsure, it is always advisable to collect more information. A client deserves no less.

Figure 7.1   *Standardized Mini–Mental State Examination (SMMSE)*

I am going to ask you some questions and give you some problems to solve. Please try to answer as best as you can.

	Max Score

1. **(Allow 10 seconds for each reply)**
   a) What year is this? (accept exact answer only) — 1
   b) What season is this? (during last week of the old season or first week of a new season, accept either season) — 1
   c) What month of the year is this? (on the first day of new month, or last day of the previous month, accept either) — 1
   d) What is today's date? (accept previous or next date, e.g., on the 7th accept the 6th or 8th) — 1
   e) What day of the week is this? (accept exact answer only) — 1

2. **(Allow 10 seconds for each reply)**
   a) What country are we in? (accept exact answer only) — 1
   b) What province/state/county are we in? (accept exact answer only) — 1
   c) What city/town are we in? (accept exact answer only) — 1
   d) **(In clinic)** What is the name of this hospital/building? (accept exact name of hospital or institution only) — 1
      (In home) What is the street address of this house? (accept street name and house number or equivalent in rural areas)
   e) **(In clinic)** What floor of the building are we on? (accept exact answer only) — 1
      (In home) What room are we in?

3. I am going to name 3 objects. After I have said all three objects, I want you to repeat them. — 3
   Remember what they are because I am going to ask you to name them again in a few minutes.
   (say them slowly at approximately 1 second intervals)

Ball	Car	Man

   For repeated use:

Bell	Jar	Fan
Bill	Tar	Can
Bull	War	Pan

   Please repeat the 3 items for me. (score 1 point for each correct reply on the first attempt) Allow 20 seconds for reply; if subject did not repeat all 3, repeat until they are learned or up to a maximum of 5 times

4. Spell the word WORLD. (you may help the subject to spell world correctly) Say **now spell it backwards please.** Allow 30 seconds to spell backwards. (If the subject cannot spell world even with assistance—score 0). — 5

5. Now what were the 3 objects that I asked you to remember? — 3

Ball	Car	Man

   Score 1 point for each correct response regardless of order, allow 10 seconds.

6. Show wristwatch. Ask: what is this called? Score 1 point for correct response. Accept "wristwatch" or "watch". Do not accept "clock", "time", etc. (allow 10 seconds). — 1

7. Show pencil. Ask: what is this called? Score 1 point for correct response, accept pencil only— Score 0 for pen. — 1

8. I'd like you to repeat a phrase after me: "no, if's, and's, or but's." (allow 10 seconds for response. Score 1 point for a correct repetition. Must be **exact**, e.g., no if's or but's—score 0) — 1

9. Read the words on this page and then do what it says: Hand subject the laminated sheet with CLOSE YOUR EYES on it.   1
    CLOSE YOUR EYES.
    If subject just reads and does not then close eyes—you may repeat: read the words on this page and then do what it says to a maximum of 3 times. Allow 10 seconds, score 1 point **only** if subject closes eyes. Subject does not have to read aloud.

10. Ask if the subject is right or left handed. Alternate right/left hand in statement, e.g., if the subject is right handed, say **Take this paper in your left hand . . .** Take a piece of paper—hold it up in front of subject and say the following: 3

    "Take this paper in your right/left hand, fold the paper in half once with both hands, and put the paper down on the floor."

    Takes paper in correct hand
    Folds it in half
    Puts it on the floor
    Allow 30 seconds. Score 1 point for each instruction correctly executed.

11. Hand subject a pencil and paper. **Write any complete sentence on that piece of paper.**   1
    Allow 30 seconds. Score 1 point. The sentence should make sense. Ignore spelling errors.

12. Place design, pencil, eraser and paper in front of the subject. Say: **copy this design please.** Allow   1
    multiple tries until patient is finished and hands it back. Score 1 point for correctly copied diagram. The subject must have drawn a 4-sided figure between two 5-sided figures. Maximum time—1 minute.

Total Test Score   30

Source: From D. W. Molloy, E. Alemayehu, and R. Roberts, "Reliability of a *Standardized Mini–Mental State Examination* compared with the traditional mini–mental examination." *American Journal of Psychiatry,* January 1991; *148,* 102–105. Copyright © 1991 American Psychiatric Association.

COUNSELING, DIAGNOSIS, AND THE *DSM-IV-TR*

The roots and tradition of counseling lie in vocational guidance and human development (Herr, 1998). However, recent societal and mental health practices have given rise to a mental health role for professional counselors regardless of work setting. Mental health counselors, substance abuse counselors, marriage and family counselors, geriatric counselors, and community counselors provide mental health counseling in clinics, agencies, and private practice in numerous states around the country—and in numerous countries around the world. Even professional school counselors and career counselors, two professions that have maintained the closest ties to counseling's developmental roots and that seldom view clinical diagnosis as a part of their job functions, provide treatment to clients or students who have been (or could be) diagnosed with mental or emotional disorders.

Mental and emotional disorders are becoming more prevalent in society, particularly among children and adolescents, and professional counselors must be knowledgeable about diagnosis and clinical assessment in order to gain respect and parity in the mental health community. A review of the extant literature finds numerous examples of increased need for clinical diagnostic and treatment services, a need that contemporary professional counselors are helping to meet. In any given year, serious mental illness can be diagnosed in about 5–7% of an adult population (New Freedom Commission on Mental Health, 2003). Diagnosable mental and emotional disorders significant enough to warrant treatment can be found in 15–22% of school-aged students (SAMHSA, 1998), but only about one in five of these impaired students actually gets help. Clients with serious mental health concerns seeking help at university counseling centers are increasing (Pledge, Lapan, Heppner, Kivlighan & Roehlke, 1998). Substance abuse, poverty, and community and domestic violence are on the rise (Dryfoos, 1994; Lockhart & Keys, 1998). Various estimates of depression among adolescents include 3 to 6 million students (American Psychiatric Association, 1994) or nearly 18% (Essau, Condradt, & Peterman, 2000). On a related note, 10,000 to 20,000 adolescents attempt suicide, while more than 2,000 adolescents commit suicide annually (Brown, 1996). This makes suicide the second leading cause of death among adolescents. Diagnosis of childhood disorders requires a great deal of improvement as certain common disorders (e.g. AD/HD) appear to be overdiagnosed in childhood (McClure, Kubiszyn, & Kaslow, 2002), quite a feat given that community prevalence estimates indicate that perhaps 50% of children and adolescents referred to mental health clinics can be diagnosed with behavior disorders, including Conduct Disorder and AD/HD (Erk, 1995).

While the above statistics paint a picture of a tremendous societal need for clinical services, they also underscore the necessity of high-level training in diagnosis and treatment of mental and emotional disorders. Nearly all clinical decisions, whether diagnostic or treatment related, are predicated on informal or formal assessment procedures. Thus the more one consciously integrates assessment procedures and outcomes research into one's practice, the more objective and informed one's practice becomes. The mental health role of the professional counselor is here to stay; diagnosis and use of the *DSM* is becoming a necessary part of training for all clinicians (Seligman, 1998), just as the *International Classification of Diseases—Tenth Revision* (*ICD-10*) is used in the health professions.

The usefulness of diagnostic systems is widely debated (see Murphy and Davidshofer, 2001). The fact of the matter is that insurance companies and employers are requiring competence in diagnosis as a condition for payment or employment, and state licensing agencies are increasingly requiring coursework and training in clinical diagnosis to obtain licensure (Hohensil, 1993; 1996). In the mental health arena, the diagnostic resource most commonly used by psychiatrists, psychologists, social workers, and professional counselors is the *Diagnostic and Statistical Manual of Mental Disorders—Fourth Edition—Text Revision* (*DSM-IV-TR*) (APA, 2000). In fact, a recent survey found that 91% of mental health counselors used the *DSM* (Mead, Hohensil, & Singh, 1997).

The ***DSM-IV-TR*** provides specific criteria through which reliable diagnoses can be made. It also provides a nomenclature, or common language, through which mental health professionals can communicate with each other to describe (*not* label) a client's condition. Such diagnostic language has the purpose of succinctly communicating categorical mental conditions so that common symptoms may be indicated and commonly agreed-upon treatments may ensue. Such a categorical reference is necessary to help organize the diagnostic and treatment outcome literature. For example, to move a field forward, it is essential for all clinicians, educators, and researchers to know exactly what is meant by the term Major Depressive Disorder so that all resources aimed at understanding the identification, treatment alternatives, and treatment outcomes of this disorder can be focused most efficiently. The *DSM-IV-TR* provides this common language. Even if some professional counselors (e.g., professional school counselors and career counselors) do not make diagnoses in their work settings, understanding what, for example, Major Depressive Disorder entails is essential for proper assessment, referral, and facilitation or coordination of treatment. For example, would a professional school counselor interviewing the mother of a 7-year-old who complains of her son's problems with disobedience, defiance, and negativity be serving the best interest of the student or family if he or she were unfamiliar with the term Oppositional Defiant Disorder (ODD). An awareness of the diagnostic criteria for ODD would streamline the assessment process and allow for efficient referral or treatment. A working knowledge of the *DSM-IV-TR* makes any professional counselor more efficient and valuable. While there is no substitute for a careful perusal of the *DSM-IV-TR,* the remainder of this chapter briefly reviews the multiaxial assessment system of the *DSM-IV-TR,* major diagnostic categories, and several instruments that are particularly helpful in the clinical assessment process.

Using the *DSM-IV-TR*—Multiaxial Diagnosis

The *DSM-IV-TR* (APA, 2000) is the latest in a series of diagnostic resource guides. The *DSM-IV-TR* is a text revision of the *DSM-IV* (APA, 1994), with editorial changes primarily to the information supplied in the text, rather than to the diagnostic criteria sets for the specified disorders. The *DSM-IV-TR* describes nearly 300 diagnostic categories that enable mental health professionals to diagnose, treat, research, and efficiently discuss mental and emotional disorders.

The diagnostic process calls for a **multiaxial classification system** to describe the condition of the client. Five axes, or different facets, are included:

- Axis I—Clinical disorders and other conditions that may be a focus of clinical attention
- Axis II—Personality disorders and mental retardation
- Axis III—General medical conditions
- Axis IV—Psychosocial and environmental problems
- Axis V—Global assessment of functioning

The systematic multiaxial approach provides a shorthand notation of a comprehensive process, conveying a tremendous amount of information about the current mental status of a client, including mental disorders, concurrent medical issues, and adaptive functioning. APA (2000, p. xxxi) defines a **mental disorder** as a

clinically significant behavior or psychological syndrome or pattern that occurs in an individual and that is associated with present distress (e.g., a painful symptom) or disability (i.e., impairment in one or more areas of functioning) or with a significantly increased risk of suffering death, pain, disability, or an important loss of freedom.

Axes I and II include the mental disorders that make up the classification system. Axis II includes personality disorders and mental retardation, while Axis I is used to document the existence of all other mental disorders. The behavioral effects of physical and medical disorders are listed on Axis III. The listing of occupational, familial, financial, legal, and other social and emotional effects is noted on Axis IV. And the professional counselor's assessment of how well the client is, or has been, adapting to the stresses of everyday life is recorded on Axis V.

The *DSM-IV-TR* provides comprehensive information about mental disorders by describing essential diagnostic features, associated features and disorders, specific age and gender features, prevalence, course of the disorder, familial pattern, and differential diagnosis. Most importantly, the diagnostic code and criteria for each disorder are provided. These criteria enhance the reliability and validity of the diagnostic system by providing specific descriptions of symptoms and conditions relevant to diagnosis. The criteria are meant to be so specific that, regardless of the clinician assessing the client, a similar diagnostic outcome should emerge. As examples, Table 7.4 contains the diagnostic criteria for Posttraumatic Stress Disorder (PTSD) (APA, 2000, pp. 467-468) and Table 7.5 for Attention-Deficit Hyperactivity Disorder— Combined Type (AD/HD) (APA, 2000, p. 92; symptom criteria only).

Note how the specificity of the criteria allows for clinicians to reliably determine whether the disorder applies to a given client. This allows numerous clinicians assessing the same client to arrive at a consistent determination as to whether a client meets the specified diagnostic criteria. Accurate diagnosis occurs to a large extent because professional counselors ask specific questions about client symptoms as necessary. It is better to ask a specific question or seek information of a specific nature and receive a negative reply than to not ask and therefore not know whether a client presents with a given disorder. Clinical diagnosis is a process in which it is generally good advice and good practice to leave no stone left unturned.

It is essential that professional counselors adhere closely to the diagnostic criteria provided in the *DSM-IV-TR,* as short- and long-term damage to clients can result from misdiagnosis. In the short term, misdiagnosis can cause a client to receive an inappropriate treatment and accrue unnecessary expense and wasted time. In the long term, an incorrect diagnosis can follow a client, as insurance companies and healthcare professionals may make future decisions about treatment based on faulty past information. These entities also may not always keep such private information confidential.

The remainder of this chapter provides an orientation to diagnosis and classification using the multiaxial framework. Professional counselors wanting additional training and practice with clinical diagnosis are encouraged to take graduate coursework in which the *DSM-IV-TR* diagnostic system is prominently featured and supervised training is provided. In addition, other text resources are available, including the *DSM-IV Casebook* (Spitzer, Gibbon, Skodol, Williams, & First, 1994) and the *DSM-IV Guide* (Frances, First, & Pincus, 1995).

Table 7.4 Diagnostic criteria for Posttraumatic Stress Disorder (PTSD)

A. The person has been exposed to a traumatic event in which both of the following were present:
   (1) the person experienced, witnessed, or was confronted with an event or events that involved actual or threatened death or serious injury, or a threat to the physical integrity of self or others
   (2) the person's response involved intense fears, helplessness or horror. *Note:* In children, this may be expressed instead by disorganized or agitated behavior
B. The traumatic event is persistently reexperienced in one (or more) of the following ways:
   (1) recurrent and intrusive distressing recollections of the event, including images, thoughts, or perceptions. *Note:* In young children, repetitive play may occur in which themes or aspects of the trauma are expressed
   (2) recurrent distressing dreams of the event. *Note:* In children, there may be frightening dreams without recognizable content
   (3) acting or feeling as if the traumatic event were recurring (includes a sense of reliving the experience, illusions, hallucinations, and dissociative flashback episodes, including those that occur on awakening or when intoxicated). *Note:* In young children, trauma specific reenactment may occur
   (4) intense psychological distress at exposure to internal or external cues that symbolize or resemble an aspect of the traumatic event
   (5) physiological reactivity on exposure to internal or external cues that symbolize or resemble an aspect of the traumatic event
C. Persistent avoidance of stimuli associated with the trauma and numbing of general responsiveness (not present before the trauma), as indicated by three (or more) of the following:
   (1) efforts to avoid thoughts, feelings, or conversations associated with the trauma
   (2) efforts to avoid activities, places, or people that arouse recollections of the trauma
   (3) inability to recall an important aspect of the trauma
   (4) markedly diminished interest or participation in significant activities
   (5) feeling of detachment or estrangement from others
   (6) restricted range of affect (unable to have loving feelings)
   (7) sense of foreshortened future (e.g., does not expect to have career, marriage, children, or a normal lifespan)
D. Persistent symptoms of increased arousal (not present before the trauma), as indicated by two (or more) of the following:
   (1) difficulty falling or staying asleep
   (2) irritability or outbursts of anger
   (3) difficulty concentrating
   (4) hypervigilance
   (5) exaggerated startle response
E. Duration of the disturbance (symptoms in Criteria B, C, and D) is more than 1 month.
F. The disturbance causes clinically significant distress or impairment in social, occupational, or other important areas of functioning.
Specify if:
   Acute: if duration of symptoms is less than 3 months
   Chronic: if duration of symptoms is 3 months or more
Specify if:
   With Delayed Onset: if onset of symptoms is at least 6 months after the stressor

Source: Reprinted with permission from the *Diagnostic and Statistical Manual of Mental Disorders,* (4th ed., text rev.), American Psychiatric Association. Copyright 2000, Washington, DC: Author.

Table 7.5   Diagnostic criteria for Attention-Deficit Hyperactivity Disorder—
Combined Type (inattentive and hyperactive impulsive symptoms only)

A. Either (1) or (2):

   (1) six (or more) of the following symptoms of **inattention** have persisted for at least 6
   months to a degree that is maladaptive and inconsistent with developmental level:

   Inattention

   (a) often fails to give close attention to details or makes careless mistakes in
   schoolwork, work, or other activities

   (b) often has difficulties sustaining attention in tasks and play activities

   (c) often does not seem to listen when spoken to directly

   (d) often does not follow through on instructions and fails to finish schoolwork,
   chores, or duties in the workplace (not due to oppositional behavior or failure to
   understand instructions)

   (e) often has difficulty organizing tasks and activities

   (f) often avoids, dislikes, or is reluctant to engage in tasks that require sustained mental
   effort (such as schoolwork or homework)

   (g) often loses things necessary for tasks or activities (e.g., toys, school assignments,
   pencils, books, or tools)

   (h) is often easily distracted by extraneous stimuli

   (i) is often forgetful in daily activities

   (2) six (or more) of the following symptoms of **hyperactivity-impulsivity** have persisted for
   at least 6 months to a degree that is maladaptive and inconsistent with developmental
   level:

   Hyperactivity

   (a) often fidgets with hands or feet or squirms in seat

   (b) often leaves seat in classroom or in other situations in which remaining seated is
   expected

   (c) often runs about or climbs excessively in situations in which it is inappropriate (in
   adolescents or adults, may be limited to subjective feelings of restlessness)

   (d) often has difficulty playing or engaging in leisure time activities quietly

   (e) is often "on the go" or acts as if "driven by a motor"

   (f) often talks excessively

   Impulsivity

   (g) often blurts out answers before questions have been completed

   (h) often has difficulty awaiting turn

   (i) often interrupts or intrudes on others (e.g., butts into conversations or games)

Source: Reprinted with permission from the *Diagnostic and Statistical Manual of Mental Disorders,* (4th ed.,
text rev.), American Psychiatric Association. Copyright 2000, Washington, DC: Author.

Axis I Disorders—Clinical Disorders and Other Conditions
That May Be a Focus of Clinical Attention

Axis I disorders include all of the disorders from the *DSM-IV-TR* except for mental
retardation and personality disorders (see Table 7.6). It is essential to understand
from the outset that a minority of clients actually enter the clinical arena with only

Table 7.6 *DSM-IV-TR* Axis I clinical disorders and other conditions that may be a focus of clinical attention

---

Disorders usually first diagnosed in infancy, childhood, or adolescence
1. Delirium, dementia, and amnestic and other cognitive disorders
2. Mental disorders due to a general medical condition
3. Substance-related disorders
4. Schizophrenia and other psychotic disorders
5. Mood disorders
6. Anxiety disorders
7. Somatoform disorders
8. Factitious disorders
9. Dissociative disorders
10. Sexual and gender identity disorders
11. Eating disorders
12. Sleep disorders
13. Impulse-control disorders not elsewhere classified
14. Adjustment disorders
15. Other conditions that may be a focus of clinical attention

---

a single well-defined problem. It is common for a client to obtain multiple diagnoses on Axis I and/or Axis II, referred to as *comorbidity*. Clark, Watson, and Reynolds (1995) found that 60–80% of clients present with comorbidity, while only about 20–40% present with a singular diagnosis. This reality makes diagnosis of the typical client somewhat complicated. Therefore, professional counselors must start by looking at the big picture of all characteristics and symptoms, then refine the questioning to arrive at more specific categorical decisions. This diagnostic decision-making process is explained in more detail at the end of this chapter. Sometimes a client may not meet all criteria for a given disorder, so each Axis I disorder allows for the designation "Not Otherwise Specified" (NOS) to be used; however, this designation should be used with caution because it may lead to misdiagnosis and inappropriate treatment if misused.

Report all applicable disorders on Axis I, specifying the primary diagnosis by listing it first and designating that it was the difficulty that prompted the office visit (in an outpatient setting, state "reason for visit") or inpatient stay (state "principle diagnosis"). Finally, severity specifiers may follow the disorder to denote the nature of the disorder. Course specifiers and descriptors include Mild, Moderate, Severe, In Partial Remission, In Full Remission, and Prior History (APA, 2000). Each of these is explained in detail. For example, Severe is described as "many symptoms in excess of those required to make the diagnosis, or several symptoms that are particularly severe, are present, or the symptoms result in marked impairment in social or occupational functioning" (p. 2).

Numerous other conditions are included in the *DSM-IV-TR* that present with clinical relevance deserving of attention, but are *not* considered a mental disorder. Many of these more developmental conditions are referred to as "V-Codes" and all

Table 7.7   Other conditions that may be the focus of clinical attention

Psychological factors affecting medical conditions
- Mental disorders
- Psychological symptoms
- Personality traits or coping style
- Maladaptive health behaviors
- Stress-related physiological response

Medication-induced movement disorders
- Neuroleptic-induced
- Parkinsonism
- Malignant syndrome
- Acute dystonia
- Acute akathisia
- Tardive dyskinesia
- Medication-induced postural tremor

Other Medication-induced disorder
- Adverse effects of medication NOS

Relational problems
- Relational problem related to a mental disorder or general medical condition
- Parent-child relational problem
- Partner relational problem
- Sibling relational problem

Problems related to abuse or neglect
- Physical abuse of child
- Sexual abuse of child
- Neglect of child
- Physical abuse of adult
- Sexual abuse of adult

Additional conditions that may be a focus of clinical attention
- Noncompliance with treatment
- Malingering
- Adult antisocial behavior
- Child or adolescent antisocial behavior
- Borderline intellectual functioning
- Age-related cognitive decline
- Bereavement
- Academic problem
- Occupational problem
- Identity problem, religious or spiritual problem
- Acculturation problem
- Phase-of-life problem

---

are coded on Axis I (except Borderline Intellectual Functioning). Fortunately, most of the conditions have titles that are self-explanatory, so rather than expanding on each, we present all of these conditions in Table 7.7.

Axis II Disorders—Personality Disorders and Mental Retardation

Axis II disorders are inflexible and enduring conditions that cause significant impairment in social, occupational, academic, or other adaptive functioning. While most clients will seek or be referred for treatment because of more acute problems or mental disorders on Axis I, Axis II disorders may also be present, though not necessarily responsible for prompting the referral. Personality disorders also often exacerbate Axis I conditions. Importantly, clients presenting with Axis II disorders are frequently less capable of accurate symptom self-report. This, coupled with generally less precise diagnostic criteria, makes diagnosis of personality disorders a challenging endeavor (Fong, 1995). Axis II disorders include mental retardation and personality disorders.

Personality disorders have been categorized according to the following clusters:

- Cluster A: Paranoid Personality Disorder, Schizoid Personality Disorder, Schizotypal Personality Disorder
- Cluster B: Antisocial Personality Disorder, Borderline Personality Disorder, Histrionic Personality Disorder, Narcissistic Personality Disorder
- Cluster C: Avoidant Personality Disorder, Dependent Personality Disorder, Obsessive-Compulsive Personality Disorder

Such a clustering scheme does not preclude an individual from having co-occurring personality disorders across two or more clusters. In addition, the *DSM-IV-TR* allows diagnosis of Personality Disorder—NOS for individuals who display characteristics of one or more personality disorder but do not fulfill all specific criteria in a given classification.

Axis III—Current Medical Conditions

Axis III is utilized for the report of current general medical conditions of potential relevance to a client's current mental disorders or conditions and treatment (APA, 2000). If a medical condition causes the disorder, it should not be listed on Axis III, as it should already be included on Axis I (e.g., Personality Change Due to a General Medical Condition). However, if the general medical condition is a direct physiological result of a mental disorder, then Mental Disorder Due to a General Medical Condition should be listed on Axis I, with the general medical condition noted on both Axis I and Axis III. In other words, the purpose of Axis III is to allow description of medical conditions that are not the direct cause of a mental disorder, but which must be considered when planning a client's treatment. For example, if a client presents with depressive symptoms that are believed to give rise to a client's hypothyroidism, the Axis I diagnosis should be Mood Disorder Due to Hypothyroidism, With Depressive Features, and Hypothyroidism should again be included on Axis III. The general medical conditions used on Axis III are those not included in the chapter on Mental Disorders in the *International Classification of Diseases (ICD-9-CM)* and are important to include in a multiaxial diagnosis because these conditions may affect a managed care organization's decision to continue

Table 7.8   Categories of psychosocial and environmental problems

- Problems with primary support
- Problems related to the social environment
- Educational problems
- Occupational problems
- Housing problems
- Economic problems
- Problems with access to healthcare services
- Problems related to interaction with the legal system or crime
- Other psychosocial and environmental problems

treatment. If no Axis III diagnosis is evident, clinicians should provide the designation "None." If the Axis III diagnosis will be made pending further evaluation, clinicians should provide the designation "Deferred."

Axis IV—Psychosocial and Environmental Problems

Axis IV is used to report environmental and psychosocial problems that may be influencing diagnosis, treatment planning, and eventual prognosis of a client's mental disorder(s). Examples include the death or loss of a family member, close friend, or job; estrangement, separation, or divorce; academic problems; poverty, homelessness, or inadequate healthcare. For convenience, Table 7.8 lists the common categorical designations included in the *DSM-IV-TR* (APA, 2000). While these problems are typically listed on Axis IV, if these problems constitute the reason the client is seeking treatment, it is appropriate to list them on Axis I while specifying "Other Conditions That May Be the Focus of Clinical Attention."

Axis V—Global Assessment of Functioning (GAF)

Axis V allows the clinician to provide an assessment of the client's overall level of functioning, using what APA (2000) refers to as the **Global Assessment of Functioning (GAF)**. This assessment reflects one's professional judgment and is useful in treatment planning and outcome assessment. The GAF indicates a client's current level of functioning unless otherwise noted; at times, the clinician may want to indicate the client's highest level of overall functioning during the past three months or even the previous year. The GAF should not involve a reflection of the client's physical or environment problems or limitations, only the client's functioning in the social, occupational, or psychological areas. Reported as "GAF = ###" on Axis V, the GAF scale ranges from 0 to 100, subdivided by sublevels of ten 10-point ranges. The higher the GAF, the higher the client's level of functioning. Table 7.9 contains the GAF scale descriptors (APA, 2000). Each is explained in greater detail. For example, a GAF between 41 and 50 indicates "Serious symptoms (e.g., suicidal ideation, severe obsessional rituals, frequent shoplifting) *or* any serious impairment in social, occupational, or school func-

Table 7.9   Global Assessment of Functioning (GAF) designations

91–100	Superior functioning
81–90	Absent or minimal symptoms
71–80	Transient and expectable reactions
61–70	Mild symptoms
51–60	Moderate symptoms
41–50	Serious symptoms
31–40	Some impairments in reality testing or communication
21–30	Delusions, hallucinations, or serious impairment in judgment
11–20	Some danger to self or others
1–10	Persistent danger to self or others
0	Inadequate information

Source: Reprinted with permission from the *Diagnostic and Statistical Manual of Mental Disorders,* (4th ed., text rev.), p. 34. American Psychiatric Association. Copyright 2000, Washington, DC: Author.

tioning (e.g., no friends, unable to keep a job)," while a GAF between 51 and 60 indicates Moderate symptoms (e.g., flat affect and circumstantial speech, occasional panic attacks) or moderate difficulty in social, occupational, or school functioning [e.g., few friends, conflicts with peers or co-workers (p.34)]."

For instances in which a clinician might wish to separately assess individual components of functioning, rather than an overall level, APA (2000) provides a Social and Occupational Functioning Assessment Scale (SOFAS), a Global Assessment of Relational Functioning (GARF), and a Defensive Functioning Scale (DFS).

Diagnostic Decision Making Using the *DSM-IV-TR*

The five axes reviewed above can be combined to construct a systematic and comprehensive *DSM-IV-TR* multiaxial assessment system (APA, 2000) that describes a client's mental disorder(s), medical condition(s), environmental and psychosocial factors, and overall level of functioning. The multiaxial system is designed to provide organized, substantive communication about complex diagnostic situations. Professional counselors are encouraged to provide the complete five-axial diagnosis for every client in order to effectively communicate the diagnosis to other professionals and plan an effective treatment regimen (Fong, 1995).

Multiaxial diagnosis is a complicated process, and mastery requires substantial education, training, and practice under supervision. While master clinicians can sometimes reach reliable and accurate diagnostic decisions based on clinical experience, many clinicians find it helpful to use a structured decision-making process. Figure 7.2 presents a structured process clinicians may find helpful in guiding diagnostic decision making. This flow chart guides the clinician through a process in which very general questions can lead to deeper examination using the decision trees provided in the *DSM-IV-TR*. For example, consider the case of an adult undergoing a stressful divorce and employed by a company undergoing downsizing who presents with symptoms of depression. These symptoms have been occurring for about four weeks and have led to intense feelings of hopelessness, weight loss, and insomnia. On the flow chart, this case would be tracked through the Axis I Disorders category and pursued with the *DSM-IV-TR* decision tree for differential diagnosis of Mood Disorders, eventually resulting in a probable diagnosis of Major Depressive Disorder, Single Episode (assuming this was the first time depressive symptoms were displayed to this degree). If the client has no enduring personality disorders or complicating medical conditions, this client's symptoms may result in the following multiaxial diagnosis:

- Axis I   296.22—Major Depressive Disorder, Single Episode, Moderate Without Psychotic Features
- Axis II   None
- Axis III   None
- Axis IV   Disruption of family by divorce, threat of job loss
- Axis V   GAF = 55 (current)

Note that in the example above, the initial question involved whether a client's symptoms constituted a possible mental disorder. If the answer had been no, the process would have stopped right there because the *DSM-IV-TR* is helpful only in diagnosing mental disorders, and no diagnosis would have been warranted. Also, note that the depressive symptoms were relatively recent and acute, not enduring, persistent, and inflexible. Thus it was judged that a Personality Disorder (or Mental Retardation) was not evident and that the condition was likely a mental disorder located on Axis I. If a Personality Disorder was indicated, exploration of these disorders would commence, followed by a return to consideration of Axis I disorders to address the more acute symptoms. When pursuing an Axis I diagnosis, the clinician needs to address each query in the remainder of the flow chart (and subsequent decision trees, if necessary) to ensure a comprehensive diagnosis. As mentioned above, most clients present with more than one condition, so the experienced clinician approaches each client's diagnosis with an eye toward "leaving no stone unturned." While this complicates the diagnostic process, a comprehensive diagnosis generally improves the prospects for treatment, because multimodal treatment strategies can be undertaken to address all areas of concern. Note that the *DSM-IV-TR* has numerous other mental disorders that are not accounted for by the flow chart until the final "catchall" box on the decision tree. The burden for comprehensive diagnostic work always relies on the competence and experience of the clinician. For further discussions and applications of multiaxial diagnosis, the reader is referred to the *DSM-IV Casebook* (Spitzer et al., 1994).

Finally, cultural considerations must always be monitored throughout the diagnostic and treatment processes and are ultimately the responsibility of the clinician. The *DSM-IV-TR* provides discussions of relevant cultural considerations for most of the disorders, and Appendix I of the *DSM-IV-TR* contains a glossary of culture-bound syndromes, including descriptions and relevance to psychopathology.

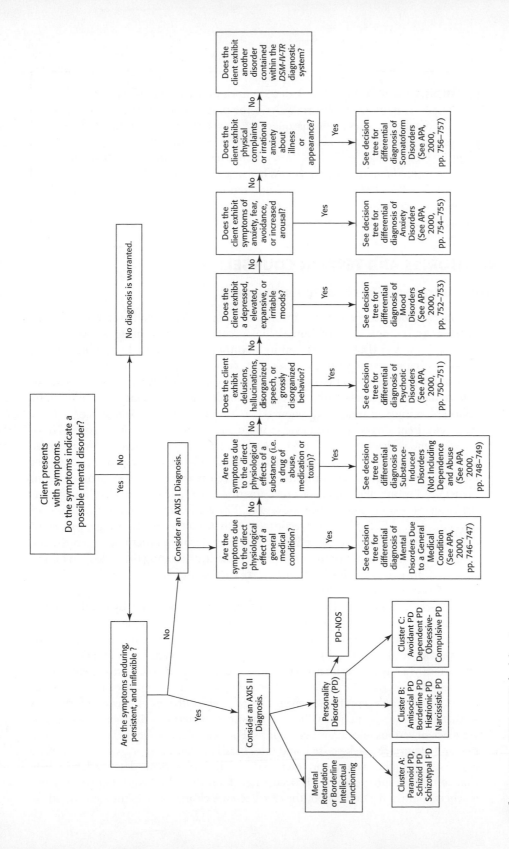

Figure 7.2 *DSM-IV-TR* decision tree

> **Think About It 7.3**   Think of a client or associate who is experiencing a mental or emotional problem. What is the problem, its severity, and its environmental influences and consequences? How can you explain the difficulties from a developmental perspective? What approach(es) could you use to help? Next, using the *DSM-IV-TR,* attempt to understand the individual's issue using the multiaxial system. What treatment approach(es) could be used? Finally, what similarities and differences did you note between the developmental and clinical approaches employed?

USING CLINICAL INVENTORIES AND TESTS IN COUNSELING

Information Sources for Clinical and Personality Assessment

Piedmont (2006) suggested that information on clients be gathered through four different and complementary sources: life outcomes, observer rating, self-report ratings, and test data (LOST). Each information source has strengths and limitations, but accessing information from each source frequently provides a synergistic effect that offers a balanced and confirmatory approach to a comprehensive evaluation. **Life outcomes** data include the factual information about a client that can often be collected during an intake interview: "Has the client ever been married?" "How many children?" "Has the client ever received counseling services in the past?" "If so, for what and with what result?" Each question reveals certain factual information the professional counselor needs to understand the client's life history, properly diagnose or understand current complaints, and develop an effective treatment plan. Generally, life outcome data are factual, unambiguous, and objective, although confirmation of client report is always advisable. These data can be obtained from school or medical records, legal or civic records, directly from the client during a written or oral intake interview, or through direct assessment during a structured or semi-structured clinical interview. Comprehensive attempts at structuring the collection of personal histories include the *Personal History Checklist* (Schinka, 1989) and *Mental Status Checklist* (Schinka, 1988).

Observer ratings involve the report of observations of clients by significant and informed people in their lives. Parents and teachers are often in a good position to rate and evaluate the behaviors of children. Likewise, spouses and some friends or peers make be able to provide helpful insight and observations on an adult client. Importantly, a rating scale is an attempt to objectify someone's subjective perceptions. As such, caution over the veracity and honesty of the ratings must be taken into account. The key is to capture the perceptions of several different sources of information so that a clinician can perform cross-validation and determine the robustness or convergence of various informant perceptions. For example, if a client is referred for depression, reports she is depressed, and rates herself as depressed, she may very well be depressed. But if her parents and teachers do not rate her as being depressed, it is likely that something more complex is occurring. If, on the other hand, her parents and teachers confirm her depression, the case becomes clearer. Such is the value of other-report observer ratings. While observer ratings can be just as biased as self-report ratings, the bias is of a different type and therefore usually adds more clarity than confusion. Indeed, McCrae & Costa (1987) and Piedmont (1994) reported convergence of perspectives of observers to be robust and helpful in confirming personality traits. Many clinical and personality tests have observer report versions, and more of these include validity scales to help clinicians determine the veracity of results.

Self-report ratings are most commonly used in clinical and personality assessment because professional counselors nearly always have direct access to the client. and client perspectives are essential to effective treatment planning, even in cases when they are less than cooperative. Self-report instruments are frequently referred to as objective tests, even though, like observer ratings, professional counselors are best advised to view them as attempts to objectify the subjective perceptions of clients. Some clients present themselves in a biased manner, and clinicians must be wary of the impact such bias may have on test results. Many self-report scales include validity scales to help clinicians determine likely inaccuracies of self-perception and outright dishonesty in a client's self-presentation. In spite of the potential limitation of bias, self-report rating scales have two major strengths. They allow: (1) comparison of a client's self-ratings to a norm sample (i.e., are norm referenced), and (2) direct assessment of client thoughts, feelings, and behaviors, which are all facets of a client's mental state and personality functioning (Piedmont, 2006). Many of the tests reviewed throughout the remainder of this chapter are self-report inventories.

Test data involve the use of instruments to directly assess client functioning. Importantly, such instrumentation measures information that clients either do not know they are producing, or are unaware of how the information will be interpreted. Physiological measures fall into this category (e.g., galvanic skin response, electrocardiogram). In clinical and personality assessment, projective tests are examples of collecting test data. In general, projective tests present a client with ambiguous stimuli, such as inkblots, incomplete sentences, or pictures about which a client tells a story. The client, unaware of the purpose of the activity or the meaning of responses, projects thoughts and feelings onto the stimuli. Clinicians then interpret these responses to understand the client's underlying needs, drives, motivations, thoughts, and emotions. Test data have the advantage of being difficult to "fake," thus reducing the opportunity to bias the results. While projective test data are certainly used by some clinicians for diagnostic purposes, the psychometric properties of most projective tests do not support their use for this purpose. On the other hand, rich description and understanding of client personality can often be derived from projective techniques by skilled professional counselors. Thus an expanded discussion of projective assessment and commonly used projective tests will be provided at the end of this chapter within the context of personality assessment.

How Clinical and Personality Test Content Is Developed

Clinical and personality inventories are generally multidimensional tests composed of several to numerous scales. Each of these scales is supposed to provide a helpful addition to the overall test, usually measuring some unique or important facet of the overall construct being measured. Four primary methods are used to construct clinical and personality inventories: content validation, theory, empirical-criterion keying, and factor analysis. *Content validation* relies on the logical process of deductive reasoning to determine the items that are assigned to a given scale. Each item under consideration may be included on the scale if the test developer determines (through logical analysis) that it contributes to the measurement of the concept under study (e.g. Major Depression, Schizophrenia, General Anxiety Disorder). Scales such as the *Woodworth Personal Data Sheet* and the *Edwards Personal Preference Schedule* were constructed using the content validation method.

Theories are sometimes used to develop test items and scales. The theory guides item development and categorical assignments to potential subscales. An example of a popular test designed using an underlying theory is the *Myers-Briggs Type Indicator* (*MBTI*), which is based on Jung's theory. To be fair, many other inventories also use content validation of a theory at an early phase of test development but subsequently use one of the next two procedures to complete the instrument design (see the discussion of bootstrapping included in Chapter 6).

Empirical-criterion keying is a procedure in which selected items are administered to both nonclinical samples (individuals without the diagnosis) and clinical samples (individual with the diagnosis). While this process can sometimes use complex analyses, simply put, the items that identify the clinical group and not the nonclinical group are selected to comprise that particular clinical scale. The *MMPI-2, MMPI-A,* and *California Personality Inventory* are among the better-known tests using the empirical-criterion key method. For example, the *MMPI-2* Depression clinical scale (D), is comprised of 57 items, many of which are obviously related to depression (i.e., have face validity) and some that leave examiners wondering how the item could possibly be related to depression. What is the "rational" or "logical" connection? The connection is that the individuals with depression comprising the clinical sample endorsed the item significantly more frequently that the nonclinical sample of individuals without depression. Thus the "logic" is that there is something about the item that makes it relate to responses of individuals with depression, even though the link may not be obvious or rationally determined.

Factor analysis has risen in prominence as a procedure for scale construction over the past half century due to the advent of high-speed computers. As described in Chapter 6, factor analysis is an item-sorting technique based on item intercorrelations, and the subsequent correlation between each item and derived dimensions or components, called *factors.* The factors are subsequently named and may or may not be "pure measures" of any given clinical diagnosis or personality trait. Each factor is a statistical entity that has been empirically derived and which can be studied and refined through further research and test development. The *16PF* and *NEO-PI-R* are examples of empirically derived tests constructed through the use of factor analysis. Factor analysis has contributed to an explosion of clinical and personality inventories. Of course, the primary criticism of the use of factor analysis is that it derives statistical models of item relationships, rather than theoretical models of item relationships. That is, many test developers put too much faith in factor analysis and actually use it to design the test, rather than constructing the test using a theoretical model and using factor analysis to explore the dimensions underlying the test and confirming the original design.

As mentioned earlier, some clinical and personality inventories use one or more of these three design methodologies. Regardless of the test development procedure, numerous studies must be undertaken to explore the reliability and validity of test scores across various samples and for various purposes before the test is ready for widespread use in clinical decision making.

SOME COMMONLY USED CLINICAL ASSESSMENT INVENTORIES

Professional counselors in clinical practice may rely heavily on objective clinical inventories when exploring a client's presenting problem, diagnosing client symptoms, developing a treatment plan, and determining the effectiveness of therapeutic interventions. Numerous clinical inventories have been developed, and this section presents a basic review of more than 15 of those most commonly used by professional counselors in clinical practice. As with any of the tests reviewed throughout this book, more in-depth information on administration, scoring, interpretation, and technical characteristics can be found in the test manual, *Mental Measurements Yearbook* reviews, and the extant literature.

Minnesota Multiphasic Personality Inventory—Second Edition (MMPI-2)

The *Minnesota Multiphasic Personality Inventory—Second Edition* (*MMPI-2* (Butcher et al., 1989) is a 567-item, true-false, self-report inventory designed to assess some of the major patterns of personality in adults ages 18–90 years. Items measure 6 validity indicators, 10 clinical scales (see Table 7.10), and numerous supplementary, clinical component, content scales, and clinical subscales (see Table 7.11). Some advocate for the use of Clinical scale patterns to provide quick insight into client diagnosis and personality, rather than relying on interpretation of individual scales. Patterns are represented by reporting the Clinical Scale numeric designation for the two or three highest scale scores. For example, if the client's highest score is on scale 2 (Depression), and the client's second highest score is on scale 7 (Psychasthenia), the pattern would be "27." Numerous books written about the *MMPI* and *MMPI-2* provide interpretive suggestions applicable to pattern analysis.

The restandardization sample (*n* = 2,600) consisted of paid volunteer adults (1,138 men and 1,462 women) recruited from seven states, a federal Indian reservation, and four military bases via random mailings and advertisements. Biographical data and information about recent stressful life events were also collected (Nichols, 1992). Hispanic and Asian American subgroups were underrepresented in the normative sample, whereas Native Americans were overrepresented (Butcher et al., 2001).

The *MMPI-2* takes about 60 to 90 minutes to complete and can be scored by hand in 30 to 60 minutes, or in about 5 minutes by computer. Sample items include "Spirits sometimes speak to me," "I am as happy as others seem to be," and "I dread the thought of a hurricane." Convenient score profiles are available to plot and transform raw scores into T scores. Test-retest coefficients based on 82 males and 111 females with a median interval of seven days ranged from 0.54 (females on the Sc scale) to 0.93 (males on the Si scale) on the Clinical scales, 0.77 (males on the BIZ scale) to 0.91 (males and females on the SOD scale) on the Content scales, and 0.63 (males on the MAC-R scale) to 0.91 (males and females on the A scale) on Supplementary scales. Internal consistency estimates ranged from 0.56 to 0.87 (except for the Pa scale, which yielded coefficients 0.34 for males and 0.39 for females) on the Clinical scales and 0.68 (females on the TPA scale) to 0.86 (males and females on the CYN and DEP scales, respectively) on the Content scales (Butcher et al., 2001).

In general, caution is warranted when using the *MMPI-2* for diagnostic purposes. Low scale reliabilities (<0.90) make the *MMPI-2* more helpful as a test for understanding individual pathology and exploring intrapersonal hypotheses than for making diagnoses. The *MMPI-2* is a Level C instrument and requires proficiency in reading English at the 8th-grade level. The clinician should note the inclusion of several helpful validity scales. The L scale identifies individuals presenting themselves in a favorable light, the K scale is a measure of defensiveness, and the F scale is designed to detect clients who randomly respond, cannot understand the items, or are attempting to fake bad (Erford, 2006). The VRIN and TRIN (validity scales) help determine if a subject responded in an inconsistent or contradictory way. Although the *MMPI-A* (Adolescent version) is designed for adolescents ages 14–18 years, the *MMPI-2* is more appropriate for 18-year-olds living independently from their parents (Butcher et al., 2001). Clinicians should also note that Hispanics, Asian Americans, and older women were underrepresented in the restandardization of the

Table 7.10 *MMPI-2* Clinical scale descriptions

Clinical scale designations			Description
1	Hs	Hypochondriasis	Excessive health concerns, somatic complaints, narcissism, self-centeredness
2	D	Depression	Depression, brooding, discouragement, pessimism, hopelessness
3	Hy	Hysteria	Sensory or physical complaints of no organic cause, immaturity, physical complaints, denial of aggression, need for affection
4	Pd	Psychopathic deviation	Antisocial/Asocial behavior, impulsivity, immaturity, lack of concern over social and moral standards of conduct
5	Mf	Masculinity/Femininity	Masculine and feminine interests
6	Pa	Paranoia	Paranoia, suspicion, hostility, psychotic behavior, cynicism, excessive moral virtue
7	Pt	Psychasthenia	Anxiety, obsessions, compulsions, exaggerated fears, difficulty concentrating, physical complaints
8	Sc	Schizophrenia	Withdrawal, social/emotional alienation, thought disturbance, bizarre sensory experiences, lack of ego mastery
9	Ma	Hypomania	High energy, elated mood, low frustration tolerance, denial of social anxiety
0	Si	Social introversion	Introversion, shyness, neurotic maladjustment, self-depreciation

Source: Manual for Administration, Scoring, and Interpretation of the Minnesota Multiphasic Personality Inventory—Third Edition by Butcher et al., (2001). Minneapolis: University of Minnesota Press.

Table 7.11   Scales and subscales derived from *MMPI-2* items

Validity scales
—Cannot Say (?) (reported as a raw score only, not plotted)
VRIN—Variable response inconsistency
TRIN—True response inconsistency
F—Infrequency
F_B—Back F
F_P—Infrequency–Psychopathology
L—Lie
K—Correction
S—Superlative self-presentation

Superlative self-presentation subscales
S_1—Beliefs in human goodness
S_2—Serenity
S_3—Contentment with life
S_4—Patience/Denial of irritability
S_5—Denial of moral flaws

Clinical scales
1 Hs—Hypochondriasis
2 D—Depression
3 Hy—Hysteria
4 Pd—Psychopathic deviate
5 Mf—Masculinity–Femininity
6 Pa—Paranoia
7 Pt—Psychasthenia
8 Sc—Schizophrenia
9 Ma—Hypomania
0 Si—Social introversion

RC (Restructured clinical) Scales
RCd—dem—Demoralization
RC1—som—Somatic complaints
RC2—lpe—Low positive emotions
RC3—cyn—Cynicism
RC4—asb—Antisocial behavior
RC6—per—Ideas of persecution
RC7—dne—Dysfunctional negative emotions
RC8—abx—Aberrant experiences
RC9—hpm—Hypomanic activation

Clinical subscales
Harris-Lingoes subscales
D1—Subjective depression
D2—Psychomotor retardation
D3—Physical malfunctioning

D4—Mental dullness
D5—Brooding
Hy1—Denial of social anxiety
Hy2—Need for affection
Hy3—Lassitude-Malaise
Hy4—Somatic complaints
Hy5—Inhibition of aggression
Pd1—Familial discord
Pd2—Authority problems
Pd3—Social imperturbability
Pd4—Social alienation
Pd5—Self-alienation
Pa1—Persecutory ideas
Pa2—Poignancy
Pa3—Naïveté
Sc1—Social alienation
Sc2—Emotional alienation
Sc3—Lack of ego mastery–cognitive
Sc4—Lack of ego mastery–conative
Sc5—Lack of ego mastery–defective inhibition
Sc6—Bizarre sensory experiences
Ma1—Amorality
Ma2—Psychomotor acceleration
Ma3—Imperturbability
Ma4—Ego inflation

Social introversion subscales
Si1—Shyness/Self-consciousness
Si2—Social avoidance
Si3—Alienation – self and others

Content scales
ANX—Anxiety
FRS—Fears
OBS—Obsessiveness
DEP—Depression
HEA—Health concerns
BIZ—Bizarre mentation
ANG—Anger
CYN—Cynicism
ASP—Antisocial practices
TPA—Type A
LSE—Low self-esteem
SOD—Social discomfort
FAM—Family problems
WRK—Work interference
TRT—Negative treatment indicators

continued

Table 7.11   continued

Content component scales	*Negative treatment indicators*
Fears subscales	TRT1—Low motivation
FRS1—Generalized fearfulness	TRT2—Inability to disclose
FRS2—Multiple fears	
Depression subscales	***Supplementary scales***
DEP1—Lack of drive	*Personality psychopathology five scales (PSY-5)*
DEP2—Dysphoria	AGGR—Aggressiveness
DEP3—Self-depreciation	PSYC—Psychoticism
DEP4—Suicidal ideation	DISC—Disconstraint
	NEGE—Negative emotionality/Neuroticism
Health concerns subscales	INTR—Introversion/Low positive emotionality
HEA1—Gastrointestinal symptoms	
HEA2—Neurological symptoms	*Broad personality characteristics*
HEA3—General health concerns	A—Anxiety
	R—Repression
Bizarre mentation subscales	Es—Ego strength
BIZ1—Psychotic symptomatology	Do—Dominance
BIZ2—Schizotypal characteristics	Re—Social responsibility
Anger subscales	*Generalized emotional distress*
ANG1—Explosive behavior	Mt—College maladjustment
ANG2—Irritability	PK—Post-Traumatic Stress Disorder–Keane
	MDS—Marital distress
Cynicism subscales	
CYN1—Misanthropic beliefs	*Behavioral dyscontrol*
CYN2—Interpersonal suspiciousness	Ho—Hostility
	O-H—Overcontrolled hostility
Antisocial practices subscales	MAC-R—MacAndrew–revised
ASP1—Antisocial attitudes	AAS—Addiction admission
ASP2—Antisocial behavior	APS—Addiction potential
Type A subscales	*Gender Role*
TPA1—Impatience	GM—Gender role—masculine
TPA2—Competitive drive	GF—Gender role—feminine
Low self-esteem subscales	
LSE1—Self-doubt	***Special Indices***
LSE2—Submissiveness	Welsh Code
	F–K Dissimulation Index
Social discomfort	Percent True and Percent False
SOD1—Introversion	Average Profile Elevation
SOD2—Shyness	Megargee Offender Classification System
	P-A-I-N Classification
Family problems	
FAM1—Family discord	
FAM2—Familial alienation	

MMPI-2. Likewise, clients who fit within the lowest educational and occupational levels might not be appropriate candidates for the *MMPI-2* because of their under-representation within the normative restandardization sample (Nichols, 1992). The *MMPI-2* is available on audiocassette and computer-adapted software and in Spanish, French, and the Hmong languages.

Minnesota Multiphasic Personality Inventory–Adolescent (MMPI-A)

The *Minnesota Multiphasic Personality Inventory—Adolescent* (*MMPI-A*) (Butcher et al., 1992) is a 478-item true-false, self-report inventory designed for use with adolescents ages 14–18 years to assess some of the major patterns of personality and emotional disorders. The derived scales are very similar to the *MMPI-2* scales listed in Table 7.10. Items measure 6 Validity Scales, 10 Clinical Scales, 15 Content Scales, 6 Supplementary Scales, and about 30 Harris-Lingoes scales. Table 7.12 provides a sample computerized interpretive report from the Pearson software package. As with any test, it is essential that any statements from computerized sources be validated with other clinical information. The normative sample (*n* = 1,620) was very diverse, although it may have oversampled a more educated population. It consisted of male (*n* = 805) and female (*n* = 815) adolescents ages 14–18 years living in eight U.S. states; one state's sample was from an American Indian reservation. There was also a large adolescent clinical population (*n* = 703). Most of these subjects were paid to complete the test (Butcher et al., 1992). This inventory requires a 6th-grade English reading level.

Raw scores are converted to Uniform T percentile-comparable scores for interpretation through use of convenient profile forms. Different scoring keys are used according to gender. The *MMPI-A* may take up to three hours to complete and can be scored by hand or computer. It is a Level C instrument. Sample items include "I'm afraid to go home," "Others do not really love me," and "I feel uneasy outdoors." Test-retest reliability results range from 0.65 to 0.84 for the Clinical scales (Butcher et al., 1992). Strong internal consistency coefficients were reported for 4 of the 15 basic and clinical scales (*r* = 0.80+); 7 of 15 were between *r* = 0.60 and 0.80. Two response set indicators (VRIN and TRIN) are validity scales that show a respondent's patterns of responding in an inconsistent or contradictory manner (Butcher et al., 1992). The *MMPI-A* is one of the only adolescent clinical inventories to comprehensively incorporate a number of validity scales to evaluate client response sets (Archer & Krishnamurthy, 2002). Unfortunately, fewer *MMPI-A* items demonstrate the same discriminative value in differentiating clients from normal and clinical samples than the adult version of the test (Archer & Handel, 2001).

Bright 12- and 13-year-olds can also be tested, as well as 18-year-olds who have completed high school (Lanyon, 1995). As a Level C instrument, examiners are required to undergo training and supervision prior to administration, scoring, and interpretation of this test (Butcher et al., 1992). The *MMPI-A* has a number of unique features appropriate for its intended use with adolescents, yet several of the scale labels seem outdated and/or offensive (i.e., Masculine-Feminine, Hypomania, Hysteria, and Psychopathic Deviate) (Claiborn, 1995). "Clinicians should recognize that not all adolescents have the necessary skills to complete the *MMPI-A*" if their reading comprehension skills are inadequate or if their cultural background and life experiences are out of the range of the test (Butcher et al., 1992, p. 27). (Special learning problems and English as a second language may prohibit the prerequisite reading comprehension, including idioms or other cultural meanings.) It may be prudent to break the testing up into smaller sessions because some adolescents may

Table 7.12   *MMPI-A* The Minnesota Report: Adolescent System Interpretive Report by Butcher & Williams for Rachel, female, age 15, outpatient mental health center

Validity Considerations

She had a tendency to inconsistently respond True without adequate attention to item meaning. Although her TRIN score is not elevated enough to invalidate her *MMPI-A,* caution is suggested in interpreting and using the resulting profiles (see Figure 7.3).

Symptomatic Behavior

This adolescent is immature, impulsive, and hedonistic, and she frequently rebels against authority. She may be hostile, aggressive, and frustrated. She seems unable to learn from punishing experiences and repeatedly gets into the same type of trouble. Many young people with this clinical profile develop severe acting-out problems and have legal, family, or school difficulties. This individual's nonconforming and impulsive lifestyle probably includes alcohol or drug problems.

Many externalizing behavior problems are likely. Her friends are frequently in trouble. They may cheat others and lie to avoid problems. They show little remorse for their misbehavior. If their difficulties pile up, they may run away.

The highest clinical scale (see Figure 7.4) in her *MMPI-A* clinical profile, Pd, occurs with very high frequency in adolescent alcohol/drug or psychiatric treatment units. Over 24% of girls in treatment settings have this well-defined peak score (i.e., with the Pd scale at least 5 points higher than the next scale). The Pd scale is among the least frequently occurring peak elevations in the normative girls' sample (about 3%).

Her *MMPI-A* Content scales profile (see Figure 7.5) reveals important areas to consider in her evaluation. She endorsed a number of very negative opinions about herself. She reported feeling unattractive, lacking self-confidence, feeling useless, having little ability and several faults, and not being able to do anything well. She may be easily dominated by others.

She reported numerous problems in school, both academic and behavioral. She has limited expectations of success in school and is not very interested or invested in succeeding. She reported several symptoms of anxiety, including tension, worries, and difficulties sleeping. Symptoms of depression were reported.

Interpersonal Relations

She may appear charming and tends to make a good first impression, but she is selfish, hedonistic, and untrustworthy in interpersonal relations. She seems interested only in her own pleasure and is insensitive to the needs of others. She seems unable to experience guilt over causing others trouble.

Because she is unable to form stable, warm relationships, her current relationships are likely to be quite strained. In addition, she is likely to be openly hostile and resentful at times.

Some interpersonal issues are suggested by her *MMPI-A* Content scales profile. Family problems are quite significant in this person's life. She reports numerous problems with her parents and other family members. She describes her family in terms of discord, jealousy, fault finding, anger, serious disagreements, lack of love and understanding, and very limited communication. She looks forward to the day when she can leave home for good, and she does not feel that she can count on her family in times of trouble. Her parents and she often disagree about her friends. She indicates that her parents treat her like a child and frequently punish her without cause. Her family problems probably have a negative effect on her behavior in school. She feels uncomfortable emotional distance from others. She may believe that other people do

continued

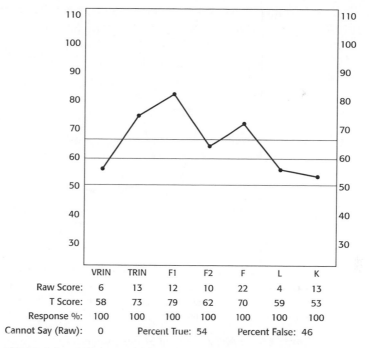

	VRIN	TRIN	F1	F2	F	L	K
Raw Score:	6	13	12	10	22	4	13
T Score:	58	73	79	62	70	59	53
Response %:	100	100	100	100	100	100	100

Cannot Say (Raw): 0   Percent True: 54   Percent False: 46

Figure 7.3   *MMPI-A* validity pattern

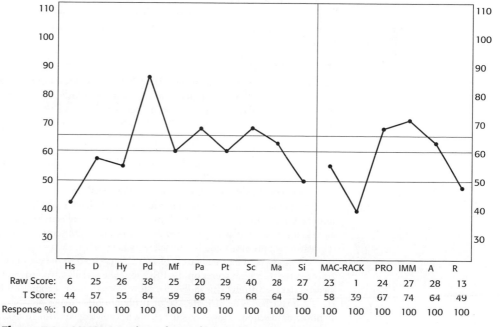

	Hs	D	Hy	Pd	Mf	Pa	Pt	Sc	Ma	Si	MAC-RACK	PRO	IMM	A	R
Raw Score:	6	25	26	38	25	20	29	40	28	27	23	1	24	27	28	13
T Score:	44	57	55	84	59	68	59	68	64	50	58	39	67	74	64	49
Response %:	100	100	100	100	100	100	100	100	100	100	100	100	100	100	100	100

Figure 7.4   *MMPI-A* Basic and Supplementary Scales profile

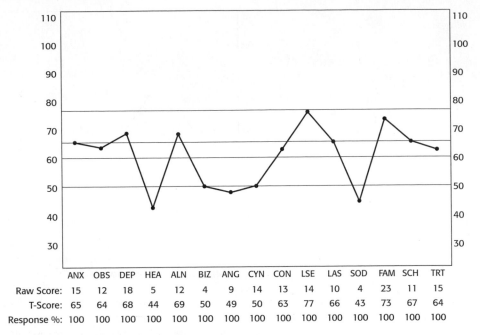

	ANX	OBS	DEP	HEA	ALN	BIZ	ANG	CYN	CON	LSE	LAS	SOD	FAM	SCH	TRT
Raw Score:	15	12	18	5	12	4	9	14	13	14	10	4	23	11	15
T-Score:	65	64	68	44	69	50	49	50	63	77	66	43	73	67	64
Response %:	100	100	100	100	100	100	100	100	100	100	100	100	100	100	100

Figure 7.5   *MMPI-A Content Scales profile*

Table 7.12   continued

not like, understand, or care about her. She reports having no one, including parents or friends, to rely on.

Behavioral Stability
The relative elevation of the highest scale (Pd) in her clinical profile shows very high profile definition. Her peak scores are likely to remain very prominent in her profile pattern if she is retested at a later date. Her clinical profile tends to be associated with long-standing behavior problems.

Diagnostic Considerations
A diagnosis of one of the disruptive behavior disorders is highly likely given her elevations on Pd and A-con.

Given her elevation on the School Problems scale, her diagnostic evaluation could include assessment of possible academic skills deficits and behavior problems. Academic underachievement, a general lack of interest in any school activities, and low expectations of success are likely to play a role in her problems. Her endorsement of a significant number of depressive symptoms should be considered when arriving at a diagnosis.

She appears to be having difficulties that may involve the use of alcohol or other drugs. Adolescents with high scores on the PRO scale are usually involved with a peer group that uses alcohol or other drugs. This individual's involvement in an alcohol- or drug-using lifestyle should be further evaluated. Her use of alcohol or other drugs may be contributing to problems at home or in school. However, she has not acknowledged through her item responses that she has problems with alcohol or other drugs.

Treatment Considerations

Her serious conduct disturbance should figure prominently in any treatment planning. Her Clinical scales profile suggests that she is a poor candidate for traditional, insight-oriented psychotherapy. A behavioral strategy is suggested. Clearly stated contingencies that are consistently followed are important for shaping more appropriate behaviors. Punishment techniques seem to have more limited success than positive rewards for appropriate behaviors. Treatment in a more controlled setting may need to be considered if there is no improvement in her behavior.

Her very high potential for developing alcohol or drug problems requires attention in therapy if important life changes are to be made. However, her relatively low awareness of or reluctance to acknowledge problems in this area might impede treatment efforts.

She should be evaluated for the presence of suicidal thoughts and any possible suicidal behaviors. If she is at risk, appropriate precautions should be taken.

Her family situation, which is full of conflict, should be considered in her treatment planning. Family therapy may be helpful if her parents or guardians are willing and able to work on conflict resolution. However, if family therapy is not feasible, it may be profitable during the course of her treatment to explore her considerable anger at and disappointment in her family. Alternate sources of emotional support from adults (e.g., foster parent, teacher, other relative, friend's parent, or neighbor) could be explored and facilitated in the absence of caring parents.

There are some symptom areas suggested by the Content scales profile that the therapist may wish to consider in initial treatment sessions. Her endorsement of internalizing symptoms of anxiety and depression could be explored further.

She endorsed some items that indicate possible difficulties in establishing a therapeutic relationship. She may be reluctant to self-disclose, she may be distrustful of helping professionals and others, and she may believe that her problems cannot be solved. She may be unwilling to assume responsibility for behavior change or to plan for her future.

This adolescent's emotional distance and discomfort in interpersonal situations must be considered in developing a treatment plan. She may have difficulty self-disclosing, especially in groups. She may not appreciate receiving feedback from others about her behavior or problems.

Note: This *MMPI-A* interpretation can serve as a useful source of hypotheses about adolescent clients. This report is based on objectively derived scale indexes and scale interpretations that have been developed with diverse groups of clients from adolescent treatment settings. The personality descriptions, inferences, and recommendations contained herein need to be verified by other sources of clinical information because individual clients may not fully match the prototype. The information in this report should most appropriately be used by a trained, qualified test interpreter. The information contained in this report should be considered confidential.

---

be too easily distracted or unable to complete the test in one sitting (Butcher et al., 1992). The *MMPI-A* is a good tool that can help to measure psychopathology in adolescents (Archer & Krishnamurthy, 2002; Claiborn, 1995) and is very useful in planning, directing, and evaluating treatment (Lanyon, 1995).

Millon Clinical Multiaxial Inventory—III (MCMI-III)

The *Millon Clinical Multiaxial Inventory—III* (*MCMI-III*) (Millon, Davis, & Millon, 1997) is a 175-item, true-false, self-report inventory designed to provide diagnostic and treatment information to clinicians in the areas of personality disorders and clinical syndromes. Scale items measure 1 type of Clinical Personality Pattern (Schizoid, Avoidant, Depressive, Dependent, Histrionic, Narcissistic, Antisocial, Aggressive [Sadistic], Compulsive, Passive-Aggressive [Negativistic], Self-Defeating); 3 Severe Personality Pathologies (Schizotypal, Borderline, Paranoid); 7 Clinical Syndromes (Anxiety, Somatoform, Bipolar: Manic, Dysthymia, Alcohol Dependence, Drug Dependence, Post-Traumatic Stress Disorder); 3 Severe Clinical Syndromes (Thought Disorder, Major Depression, Delusional Disorder), and 4 Modifying Indices (Disclosure, Desirability, Debasement, Validity). These scales are grouped to reflect distinctions between acute clinical disorders pertinent to the *DSM-IV* Axis I and the enduring personality characteristics found on *DSM-IV* Axis II (Millon et al., 1997). The total normative population (*n* = 998) consisted of male and female volunteer adults ages 18–88 years from 26 states and Canada (development sample *n* = 600 and cross-validation sample *n* = 398).

Except for Scale V (Validity) raw scores, raw scores are converted to *Base Rate* (*BR*) *scores* for interpretation. Different BR transformation tables are used for males and females and provide cutoff points on the continuums for the 24 clinical scales (BR 0 = raw score 0, BR 60 = median raw score, BR 115 = highest raw score). A BR score of 75 or higher is an indication of psychopathology (Millon et al., 1997; Erford, 2006). The *MCMI-III* usually requires about 20 to 30 minutes to complete and can be scored by hand and interpreted in about 20 to 40 minutes. It can also be sent to the publisher by mail, or scored by onsite computer software in about 5 minutes (Erford, 2006). Sample items include "I've become very anxious lately," "I often feel tired," and "I often make people angry." Internal consistency reliabilities range from 0.66 for the Compulsive scale to 0.90 for the Major Depression scale. Twenty of the 24 scales have reliabilities of 0.80 or higher. Test-retest reliability results range from 0.82 to 0.96 for a 5- to 14-day interval (Millon et al., 1997). The median stability coefficient is 0.91, which provides high stability for use of the test over short periods. Criterion-related validity correlations are moderate in magnitude (Erford, 2006).

The *MCMI-III* is designed for adults 18 years and older who are seeking, or are in, mental health treatment. Since the *MCMI-III* is a Level C instrument, examiners are required to have "a graduate degree in psychology or a related field, or appropriate licensure, a course in testing theory, coursework in personality theory, or abnormal psychology, and appropriate experience under supervision" (Erford, 2006, p. 41). The *MCMI-III*'s theoretical conceptualization and prototypes are familiar to many clinicians because they are often covered in graduate coursework and clinical literature. "Because it also offers scales measuring clinical syndromes (Axis I of the *DSM-IV*), the diagnostician does not have to resort to a different instrument in order to assess those areas of functioning" (Choca, 2001, p. 766). Clinicians can also make adjustments to the cutoff scores that place a client along a continuum of pathology based on estimates of the prevalence rate within a particular setting or local area (Widiger, 2001). Weaknesses of the *MCMI-III* include the complex hand scoring process, overrepresentation of Whites and people who differ in levels of educational experience, and underrepresentation of most minority groups (Erford, 2006). Use with various cultures (e.g., Korean) must be undertaken with caution (Erford, 2006; Gunsalus & Kelly, 2001). Table 7.13 provides a computerized interpretive report for the protocol of a 44-year old, divorced, White female outpatient. As always, information from a computerized report must be validated by other clinical information.

Table 7.13   *MCMI-III* sample computerized interpretive report of a female, age 44, White, divorced outpatient never hospitalized (Millon)

Capsule summary
MCMI-III reports are normed on patients who were in the early phases of assessment or psychotherapy for emotional discomfort or social difficulties. Respondents who do not fit this normative population or who have inappropriately taken the *MCMI-III* for nonclinical purposes may have distorted reports. The *MCMI-III* report cannot be considered definitive. It should be evaluated in conjunction with additional clinical data. The report should be evaluated by a mental health clinician trained in the use of psychological tests. The report should not be shown to patients or their relatives.

Interpretive considerations
The client is a 44-year-old divorced White female. She is currently being seen as an outpatient, and she did not identify specific problems and difficulties of an Axis I nature in the demographic portion of this test.

This patient's response style may indicate a tendency to magnify illness, an inclination to complain, or feelings of extreme vulnerability associated with a current episode of acute turmoil. The patient's scale scores may be somewhat exaggerated, and the interpretations should be read with this in mind.

Profile severity
On the basis of the test data, it may be assumed that the patient is experiencing a severe mental disorder, further professional observation and inpatient care may be appropriate. The text of the following interpretive report may need to be modulated upward given this probable level of severity.

Possible diagnoses
She appears to fit the following Axis II classifications best: Negativistic (Passive-Aggressive) Personality Disorder, and Borderline Personality Disorder, with Dependent Personality Traits, and Depressive Personality Traits.

Axis I clinical syndromes are suggested by the client's *MCMI-III* profile in the areas of Major Depression (recurrent, severe, without psychotic features), Generalized Anxiety Disorder, and Psychoactive Substance Abuse NOS (see Figure 7.6).

Therapeutic considerations
Inconsistent and pessimistic, this patient may expect to be mishandled, if not harmed, even by well-intentioned therapists. Sensitive to messages of disapproval and lack of interest, she may complain excessively and be irritable and erratic in her relations with therapists. Straightforward and consistent communication may moderate her dependent/negativistic attitude. Focused, brief treatment approaches are likely to overcome her initial oppositional outlook.

continued

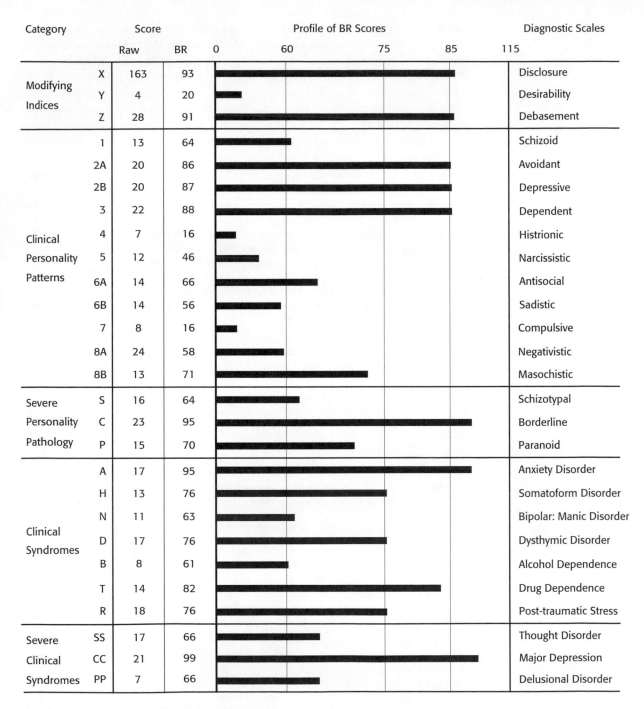

Category		Score		Profile of BR Scores					Diagnostic Scales
		Raw	BR	0	60	75	85	115	
Modifying Indices	X	163	93						Disclosure
	Y	4	20						Desirability
	Z	28	91						Debasement
Clinical Personality Patterns	1	13	64						Schizoid
	2A	20	86						Avoidant
	2B	20	87						Depressive
	3	22	88						Dependent
	4	7	16						Histrionic
	5	12	46						Narcissistic
	6A	14	66						Antisocial
	6B	14	56						Sadistic
	7	8	16						Compulsive
	8A	24	58						Negativistic
	8B	13	71						Masochistic
Severe Personality Pathology	S	16	64						Schizotypal
	C	23	95						Borderline
	P	15	70						Paranoid
Clinical Syndromes	A	17	95						Anxiety Disorder
	H	13	76						Somatoform Disorder
	N	11	63						Bipolar: Manic Disorder
	D	17	76						Dysthymic Disorder
	B	8	61						Alcohol Dependence
	T	14	82						Drug Dependence
	R	18	76						Post-traumatic Stress
Severe Clinical Syndromes	SS	17	66						Thought Disorder
	CC	21	99						Major Depression
	PP	7	66						Delusional Disorder

Figure 7.6   *MCMI-III* profile for female, age 44

Table 7.13   continued

Response tendencies

This patient's response style may indicate a broad tendency to magnify the level of experience illness or a characterological inclination to complain or to be self-pitying. On the other hand, the response style may convey feelings of extreme vulnerability that are associated with a current episode of acute turmoil. Whatever the impetus for the response style, the patient's scale scores, particularly those on Axis I, may be somewhat exaggerated, and the interpretation of this profile should be made with this consideration in mind.

The BR scores reported for this individual have been modified to account for the high self-revealing inclinations indicated by the high raw score on Scale X (Disclosure) and the psychic tension and dejection indicated by the elevations on Scale A (Anxiety) and Scale D (Dysthymia).

Axis II: Personality patterns

The following paragraphs refer to those enduring and pervasive personality traits that underlie this woman's emotional, cognitive, and interpersonal difficulties. Rather than focus on the largely transitory symptoms that make up Axis I clinical syndromes, this section concentrates on her more habitual and maladaptive methods of relating, behaving, thinking, and feeling.

There is reason to believe that at least a moderate level of pathology characterizes the overall personality organization of this woman. Defective psychic structures suggest a failure to develop adequate internal cohesion and a less than satisfactory hierarchy of coping strategies. This woman's foundation for effective intrapsychic regulation and socially acceptable interpersonal conduct appears deficient or incompetent. She is subjected to the flux of her own enigmatic attitudes and contradictory behavior, and her sense of psychic coherence is often precarious. She has probably had a checkered history of disappointments in her personal and family relationships. Deficits in her social attainments may also be notable as well as a tendency to precipitate self-defeating vicious circles. Earlier aspirations may have resulted in frustrating setbacks, and efforts to achieve a consistent niche in life may have failed. Although she is usually able to function on a satisfactory basis, she may experience periods of marked emotional, cognitive, or behavioral dysfunction.

The *MCMI-III* profile of this woman suggests her marked dependency needs, deep and variable moods, and impulsive, angry outbursts. She may anxiously seek reassurance from others and is especially vulnerable to fear of separation from those who provide support, despite her frequent attempts to undo their efforts to be helpful. Dependency fears may compel her to be alternately overly compliant, profoundly gloomy, and irrationally argumentative and negativistic. Almost seeking to court undeserved blame and criticism, she may appear to find circumstances to anchor her feeling that she deserves to suffer.

She strives at times to be submissive and cooperative, but her behavior has become increasingly unpredictable, irritable, and pessimistic. She often seeks to induce guilt in others for failing her, as she sees it. Repeatedly struggling to express attitudes contrary to her feelings, she may exhibit conflicting emotions simultaneously toward others and herself, most notable are love, rage, and guilt. Also notable may be her confusion over her self-image, her highly variable energy levels, easy fatigability, and her irregular sleep-wake cycle.

She is particularly sensitive to external pressure and demands, and she may vacillate between being socially agreeable, sullen, self-pitying, irritably aggressive, and contrite. She may make irrational and bitter complaints about the lack of care expressed by others and about being treated unfairly. This behavior keeps others on edge, never knowing if she will react to them in a cooperative or a sulky manner. Although she may make efforts to be obliging and submissive to others, she has learned to anticipate disillusioning relationships, and she often creates the

continued

Table 7.13   continued

expected disappointment by constantly questioning and doubting the genuine interest and support shown by others. Self-destructive acts and suicidal gestures may be employed to gain attention. These irritable testing maneuvers may exasperate and alienate those on whom she depends. When threatened by separation and disapproval, she may express guilt, remorse, and self-condemnation in the hope of regaining support, reassurance, and sympathy.

Axis I: Clinical syndromes

The features and dynamics of the following Axis I clinical syndromes appear worthy of description and analysis. They may arise in response to external precipitants but are likely to reflect and accentuate several of the more enduring and pervasive aspects of this woman's basic personality makeup.

Testy and demanding, this woman evinces an agitated, major depression that can be noted by her daily moodiness and vacillation. She is likely to display a rapidly shifting mix of disparaging comments about herself, anxiously expressed suicidal thoughts, and outbursts of bitter resentment interwoven with a demanding irritability toward others. Feeling trapped by constraints imposed by her circumstances and upset by emotions and thoughts she can neither understand nor control, she has turned her reservoir of anger inward, periodically voicing severe self-recrimination and self-loathing. These signs of contrition may serve to induce guilt in others, an effective manipulation in which she can give a measure of retribution without further jeopardizing what she sees as her currently precarious, if not hopeless, situation.

Failing to keep deep and powerful sources of inner conflict from overwhelming her controls, this characteristically difficult and conflicted woman may be experiencing the clinical signs of an anxiety disorder. She is unable to rid herself of preoccupations with her tension, fearful presentiments, recurring headaches, fatigue, and insomnia, and she is upset by their uncharacteristic presence in her life. Feeling at the mercy of unknown and upsetting forces that seem to well up within her, she is at a loss as to how to counteract them, but she may exploit them to manipulate others or to complain at great length.

Abuse of either legal or street drugs or both is indicated in the *MCMI-III* protocol of this woman, who is often erratic, irritable, and negativistic. Her use of drugs may be both a statement of resentful independence from the constraints of conventional life and a means of disjoining her conflicts and liberating her uncharitable impulses toward others. An act of assertive defiance that has undertones of self-destruction, her drug abuse may be employed with a careless indifference to its consequences.

Related to but beyond her characteristic level of emotional responsivity, this woman appears to have been confronted with an event or events in which she was exposed to a severe threat to her life, a traumatic experience that precipitated intense fear or horror on her part. Currently, the residuals of this even resemble or symbolize an aspect of the traumatic event. Where possible, she seeks to avoid such cues and recollections. Where they cannot be anticipated and actively avoided, as in dreams or nightmares, she may become terrified, exhibiting a number of symptoms of intense anxiety. Other signs of distress might include difficulty falling asleep, outbursts of anger, panic attacks, hypervigilance, exaggerated startle response, or a subjective sense of numbing and detachment.

This moody and conflicted woman's bodily preoccupations and concerns are likely to be produced by both physical and psychological factors, resulting in a syndrome of features suggestive of a somatoform disorder. Enmeshed in an erratic pattern of resentment and brittle emotions, her anxious concerns about her somatic state aggravate her characteristic sullenness, leading her to demand attention and special treatment. Not only does she exploit her ailments to control the lives of others, but she is also likely to complain of her discomfort in ways that induce others to feel guilty.

Possible DSM-IV *multiaxial diagnoses*

The following diagnostic assignments should be considered judgments of personality and clinical prototypes that correspond conceptually to formal diagnostic categories. The diagnostic criteria and items used in the *MCMI-III* differ somewhat from those in the *DSM-IV*, but there are sufficient parallels in the *MCMI-III* items to recommend consideration of the following assignments. It should be noted that several *DSM-IV* Axis I syndromes are not assessed in the *MCMI-III*. Definitive diagnoses must draw on biographical, observational, and interview data in addition to self-report inventories such as the *MCMI-III*.

Axis I: Clinical syndrome

The major complaints and behaviors of the patient parallel the following Axis I diagnoses, listed in order of their clinical significance and salience.

> 296.33 Major Depression (recurrent, severe, without psychotic features)
> 300.02 Generalized Anxiety Disorder
> 305.90 Psychoactive Substance Abuse NOS

Axis II: Personality disorders

Deeply ingrained and pervasive patterns of maladaptive functioning underlie Axis I clinical syndromal pictures. The following personality prototypes correspond to the most probable *DSM-IV* diagnoses (Disorders, Traits, Features) that characterize this patient.
Personality configuration composed of the following:

> 301.84 Negativistic (Passive-Aggressive) Personality Disorder
> 301.83 Borderline Personality Disorder with Dependent Personality Traits and Depressive Personality Traits

Course: The major personality features described previously reflect long-term or chronic traits that are likely to have persisted for several years prior to the present assessment. The clinical syndromes described previously tend to be relatively transient, waxing and waning in their prominence and intensity depending on the presence of environmental stress.

Axis IV: Psychosocial and environmental problems

In completing the *MCMI-III*, this individual identified the following problems that may be complicating or exacerbating her present emotional state. They are listed in order of importance as indicated by the client. This information should be viewed as a guide for further investigation by the clinician.

> None identified

Treatment guide

If additional clinical data are supportive of the *MCMI-III's* hypotheses, it is likely that this patient's difficulties can be managed with either brief or extended therapeutic methods. The following guide to treatment planning is oriented toward issues and techniques of a short-term character, focusing on matters that might call for immediate attention, followed by time-limited procedures designed to reduce the likelihood of repeated relapses.

As a first step, it would appear advisable to implement methods to ameliorate this patient's current state of clinical anxiety, depressive hopelessness, or pathological personality functioning by the rapid implementation of supportive psychotherapeutic measures. With appropriate consultation, targeted psychopharmacologic medications may also be useful at this initial stage.

Worthy of note is the possibility of a troublesome alcohol and/or substance-abuse disorder. If verified, appropriate short-term behavioral management or group therapy programs should be rapidly implemented.

continued

Table 7.13   continued

Once this patient's more pressing or acute difficulties are adequately stabilized, attention should be directed toward goals that would aid in preventing a recurrence of problems, focusing on circumscribed issues and employing delimited methods such as those discussed in the following paragraphs.

A primary short-term goal of treatment with this patient is to aid her in reducing her intense ambivalence and growing resentment of others. With an empathic and brief focus, it should be possible to sustain a productive, therapeutic relationship. With a therapist who can convey genuine caring and firmness, she may be able to overcome her tendency to employ maneuvers to test the sincerity and motives of the therapist. Although she will be slow to reveal her resentment because she dislikes being viewed as an angry person, it can be brought into the open, if advisable, and dealt with in a kind and understanding way. She is not inclined to face her ambivalence, but her mixed feelings and attitudes must be a major focus of treatment. To prevent her from trying to terminate treatment before improvement occurs or to forestall relapses, the therapist should employ brief and circumscribed techniques to counter the patient's expectation that supportive figures will ultimately prove disillusioning.

Circumscribed interpersonal approaches (e.g., Benjamin, Kiesler) may be used to deal with the seesaw struggle enacted by the patient in her relationship with her therapist. She may alternately exhibit ingratiating submissiveness and a taunting and demanding attitude. Similarly, she may solicit the therapist's affections, but when these are expressed, she may reject them, voicing doubt about the genuineness of the therapist's feelings. The therapist may use cognitive procedures to point out these contradictory attitudes. It is important to keep these inconsistencies in focus or the patient may appreciate the therapist's perceptiveness verbally but not alter her attitudes. Involved in an unconscious repetition-compulsion in which she recreates disillusioning experiences that parallel those of the past, the patient must not only come to recognize the expectations cognitively but may be taught to deal with their enactment interpersonally.

Despite her ambivalence and pessimistic outlook, there is good reason to operate on the premise that the patient can overcome past disappointments. To capture the love and attention only modestly gained in childhood cannot be achieved, although habits that preclude partial satisfaction can be altered in the here and now. Toward that end, the therapist must help her disentangle needs that are in opposition to one another. For example, she both wants and does not want the love of those upon whom she depends. Despite this ambivalence, she enters new relationships, such as in therapy, as if an idyllic state could be achieved. She goes through the act of seeking a consistent and true source of love, one that will not betray her as she believes her parents and others did in the past. Despite this optimism, she remains unsure of the trust she can place in others. Mindful of past betrayals and disappointments, she begins to test her new relationships to see if they are loyal and faithful. In a parallel manner, she may attempt to irritate and frustrate the therapist to check whether he or she will prove to be as fickle and insubstantial as others have in the past. It is here that the therapist's warm support and firmness can play a significant short-term role in reframing the patient's erroneous expectations and in exhibiting consistency in relationship behavior.

Although the rooted character of these attitudes and behavior will complicate the ease with which these therapeutic procedures will progress, short-term and circumscribed cognitive and interpersonal therapy techniques may be quite successful. A thorough reconstruction of personality may not be necessary to alter the patient's problematic pattern. In this regard, family treatment methods that focus on the network of relationships that often sustain her problems may prove to be a useful technique. Group methods may also be fruitfully employed to help the patient acquire self-control and consistency in close relationships.

It is advisable that the therapist not set goals too high because the patient may not be able to tolerate demands or expectations well. Brief therapeutic efforts should be directed to build the patient's trust, to focus on positive traits, and to enhance her confidence and self-esteem.

Millon Adolescent Clinical Inventory (MACI)

The *Millon Adolescent Clinical Inventory* (*MACI*) (Millon, Millon, & Davis, 1993) is a 160-item inventory that requires a 6th-grade reading level. The *MACI* is designed to assess an adolescent's personality, along with self-reported concerns and clinical syndromes using 27 content scales and 4 response bias scales: Personality Patterns, Expressed Concerns, Clinical Syndromes, and Modifying Indices. For further breakdown of the scales, see Table 7.14. These scales coordinate with descriptive characteristics in recent *DSM* classifications (Millon et al., 1993). The test was normed using13- to19-year-olds. The development sample (*n* = 579) was 54% male and 46% female. The two cross-validation samples (*n* = 139, *n* = 194) were 53% and 65% male, respectfully, and 47% and 35% female, respectively (Millon et al., 1993). Over 1,000 adolescents and their clinicians from 28 states and Canada were involved in the development of the *MACI*.

The *MACI* usually requires about 20 to 40 minutes to complete and can be scored by hand in about 20 minutes, sent to the publisher by mail, or scored by computer onsite in about 5 minutes (Erford, 2006). Sample items include "I have an attractive body," "I go on eating binges frequently," and "I enjoy fighting." Internal consistency reliabilities for the Development Sample range from 0.73 for the Scales D (Sexual Discomfort) and Y (Desirability) to 0.91 for Scale B (Self-Devaluation). Except for Scale VV (Reliability) scores, raw scores are converted to Base Rate Scores (BRS) for interpretation. Different BR transformation tables are used depending on the age and gender of the adolescent and are adjusted to a value that falls between 1 and 115 (Millon et al., 1993). Internal consistencies for the two cross-validation samples combined ranged from 0.69 for Scale D (Sexual Discomfort) to 0.90 for Scale B (Self-Devaluation). Internal consistency coefficients for the development sample Personality Patterns scales ranged from 0.74 for Scale 3 (Submissive) to 0.90 for Scale 8B (Self-Demeaning). Test-retest reliability results ranged from 0.57 for Scale E (Peer Insecurity) to 0.92 for Scale 9 (Borderline Tendency) for a 3- to 7-day interval. The median stability coefficient is reported as 0.82 (Millon et al., 1993). Criterion-related validity correlations are moderate in magnitude (Erford, 2006).

The *MACI* is designed for use with emotionally disturbed adolescents ages 13–19 years as an aid to help identify, predict, and understand some of the psychological difficulties this group experiences. Since this is a Level C instrument, examiners are required to have "a graduate degree in psychology or a related field, or appropriate licensure, a course in testing theory, coursework in personality theory, or abnormal psychology, and appropriate experience under supervision" (Erford, 2006,

Table 7.14   Response bias scales and content scales

Personality patterns	Expressed concerns	Clinical syndromes	Modifying indices
Scale 1—Introversive	Scale A—Identity diffusion	Scale AA—Eating dysfunctions	Scale X—Disclosure
Scale 2A—Inhibited	Scale B—Self-devaluation	Scale BB—Substance-abuse proneness	Scale Y—Desirability
Scale 2B—Doleful	Scale C—Body disapproval	Scale CC—Delinquent predisposition	Scale Z—Debasement
Scale 3—Submissive	Scale D—Sexual discomfort	Scale DD—Impulsive propensity	
Scale 4—Dramatizing	Scale E—Peer insecurity	Scale EE—Anxious feelings	**Other**
Scale 5—Egotistic	Scale F—Social insensitivity	Scale FF—Depressive affect	Scale W—Reliability
Scale 6A—Unruly	Scale G—Family discord	Scale GG—Suicidal tendency	
Scale 6B—Forceful	Scale H—Childhood abuse		
Scale 7—Conforming			
Scale 8A—Oppositional			
Scale 8B—Self-Demeaning			
Scale 9—Borderline tendency			

p. 41). Strengths of the *MACI* include ease of scoring and interpretation, personality variables mapped to *DSM* personality disorders, appropriateness of concerns frequently expressed by emotionally disturbed adolescents, and identification of important clinical syndromes (Retzlaff, 1995). Clinicians using the computer interpretive report are likely to find the response cover sheet, printout, histographic display, narrative, and list of correlated Axis I and II entities useful (Stuart, 1995). Weaknesses of the *MACI* include the underrepresentation of participants ages 18–19 years in the normative samples (Stuart, 1995). The manual clearly stated that use of the *MACI* for any population outside the 13–19 age designation would be inappropriate (Millon et al., 1993). There is a lack of item and scale specificity because 160 items attempt to score 30 scales (Retzlaff). Also, overrepresentation of Whites (78.8%) (Stuart) and males in the normative sample may make it less appropriate for use with some populations (Millon et al., 1993). Lastly, it may not be particularly useful as a screening level test for the general adolescent population because the norming sample did not include adolescents not identified as patients in treatment programs (Stuart, 1995). Overall, the best use of the *MACI* is for hypothesis generation and validation, outcomes assessment, and screening for pathology, not for diagnosis.

Achenbach System of Empirically Based Assessment (ASEBA)

The *Achenbach System of Empirically Based Assessment* (*ASEBA*) (Achenbach & Rescorla, 2001) is a series of multi-informant inventories for rating the behavior of children ages 1½–5 years and another for children ages 6–18 years. Each is designed to assess competencies, adaptive functioning, and other problems through the use of four forms: *Child Behavior Checklist* (*CBCL/1½–5*) and the *CBCL/6–18* (i.e., a parent report form), *Youth Self-Report* (*YSR* for children ages 11–18 years), and *Teacher's Report Form* (*TRF*). Items measure six *DSM*-oriented scales that include Affective Problems, Anxiety Problems, Attention Deficit/Hyperactivity Problems, Conduct

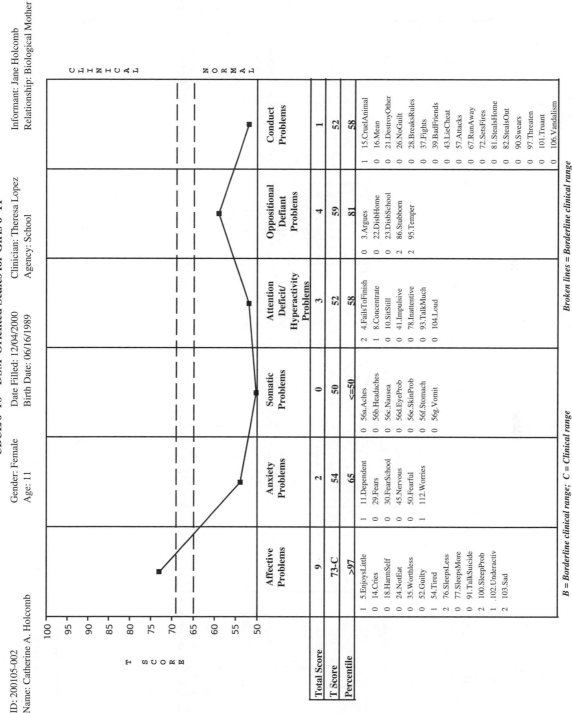

Figure 7.7 *ASEBA* Syndrome & Scale scores

Source: Reprinted by permission of Professor Thomas Achenbach.

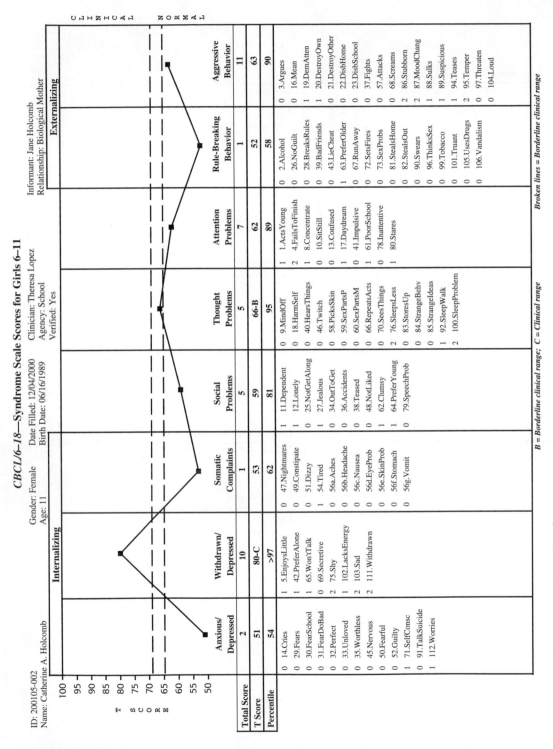

Figure 7.8   *ASEBA DSM-oriented scales*

Source: Reprinted by permission of Professor Thomas Achenbach.

Problems, Oppositional Defiant Problems, and Somatic Problems (Achenbach & Rescorla, 2001). Informants are prompted to rank items 0 (Not True), 1 (Somewhat or Sometimes True), or 2 (Very True or Often True) and are invited to describe several selections in detail. Item prompts include "Physically attacks people," "Inattentive," and "Wets the bed." The *ASEBA* can be completed by hand, on computer, or online via the *ASEBA* Web-Link (www.aseba.org), which permits access to informants in remote areas. This test takes about 15–20 minutes to complete and can be scored by hand or computer.

Test-retest reliability coefficients for intervals of 8–16 days were mostly in the 0.80s and 0.90s for subscales of the *CBCL/6–18* and ranged from 0.91 to 0.95 for Total Competence, Total Adaptive Functioning, and Total Problems (Achenbach & Rescorla, 2001). "Percentiles and normalized T scores are based on national probability samples of children who had not received mental health, substance abuse, or special education services for major behavioral, emotional, or developmental problems in the preceding 12 months" (Achenbach & Rescorla, 2001, p. 80) (see Figures 7.7 & 7.8 for sample profile forms). The *ASEBA* national normative sample (*n* = 9,052) included children from 40 states and the District of Columbia. Clinicians may find that routine use of the *ASEBA* forms for intake, screening, and evaluations gleaned from parent, teacher, and self-reports provide a broad picture of the client and can serve as a starting point, or springboard, for discussing pertinent issues in the clinical interview (Achenbach & Rescorla, 2001). Watson (2006) reported that it is a psychometrically sound instrument but has some weaknesses, especially concerning the scales for younger children. In addition, the directions and manuals are improved over the original versions.

The *ASEBA* system is one of the best behavioral assessment systems currently available (Salvia & Ysseldyke, 2004) and can be a helpful adjunct to functional behavioral analysis (FBA) (Gresham, Watson, & Skinner, 2001). While the *CBCL, TRF,* and *YSR* are the most frequently used components of *ASEBA*, additional components include the *Direct Observation Form* (*DOF*); a *Young Adult Self-Report* (*YASR*) for adults ages 18–30 years; a *Young Adult Behavioral Checklist* (parent report); and a *Semi-structured Clinical Interview for Children and Adolescents* (*SCICA*) for use with children ages 6–12 years. The *ASEBA* is a Level B instrument.

Personality Inventory for Children–Second Edition (PIC-2)

The *PIC-2* (Lachar & Gruber, 2001) is a multidimensional clinical measure of behavioral, emotional, and cognitive status for children ages 3–16 years. It is a screening instrument that is usually completed by the parent. The *PIC-2* has 275 items in its standard format and contains 12 psychological scales with various subscales. The *PIC-2* also contains an abbreviated behavioral summary of 96 items. The psychological scales include Cognitive Impairment, Impulsivity and Distractibility, Delinquency, Family Dysfunction, Reality Distortion, Somatic Concern, Psychological Discomfort, Social Withdrawal, Social Skills Deficits, as well as three Response Validity scales. Parents are asked to respond to the items with True or False answers. The standardization sample generally conformed to U.S. population demographics with the exception of an overrepresentation of Whites and underrepresentation of Hispanics. There was also an overrepresentation of biological parents and an underrepresentation of single parents (Erford & McKechnie, 2006).

No overall composite score is derived, but there are three separate composite scale scores: Externalization-Composite, Internalization-Composite, and Social Adjustment Composite. Raw scores can be converted to T scores when the Student Behavior Survey, a profile form, is completed. Test-retest reliability coefficients ranged from $r = 0.82$ to 0.92 and internal consistency coefficients ranged from $r = 0.81$ to 0.92 for the interpreted scales. Criterion validity studies were conducted but did not use other commonly used instruments (Erford & McKechnie, 2006). However, because this new version of the PIC-2 is a major revision of the original, clinicians should be cautious in making diagnostic decisions using the PIC-2 until further research and diagnostic validity studies have been conducted. The PIC-2's primary benefit continues to be the assessment of parental perceptions of childhood behavioral and clinical difficulties.

Devereux Scales of Mental Disorders (DSMD)

The DSMD (Naglieri, LeBuffe, & Pfeiffer, 1996) is used to assess behaviors related to psychopathology. It can be administered both to individuals as well as groups of children ages 5–18 years in about 15 minutes. There are two forms of the DSMD, the child form and the adolescent form, and each can be rated by parents, teachers, and other appropriate professionals. There are 110 items on this inventory, which measures nine constructs, including Conduct, Attention-Delinquency, Anxiety, Depression, Autism, Acute Problems, Internalizing Composite, Externalizing Composite, and the Critical Pathology Composite. Responses are based on a 5-point scale ranging from Never to Very Frequently. Raw scores can be converted into T scores and percentile ranks. Standardization samples generally conformed to U.S. population demographics for both children and adolescents (Cooper, 2001).

Alpha coefficients were reported at about $r = 0.90$ or higher, and test-retest reliability coefficients were in the 0.80s and 0.90s. Interrater reliability coefficients between parents and teachers were in the 0.40s and 0.50s. This is not surprising given that teachers and parents observe the child's behavior in two distinct ecological contexts (i.e., school and home). Validity studies yielded adequate results on all levels, with items showing a strong congruence to DSM-IV criteria for the specific behavior disorders in question (Peterson, 2001). There is some dispute in the composition of types of participants used in the reliability and validity study samples and as to whether the type of subjects might have caused elevated coefficients. Even so, there is substantial normative data for the DSMD, and it has emerged as a good assessment for certain antisocial behaviors in children and adolescents.

Children's Depression Inventory (CDI)

The CDI (Kovacs, 1992) is a self-report inventory used to assess children's depression. Parent and teacher versions are also available. It can be administered both individually as well as to small groups of children ages 8–17 years in about 10 to 15 minutes. This assessment contains 27 items that cover all nine symptoms for a major depressive syndrome in children as presented in the *DSM-III-R.* Children's responses are based on a 3- point scale, from 0 to 2, with 2 being the most severe (Kavan, 1992). Limited normative data are available for the *CDI* because it was not nationally standardized. The standardization sample was inadequately small and geographically restricted (Knoff, 1992). Scoring was simple and convenient, using the QuickScore™ forms.

Reliability and validity data are also questionable. Although coefficient *alphas* from two different samples reported in the manual were consistent at $r = 0.86$ and 0.87, respectively, many empirical studies yielded inconsistent results. Item–total score coefficients ranged from $r = 0.08$ to 0.62. A one-month test-retest reliability coefficient was $r = 0.43$, while a nine-week test-retest reliability coefficient was $r = 0.84$. Regarding validity, the *CDI* had adequate correlations with the *Revised Children's Manifest Anxiety Scale* but yielded low correlations with *Coopersmith Self-Esteem Inventory* (Kavan, 1992). The *CDI* has demonstrated good discrimination between clinical and nonclinical groups (Carey, Gresham, Ruggerio, Faulstich, & Engart, 1987; Hodges, 1990). It is obvious that more empirical data need to be collected with regard to the *CDI* and it should not be used as a diagnostic tool (Craighead, Curry, & Ilardi, 1995; Fristad, Emery, & Beck, 1997; Knoff, 1992). Admittedly, the construct of depression is more difficult to accurately assess in children than adults because depressive symptoms are more transient in younger clients. In spite of this, the *CDI* is easy to administer and score and may be helpful during initial clinical assessment (Kavan, 1992). It is, perhaps, the most commonly used screening tool for childhood depression (Craighead et al., 1995; Fristad et al., 1997).

Reynolds Adolescent Depression Scale–Second Edition (RADS-2)

The *Reynolds Adolescent Depression Scale—Second Edition* (*RADS-2*) (Reynolds, 2002) is a 30-item self-report inventory for adolescents ages 11–20 years and is designed to assess symptoms associated with depression. Items measure four subscales: Dysphoric Mood (DM, 8 items); Anhedonia/Negative Affect (AN, 7 items); Negative Self-Evaluation (NS, 8 items); and Somatic Complaints (SC, 7 items). Sample items include "I feel lonely," "I feel like running away," and "I feel like nothing I do helps anymore." The items are scored on a 4-point Likert scale (Almost Never, Hardly Ever, Sometimes, or Most of the Time) (Blair, 2005). The *RADS-2* is a Level B test and takes about 10 minutes to administer, score, and interpret. The normative restandardization sample ($n = 3,300$) for the *RADS-2* was comprised of an equal number of adolescent males and females living in the United States and Canada. Compared to the 2000 U.S. Census, this sample was considered ethnically diverse and heterogeneous in socioeconomic composition (Reynolds, 2002).

Raw scores are summed to derive a Depression Total score. The Depression Total and four subscales can be converted to a T score or percentile rank according to gender, age group, and gender by age group norms. More than 20 years of research supports the psychometric qualities of the *RADS-2,* and the new version is found to continue the tradition of a sound instrument (Blair, 2005). Internal consistency of the Depression Total score was $r = 0.92$ (Reynolds, 2002). Test-retest reliability (two weeks) was $r = 0.86$ for the Depression Total score (Reynolds, 2002). Criterion-related validity studies resulted in moderate to high correlations with other measures of depression and indicated the *RADS-2* is best used as a screening level test for depression (Erford, 2006). Overall, "the *RADS-2* is cost- and time-efficient, easy to use, and a reliable and valid screening instrument for adolescents with symptoms of depression" (Erford, 2006, p. 58).

The *RADS-2* is one of the only depression screening tests validated for use with adolescents (Brooks & Kutcher, 2001), and its recommended clinical cutoff of $T = 61+$ has been shown to identify clinically severe symptoms of depression on the *Hamilton Depression Rating Scale* (*HDRS*) (Reynolds & Mazza, 1998). The *RADS-2* is a screening test and should not be used to supplant use of a clinical interview (Davis, 1990) and is not a substitute for an interview of suicidal ideation (Reynolds, 2002). Volpe and DuPaul (2001) also indicated the *RADS-2* shows some usefulness in monitoring the effects of treatment and as one component in a comprehensive diagnostic approach for depression.

Symptom Checklist-90–Revised (SCL-90-R)

The *SCL-90-R* (Derogatis, 1992) portrays patterns of psychological symptoms in patients and nonpatients. The *SCL-90-R* can be administered to groups or individuals ages 13 years to adult in about 15 to 20 minutes. Symptoms are measured on 12 constructs: Somatization, Obsessive-Compulsive, Interpersonal Sensitivity, Depression, Anxiety, Hostility, Phobic Anxiety, Paranoid Ideation, Psychoticism, Global Severity Index, Positive Symptom Distress Index, and Positive Symptom Total. There are a total of 90 items on this inventory. Clients are asked to rate their level of discomfort with a particular problem 0 (Not at all) to 4 (Extremely). Norms were constructed on several standardization samples, including psychiatric outpatients, psychiatric inpatients, adult nonpatients, and adolescent nonpatients (Pauker, 1985).

Pauker (1985) and Payne (1985) asserted that the original *SCL-90* manual reported satisfactory results for internal consistency ($r = 0.77$–0.90) and test-retest reliability coefficients ($r = 0.78$–0.90, one week apart). The few validity studies conducted portrayed comparable levels to other self-report inventories; however, more research is needed in this area. Other criticisms included a lack of clarity in the manual and the possible limitations inherent in requiring an 8th-grade reading level when using an inventory with adolescents ages 13 years and older. Strengths of the *SCL-90-R* are the quick administration and scoring procedures as well as its straightforward scoring criteria.

Beck Depression Inventory–Second Edition (BDI-II)

The *Beck Depression Inventory—Second Edition* (*BDI-II*) (Beck et al., 1996) is a 21-item self-report inventory used to assess the severity of depression of individuals ages 13 years or older. Each item is formatted on a 4-point scale (i.e., ranging from 0 to 3 in terms of severity) and indicates a particular depressive symptom occurring during the past two weeks. *The BDI-II* has gone through several revisions since its original publication. The last major revision changed the instrument from the *BDI-IA* to the *BDI-II* in 1996 to correspond with the criteria for depressive disorders in the *Diagnostic and Statistical Manual of Mental Disorders—Fourth Edition* (*DSM-IV*) (American Psychiatric Association, 1994). On revision of the *BDI-II*, four items (i.e., Weight Loss, Body Image Change, Somatic Preoccupation, Work Difficulty) were replaced with four new items (i.e., Agitation, Worthlessness, Concentration Difficulty, Loss of Energy). In addition, two items (i.e., Changes in Sleeping Pattern and Changes in Appetite) were revised by creating seven optional scales representing differences between increases and decreases of severity. Paper-and-pencil record forms, scannable record forms, and Spanish record forms are available. Current cost information and online order are available on the website of Harcourt Assessment, Inc. (2004b). The *BDI-II* takes 5 to 10 minutes to complete. Although the *BDI-II* is self-administered, a trained examiner can read the questions aloud if needed. Administration and interpretation qualification is Level C (i.e., requires doctoral-level training in psychology, education, counseling, or related fields, or licensure or certification as a professional counselor or other psychological professional). Hand scoring and computer scoring are available. Summing all the responded scales yields a total score (maximum is 63). A total score of 14 or above indicates the possibility of depression. Although the responses for items 2a and 2b (i.e., Changes in Sleeping Pattern and Changes in Appetite) are not considered in calculating a total score, they should be considered in the diagnosis of depression.

The normative sample for the *BDI-II* consisted of 500 outpatient clients from four different psychiatric clinics in urban and suburban areas in the United States, and 120 students from one college in Canada (Farmer, 2001). Scores on the *BDI-II* have shown to be reliable (e.g., internal consistency, test-retest reliability) and valid (e.g., content validity, construct validity, factorial validity) (Beck et al., 1996).

Beck Anxiety Inventory (BAI)

The *Beck Anxiety Inventory* (*BAI*) (Beck et al., 1988; Beck & Steer, 1993) is a 21-item self-report instrument used to assess the severity of anxiety of individuals ages 17 years or older. Each item on the *BAI* is formatted on a 4-point scale (i.e., ranging from Not at All=1 to Severely; "I could barely stand it") and indicates symptoms related to anxiety during the past week. Paper-and-pencil record forms, scannable record forms, and Spanish record forms are available. Current cost information and online ordering information are available on the website of Harcourt Assessment, Inc. (2004b).

Like the other Beck instruments discussed, the *BAI* is self-administered, but a trained examiner can administer it verbally. The *BAI* takes 5 to 10 minutes to complete. The administration and interpretation qualifications for this instrument are also Level C. Hand scoring and computer scoring are available. Summing all responses yields a total score with a maximum of 63.

The first normative sample for the *BAI* consisted of 810 outpatient clients with affective and anxiety disorders. Subsequent studies were conducted to determine the reliability and validity of scores (for detailed development procedures, see Beck et al., 1988). Beck et al. demonstrated high internal consistency and sufficient test-retest reliability for scores on the *BAI*. The test authors also demonstrated convergent validity and discriminant validity. For example, the *BAI* was moderately correlated with the *Hamilton Anxiety Rating Scale—Revised* (*HARS-R*) and the *Cognition Checklist Anxiety* subscale (*CCL-A*). Beck et al. (1988) also demonstrated factorial validity as the *BAI* consisted of the two factors: (1) somatic symptoms and (2) subjective anxiety and panic symptoms. However, Osman, Barrios, Aukes, Osman, & Markway (1993) discovered four factors of the *BAI*: (1) Subjective, (2) Neurophysiological, (3) Automatic, and (4) Panic.

Overall, establishing an ability to discriminate between anxiety and depression (i.e., discriminant validity) is one of the most critical useful aspects of the *BAI* (Beck at al., 1988). Thus professional counselors may find this tool useful for clarifying the presenting problem and formulating effective treatment plans.

Beck Scale for Suicide Ideation (BSSI)

The *Beck Scale for Suicide Ideation* (*BSSI*) (Beck, Kovacs, & Weissman, 1979) is a 21-item self-report inventory used to assess the severity of suicide ideation of individuals ages 17 years or older. Suicide ideators are defined as "individuals who currently have plans and wishes to commit suicide but have not made any recent overt suicide attempt" (Beck, Kovacs, & Weissman, 1979, p. 344). Beck et al. (1979) first developed a 19-item *Scale for Suicide Ideation* (*SSI*) to assess suicide intention. An examiner completes the *SSI* by asking each item in a semi-structured interview format and recording the client's responses. The *SSI* was revised into the *BSSI* in 1991 through the creation of a self-report format. Paper-and-pencil record forms, scannable record forms, and Spanish record forms are now available. Current cost information and online ordering information are available on the website of Harcourt Assessment, Inc. (2004b).

The *BSSI* consists of the three parts: (1) Items 1 through 5 (i.e., attitudes toward living and dying); (2) Items 6 through 19 (i.e., suicide ideation and anticipated reaction of the ideation); and (3) Items 20 and 21 (i.e., the number of past suicide attempts and the seriousness of intention in the last suicide attempt) (Stewart, 1998). Each item is formatted on a 3-point scale ranging from 0 to 2 in terms of severity. The *BSSI* takes 5 to 10 minutes to complete. The *BSSI* is self-administered, but a trained examiner can read the items aloud if necessary. Administration and interpretation qualifications are Level C. Hand scoring and computer scoring are available. A total score is calculated, with a maximum of 42. However, because the test's authors do not provide a cutoff score, an examiner should cautiously analyze a total score and client responses to each item (called "critical item analysis") to examine suicide risk (Stewart, 1998).

The normative sample for the *BSSI* consisted of 178 adults (126 inpatient and 52 outpatient clients) who were receiving psychiatric services and were identified as suicide ideators. Although scores have been reliable only for the first 19 items, the *BSSI* has high internal consistency and moderate test-retest reliability (Stewart,

1998). Also, the *BSSI* has good construct validity. For example, the *BSSI* was significantly correlated with the *SSI* (Stewart, 1998). Although the normative sample lacked adolescents, Steer, Kumar, and Beck (1993) demonstrated in their study using adolescent inpatients that the *BSSI* was positively correlated with a history of a past suicide attempt, the *Beck Depression Inventory* (*BDI*) (Beck et al., 1996), the *Beck Hopelessness Scale* (*BHS*) (Beck & Steer, 1993), and the *Beck Anxiety Inventory* (*BAI*) (Beck, Epstein, Brown, & Steer, 1988).

Professional counselors should consider using the *BSSI* to assess the suicide risk of individuals who obtain a high score on the *BHS,* given that hopelessness may be a significant suicide indicator for adolescents and adults, rather than depression and anxiety (Beck et al., 1979; Steer at al., 1993).

Substance Abuse Subtle Screening Inventory–3 (SASSI-3)

The *Substance Abuse Subtle Screening Inventory—3* (*SASSI-3*) (Miller & Lazowski, 1999) is a self-report inventory used to assess the probability of substance dependence (e.g., alcohol or other drugs of abuse) of individuals ages 18 years or older. An adolescent version of the *SASSI* is also available. Paper-and-pencil record forms, computer versions, audiotape versions for individuals with reading problems, and the Spanish *SASSI* are available. Information on current cost and other *SASSI* products and online ordering information are available on the website of the SASSI Institute (2004).

The *SASSI-3* consists of two parts, each of which is printed on a separate side of one test form. One part contains 67 items consisting of true-false questions regarding substance dependence. The other part contains 26 items (12 for alcohol use and 14 for drug use) formatted on a Likert scale ranging from 0 (Never) to 4 (Repeatedly). For each of the Likert items, the client is asked to respond considering one of the following four time periods: entire life, past 6 months, 6 months before a critical event, or 6 months after a critical event. According to Miller (1997), the author of the *SASSI-3,* there were three main changes from the *SASSI-2* that increased accuracy: (1) A new scale, Symptoms (SYM), was created, which provides information regarding the client's substance use and the environmental impact of substance use on the client; (2) two items were eliminated because of reported discomfort by some users; and (3) the four time periods mentioned above were added to the Likert scale format. The *SASSI-3* consists of 10 subscales and takes approximately 15 minutes to administer (for details of subscales, see Juhnke et al., 2006; Pittenger, 2003). The subscales include Face Valid Alcohol, Face Valid Other Drug, Symptoms, Obvious Attributes, Subtle Attributes, Defensiveness, Supplemental Addiction Measure, Family versus Control Subjects, Correctional, and Random Answering Pattern. Administration and interpretation are Level B (master's level in psychology, counseling, or related fields, with certification or professional training in psychological assessment). An examiner scores the *SASSI-3* using a scoring key and obtains a profile by plotting a raw score for each subscale; raw scores are converted into percentile ranks and T scores ($M = 50$; $SD = 10$). Interpretation of the results is done according to decision rules provided in the test manual.

Some researchers investigated reliability and validity of *SASSI-3* scores. Lazowski, Miller, Boye, and Miller (1998) found high test-retest reliability, internal consistency, and criterion-related validity. However, there are some mixed results when using the *SASSI-3* with special populations (e.g., clients who have a traumatic brain injury) For example, Arenth, Bogner, Corrigan, and Schmidt (2001) reported lower accuracy, sensitivity, and specificity in their study investigating the utility of the *SASSI-3* to diagnose chemical dependence for individuals with brain injury. However, Arenth et al. concluded that the *SASSI-3* was promising for individuals with brain injury, given that substance abuse strongly affects brain injury. Finally, the customer support from the SASSI Institute is excellent, often providing free profile consultations using an 800 number.

Eating Disorder Inventory–3 (EDI-3)

The *Eating Disorder Inventory—3* (*EDI-3*) (Garner, 2004) is an effective self-report inventory for assessing the attitudes, behaviors, and psychological traits related to Anorexia Nervosa and Bulimia Nervosa for individuals ages 12 years or older. The *EDI-3* was revised from the original *EDI* published in 1984 and the *EDI-2* (published in 1991). Anorexia Nervosa contains symptoms such as refusal to maintain a minimally normal body weight and fear of gaining weight, whereas Bulimia Nervosa contains symptoms such as binge eating, self-induced vomiting, misuse of medications (e.g., diuretics, laxatives), and excessive exercise (APA, 2000). Paper-and-pencil record forms and computer versions are available. Current cost information and online ordering information are available on the website of Psychological Assessment Resources, Inc. (2004b).

The *EDI-3* contains 91 items, broken down into 12 scales (3 eating-disorder-specific scales and 9 general psychological scales that are highly relevant to eating disorders), each of which is formatted on a 4-point scale that helps to improve the reliability of some of the scales and provides a wider range of scores. In addition, the results yield six composite scores (Eating Disorder Risk, Ineffectiveness, Interpersonal Problems, Affective Problems, Overcontrol, and General Psychological Maladjustment) that are helpful when creating treatment plans, interventions, and treatment monitoring. The *EDI-3* takes approximately 20 minutes to complete. Administration and interpretation qualification is Level A (4-year-college or university level in psychology, counseling, or related fields with certification or professional training in psychological assessment). Each subscale score is obtained by summing all the scores for the subscale. Plotting each subscale score on a profile and comparing the profile to norms yields the potential severity of an eating disorder. Norms are available for (a) patients with Anorexia Nervosa—Restricting Type; (b) patients with Anorexia Nervosa–Binge-Eating/Purging Type; (c) patients with Bulimia Nervosa only; and (d) Eating Disorders Not Otherwise Specified (Psychological Assessment Resources, Inc., 2004b).

Scores on the *EDI-3* have been found to be reliable and valid. According to the publisher (Psychological Assessment Resources, 2004b), moderate to high composite reliabilities were reported for all the subscales except one (0.80s to 0.90s) and test-retest reliability coefficients in the 0.90s were reported for most of the subscales. Psychological Assessment Resources, Inc., reports that a relationship exists between the *EDI-3* and a wide variety of external instruments. With this new revision, a Referral Form, which is a shortened form of the entire inventory, is included. It is especially useful when trying to identify students who may be at risk for eating disorders.

SUMMARY/CONCLUSION

Clinical assessment and proper diagnosis of mental disorders relies heavily on the professional counselor's knowledge of the *DSM-IV-TR* multiaxial diagnostic system and implementing effective and efficient interviewing and clinical testing procedures. This chapter has provided a wealth of introductory material to orient the professional counselor to each of these essential dimensions.

Professional counselors generally make clinical decisions using either a statistical model (based predominately on test scores) or a clinical judgment model (based predominately on counselor experience). A great deal of helpful information can be obtained from a clinical interview. Structured interviews ask a standard set of questions and allow little variation from the standardized protocol. Such procedures often result in similar conclusions by different counselors. Unstructured interviews have no preset list of questions and allow maximum flexibility for counselor questioning and follow-up. But this flexibility means that different professional counselors using unstructured interviews frequently develop different conclusions. As a compromise, semi-structured interviews use a standardized set of questions but allow the professional counselor flexibility to pursue important information that falls outside of the more structured format. Specialized types of interviews discussed in the chapter include the intake interview and mental status exam.

Sources of information about a client usually stem from four sources and can be recalled using the acronym LOST: life outcome data, observer ratings, self-report ratings, and test data. The chapter also explored general procedures for development of clinical and personality tests. Some tests are based on theories of personality or clinical pathology, while others use empirical procedures such as factor analysis or empirical-criterion keying. This chapter has provided an overview of numerous clinical tests to familiarize the reader with instruments commonly used by professional counselors.

KEY TERMS

clinical assessment

clinical judgment

DSM-IV-TR

empirical-criterion keying

Global Assessment of Functioning (GAF)

hyperactivity-impulsivity

hypothesis confirmation bias

inattention

intake interview

life outcomes

mental disorder

multiaxial classification system

observer rating

self-fulfilling prophecy
self-report ratings
semi-structured interview
statistical decision-making model
statistical models
structured interview

test data
True Response Inconsistency (TRIN)
    scale
unstructured interview
Variable Response Inconsistency
    (VRIN) scale

CHAPTER 8

Personality Assessment

by Bradley T. Erford, Kathleen McNinch, and Carol Salisbury

T his chapter addresses the basic knowledge and skills required for personality assessment. Attention is given to trait approaches, especially the five-factor model, and to personality instruments based on trait approaches. In addition, an introduction to projective assessment is provided. Commonly used projective assessments are discussed from a classification framework, including association, picture-story construction, verbal completion, choice arrangement, and production-expression techniques.

WHAT IS PERSONALITY?

Some people are described as having so much personality that they "ooze" with it, others as having "no personality at all." Still others are diagnosed with a "personality disorder." So what is this thing that appears to be so important to people that the services of professional counselors are sought to help assess, understand, and sometimes even restructure it? You may not find it hard to imagine that experts do not agree on a definition of **personality**, what comprises it, or how best to measure it. Some believe personality is an all-encompassing construct that accounts for all of an individual's thoughts, feelings, and behaviors. Others view personality with a much narrower focus. The unfortunate (or fortunate) thing about science is that in order to study something, one needs to be able to define it. Since few agree on any one definition, the authors have chosen one that makes sense and which can serve as a springboard to a robust discussion on personality and its assessment.

Piedmont (1998) defined personality as an intrinsic, adaptive organizational structure that is consistent across situations and stable over time. Note the four essential facets of this definition. First, personality is *intrinsic*, meaning located within the individual, not imposed on the individual by the environment. Second, personality is an *adaptive, organized structure* that allows the individual to adjust (or not adjust) to environmental, contextual demands. These demands are basically competing needs and desires that may come from inside or outside of the individual. Third, personality is *consistent across situations*—that is, one's personal goals and world view remain fairly constant from one situation to the next, even though one's behaviors or thoughts can be adapted in different ways. Finally, personality is *stable over time*. This should not be understood to mean that personality does not change over time, for it certainly does. But there is some lingering connection or thread that ties together one's functioning during childhood, adolescence, and adulthood—consistent themes, needs, and motivations.

Importantly, personality should not be viewed as being good or bad, because its basic purpose is to help the individual adapt and survive in a given context. Personality is a dynamic structure that is shaped and contoured over time to allow the individual to adapt to environmental demands and contexts in such a way that individual needs, desires, and motivations can be expressed. Just as in physical development, one is born with an immature personality that grows over time and is influenced by culture and by environmental events. Personality helps one to perceive and interpret both the internal and external world and to select goals to pursue. Importantly, while personality does change over time, most of the change occurs during childhood, adolescence, and young adulthood. Indeed, there is overwhelming evidence that one's personality is essentially stable by about the age of 30 years (Piedmont, 2006), barring major transformative events (e.g., religious conversion, significant trauma, intensive psychotherapy).

THE PURPOSE OF PERSONALITY ASSESSMENT

In general terms, the purpose of **personality assessment** is to help the professional counselor and client understand the client's various attitudes, characteristics, interpersonal needs, and intrinsic motivations in order to gain insight into current events, activities, and conflicts and also to generalize this understanding to new situations clients will encounter on their own, both now and in the future. In more specific terms, personality assessment has the same purposes as most other types of assessment, as discussed in Chapter 1: screening, diagnosis, placement, treatment planning, and outcomes evaluation. While diagnosis may seem out of place in the context of personality as defined above, one should bear in mind the existence of personality disorders. Personality assessment can play a crucial role in identifying individuals with some personality disorders. Professional counselors must be cognizant of which purpose is being pursued, because of all the types of assessment instruments available to professional counselors, structured and unstructured personality instruments have the widest variability in terms of psychometric quality and usefulness; that is, some are extremely well developed and well studied, while others lack virtually any empirical support or rigor. As a result, experienced clinicians approach the task of personality assessment with great seriousness and caution.

The two most common approaches to personality assessment are the (structured) trait approach and the (unstructured) projective approach. The discussion of each approach and commonly used tests based on each approach make up the remainder of this chapter.

TRAIT APPROACHES TO PERSONALITY ASSESSMENT

Most personality tests measure traits or states (many measure both, of course), and it is sometimes helpful to consider traits and states as two ends of the same continuum. **Traits** are enduring, statistically derived dimensions used to explain personality characteristics (e.g., introversion, agreeableness), while states are generally more transient or situation-dependent facets of personal adjustment (e.g., anxiety, self-confidence). Some measures, such as the *State-Trait Anxiety Inventory for Children* (Spielberger, 1973), aim to differentiate between the presence and importance of these two ends of the continuum. Client states are important for professional counselors to understand. They are often relevant to clinical diagnosis and often serve as the impetus for clients to actually seek counseling services. For example, many clients endure a life of anxiety or sadness but will only seek treatment when they experience a panic attack or major depressive episode. Acute anxious or depressive reactions are (generally) short-lived occurrences that result from situational events and/or internal physiology, not long-term conditions that stem from personality characteristics. Thus states are important, but because of their unpredictability and transience, they provide little help to clients and professional counselors who seek to understand and predict a client's likely pattern of cognitive, affective, and behavioral functioning. Thus most structured personality assessment deals with the identification of the more enduring personality traits to understand and predict human behavior.

Unfortunately, social scientists who study traits disagree on a standard definition to about the same degree that they disagree on a definition of personality. Personality traits are certainly not physical structures, although pseudoscientific approaches during the past several centuries have espoused just that. For example, *physiognomy* is the study of personality through determining a person's physical characteristics. Thus the shape of one's nose may be used to determine personality characteristics: A pointed nose resembling a dog's snout would represent tenacity and faithfulness, and a large, rounded nose resembling a pig's snout would represent slovenly, piggish characteristics (Sax, 1997). *Phrenology* was a 19th-century system for studying the physical characteristics of the skull (i.e., protrusions or depressions), which were believed connected to functions within the brain. This theory espoused that the brain center responsible for a specific ability would "grow out" (i.e., protrude) when highly developed, or "sink in" (i.e., depress) when underdeveloped. Thus phrenologists of that era were quite confident that they could identify abilities such as concentration and secretiveness, as well as several dozen other characteristics. Additional pseudoscientific approaches include numerology, astrology, and palmistry. None has received support from the scientific community.

While the study of traits has a long history of pseudoscientific attempts, it has been studied scientifically for only a little more than half a century. In the historical evolution of our understanding of traits, Gordon Allport (1937) attempted to understand traits as rational dimensions that underlie the thousands of words people use to describe each other. In one study, Allport & Odbert (1936) searched the dictionary for descriptive words and identified more than 18,000 words that could describe human personality characteristics. They next whittled that list down to about 4,500 by eliminating synonyms and by retaining descriptors of stable characteristics (remember, traits are enduring). But 4,500 is still a huge number of personality traits. The advent of new statistical techniques (i.e., factor analysis) and high-speed computers spurred further attempts to identify and understand the number of dimensions, or component traits, that underlie personality. Today, there are hundreds of personality tests that purport to measure one or more personality traits. But until recently, there was little agreement over the number of factors or traits that explained human personality. For example, Cattell, Cattell, and Cattell (1993) developed the *16 Personality Factors* inventory (*16PF*). Others have determined that more than 100 personality traits may exist.

However, recent well-designed research and instrumentation by Costa & McCrae (1990, 1992) have helped to integrate much of the disparate research on personality traits conducted over the past half century into a model with substantial empirical support: The *five-factor model* (FFM). Costa & McCrae (1990, p. 23) defined traits as "dimensions of individual differences in tendencies to show consistent patterns of thoughts, feelings, and actions." There are two key parts to this definition. First, traits are dimensions, which are empirically verifiable concepts organizing human behavior along a continuum. Second, individuals differ or vary according to how much or how little of a particular trait they may possess. It is these differences in traits, then, that describe an individual's "personality." Costa and McCrae identified five primary traits along which individuals differ—not dozens or hundreds; just five: Neuroticism, Extraversion, Openness, Agreeableness, and Conscientiousness. For example, the trait of Extraversion involves the intensity of interpersonal relationships. An individual can be described as introverted (i.e., shy, aloof, withdrawn) on one end of the continuum, extraverted (i.e., sociable, outgoing, adventurous, enthusiastic) on the other end of the continuum, or somewhere in between (i.e., ambiverted). Most importantly, the amount of the trait an individual possesses can be measured and compared to some norm group to determine whether the individual displays an average, significantly higher, or significantly lower amount of the trait than other individuals with like characteristics (e.g., age, sex). The amount of a trait a client exhibits helps professional counselors understand and predict client actions now and in the future.

Costa and McCrae and other researchers have accumulated substantial evidence that these factors can be found on most multifaceted personality inventories available today (see Piedmont, 2006). The FFM has emerged as a fairly comprehensive taxonomy, useful in classifying and understanding personality traits. The FFM traits and facets are closely aligned with those of the *Revised NEO Personality Inventory* (*NEO-PI-R*) (Costa & McCrae, 1992), which will also be reviewed later in this chapter.

Because traits are often described as existing on a continuum (e.g. introversion-extraversion, agreeable-disagreeable, conscientiousness-carelessness), some researchers and test developers have found it helpful to juxtapose these continua in order to categorize or label people according to some typology—for example, juxtaposing the Extraversion and Neuroticism traits results in four "types" of clients. A client who is high on both traits (i.e., high extraversion, high neuroticism) may be hot tempered, impulsive, or easily influenced. Someone who is low on both traits (i.e., low extraversion, low neuroticism) may be calm, impassive, and reliable. One who is high on extraversion and low on neuroticism may be easygoing, talkative, and optimistic. One who is low on extraversion and high on neuroticism may be pessimistic, sad, and sober. Note the consistent use of the phrase "may be," for these characteristics are certainly not representative of all individuals of a given type under all circumstances. Still, research (and common sense) indicates that the more of a given trait one possesses, the more stable the categorization, and the greater the predictive validity.

While juxtaposing two or more continua can be done with virtually any set of traits, some tests and theories are predicated on such a system. For example, the *Myers-Briggs Type Indicator—Form M (MBTI)* (Myers, McCaulley, Quenk & Hammer, 1998), a very commonly used personality inventory, was based upon the theory of Carl Jung (1923). With the exception of the *MBTI,* the development and use of tests based on typologies has been on the decline over the past several decades, ostensibly due to increased societal sensitivity to stereotyping of people. Likewise, numerous cautionary chimes have been sounded regarding the potential dangers of using personality instruments with clients from culturally diverse backgrounds (Anderson, 1995; Campos, 1989; Hinkle, 1994). In the final analysis, the focus among structured personality assessment today is firmly on the objective measurement and analysis of personality traits for their descriptive and predictive value.

Strengths and Limitations of the Trait Approach

Traits have substantial potential value when used judiciously by professional counselors. Piedmont (2006) suggested that professional counselors can use traits approaches in six primary ways: (1) understanding the client; (2) making differential diagnoses; (3) establishing empathy and rapport; (4) giving feedback and insight; (5) anticipating the course of therapy; and (6) matching treatments to clients.

Structured trait approaches to personality assessment have several noteworthy strengths. Trait inventories are relatively easy to administer, score, and interpret, either by hand or by computer. Most trait inventories are also norm referenced, allowing comparison of an individual's scores to a norm group. This allows examiners to determine whether clients have an average amount of a given trait, higher than average amounts, or lower than average amounts. Remember that knowing how much of a given trait an individual possesses is often useful in predicting client actions and outcomes.

Perhaps the greatest strength of trait approaches to personality assessment is that they focus on normal, healthy personality functioning, not just the clinical or pathological aspects of personality. In this way, they help us to understand a client's strengths and protective factors, rather than providing a myopic focus on a client's weaknesses and vulnerabilities.

Because traits are empirically derived constructs, they actually do exist in nature and can be observed and measured reliably. Traits also usually have robust predictive validity that can be empirically verified. In fact, research on the FFM has shown traits can predict a significant amount of variance across a wide range of clinical outcomes. Thus professional counselors can rely on knowledge of client traits to develop rapport, communicate in the most effective therapeutic manner, and, in general, structure treatment in the most efficacious manner.

Trait inventories are also amenable to computer scoring and interpretation, which can save professional counselors time and clients money. The standardized programming of computerized reports also tends to minimize scoring errors and examiner bias in judgment and interpretation. In addition, predictions and narrative written into the program usually are based on empirical evidence. This is in contrast to constructed commentary by examiners who vary substantially in experience and expertise. On the flip side, computer programs are frequently criticized for promoting a loss of individuation (i.e., every report sounds the same). Because examiners almost never have access to the programming language, it is usually impossible to evaluate the source and veracity of narrative statements generated by the report, or even the standard scores derived by internal scoring and conversion programs (Note: Fortunately, norm tables for most computerized interpretive tables are still published in hard-copy formats so clinicians can verify score accuracy by hand if necessary). Finally, given the boilerplate statements generated by many computerized programs, some professional counselors may question the accuracy of interpretive statements for the actual client being assessed. Several of the tests reviewed below and in the previous section have examples of computer-generated reports.

While very helpful, trait approaches do not escape substantial criticism. Some of the criticism is more theoretical or philosophical, while some involves more practical aspects. In regard to the theoretical and practical issues, some question how useful and helpful descriptions of personality can possibly be without some overriding theory to hold them together and bring meaning in some holistic manner. Indeed, little explanation or rationale has been offered as to why the traits even exist, how they develop and become differentiated over time, or even the degree to which each is genetically determined or environmentally influenced. On a more philosophical level, trait approaches are sometimes criticized for being tautological (redundant) in nature; that is, we know that outgoing, energetic, and sociable people are extraverted because extraverted people are outgoing, energetic, and sociable (Piedmont, 2006).

Another criticism is that different models predict different numbers of primary traits. While this may be expected on the basis of one's theoretical orientation, please recall that there is no theoretical orientation. These models are statistically derived subjected to empirical validation (i.e., "I exist (statistically); therefore I am"). Much of the recent evidence supports the five-factor model. But are there more than five factors? Costa and McCrae do not deny the possibility, and a research associate of theirs, Ralph Piedmont (2006), has identified a sixth factor, spirituality, using the same methodology that Costa and McCrae used to derive the original five factors. A holistic, integrative explanation based in theory is a critical next step in making trait approaches more explanatory (note the tautological emphasis).

There are several criticisms of trait approaches grounded more in the realm of pragmatics. First, self-report instruments usually only measure superficial portions of personality functioning that a client or observer of the client could also readily identify through an effective interview process. In a related criticism, trait approaches often lack the explanatory depth of projectives (psychoanalysis) and provide less insight into the client's internal world. Relatedly, professional counselors must ensure that all personality assessment is conducted according to the highest degree of ethical practice and guard against an invasion of privacy or inappropriate disclosure of information to others who may misunderstand or misuse the results (e.g., discriminate against clients with "undesirable" characteristics by limiting their opportunities).

Finally, a primary criticism continues to be that self-report trait inventories are a relatively transparent means of obtaining information about clients. As such, trait-based inventories are susceptible to client response sets and faking (e.g., acquiescence, nonacquiescence, malingering, socially desirable responses). It is inevitable that some clients will answer in a guarded manner, while others will be too self-critical. More and more structured inventories are including validity scales to allow professional counselors to identify clients who may be presenting with a response set that could invalidate interpretations.

SOME COMMONLY USED STRUCTURED PERSONALITY ASSESSMENT INVENTORIES

Revised NEO Personality Inventory (NEO-PI-R)

The *Revised NEO Personality Inventory* (*NEO-PI-R*) (Costa & McCrae, 1992) is a 240-item inventory designed to measure the five major dimensions of personality and is best used as a basic research instrument (Botwin, 1995; Digman, 1990; Goldberg, 1992; Piedmont, 2006). The *NEO-PI-R* usually requires about 25 to 35 minutes for an adult to complete, and hand scoring can be done quickly. Scale items measure Neuroticism, Extraversion, Openness to Experience, Agreeableness, and Conscientiousness, and each of these scales has six subscales (Botwin, 1995). Table 8.1 contains factor facets and descriptions from the *NEO-PI-R* (Costa & McCrae, 1992). These scales use both a self-report and an observer-rater form and can be individually or group administered. Scores are derived from a 5-point Likert scale ranging from Strongly Agree (1) to Strongly Disagree (5), and are translated into T scores for interpretation. Sample items include "Watching sports bores me," "I often feel calm and relaxed," and "It is easy for me to take charge of situations."

The self-rating, stratified sample consisted of 500 men and 500 women (screened from a larger pool of 2,273 people) and was selected demographically to match 1995 U.S. Census projections. The attention to sample selection is an improvement over the *NEO-PI* (Botwin, 1995). Observer rating norms were obtained from 143 ratings of 73 men and 134 ratings of 69 women from both spouses and multiple peer ratings (Costa & McCrae, 1992; Piedmont, 2006). Internal consistencies for individual facet scales ranged from $r = 0.56$ to $r = 0.81$ in self-reports and from $r = 0.60$ to $r = 0.90$ in observer ratings (Costa & McCrae, 1992). Test-retest reliabilities for facet scales on the original *NEO* ranged from $r = 0.66$ to $r = 0.92$ (McCrae & Costa, 1983). The *NEO-PI-R* correlated with similar scales, and construct, convergent and divergent validity were found to be adequate.

Table 8.1   *NEO-PI-R descriptions of traits and facets*

Domains

N: Neuroticism	General tendency to experience negative affects
E: Extraversion	Sociability, assertiveness, activeness, talkativeness
O: Openness	Active imagination, aesthetic sensitivity, attentiveness to inner feelings, preference for variety, intellectual curiosity, independence of judgment
A: Agreeableness	Interpersonal tendencies, altruism, sympathy, eagerness to help
C: Conscientiousness	Control of impulses, management of desires

Neuroticism facets

N1: Anxiety	Apprehensive, fearful, prone to worry, nervous, tense, jittery
N2: Angry Hostility	Tendency to experience anger and related states
N3: Depression	Tendency to experience depressive affect
N4: Self-Consciousness	Emotions of shame and embarrassment, uncomfortable around others
N5: Impulsiveness	Inability to control cravings and urges
N6: Vulnerability	Vulnerability and inability to cope with stress

Extraversion facets

E1: Warmth	Issues of interpersonal intimacy
E2: Gregariousness	Preference for other people's company
E3: Assertiveness	Tendency toward dominance, forcefulness, and social ascendancy
E4: Activity	Tendency toward rapid tempo and vigorous movement (energy)
E5: Excitement seeking	Tendency to crave excitement and stimulation
E6: Positive emotions	Tendency to experience positive emotions

Openness facets

O1: Fantasy	Intensity of imagination and fantasy life
O2: Aesthetics	Appreciation for and interest in art and beauty
O3: Feelings	Openness to feelings, receptivity to one's own inner feelings, evaluation of emotion as an important part of life
O4: Actions	Behavioral willingness to try different activities, etc.
O5: Ideas	Intellectual curiosity, open-mindedness, willingness to consider new things, ideas
O6: Values	Readiness to reexamine social, political, and religious values

Agreeableness facets

A1: Trust	Tendency to trust or distrust others
A2: Straightforwardness	Frankness, sincerity, and ingenuousness relative to others
A3: Altruism	Concern for others' welfare, generosity, consideration of others
A4: Compliance	Characteristic reactions to interpersonal conflict
A5: Modesty	Humbleness, self-efficacy
A6: Tender-mindedness	Attitudes of sympathy and concern for others

Conscientiousness facets

C1: Competence	Sense that one is capable, sensible, prudent, and effective
C2: Order	Tidiness, level of organization
C3: Dutifulness	Governed by conscience
C4: Achievement striving	Levels of aspiration and hard work toward goals
C5: Self-discipline	Ability to begin tasks and carry them through to completion
C6: Deliberation	Tendency to think carefully before acting

Source: Revised NEO Personality Inventory (NEO-PI-R) and NEO Five-Factor Inventory (NEO-FFI) Professional Manual by P. T Costa Jr. & R. R. McCrae, (1992). Odessa, FL: Psychological Assessment Resources.

Think About It 8.1   Using Table 8.1, describe your own personality using the five-factor model.

16 Personality Factors (16PF) Questionnaire

The *16PF Questionnaire* (Cattell et al., 1993) is a 185-item self-report inventory for clients ages 16 years to adult and is designed to measure normal personality characteristics, problem-solving abilities, and preferred work activities and to identify problems in areas known to be problematic to adults. Items of the *16PF* measure Anxiety, Extraversion, Independence, Self-Control, and Tough-Mindedness (Erford, 2006) and can be used to predict vocational interest as classified by Holland's occupational typology (Conn & Rieke, 1994). The *16PF* may prove helpful as a career counseling tool and as a work behavior and work attitude device (Vansickle & Conn, 1996). Administration of the *16PF* requires a 5th-grade reading level and can be conducted for individuals or groups by paper and pencil in 30 to 50 minutes, or in 25 to 35 minutes by computer (Russell & Karol, 1994). Scoring can be done by hand using four scoring keys, a norm table, and an Individual Record form, or by computer through a mail-in scoring service or the Institute for Personality and Ability Testing's (IPAT) OnSite System software. Raw scores are converted into standardized (sten) scores that are based on a 10-point scale (M = 5.5; SD = 2) (Russell & Karol, 1994). Sample items include "I often like to watch team games. a) true; b) false," and "I prefer friends who are: a) quiet; b) ?; c) lively." A portion of a sample computerized *16PF* Basic Interpretive Report from IPAT is provided in Table 8.2. Professional counselors may also be interested in the *Karson Clinical Report* (*KCR*) and *Cattell Comprehensive Personality Interpretation* (*CCPI*). Sample reports can be viewed at www.ipat.com.

The stratified normative sample (n = 2,500) consisted of approximately equal numbers of males and females from every U.S. state and the District of Columbia, closely representing the demographic variables of gender, race, age, and education in the 1990 U.S. census. Reliability reports of scores on the *16PF* are low, with only the Social Boldness scale consistently above r = 0.80 (Erford, 2006). Clinicians should be cautious when using this inventory for high school graduates and people over age 65, because these were underrepresented in the normative sample (McLellan, 1995). While the *16PF* may prove helpful in developing or confirming hypotheses about client personality characteristics, score reliability and validity are generally inadequate for decision-making purposes, unless used in conjunction with multiple sources of information.

One of the primary criticisms of the *16PF* continues to be the identification of too many primary factors (Chernyshenko, Stark, & Chan, 2001; Digman & Inouye, 1986), and second-order factor analytic studies indicate that about 4 to 6 factors explain the items' variance to a more substantial degree; after all, many of the 16 factors are highly intercorrelated. The addition of impression management scales are a benefit in interpretation (Schueger, 1992).

Table 8.2   *16PF* Basic Interpretive Report for a 33-year-old female.

RESPONSE STYLE INDICES

Index	Raw Score
Impression Management	19 within expected range
Infrequency	0 within expected range
Acquiescence	51 within expected range

All response style indices are within the normal range.

16PF **PROFILE**

Sten	Factor	Left meaning	Low	Average	High	Right meaning
			1 2 3		8 9 10	
6	Warmth (A)	Reserved				Warm
9	Reasoning (B)	Concrete				Abstract
7	Emotional Stability (C)	Reactive				Emotionally Stable
6	Dominance (E)	Deferential				Dominant
5	Liveliness (F)	Serious				Lively
6	Rule-Consciousness (G)	Expedient				Rule-Conscious
8	Social Boldness (H)	Shy				Socially Bold
7	Sensitivity (I)	Utilitarian				Sensitive
4	Vigilance (L)	Trusting				Vigilant
7	Abstractedness (M)	Grounded				Abstracted
4	Privateness (N)	Forthright				Private
6	Apprehension (O)	Self-Assured				Apprehensive
9	Openness to Change (Q1)	Traditional				Open to Change
4	Self-Reliance (Q2)	Group-Oriented				Self-Reliant
4	Perfectionism (Q3)	Tolerates Disorder				Perfectionistic
6	Tension (Q4)	Relaxed				Tense

GLOBAL FACTORS

Sten	Factor	Left meaning	Low	Average	High	Right meaning
			1 2 3 4 5	6 7	8 9 10	
7	Extraversion	Introverted				Extroverted
5	Anxiety	Low Anxiety				High Anxiety
2	Tough-Mindedness	Receptive				Tough-Minded
7	Independence	Accommodating				Independent
5	Self-Control	Unrestrained				Self-Controlled

TOUGH-MINDEDNESS

Tough-Mindedness is low. Ms. Female tends to value breadth and variety of experience, including openness to different ideas, people, or situations. When approaching problems, she may focus on subjective or emotional considerations rather than cold, hard facts.

- Ms. Female can be sensitive to emotional and aesthetic considerations.
- She often gets absorbed in ideas and thoughts.
- She is open to change and enjoys pursuing new ideas, opinions, and experiences.

EXTRAVERSION

Extraversion is high-average. Ms. Female is socially participative and probably enjoys activities involving others. Her attention is generally directed toward other people.

- Because this person is often socially bold, she is unlikely to feel intimidated in group settings. She may be relatively unaffected by insults or threats.
- When Ms. Female chooses to reveal personal matters to others, she tends to be forthright and genuine.
- Ms. Female shows a tendency to do things and make plans with others rather than alone.

INDEPENDENCE

Independence is high-average. Generally, Ms. Female prefers to lead an independent and self-directed life. Although she can sometimes be accommodating to others' wishes, she may often assert control or be persuasive.

- This person is venturesome and expressive, especially in front of others. Extreme boldness sometimes can be associated with a high desire for influence and attention.
- Vigilance does not appear to shape her stance on influencing or persuading others. She tends to trust other people's motivations rather than to question them.
- She is experimenting and has an inquiring, critical mind. She tends to question traditional methods and to press for new approaches.

ANXIETY

At the present time, Ms. Female presents herself as no more or less anxious than most people.

- Usually, Ms. Female meets challenges with calm and inner strength.
- She shows a tendency to be trusting and accepting of other people and their motives.

SELF-CONTROL

Self-Control is average. At times, Ms. Female may show the self-discipline and conscientiousness needed to meet her responsibilities. At other times, she may be less restrained, following her own wishes.

- Because this individual tends to be preoccupied with ideas, she may disregard the practical aspects of a situation.
- This individual seems to balance casualness and a tolerance for disorder with the need for organization and structure. She may function best in an unexacting, flexible setting rather than in a rigid system.

SELF-ESTEEM AND ADJUSTMENT

Overall, this individual tends to view herself positively, having a strong sense of self-worth and competence. She is likely to be capable of obtaining most of her personal goals. Self-Esteem is high-average (7).

The degree of emotional stability shown by Ms. Female is typical of most adults. That is, most of the time she tends to be calm and relaxed, but in demanding situations, she may be reactive or upset. Emotional Adjustment is average (6).

Not only is Ms. Female likely to feel quite comfortable in social gatherings, but she may initiate contact, lead conversations, and draw attention to herself. She probably will not hesitate to express what she needs from others. Social Adjustment is high (8).

SOCIAL SKILLS

The following six scales pertain to the ways in which information is communicated in social environments. The scales are broadly divided into two categories: nonverbal communication (Emotional Scales) and verbal communication (Social Scales). Within each category, communication skills are discussed at three more specific levels: the ability to send information (Expressivity), to receive and interpret messages (Sensitivity), and to control information (Control). Although a person may be more or less skilled in certain areas, overall social competence is reflected in a general balance among the six scales below.

Ms. Female's communication is predicted to be demonstrative and forceful. That is, her emotional displays are probably uninhibited and genuine. Her emotions are likely to be easily perceived by others, and thus are likely to influence the emotional states of those around her. Emotional Expressivity is high (8).

continued

Table 8.2   *continued*

This person may enjoy observing other people's gestures, moods, and nonverbal interactions. Thus, she may feel comfortable interpreting people's emotional and other nonverbal messages. Emotional Sensitivity is high-average (7).

At times, Ms. Female may adapt her emotional displays to the given situation. At other times, she may be unable to suppress a strongly felt emotion. Emotional Control is average (5).

This person is probably outgoing and articulate and would often make a good first impression. She may feel comfortable with verbal disclosure and could probably join in most discussions with relative ease. Social Expressivity is high-average (7).

Ms. Female may not be very concerned about monitoring or interpreting others' social behavior or mannerisms. Ms. Female's self-comfort may mean that she is not overly concerned about the appropriateness of her own actions. Social Sensitivity is low-average (4).

This person projects a comfortable social presence. That is, she probably presents herself well in just about any type of social situation and is likely to participate with any social group. She may consider the appropriateness of when to speak up and when to withhold comment according to the demands of a given situation. Social Control is high (9).

This person is attentive to other people and is likely to be sensitive to their feelings. She is probably willing to consider another person's point of view. As a consequence, others may seek her out for sympathy and support. Ms. Female should be careful not to allow the problems of others to override her own. Empathy is high (8).

LEADERSHIP AND CREATIVITY

In a group of peers, potential for leadership is predicted to be average (6).

At the client's own level of abilities, potential for creative functioning is predicted to be high (8). She probably has the sense of adventure, assertiveness, and orientation toward ideas that are necessary for pursuing creative interests.

Ms. Female shows characteristics somewhat similar to persons who invest a lot of time producing novel or original works. Should this individual choose to pursue creative endeavors, her rate of output is predicted to be above average (7).

VOCATIONAL ACTIVITIES

Different occupational interests have been found to be associated with different personality qualities. The following section compares Ms. Female's personality to these known associations. The information below indicates the degree of similarity between Ms. Female's personality characteristics and each of the six Holland Occupational Types (*Self-Directed Search;* Holland, 1985). Those occupational areas for which Ms. Female's personality profile shows the highest degree of similarity are described in greater detail. Descriptions are based on item content of the Self-Directed Search as well as the personality predictions of the Holland types as measured by the *16PF.*

Remember that this information is intended to expand Ms. Female's range of career options rather than to narrow them. All comparisons should be considered with respect to other relevant information about Ms. Female, particularly her interests, abilities, and other personal resources.

HOLLAND THEMES

Sten	Factor	1 2 3 4 5 6 7 8 9 10
9	Artistic	————————◆
7	Investigative	——————◆
7	Social	——————◆
6	Enterprising	—————◆
5	Realistic	————◆
4	Conventional	———◆

Artistic = 9

Ms. Female shows personality characteristics similar to Artistic persons, who are self-expressive, typically through a particular mode such as art, music, design, writing, acting, composing, etc. Like Artistic persons, Ms. Female may be venturesome and open to different views and experiences. Sometimes she may be preoccupied with thoughts and ideas, which may relate to the overall creative process. She may do her best work in an unstructured, flexible environment. It may be worthwhile to explore whether Ms. Female appreciates aesthetics and possesses artistic, design, or musical talents.

Occupational Fields: Art
Music
Design
Theater
Writing

Investigative = 7

Ms. Female shows personality characteristics similar to Investigative persons. Such persons typically have good reasoning ability and enjoy the challenge of problem solving. They tend to have critical minds, are curious, and are open to new ideas and solutions. Investigative persons tend to be reserved and somewhat impersonal; they may prefer working independently. They tend to be concerned with the function and purpose of materials rather than aesthetic principles. Ms. Female may enjoy working with ideas and theories, especially in the scientific realm. It may be worthwhile to explore whether Ms. Female enjoys doing research, reading technical articles, or solving challenging problems.

Occupational Fields: Science
Math
Research
Medicine and Health
Computer Science

Social = 7

Ms. Female shows personality characteristics similar to Social persons, who indicate a preference for associating with other people. Such interactions are distinguished by a nurturing, sympathetic quality. Ms. Female may find it very easy to relate to all kinds of people. In addition to being warm and friendly, Social persons are typically receptive to different views and opinions. They feel most comfortable in positions that allow for regular social interaction. It might be worthwhile to explore whether Ms. Female enjoys working with others and having them seek her out for advice or comfort.

Occupational Fields: Teaching
Counseling
Psychology
Social Work
Health Services

Source: Copyright © 1994, The Institute of Personality and Ability Testing, Inc., Champaign, IL. All rights reserved. Reproduced with permission of the Institute of Personality and Ability Testing, Inc.

Note: The original *16PF Basic Interpretive Report* included graphical score displays for each interpreted factor. These graphs have been removed to conserve space. The *16PF Basic Interpretive Report* usually generates a 10-page report.

Myers-Briggs Type Indicator—Form M (MBTI)

The *Myers-Briggs Type Indicator—Form M* (*MBTI*) (Myers, McCaulley et al., 1998) is a 93-item self-report inventory for clients ages 14 years and older. Based on Jungian theory, items measure four different bipolar continua: Extraversion-Introversion (E-I), Sensing-Intuition (S-N), Thinking-Feeling (T-F), and Judging-Perceiving (J-P). These scales result in four-letter combinations that identify and describe 16 personality types (see Table 8.3). Sample items include "Are you: easy to get to know, or hard to get to know?" and "Can you: talk easily to almost anyone for as long as you

Table 8.3   Examples of associated traits with *MBTI* typologies

Example Typology 1: Introverted-Intuition-Thinking-Judging (INTJ)
Have original minds and great drive for implementing their ideas and achieving their goals. Quickly see patterns in external events and develop long-range explanatory perspectives. When committed, organize a job and carry it through. Skeptical and independent, have high standards of competence and performance – for themselves and others.

Example Typology 2: Extroverted-Sensing-Feeling-Perceiving (ESFP)
Outgoing, friendly, and accepting. Exuberant lovers of life, people, and material comforts. Enjoy working with others to make things happen. Bring common sense and a realistic approach to their work, and make work fun. Flexible and spontaneous, adapt readily to new people and environments. Learn best by trying a new skill with other people.

Source: Introduction to type (6th ed.) by I. B. Myers, L. K. Kirby, & K. D. Myers, (1998), p. 13. Palo Alto, CA: Consulting Psychologists Press.

have to, or find a lot to say only to certain people or under certain conditions?" The *MBTI* requires a 7th-grade reading level and takes about 15 to 25 minutes to administer. This inventory can be hand-scored or computer-scored. Forced-choice items produce responses that are weighted in points. The normative sample ($n = 3,009$) consisted of U.S. adults ages 18 years and older, generally representing sex and ethnicity consistent with the 1990 U.S. Census, although White women were overrepresented and Black men were underrepresented (Myers, McCaulley, et al., 1998).

Split-half reliability falls above an acceptable range of 0.90 for the national sample. Test-retest reliability (4-week interval), ranged from $r = 0.83$ to $r = 0.97$, and internal consistency (coefficient *alpha*) for males and females ranged from $r = 0.90$ to $r = 0.93$ (Myers, McCaulley et al., 1998). Validity of the *MBTI* is moderate to high when correlated with the five-factor model as portrayed in the *NEO PI-R* (Erford, 2006). Construct validity was found for each of the four dichotomies (Erford, 2006; Myers, McCaulley et al., 1998). More than 3 million people are administered the *MBTI* each year (Michael, 2003). This inventory can be used to increase insight (Fleener, 2001), to assist in career counseling in conjunction with human resource issues (Capraro & Capraro, 2002), and to identify obstacles to career development (Healy & Woodward, 1998). Clinicians should note that the artificial manner with which the *MBTI* types people may not lead to meaningful descriptions (Vacha-Haase & Thompson, 1999), and clients may feel restricted by reporting specific behaviors, attitudes, career choices, or interests (Watkins & Campbell, 2000) because of the forced-choice test construction. While the *MBTI* does appear to measure at least four important personality dimensions, the evidence does not support the establishment of 16 unique personality types (Johnson, Mauzey, Johnson, Murphy, & Zimmerman, 2002). Finally, as with all self-report instruments, it is difficult to confirm the accuracy of self-perceptions constituting an *MBTI* client typology (Gailbreath, Wagner, Moffett, & Hein, 1997; Gardner & Martinko, 1996), especially when no response validity measures are provided.

Millon Index of Personality Styles Revised (MIPS Revised)

The *Millon Index of Personality Styles Revised* (*MIPS Revised*) (Millon, 2003) is a 180-item true-false Level B self-report instrument for adults ages 18 years and older and is designed to measure personality styles of normally functioning adults. Scale names and the profile display of the original *MIPS* were updated to provide administrators with a better, more intuitive approach to interpreting test results. This inventory measures three dimensions of normal personality using 6 Motivating Style scales (Pleasure-Enhancing, Pain-Avoiding, Actively Modifying, Passively Accommodating, Self-Indulging, Other-Nurturing); 8 Thinking Style scales (Externally Focused, Internally Focused, Realistic/Sensing, Imaginative/Intuitive, Thought-Guided, Feeling-Guided, Conservation-Seeking, Innovation-Seeking); 10 Behaving Style scales (Asocial/Withdrawing, Gregarious/Outgoing, Anxious/Hesitating, Confident/Asserting, Unconventional/Dissenting, Dutiful/Conforming, Submissive/Yielding, Dominant/Controlling, Dissatisfied/Complaining, Cooperative/Agreeing); and 4 Validity Indices that provide information about Positive Impression, Negative Impression, Consistency, and Clinical Index. The *MIPS Revised* takes about 30 minutes to complete using either the paper-and-pencil or computer format. An 8th-grade reading level is required, and it is important to designate age and gender to obtain an accurate report. The *MIPS Revised* can be scored by hand, computer, mail-in, or optical scanning methods.

The *MIPS Revised* test offers separate norms for adults and college students, and for both separate and combined genders. The adult sample consisted of 1,000 individuals (500 females, 500 males) ages 18–65 years and is stratified according to the U.S. population by age, race or ethnicity, and education level (Millon, 2003). The college sample consisted of 1,600 students (800 males, 800 females) selected from 14 colleges and universities to be representative of a college student population in terms of ethnicity, age, year in school, major area of study, region of the county, and type of institution. The *MIPS Revised* can be used as a screening tool in employee selection; for employee assistance programs and leadership and employee development programs; in career planning for high school and college students; in the curriculum for college courses in psychological testing; and in relationship, premarital, marriage, and individual counseling.

Personality Assessment Inventory (PAI)

The *Personality Assessment Inventory* (*PAI*) (Morey, 1991) is used to assess behaviors related to psychopathology as well as to provide information for screening, clinical diagnosis, and treatment. It can be administered in individual or group formats to clients ages 18 years to adult in about 40 to 50 minutes. There are 344 items on this self-reported inventory, and responses are based on a 4-point scale (Not at All True, Slightly True, Mainly True, and Very True). The *PAI* requires a 4th-grade reading level. There are 22 nonoverlapping scales, including 4 validity scales (Inconsistency, Infrequency, Negative Impression, Positive Impression); 11 clinical scales (Somatic

Complaints, Anxiety, Anxiety-Related Disorders, Depression, Mania, Paranoia, Schizophrenia, Borderline Features, Antisocial Features, Alcohol Problems, Drug Problems); 5 treatment scales (Aggression, Suicidal Ideation, Stress, Nonsupport, Treatment Rejection); and 2 interpersonal scales (Dominance, Warmth). Answers can be scored by hand or by optical scanning, and raw scores can be converted into T scores (Boyle, 1995).

Standardization samples conformed to U.S. population demographics with respect to the test's diagnostic groups (Kavan, 1995). Reliability of scores seems questionable based on the wide range of coefficients for different variables. Internal consistency coefficients for the 22 scales ranged from $r = 0.45$ to $r = 0.90$, with a median of 0.81 (normative sample); from $r = 0.22$ to $r = 0.89$, with a median of 0.82 (college sample); and from $r = 0.23$ to $r = 0.94$, with a median of 0.86 (clinical sample). Median *alphas* were consistent between various races, ages, and genders in the mid to high 0.70s. Test-retest reliability coefficients (3- to 4-week interval) ranged from $r = 0.31$ to $r = 0.92$, with a median of 0.82 (Boyle, 1995). Correlation studies with the *Minnesota Multiphasic Personality Inventory* (*MMPI*) and the *Marlowe-Crowne Social Desirability Scale* yielded mixed validity results. Even with the disputed reliability and validity information, Kavan (1995) viewed the *PAI* as a competitor of the *MMPI-2* that is easier to administer, score, and interpret.

California Psychological Inventory (CPI)

The *California Psychological Inventory* (*CPI*) (Gough & Bradley, 1996) is a 434-item inventory designed to assess personality characteristics and to predict what people will say and do in specified contexts. The *CPI* has numerous questions that overlap with the original *MMPI* but was designed for a different population and purpose than the *MMPI* (i.e., personality descriptions of a nonclinical population). Scale items measure 20 Folk scales (Dominance, Capacity for Status, Sociability, Social Presence, Self-Acceptance, Independence, Empathy, Responsibility, Socialization, Self-Control, Good Impression, Communality, Well-Being, Tolerance, Achievement via Conformity, Achievement via Independence, Intellectual Efficiency, Psychological-Mindedness, Flexibility, and Femininity-Masculinity); 3 Vector scales (Internality-Externality, Norm-Questioning-Favoring, and Self-Realization); and 13 Special Purpose scales. These scales are for clients ages 13 years and older, are written at a 5th-grade reading level, and take about 45 to 60 minutes to administer (Atkinson, 2003). The *CPI* is self-administered and can be done using either pencil and paper or a computer. Forms are scanned for automated data entry. Using the scores from the three Vector scales, a cuboidal personality typology is developed, which helps to classify individuals into four categories (Atkinson, 2003).

The normative sample ($n = 6,000$; 3,000 of each gender) was reported as not being representative or random because of use of primarily high school students (50%) and undergraduate students (16.7%), so these are probably the best populations for which to use the instrument, though the manual provides useful reference tables for comparing students of various ages (Hattrup, 2003). The test produced internal consistency Cronbach's *alpha* estimates on the 20 Folk scales ranging from

$r = 0.43$ to $r = 0.85$, with a median of 0.76. For the three Vector scales, the internal consistency estimates ranged from $r = 0.77$ to $r = 0.88$. Cronbach's *alpha* for the 13 specialty scales ranged from $r = 0.45$ to $r = 0.88$. *Alpha* reliabilities of the *CPI* scales ranged from $r = 0.62$ to $r = 0.84$ in the total sample, with a median of 0.77. Test-retest reliabilities were based on samples of 108 males and 129 females who were retested after a 1-year interval, and samples of 91 females and 44 males who were retested after 5- and 25-year intervals, respectively. For the 1-year retest, scale reliabilities ranged from $r = 0.51$ to $r = 0.84$, with a median of 0.68. For the 5-year and 25-year retest, reliabilities ranged from $r = 0.36$ to $r = 0.73$, and $r = 0.37$ to $r = 0.84$, respectively. Test-retest reliability estimates among high school students were between 0.60 and 0.80 for a 1-year period. The Folk and Vector scales had moderate to strong construct validity correlation scores (0.40 to 0.80), but the predictive power regarding individual behavior in a given situation was weak.

Jackson Personality Inventory–Revised (JPI-R)

The *Jackson Personality Inventory-Revised* (*JPI-R*) (Jackson, 1994) is an inventory consisting of 300 true-false statements designed to produce "a set of measures of personality reflecting a variety of interpersonal, cognitive, and value orientations" (Jackson, 1994, p. 1). Scale items represent 15 separate personality traits: Analytical (Complexity, Breadth of Interest, Innovation, Tolerance); Emotional (Empathy, Anxiety, Cooperativeness); Extroverted (Sociability, Social Confidence, Energy Level); Opportunistic (Social Astuteness, Risk Taking); and Dependable (Organization, Traditional Values, Responsibility). This inventory is used for adolescents and adults and takes approximately 35 to 45 minutes to administer. Raw scores range from 0 to 20 and are converted to a profile sheet that references gender-specific norms using a vertical grid. Scoring can be done by hand in 3 minutes or can be done by mail, computer, or online to produce a comprehensive client report. Sample items include "I usually read several books at the same time," "I enjoy taking risks," and "I am seldom at a loss for words." The *JPI-R* is a Level B instrument.

Internal consistency reliability estimates for the *JPI-R* were obtained from four college volunteer samples using the Cronbach *alpha* estimate (Jackson, 1994). In the largest college normative sample ($n = 1,107$), *alpha* estimates ranged from $r = 0.66$ for the Complexity, Tolerance, and Social Astuteness scales to $r = 0.87$ for the Innovation scale. In all four samples, the reliability estimates range from $r = 0.62$ for Social Astuteness to $r = 0.88$ for Social Confidence. In two studies, median internal consistency reliabilities (Bentler's Theta) were 0.90 and 0.93. Tables in the manual provide validity correlations for the *JPI-R* with other psychological variables and scales, including the *Minnesota Multiphasic Personality Inventory* (*MMPI*), the *Survey of Work Styles* (*SWS*), and the *Jackson Vocational Interest Survey* (*JVIS*). Counselors will find the manual instructions for administration and scoring easy to follow and are cautioned that the *JPI-R* cannot be used to diagnose pathology (Pittenger, 1998). The *JPI-R* is a helpful measure of client dispositions and can be used to help clients develop insight and understand sources of resiliency. Table 8.4 provides a sample computerized interpretive report for the *JPI-R*.

Table 8.4 *Jackson Personality Inventory—Revised (JPI-R) Basic Report for Sam Sample, a 30-year-old male*

Your *JPI-R* Scale Profile

The profile below is based on your responses to the *JPI-R*. For a better understanding of your scores, study the definitions and scale descriptions and follow the profile.

Scale	Raw	Combined %ile	Female %ile	Male %ile	Male Percent Graph 0 10 20 30 40 50 60 70 80 90 100
Complexity	14	90	88	92	
Breadth of Interest	19	96	96	96	
Innovation	18	86	90	84	
Tolerance	17	93	93	95	
Empathy	11	38	24	54	
Anxiety	2	2	1	4	
Cooperativeness	1	4	3	4	
Sociability	12	69	66	73	
Social Confidence	18	86	86	86	
Energy Level	18	92	96	88	
Social Astuteness	12	73	76	69	
Risk Taking	17	97	99	95	
Organization	14	66	66	69	
Traditional Values	3	4	3	4	
Responsibility	14	50	38	58	

RAW SCORE	Your raw score for each scale is based on your responses to the statements that make up that scale. A high raw score indicates that you endorsed many of that scale's statements.
COMBINED PERCENTILE	This score is determined by comparing your raw score for each scale with the corresponding scores of a representative group consisting of both men and women. Your score is the percentage of the people in the representative group who received a score equal to or less than your score.
FEMALE PERCENTILE	This score is the percentage of women in the representative group who received a raw score equal to or less than your score. Use this score to determine how you compare to members of the opposite sex.
MALE PERCENTILE	This score shows how you compare to members of your own sex. Your score is the percentage of men in the representative group who received a raw score equal to or less than yours. The bar graph at the right of your profile is based on this score.

[Examples of Selected Scale Descriptions]

COMPLEXITY

Your percentile rank on the **Complexity** scale is 92, placing you in the extremely high range.

Higher Scorer	Seeks intricate solutions to problems; is impatient with oversimplications; is interested in pursuing topics in depth regardless of their difficulty; enjoys abstract thought; enjoys intricacy.
Low Scorer	Prefers concrete to abstract interpretations; avoids contemplative thought; uninterested in probing for new insight.

ANXIETY

Your percentile rank on the **Anxiety** scale is 4, placing you in the extremely low range.

Higher Scorer	Tends to worry over inconsequential matters; more easily upset than the average person; apprehensive about the future.
Low Scorer	Remains calm in stressful situations; takes things as they come without worrying; can relax in difficult situations; usually composed and collected.

Your *JPI-R* Cluster Profile

Scale	Raw	Combined %ile	Female %ile	Male %ile	Male percent graph 0 10 20 30 40 50 60 70 80 90 100
Analytical	68	97	97	97	
Emotional	14	4	1	7	
Extroverted	48	90	92	88	
Opportunistic	29	96	99	90	
Dependable	31	24	18	31	

JPI-R Cluster Descriptions

The following cluster descriptions list the *JPI-R* scales that make up each cluster, as well as some of the traits found in high and low scorers. Also listed is the range into which your cluster score falls. Use this range to determine how strongly the high and/or low score traits apply to you. For more information on the scale scores that make up each of your cluster scores, refer back to the profile at the beginning of this report.

ANALYTICAL

Your percentile rank on the **Analytical** cluster is 97, placing you in the extremely high range.

Your score on this cluster is derived from your scores on the *JPI-R* COMPLEXITY, BREADTH OF INTEREST, INNOVATION, and TOLERANCE scales. If you score high on this cluster of four scales, you might be expected to consider arguments from multiple points of view and may be inclined towards drawing distinctions among otherwise related elements of information. On the other hand, if you score low on this cluster, you might be expected to think of things in more black-and-white terms and to prefer straightforward, linear interpretations of events.

EMOTIONAL

Your percentile rank on the **Emotional** cluster is 7, placing you in the extremely low range.

This second cluster includes the *JPI-R* EMPATHY, ANXIETY, and COOPERATIVENESS scales. A high score on this cluster indicates that you may express your feelings readily and that you may have difficulty hiding your emotions, especially under stressful conditions. If your score is low, you may be relatively unaffected by emotionally arousing situations and by social pressure.

EXTROVERTED

Your percentile rank on the **Extroverted** cluster is 88, placing you in the very high range.

The *JPI-R* SOCIABILITY, SOCIAL CONFIDENCE, and ENERGY LEVEL scales make up this cluster. A high score on this cluster suggests that you are outgoing, sociable, and active. A low score indicates that you may be more introverted and less active.

OPPORTUNISTIC

Your percentile rank on the **Opportunistic** cluster is 90, placing you in the very high range.

Your score on this cluster is based on your scores on the *JPI-R* SOCIAL ASTUTENESS and RISK TAKING scales. If you scored high on this cluster, you may be described as diplomatic, persuasive, skeptical, worldly, and charming. A low score suggests that you may be more direct, less adventurous, and less uncritical of the self-serving intentions of others.

DEPENDABLE

Your percentile rank on the **Dependable** cluster is 31, placing you in the low range.

This cluster includes the *JPI-R* ORGANIZATION, TRADITIONAL VALUES, and RESPONSIBILITY scales. If your score on this cluster is high, you may tend to be methodical, predictable, systematic, conservative and mature in your attitudes. Should you score low, you may be considered to be more liberal-minded and flexible in your thinking, but less organized in your work habits.

Source: Reproduced by permission of Sigma Assessment Systems, Inc., P.O. Box 610984, Port Huron, MI 48061-0984.

Piers-Harris Children's Self-Concept Scale—Second Edition (Piers-Harris-2)

The *Piers-Harris Children's Self-Concept Scale, Second Edition* (*Piers-Harris-2*) (Piers & Herzberg, 2002) is a 60-item self-report inventory used for children ages 7–18 years who are able to read at a 2nd-grade reading level. The *Piers-Harris-2* is designed to aid in the assessment of self-concept in children and adolescents. This inventory measures six cluster scales of Behavioral Adjustment (BEH), Intellectual and School Status (INT), Physical Appearance and Attributes (PHY), Freedom from Anxiety (FRE), Popularity (POP), and Happiness and Satisfaction (HAP). Sample items include "I am smart," "I feel left out of things," and "I think bad thoughts." The *Piers-Harris-2* takes about 10 to 15 minutes to complete using paper and pencil or computer and is available in Spanish. The inventory requires children to circle either Yes or No to indicate whether the statement describes the way they feel about themselves. Raw scores (total number of responses marked in the positive direction) can be converted to percentiles, stanines, and T scores and are available in the form of an overall self-concept score or as a profile of six cluster scores. Scoring can be accomplished by mail, fax, or computer (Piers & Herzberg, 2002).

Restandardization of the *Piers-Harris-2* utilized a sample of 1,387 students ranging from 7 to 18 years of age. These students were recruited from school districts all across the United States closely representing the ethnic composition of the U.S. population according to the 2001 Bureau of the Census. *Alpha* coefficients for the *Piers-Harris-2* cluster scale restandardization sample ranged from $r = 0.74$ for the Popularity scale to $r = 0.81$ for the three scales of Behavioral Adjustment, Intellectual and School Status (INT), and Freedom from Anxiety (FRE) (Piers & Herzberg, 2002). Although test-retest reliability for the *Piers-Harris-2* is not available, data for the original 80-item *Piers-Harris* reported reliability of $r = 0.77$ (2-month interval) and $r = 0.77$ (4-month interval) (Piers & Herzberg, 2002). Hattie (1992) reported a test-retest study (4-week interval) for the *Piers-Harris* total score and the six cluster scales using a sample of 135 Australian students in grades 10 through 12. Reliability coefficients ranged from $r = 0.65$ for the Happiness and Satisfaction scale to $r = 0.88$ for the Physical Appearance and Attributes scale (Piers & Herzberg, 2002). The psychometric properties of the original *Piers-Harris* were also reviewed favorably (e.g., Chiu, 1988; Epstein, 1985; Jeske, 1985). The self-report feature was also viewed as a positive (Gans, Kenny, & Ghany, 2003; Riddle & Bergin, 1997). Professional counselors should note that the *Piers-Harris-2* is not recommended for children who are unwilling or unable to cooperate in completing the questionnaire. It is also not recommended for children who are overtly hostile, uncooperative, uncommunicative, prone to exaggeration or other distortions, or disorganized in their thinking. Children with poor English-language verbal ability will have difficulty completing the scale. Spanish-speaking children should use the Spanish version of the *Piers-Harris-2*.

Factor analysis of the *Piers-Harris* basically confirmed the original factor structure (Alexopoulos & Foudoulaki, 2002). Lower subscale reliabilities mean interpretation of profile strengths and weaknesses should be undertaken with caution (Cooley & Ayres, 1988; Erford, 2006). The scale's question-and-response format has been criticized by Strein (1995) because a Yes and No response format does not allow a child to indicate the degree of agreement or disagreement. Marsh and Holmes (1990) noticed many children struggling to respond accurately to questions that were scored in the negative (e.g., "My family is disappointed in me"), thus throwing into question the validity of some scores.

The *Piers-Harris-2* is cost-effective, time-efficient, and easy to use and yields reliable and valid scores in the measurement of children's self-concept (Erford, 2006). Jeske (1985, p. 1170) indicated the original *Piers-Harris* "appears to be the best children's self-concept measure currently available." This has not changed in the interim, as verified by Kelley (2005).

Coopersmith Self-Esteem Inventories

The *Coopersmith Self-Esteem Inventories* (Coopersmith, 1981) are individual- or group-administered questionnaires used to determine personal valuation of self (Peterson, 1985). The two forms (School Form and Adult Form) were developed based on the assumption that self-esteem is associated with effective functioning (Sewell, 1985). The School Form is a 58-item form used with students ages 8–15 years. Built into the form is a Lie scale, which consists of eight questions that are scored separately from the self-esteem inventory. The Lie scale is used to determine defensiveness in the client's responses (Coopersmith, 1989). There is also a School Short Form that consists of 25 questions, on which the Adult Form is based. The Adult Form is used for clients over 15 years of age. The standardization sample information is not adequate, but several researchers have collected supplemental samples since the original inventory was standardized (Coopersmith, 1989). The reliability information indicates internal consistency coefficients ranged from 0.87 to 0.92 for 4th- through 8th-graders for the total score (Sewell, 1985). Validity was reported as being sufficient, but conclusive evidence was not presented, and very little reliability or validity information is presented for the Adult Form. The Adult norm sample was composed of 226 college students from northern California, and the reliability scores ranged from 0.78 to 0.85, but no further information was provided (Coopersmith, 1989). While internal consistency estimates appear to indicate the two forms may have some value as screening-level tests, the difficulty in defining and measuring the concept of self-esteem remains problematic. For example, according to the manual, there are no clearly defined criteria for determining low, medium, or high levels of self-esteem, although higher scores are indicative of higher self-esteem. The manual has a section for building self-esteem in students and provides some suggestions and techniques. Researchers are divided about whether to recommend the use of the inventory, but it is one of the most widely used measures of its kind (Peterson, 1985; Sewell, 1985).

Tennessee Self-Concept Scale—Second Edition (TSCS-2)

The *Tennessee Self-Concept Scale—Second Edition* (*TSCS-2*) (Fitts & Warren, 1996) is one of the most commonly used self-report measures of self-concept and can be used for children and adults. The test was standardized on 3,000 subjects, ages 7–90

Table 8.5 Scales on the *Tennessee Self-Concept Scale—Second Edition*

Self-concept scores	Supplementary scores
Physical	Identity
Moral	Satisfaction
Personal	Behavior
Family	**Validity scores**
Social	
Academic/Work	Inconsistent
Summary scores	Responding
	Self-criticism
Total self-concept	Faking good
Conflict	Response distribution

years, and can be administered to individuals or groups in about 10 to 20 minutes. The Adult Form is designed for clients ages 13 years or older and has 82 items. The Child Form is designed for students ages 7–14 years and has 76 items. A Short Form consisting of the first 20 items of either form can be used as well. Items comprise 15 subscales and a total Self-Concept score (see Table 8.5). The items are rated on a 5-point Likert scale ranging from Always False to Always True. The *TSCS-2* can be hand-scored in approximately 10 minutes, or computer-scored (Western Psychological Services, 2003c). Reliability is adequate, with lower internal consistencies on subscales than Total Self-Concept, ranging from $r = 0.73$ to $r = 0.93$. Test-retest reliability scores ranged from $r = 0.47$ to $r = 0.83$ (Brown, 1998). Fitts and Warren (1996) reported acceptable levels of score validity for the *TSCS-2*.

Think About It 8.2   Using the self-concept scales from Table 8.5, discuss with an acquaintance his or her levels of self-concept in each category. Notice whether there is consistency among the categories. What causes these consistencies or inconsistencies?

PROJECTIVE APPROACHES TO ASSESSMENT

In contrast to structured assessments of personality, which limit possible client responses, **projective assessments** present clients with unstructured, ambiguous stimuli and allow a virtually unlimited range of potential responses. Personality assessment using projective techniques is based on the **projective hypothesis**, the assumption that essential information about a client's personality characteristics, needs, conflicts, and motivations will be transferred onto ambiguous stimuli. Projective techniques are disguised and vague by design and provide clients only minimal instructions in order to reduce external structure and force clients to impose structure according to internal (intrapersonal) characteristics.

Projective personality assessment is based on the psychoanalytic notion of the *unconscious,* that portion of one's personality that is beyond awareness and control. According to Freud (1961, 1923, 1924), valuable understanding of one's true nature is obtained from the dark recesses of one's unconscious emotional and thought processes, not what is present or spoken from one's conscious mind. Freud also believed in the prominence of *drive* and *instinct,* which lead one to gratify needs while reducing tension over unfulfilled needs. Freud's concept of *psychic determinism*—that every action undertaken is done so for a reason or particular purpose—is also a key to understanding personality. Altogether, then, Freud's psychoanalytic theory proposes that when a client is presented with ambiguous stimuli and asked to respond to the stimuli in some way (and there is not necessarily a right or wrong way to respond), the client cannot help but exhibit actions and responses driven by unconscious processes that reveal internal emotional or thought processes, representing needs and desires requiring expression and gratification. Therefore, the key is to develop techniques that will help clinicians gain access to a client's unconscious, allowing inferences to be made about the client's personality and personal adjustment. Such techniques are called projective techniques.

If a professional counselor places a client in an unstructured, ambiguous circumstance, the client will attempt to bring order and meaning to chaos. And how the client brings structure to the disorder yields valuable insights into the client's unconscious processes and serves as an indirect glimpse into the client's inner world. There are many projective techniques available for use by professional counselors, depending upon education, licensure, and professional training and experience. These techniques vary in degree of standardization, with some having rather specific directions for administration and scoring. Often the interpretation of these techniques is less standardized, leading to subjective judgments based upon the professional counselor's theoretical orientation and clinical experience. Projective techniques are classified according to the nature of the ambiguous task and how clients are required to respond. The following five types of projective techniques represent a comprehensive categorization: (1) association techniques; (2) picture-story construction techniques; (3) verbal completion techniques; (4) choice arrangement techniques; and (5) production-expression techniques.

The *Rorschach Inkblot Test* is an example of an **association technique** and is quite possibly the best-known projective test ever developed. The *Rorschach* is reviewed in greater detail below, but Figure 8.1 presents a sample inkblot of the type included on the *Rorschach*. Proponents of association techniques propose that such procedures reveal details of the unconscious realm, similar to the way x-rays reveal the inner realm of the body. Clients project their inner organization onto the inkblot, and examiners interpret these attempts to organize the vague stimuli. A second example of an association task is *word association.* For this task, examiners present a list of neutral (e.g., wood, spoon) or emotionally laden (e.g., father, sex) words one at a time, and the client responds with the first idea, image, or word that comes to mind. Examiners generally record the response; the amount of time required to respond (i.e., latency effects, with lengthier time periods supposedly revealing the degree of inner conflict/turmoil); and expressions of emotion while responding (e.g., anger, embarrassment). Responses to association technique stimuli are usually compared

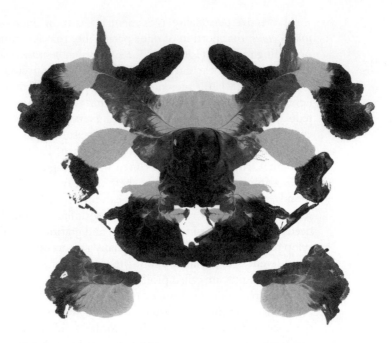

Figure 8.1   Sample inkblot

with responses of nonclinical individuals to determine whether responses are "normal" or pathological. Interpretation of themes and content categorizations is then conducted to reveal insights into personality functioning, inner needs, and conflicts.

Picture-story construction techniques usually involve showing a client a picture or other visual stimulus and requiring the client to construct a story about the picture. The stimulus pictures vary in terms of scenery, people, and social situations. The most commonly used construction technique is the *Thematic Apperception Test* (*TAT*). A sample picture stimulus similar to a *TAT* card is presented in Figure 8.2. The *Children's Apperception Test* (*CAT*) and *Robert's Apperception Test for Children* (*RATC*) are examples of picture-story construction techniques commonly used with children and adolescents. For Hispanic clients, another example would be the *Tell Me a Story* (*TEMAS*). Each of these tests is reviewed in greater detail below. The common strand through picture-story construction techniques is that the client is shown a stimulus picture and then asked to tell a good story about the picture. The story should describe what led up to the depicted scene, what is currently happening, and what the likely outcome of the story will be. While some of the pictures may "pull" for different content and emotion, most are neutral and simply reflect the unconscious process of the client. In other words, the client is given no reason to tell a particular story about a given card in a particular manner. The assumption is that the story the client tells, and the manner in which the client tells it, reflect some inner need that surfaces in response to that given stimulus picture. In this way,

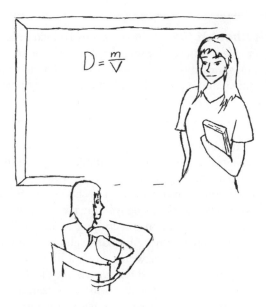

$$D = \frac{m}{V}$$

Figure 8.2   Sample picture-story card

clients convey inner thoughts and emotions and provide the content for clinicians to interpret and contextualize.

Verbal completion techniques consist of verbal content presented in an incomplete format, requiring the client to complete the stimulus. Sentence and story completion tasks are among the more commonly used completion techniques. For example, a client may be presented with a sentence stem (e.g., "I think . . ." or "Other people treat me like . . .") and be asked to complete the stem. As with any projective technique, the client is given no reason to provide any specific response. The assumption is that some internal need, emotion, or thought is being expressed in the face of a vague, ambiguous stimulus (e.g., "I think dogs are cute" versus "I think men are horrid creatures," or "Other people treat me like a princess" versus "Other people treat me like I am invisible"). The *Forer Structured Sentence Completion Test* is a good example of this type of projective assessment and is reviewed in greater detail below. A *story completion test* presents the client with the start of a story and requires the client to finish the story. For example, the professional counselor may begin by saying, "A woman leans over to kiss a man on the cheek. The man suddenly pulls away and looks angry. Why?" The content of client responses is recorded verbatim and thematically analyzed. An example of a story completion task that also uses pictures is the *Rosenzweig's Picture-Frustration Study* (Rosenzweig, 1949), in which 24 cartoons depicting a potentially frustrating situation are presented to a client. Each cartoon has a situation written in one of the "thought bubbles," and the other bubble is blank. The client indicates a verbal reaction (orally or in writing) to each stimulus. Responses are scored in one of three ways: (1) evasion of frustration; (2) frustration directed at other people or objects; or (3) frustration directed at self.

> **Think About It 8.3**   Construct 5 to 10 incomplete sentences and "administer" them to several associates. What theme or patterns emerged? Do statements phrased in certain ways lead to certain more predictable results? How could you use projective techniques in your practice as a professional counselor.

Choice arrangement techniques make up a diverse category, the commonality being that clients are given several to numerous options to rank-order or select from. Young children are often given the choice of which toys or dolls to play with in therapy. Again, the child is given no reason to choose any given puppet, doll, or other toy, or to play with or tell stories using it in the particular manner he or she does. It is assumed that the child's selection and ensuing actions and verbalizations are the expression of some inner motivation. Alternative choice arrangement projective techniques include arranging pictures or words along a like-dislike continuum or a multiple-choice response format designed for a *Rorschach*-like inkblot test. Of course, when an examiner uses a choice arrangement format, the examinee's potential range of choices becomes restricted. In some ways, this defeats the purpose of a projective technique, which is to allow clients maximum leeway to respond from the unconscious. Importantly, research supporting the use of choice techniques for assessment is very sparse when compared with that available for other types of projective assessment.

Production-expression techniques require clients to actively participate in the assessment by creating some product that can be analyzed and interpreted to reveal facets of the client's personality. Commonly used techniques include drawings (e.g., *House-Tree-Person, Human Figure Drawing, Kinetic Family Drawing, Kinetic School Drawing*), painting or coloring, or a dramatic performance (e.g., psychodrama). **Drawing techniques** are by far the most commonly used assessment devices from this category. Importantly, how clients act and respond to verbal queries while engaging in this task is just as important as any characteristics of the final product, and professional counselors using these techniques are strongly encouraged to observe, and ask follow-up questions of, clients creating expression products. When using a drawing technique, such as the *Human Figure Drawing,* clients are usually given a blank sheet of paper and pencil (or pens, colored pencils, crayons, etc.) and asked to draw a picture of a person. Interpretation of these drawings varies widely, depending on the professional counselor's theoretical orientation, training, and focus.

Some test manuals and textbooks offer specific guidance for interpreting drawing characteristics, or even specific objects within a drawing. For example, aggression may be indicated by heavy, dark lines; low self-esteem may be indicated by a small drawing. Handler (1996) suggested that particular attention be paid to erasures, placement of the figure on the paper, too much or too little detail, shading and heavy or pressured lines, among other things. Of critical importance is that examiners not give too much emphasis to any one sign. Also, the professional counselor should never rely solely on the drawn product for interpretive insights. It is excellent practice to query the client about a drawing in order to understand what the drawing might represent to the client. The best use of drawing characteristics and behaviors is for generating hypotheses to be tested out using more structured and systematic methods. Figures 8.3 through 8.5 display examples of various projective drawing techniques.

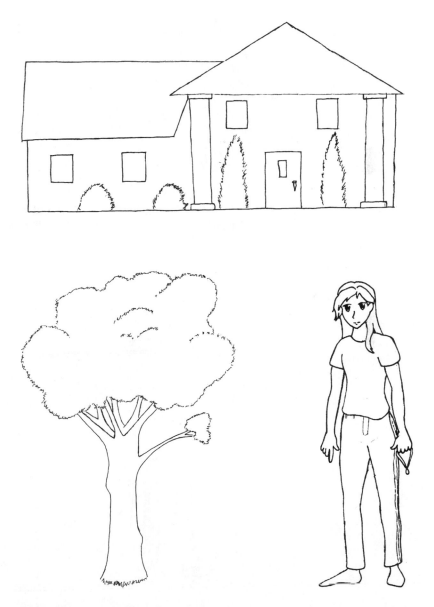

Figure 8.3   *House-Tree-Person* drawings by a selfconscious, perfectionistic teenage girl

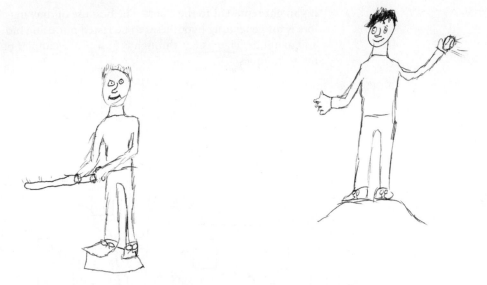

Figure 8.4   Kinetic Family Drawing by a 12-year-old boy with a fine-motor Coordination Disorder and AD/HD—Predominantly Inattentive Type

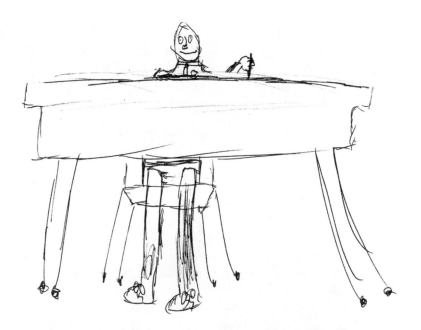

Figure 8.5   Kinetic School Drawing by a 12-year-old boy with a fine-motor Coordination Disorder and AD/HD—Predominantly Inattentive Type

Strengths and Weaknesses of Projective Techniques

Projective techniques have a number of noteworthy positive points and have remained popular over the past half century (Bellak, 1992; Piotrowski & Zalewski, 1993; Watkins, 1991). Some clinicians believe that projective techniques are great icebreakers and rapport builders when beginning an evaluation or counseling relationship with children or adolescents, because these techniques are generally perceived as nonthreatening, and clients need not worry about whether a particular answer was right or wrong. Clients generally are not limited in the number or type of responses they can make. This allows the unconscious processes maximum leeway in projecting inner needs and motivations onto the stimulus. Also, because clients are not generally familiar with the scoring and interpretive strategies of projective techniques, many clinicians believe responses to projective tests are more difficult to fake than for structured tests, although this is not necessarily the case (Masling, 1960).

Projective techniques may have valuable cross-cultural applications, especially when the stimulus involves inkblots, drawings, or brief verbal stems. Most projectives require no or very little reading ability, so they may be helpful in the assessment of young clients and clients with poor literacy skills. Likewise, because some projective techniques require a minimum of verbal input and output, they may be helpful techniques for use with young clients, clients from diverse cultures, or clients with speech and language disorders. Finally, because projective techniques are based on psychoanalytic theory, complex, multidimensional themes may emerge and provide valuable insights into the client's personality.

Projective assessment techniques also have numerous limitations. Projective techniques must be administered individually by highly educated and trained individuals and therefore are expensive to administer, score, and interpret. Subjective scoring and interpretive procedures make results difficult to replicate. Interpretation is often the most subjective part of the process. Indeed, many projective devices appear to allow wide-ranging judgments on the part of the examiner when scoring and interpreting a client's results.

Subjectivity in scoring and interpretation inevitably leads to concerns over reliability and validity of scores. Indeed, projective techniques display poor psychometrics. Scorer reliability, test-retest, and internal consistency coefficients tend to be unacceptably low. As stated earlier, low reliability leads to low score validity, and the research on projective score validity is, at best, inconclusive (Anastasi & Urbina, 1997).

Most projective tests have either absent or inadequate norms. When norms are provided, the samples are often described in vague terms. In addition, often the comparison groups are not normal samples, but clinical populations, negating a valuable comparison group for the determination of potential pathology; that is, if a client's responses are compared with clinical patients and not "normal" individuals, how can a clinician decide whether the client's responses are normal? Still, projective techniques help to "flesh out" our understanding of clients in an open-ended manner that is often missing in objective personality inventories.

Projective techniques have been shown to be susceptible to outside influences, such as examiner characteristics, examiner bias (i.e., theoretical orientation), or variations in administration directions. In addition, the validity of the "projective hypothesis" itself has been called into question because responses may reflect state-dependent characteristics rather than enduring personality characteristics. This is a critical point, because the whole idea behind projective assessment is to access the unconscious in order to understand the client's psychic determinism. If the client's "present state of mind" is being measured rather than some enduring personality structure, the goal of accessing the unconscious processes of the client's personality is thwarted. The final limitation involves the difficulty (or impossibility) of actually scientifically studying Freud's psychoanalytic developmental theory, given its emphasis on unconscious psychological processes. As psychoanalytic theory forms the basis of projective testing, this limitation is quite significant.

As a final comment on projective techniques, Anastasi and Urbina (1997) suggested projective techniques are better used as clinical tools rather than as tests per se. Given the low standard of psychometric rigor, such a guarded approach is warranted. Projectives are quite helpful when used for hypothesis generation and for helping clients gain insight into unconscious needs and motivations, as well as aids for qualitative interviewing, but their technical limitations mitigate against use for diagnostic purposes.

SOME COMMONLY USED PROJECTIVE TECHNIQUES

Rorschach Inkblot Test

The *Rorschach Inkblot Test* (Rorschach, 1921/1998), originally developed by Hermann Rorschach in 1921, is the best-known and most used projective test. The test's purpose is to assess how a client perceives and organizes thoughts about the world. The test is a Level C instrument and is individually administered to clients ages 5 and older, in about 20 to 30 minutes (Hess, Zachar, & Kramer, 2001). It consists of 10 plates of bilaterally symmetrical inkblots (Janda, 1998): 5 are black and white; 2 are black, white, and red; and the remaining 3 are comprised of pastel colors (Hess et al., 2001). Clients are presented with the cards and asked what they think of the inkblot or what it might be. In the second part of administration, clients are asked to explain their original answers. Scoring and interpretation are frequently completed using a scoring system originally developed by John Exner in the 1970s called the *Comprehensive System for Administering, Scoring, and Interpreting the Rorschach* (Exner, 2002). Exner's multifaceted system involves interpretation of three aspects of responses: Location (W for the entire blot, D major portion of the blot, and Dd for uncommon responses); Determinants (there are nearly two dozen having to do with shape, activity of humans, chromatic features, etc.); and Content (there are 26 categories used to interpret the content of the story). A Structural Summary is composed based on an interpretive rating scale developed by Exner (Janda, 1998).

As with many projective tests, it is often hard to find concrete empirical data on the *Rorschach*. Subjectivity is such a part of interpretation, and there can be definite diversity in administration procedures depending on testing purpose and clinician training. It has been noted that well-trained users of Exner's scoring system agree on the major variables over 88% of the time (Hess et al., 2001). Still, there is substantial debate over the interrater reliability of Exner's system. Exner purports that test-retest reliability estimates are at or above $r = 0.70$ at both 1-year and 3-year intervals. According to Hess et al. (2001), validity data of the *Rorschach* also yield many questions and concerns. Various questions of subjectivity arise based on administration, scoring, and interpretation procedures. Still even with the lack of standardization and empirical data, the *Rorschach* used in conjunction with Exner's *Comprehensive System* (2002) is a better personality test than most opponents will acknowledge (Hess et al.). Critics of the *Rorschach* point out that statistical prediction is usually more accurate than clinical prediction (i.e., judgment), and the *Rorschach* relies primarily on clinical prediction to measure personality. Far more psychometric research needs to be done using the *Rorschach*, but it has the potential to generate meaningful personality data (Hess et al., 2001).

Thematic Apperception Test (TAT)

The *Thematic Apperception Test* (*TAT*) (Murray & Bellak, 1973) is used to measure various aspects of a client's personality. Clients are presented with 31 picture cards and are asked to create stories based on the images. There is no time limit for this assessment, and it can be administered to children and adult clients. Specific scoring criteria are provided in the scoring protocol and assessment booklet. Many administrators choose 8 to 12 cards to use with a client. Six elements are considered when examining stories: (1) the hero; (2) the needs or motives and feelings; (3) presses or environmental forces; (4) outcomes; (5) recurring themes in the story; and (6) interests and sentiments (Janda, 1998).

According to Janda (1998), although several clinicians have determined new scoring criteria for the *TAT*, most adhere to Murray's original scoring format. Janda reported that this method can often be unstructured and biased, leading to inadequate score reliability and validity.

Children's Apperception Test–1991 Revision (CAT)

The *CAT* (Bellak & Bellak, 1992) assesses personality by interpreting story responses to presented picture stimuli. The *CAT* is administered to children ages 3–10 years in about 15 to 20 minutes. The child is presented with stimulus cards that show animals engaged in human relationship–oriented interactions. The client then gives perceptions, interpretations, and responses, and must solve developmental problems (Knoff, 1998). The 10 stimulus cards address the following: feeding problems; oral problems; sibling rivalry; attitudes toward parents; relationships to parents as (sexual) couples; jealousy toward same-gender parent figures; fantasies about aggression; acceptance by the adult world; fear and loneliness at night; and toileting behavior and parents' responses to it. There are 10 variables that are used to analyze responses: Main Theme; Main Hero; Main Needs and Drives of the Hero; the child's

Conception of the Environment; how the child sees and reacts to the figures in the cards; Significant Conflicts described; the Nature of the Child's Main Anxieties; the Child's Main Defenses; the Adequacy of the Superego as Manifested by Punishment for Crime; and the Integration of the Child's Ego (Knoff, 1998). The assessment comes with 10 additional cards that can supplement the *CAT* (Reinehr, 1998). Specific scoring and interpretive instructions are included in the interpretive manual (Knoff, 1998).

The authors state that there is no need for standardization or empirical data for a projective test like the *CAT,* and few specifics are provided in the manual (Bellak & Bellak, 1992). Due to the lack of statistical data, clinicians should be careful not to base any clinical diagnosis or intervention on this assessment (Knoff, 1998). Reinehr (1998) agreed that there is no basis in the argument of no need for empirical data on projective assessments.

Roberts Apperception Test for Children–Second Edition (Roberts-2)

The *Roberts-2* (McArthur & Roberts, 1994) is a projective test designed to measure children's social perceptions. The test can be administered to children ages 6–15 years in about 20 to 30 minutes. The child is presented with 16 different test pictures and is asked to tell a story about each one. Scoring criteria for each picture are presented in the manual and based on the presence or absence of certain characteristics in the narrative. The three scales measured are Adaptive, Clinical, and Clinical Indicators (Cosden, 2001). There are seven main constructs on which scoring criteria are based, and each has several subconstructs. The seven main constructs are: theme overview, problem identification, outcome, available resources, emotion, resolution, and unusual or atypical responses. According to the test's publisher, new standardization studies were conducted and conformed to U.S. population demographics in terms of gender, ethnicity, and parental education, although specific information about the sample is not provided (Cosden, 2001), so generalizability is questionable.

Although minimal information is available online for the *Roberts-2,* the manual contends that validity for derived test scores is adequate. However, Waller (2001) asserted the original version of the test relies too heavily on doctoral dissertations and findings are not published in refereed journals, making it difficult to evaluate score validity. A new version of the *Roberts-2* (McArthur & Roberts, 2005) became available in 2005.

House-Tree-Person (H-T-P) Projective Drawing Technique

The *House-Tree-Person* (*H-T-P*) *Projective Drawing Technique* (Buck, 1964) is a widely used projective test that is easy to use and time-efficient (Western Psychological Services, 2003b). It can be used for clients ages 3 and older (see Figure 8.6). The client draws three objects (a house, a tree, and a person) and then describes, defines, and interprets the drawings. *House-Tree-Person* is often used as the

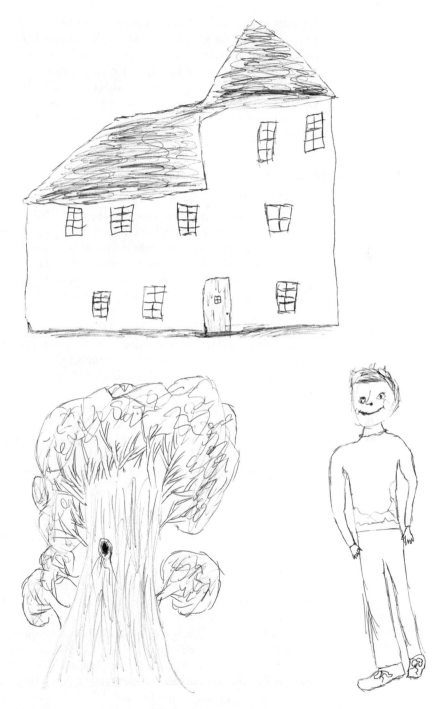

Figure 8.6   House-Tree-Person drawings by a teenager with AD/HD and fine-motor coordination difficulties

first test in an assessment for a counseling session, because drawing tends to reduce tension. It is useful for assessing personality in people from different cultures, those deprived of educational opportunities, and those developmentally delayed or non-English-speaking; in addition, it is highly sensitive to the early presence of psychopathology (Western Psychological Services, 2003b). Examiners must always be careful to validate observations from projective techniques through other assessment methods and not to overinterpret meanings of specific objects or designs drawn in a picture.

Kinetic Drawing System for Family and School (KDS)

The *Kinetic Drawing System for Family and School* (*KDS*) (Knoff & Prout, 1985) is designed to individually assess the frequency of a child's difficulties in the home and school settings. The format allows the examiner to understand the overlap of behaviors and attitudes in both settings as well as to assess the source of certain attitudes and behaviors. The *KDS* can be administered to clients ages 5–20 years. Clients are asked to draw separate pictures of both family and school situations. Examiners are asked to stress that each person in the picture should be doing something. There is no time limit for this task but most complete the task in 20 to 40 minutes. Pictures are assessed based on five categories: (1) actions of and between figures; (2) figure characteristics; (3) position and distance of figures, and barriers between them; (4) style; and (5) symbols (see Figures 8.7 and 8.8).

In a review of the manual, Cundick (1989) concluded reliability and validity data are inadequate and that the studies provided are not related to the test protocol. Weinberg (1989) stated that if administrators are well trained and scoring criteria are clearly defined, good interrater reliability coefficients can be attained; however, test-retest reliability coefficients are low. Weinberg concluded that although this test is a wonderful icebreaker and rapport-building tool, one cannot recommend this as an interpretive assessment yielding reliable and valid scores.

Forer Structured Sentence Completion Test (FSSCT)

The *Forer Structured Sentence Completion Test* (*FSSCT*) (Forer, 1967) is a 100-item test used to determine a client's attitudes and views of the world by finding out information about a client's relationships and dynamics, and the client's use of evasiveness, individual differences, and defense mechanisms (Western Psychological Services, 2003a). Separate forms are available for men, women, adolescent girls, and adolescent boys. Administration of the test takes about 15 to 20 minutes and requires a Level B qualification. A Checklist and Clinical Evaluation Form provides evaluation tools that help the examiner to group clients into one of four categories: (1) Interpersonal Figures; (2) Wishes; (3) Causes of Own (feelings and behaviors); and (4) Reactions (to others) (Benet, 2005). Reliability, validity, and normative information is not given in the manual. Example prompts might include "My father makes me feel _____"; "I like to talk to my friends about _____"; Others often think that I _____."

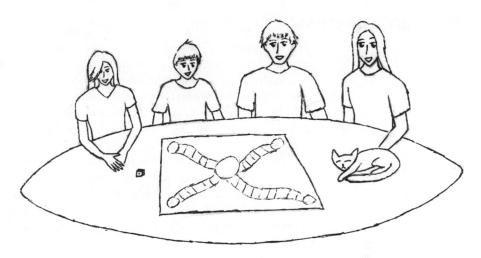

Figure 8.7   Kinetic Family Drawing by a nonclinical teenage girl

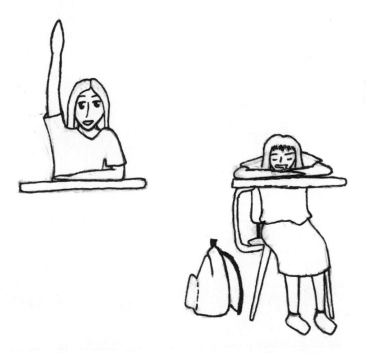

Figure 8.8   Kinetic School Drawing by a nonclinical teenage girl

SUMMARY/CONCLUSION

This chapter has provided an introduction to the information that professional counselors need to engage in personality assessment. Both objective and projective personality assessment were addressed. Objective methods typically involve trait approaches, and the five-factor model of Costa & McCrae currently enjoys popularity among personality researchers. Numerous structured personality inventories are available for use by professional counselors, including the *NEO PI-R, CPI, PAI,* and *MBTI.*

Projective assessments present clients with ambiguous stimuli, and professional counselors observe and assess how clients construct meaning and respond to these stimuli. Projective techniques generally yield lower score reliability and validity than objective personality measures. Projective techniques can be classified as association, picture-story, verbal completion, choice arrangement, and production-expression techniques.

KEY TERMS

association technique

choice arrangement techniques

drawing technique

personality

personality assessment

picture-story construction techniques

production-expression techniques

projective assessment

projective hypothesis

traits

verbal completion techniques

CHAPTER 9

Behavioral Assessment

by Carl J. Sheperis, R. Anthony Doggett, Masanori Ota,
Bradley T. Erford, and Carol Salisbury

This chapter provides a general understanding of behavioral assessment procedures for professional counselors. More specifically, the chapter provides a general definition of behavioral assessment as well as specific guidelines for conducting behavioral assessment; details the two kinds of behavioral assessment (direct behavioral assessment and nondirect behavioral assessment) and common techniques used within these two assessment categories; and gives a brief overview of the most commonly used behavioral assessment instruments.

WHAT IS BEHAVIORAL ASSESSMENT?

When children talk out loud during a class or see others become aggressive and rush to fight, professional counselors may raise the following questions: Why does this behavior occur? How can the behavior be changed? Behavioral assessment is a useful methodology to clearly answer these questions.

Behavioral assessment is generally defined as "the identification of meaningful response units and their controlling variables for the purposes of understanding and of altering behavior" (Nelson, 1985, p. 45). Because a behavior occurs through an interaction between an individual and the person's environment, professional counselors use behavioral assessment to evaluate a particular behavior and the context in which it occurs (e.g., stimuli or events affecting the behavior). Behavioral assessment, along with other traditional assessment approaches (e.g., intelligence tests, personality tests), is widely used in various applied settings, such as schools, counseling centers, and other clinical venues.

Defining Behavior

From a behavioral standpoint, all behaviors are seen as a direct result of external and environmental stimuli. Although behaviors can be indicators of internal difficulties, the professional counselor cannot readily measure or see those internal struggles. Thus a key concept in behavioral assessment is that the target behavior (i.e., the behavior the client is trying to change) must be directly observable. For example, millions of people struggle to lose weight each year, and new diets emerge on the best-seller list all the time. While the professional counselor may personally know what it is like to have an internal battle over whether to eat a certain dessert, it would be hard for a bystander to see or measure that internal struggle in a client. However, through behavioral assessment, the professional counselor can identify a certain behavior that the client is trying to change (i.e., snacking on high-fat foods), measure the number of times that the client snacks, the amount of food that is consumed, and the amount of weight that is gained or lost. The professional counselor can then develop an intervention that is clearly tied to the target behavior and accurately measure changes in the behavior.

To obtain a clear picture of what the professional counselor and client are trying to accomplish, an operational definition of a target behavior is addressed at the beginning of behavioral assessment, using observable and measurable terms. A well-developed **operational definition** contains an objective, concrete, and quantitative description, with which anyone can clearly identify the observed behavior. In other words, an operational definition must pass the "stranger test"—that is, any behavior that one defines should be clearly understandable to a stranger. That stranger should be able to pick up the definition and be able to observe someone without difficulty. For example, it is not observable or measurable to state, "Sam continually snacks on inappropriate foods," because it is not clear what "inappropriate" and "continually" specifically mean in this situation. However, it is much clearer if an inappropriate food is defined as "any food item containing more than 10 grams of carbohydrates," or "any food item containing more than 5 grams of fat." A good operational definition must also pass the "dead man test"—that is, the target behavior should not be something that only a dead man could do. If a professional counselor developed an intervention plan with the goal that Sam would not eat, that counselor would probably lose his or her license or be sued. It is impossible to ask someone not to eat. The person would have to be dead to follow this guideline. In short, behavioral goals and objectives should be MOP&D: measurable, observable, positive, and doable. Thus an operational definition is crucial to minimize inferences during observation (Sattler, 2002). To obtain reliable and valid data, it is important to maintain the same operational definition throughout the assessment process.

> **Think About It 9.1**   What behavior in your life would you like to change? How could this behavior be operationally defined? Using this definition, what new behavioral goal could you set?

Guidelines for Conducting Behavioral Assessment

It should be noted that the professional counselor does not target personality traits or psychopathology through behavioral assessment, because these things cannot readily change through intervention. For example, a professional counselor can change the frequency that a child displays tantrums (behavior) but cannot change autism (a disorder), which some people might think causes the tantrums. Thus, through behavioral assessment, the professional counselor focuses on the function of particular behaviors that are within the client's voluntary control rather than a diagnosis.

Behaviors often stem from interactions between an individual and the individual's environment. Thus, instead of examining a behavior in isolation, the professional counselor must consider environmental variables affecting the behavior (e.g., place, people, time, stimulus). Antecedents and consequences (events preceding and following a behavior, respectively) and the characteristics of behavior (e.g., function, magnitude, frequency, rate, duration, latency) are often measured in behavioral assessment. For example, a great deal of attention has been focused on school violence in recent years. On April 20, 1999, Eric Harris and Dylan Klebold killed a teacher and 12 other students, wounded 23 other people, and then killed themselves at Columbine High School in Littleton, Colorado. While it is clear that both students were disturbed, it is important to understand the environmental variables and antecedents leading to this tragedy. Harris kept a journal that helps us to understand the environment's influence on his behavior. According to *USA Today*'s online website (Killer's diary reveals plans, 2001), Harris's journal paints a picture of an isolated teen who was angry about being rejected. In his journal, Harris wrote, "I hate you people for leaving me out of so many fun things. . . . You people had my phone #, and I asked and all, but no no no no no don't let the weird looking Eric kid come along." Because one can now look at some of the ways that rejection and isolation affected Harris's behavior, schools across the country have implemented both preventive (e.g., peer counseling) and response measures (e.g., school safety plans). If we only look at Harris and Klebold as disturbed teens and ignore the environmental factors leading to the tragedy, we would be unable to prevent future crises of this nature.

In conducting behavioral assessment, it is also important to know that every behavior has its own purpose or function. When behavioral assessment is used to identify a function, it is called **functional behavioral assessment (FBA)**. In accordance with the Individuals with Disabilities Education Act Amendments of 1997, FBAs and behavior plans are specifically required in schools for children who have a special education ruling and are subject to disciplinary action.

Applied behavioral analysis researchers have identified four main variables that may maintain or reinforce the performance of target behaviors: (a) attention, (b) tangible, (c) escape, and (d) sensory stimulation (Alberto & Troutman, 2003; Iwata et al., 1994). It should be noted that even if the topographies (i.e., what a behavior looks like) of two behaviors are the same, the functions of the two behaviors might be different. For example, when a child screams more after a teacher says, "Be quiet and look at me," the function may be attention from a teacher. However, escape may be the function if a child often screams when difficult academic tasks are given during a class. Also, one behavior may have more than one function (e.g., the functions of the child's screaming may be both teacher attention and escape from difficult tasks). Thus, once a function is hypothesized in functional behavioral assessment, it should be experimentally verified through functional analysis using a single-subject research design. Functional analysis is an experimental manipulation of environmental variables (e.g., antecedents, consequences) to establish a functional relationship between a behavior and environmental variables. Discussion of functional analysis and single-subject design are beyond the scope of this chapter, so interested readers are referred to Alberto and Troutman (2003) and Miltenberger (2004).

METHODS OF BEHAVIORAL ASSESSMENT

Behavioral assessment is divided into two categories: direct assessment and indirect assessment. In **direct assessment**, the professional counselor assesses events occurring here and now through direct observation and client self-monitoring. In **indirect assessment**, the professional counselor assesses past events using behavioral interviews, and self-report and informant-report behavioral checklists and rating scales.

Direct Assessment

Through direct observation, a professional counselor observes a client's behavior in a natural setting and records it using a recording sheet. For example, a professional school counselor may observe a child to assess how many times the child leaves the seat during a class or talks to friends during a physical education period or recess on the playground. Behaviors are often recorded using the following four methods: (1) narrative recording, (2) interval recording, (3) event recording, and (4) ratings recording (Sattler, 2002). This discussion is limited to the two most prominent methods: narrative and interval recording.

Narrative recording

In **narrative recording** (see Table 9.1), the professional counselor records what is observed anecdotally. The professional counselor may observe not only a behavior, but also antecedents and consequences. Such observation, called *ABC narrative recording* (for antecedent, behavior, and consequence), is used to identify relationships between a behavior and environmental variables (Bijou, Peterson, & Ault, 1968). It can be useful to add an additional category to narrative recording: function. While it is important to know the antecedents, behaviors, and consequences, it is equally important to determine the functions of a behavior.

Interval recording

There are three primary methods of **interval recording**: (1) whole-interval recording; (2) partial-interval recording; and (3) momentary time sampling. In each interval recording method, the recording time is equally divided into intervals (e.g.,

Table 9.1   ABC narrative observation format

A	A wife asks her husband to help with the household chores.
B	Husband pouts (i.e., speaks in short sentences, complains about the task, moves slowly during the task).
C	Wife tells husband, "Forget it. I'll just do the chores."
F	Husband sought to escape task.

10-second intervals), and an observer records if a behavior occurs during each interval. Specifically, in *whole-interval recording,* an observer marks each interval on a recording sheet whenever a behavior occurs throughout the interval, whereas in *partial-interval recording,* an observer marks each interval whenever a behavior occurs at least once anytime in the interval. In *momentary time sampling,* an observer marks each interval whenever a behavior occurs at the beginning or end of the interval. It should be noted that the occurrence of a behavior may be underestimated in whole-interval recording, whereas it may be overestimated in partial-interval recording.

Although direct observation demonstrates clear descriptions of behavior, its characteristics, and environmental variables, some cautions are necessary. First, an observer may be biased. For example, if a professional counselor is attending to more than one behavior simultaneously, the professional counselor may pay more attention to some of the behaviors, but may miss others. Furthermore, because of habituation, the observer may unintentionally change the operational definition or criterion of a behavior (e.g., criterion frequency or duration), a factor called *observer drift.* To prevent observer drift, interobserver agreement should be checked (for each type of interobserver agreement and its calculation, see Kazdin, 1982). Also, an observer should have periodic trainings to recall the operational definition, criteria of a behavior, and observation procedures.

Second, clients may change a behavior if they know they are being observed, a factor called *reactivity.* For example, if children know they are being observed to determine the frequency of talking without permission during a class, they may try to remain quiet and follow the classroom rules. Clearly, in this case, an observer cannot obtain data truly reflecting the behavior (i.e., talking without permission). An observer may reduce reactivity by staying in the observation setting several times before recording observation data so that people become habituated to the observer. With cautions to the potential pitfalls associated with observation procedures, direct observation is often able to clearly draw the whole picture of behavior in natural settings. Table 9.2 provides an example of an interval recording observation with relevant operational definitions.

Self-monitoring

Self-monitoring is a method by which clients can observe and record their own behavior. Self-monitoring is an effective way to monitor infrequent behaviors (e.g., binge eating, self-injury) and internalizing problems (e.g., negative thoughts, anxiety,

Table 9.2   Sample interval recording sheet with relevant operational definitions

Sample interval recording sheet						
Behavior	10 min.	20 min.	30 min.	40 min.	50 min	60 min
Antecedents						
Targets						
Consequences						

Operational definitions for interval recording sheet

ANTECEDENTS

D: Demand—Instruction to complete educational work or an assignment given to complete ("Get to work," "Turn your books to page . . . ," teacher hands out a worksheet).

C: Command—Behavioral instruction ("Sit down," "Be quiet," "Go to your desk," "Stop talking," "Look at me").

T: Transition—Moving from one location to another in the classroom or school, switching from one assignment to another (walking from the classroom to the lunchroom, moving from a desk to the reading area, switching from a math assignment to a spelling assignment).

TARGET BEHAVIORS

OT: Off-task—Student's eyes are not directed toward the teacher for more than 5 seconds during a lecture, instruction, or assignment.

OS: Out-of-seat—Student's bottom breaks contact with the seat or floor for more than 5 seconds.

IV: Inappropriate vocalizations—Student talks to teacher or peers without permission, student argues with teacher or peers, student makes noises (whistling, howling, humming, clicking sounds).

CONSEQUENCES

E/A: Escape/avoidance—Student is allowed to refrain from working on or completing the assignment, teacher takes assignment away, teacher does not make student comply with (follow through on or complete) a command.

Teacher Attention

TP: Teacher positive attention—Smiles, praise statements, proximity following appropriate behavior, physical touch for appropriate behavior (pat on the shoulder, "Good job").

TN: Teacher negative attention—Frowns, reprimands, redirections, interruptions, proximity following problem behavior, physical touch for problem behavior ("Stop it!" "How many times have I told you to . . . ," tap on shoulder for talking without permission).

Peer Attention

PP: Peer positive attention—Smiles, praises, proximity, physical touch for appropriate behavior.

PN: Peer negative attention—Frowns, put-downs ("You're so . . ."), name calling ("dummy, butthead"), proximity following problem behavior, physical touch following problem behavior (pushing, hitting, kicking, touching).

Calculation of Performance of Behavior From Interval Recording Sheet

OT: _____ ÷ 60 × 100 =   _____ % of the intervals
OS: _____ ÷ 60 × 100 =   _____ % of the intervals
IV: _____ ÷ 60 × 100 =   _____ % of the intervals
Total Disruptive Behavior: _____ ÷ 180 × 100 =   _____ % of the intervals

fear), which are difficult for others to observe (Sattler, 2002). For example, a client who has depression may record any negative thoughts (e.g., "Although I study hard, I am not smart enough to pass this course") every 30 minutes for a certain number of hours. There are two matters to consider for self-monitoring. First, training a client to effectively monitor behavior is critical, because the client needs to identify a target behavior precisely and record it appropriately (e.g., every 1 minute). Second, to increase accuracy, it is effective for a professional counselor to monitor a client's behavior simultaneously and subsequently compare data with the client's self-monitoring. Also, periodic feedback regarding procedures and accuracy of self-monitoring may further promote accuracy.

The behavioral interview

The purpose of a *clinical interview* is to assess a client's global problems and related history (e.g., family, medical, psychological, educational) for the purpose of arriving at a diagnosis (Gresham, 1984). In contrast, the purpose of a **behavioral interview** is to identify a target behavior; to analyze environmental variables affecting the behavior; and to plan, implement, and evaluate an intervention. Thus a behavioral interview is a solution-focused interview that links assessment to intervention. A professional counselor may interview not only a client, but also significant others (e.g., parent, caregiver, spouse, employer, teacher, peer) to obtain multidimensional information about a client's problems from each individual's perspective. For example, a wife may report that her husband appears distracted and depressed at home, but peers may report that the man is upbeat and active at work. Further information from the client's children reveals that the parents have been arguing more over the last few months. While the root of the problem is not completely clear yet, it can be determined that the man's behavior is limited to one setting. Thus a professional counselor can now focus further assessment efforts around the marital relationship and design more effective interventions because of the multidimensional information derived from the interview.

Indirect Assessment

Because of their brevity, self-report and informant-report behavioral checklists and rating scales are commonly used methods of indirect assessment. In a *self-report,* a client may either respond to written questions or directly answer a professional counselor's questions regarding the nature of the client's concerns. However, in an *informant report,* significant others provide their perspective of the client's problems. For example, using a self-report, a professional counselor may ask clients to rate the quality of their relationships with immediate family members. Through an informant report, the professional counselor would ask significant others in the client's life to rate the client's relationships with immediate family members. While these questions are essentially the same, the results could be vastly different. Thus it is very useful to compare the results of a self-report and an informant report

As in a behavioral interview, eliciting useful information in a self-report or informant report often depends on the professional counselor's skills of verbal communication and strategic questions. For some clients, such as children or individuals with disabilities, the informant report plays an especially important role in obtaining useful information on the client's problems. However, for reasons of confidentiality, the client's consent is necessary before obtaining an informant report. The professional counselor should be aware that responses on a self-report or an informant report might not reflect actual problems precisely, because the responses represent human memories of past events. Intentionally or unintentionally, some clients or significant others may over- or underreport the severity of the client's problems.

Behavioral checklists and *rating scales* offer a more standardized means of indirect assessment and often have both self-report and informant-report versions available. Many of the typical checklists and rating scales have a Likert scale format (i.e., rate a behavior on a scale of 1 to 5) or some variation of this response style. For example, to the statement "I did not sleep last night," there may be three response choices, where 0 represents Not at All, 1 represents Somewhat True, and 2 represents Very True. While direct observations and interviews provide reliable information, standardized rating scales can provide normative information allowing professional counselors to compare results of an individual to the population for which the instrument was developed.

When using rating scales or checklists, professional counselors should be cautious of *halo effects* (e.g., tendency to rate a high-performing student as well-behaved regardless of actual behaviors observed), and *central tendency error* (e.g., tendency to respond with moderate or centrist descriptions rather than toward the extremes of a rating scale). For example, some people may respond more mildly or severely than their actual level (e.g., they may choose a number between 2 and 4 on a 5-point Likert scale). Clients may respond this way because they are embarrassed about certain symptoms, have ulterior motives for representing themselves in a more positive light, do not really understand the questions being presented, do not have the self-awareness to respond accurately, or view the extreme rating choices as *very* extreme. Thus, as is the case with any aspect of the assessment process, it is important for the professional counselor to provide clear instructions, adequate details about the purpose of the assessment, and information about the instrument, and to answer any questions the client or informant may have. Despite the potential weaknesses with behavioral checklists and rating scales, they are easy, inexpensive, and not time consuming. Also, some have been shown to reliably and validly screen or identify specific areas of disorders. For example, the *Child Behavior Checklist/6-18* (*CBCL/6-18*) (Achenbach & Rescorla, 2001) assesses the behavioral problems and adaptive functioning of children ages 6 to 18 years. The *CBCL/6-18* has 118 specific problem items (and an additional 20 competence items). Each item consists of a 3-point scale, on which 2 represents Very True or Often True, 1 represents Somewhat or Sometimes True, and 0 represents Not True (As Far As You Know). Normally a parent or guardian can complete the *CBCL/6-18* in approximately 15 minutes. Updated information on the *CBCL/6-18* and other Achenbach products is available on the website of the ASEBA Products (www.aseba.org/products/forms.html).

While professional counselors are strongly encouraged to follow the best practices for assessment as outlined in this text, the fact remains that assessment can be a time-consuming process. The reality is that professional counselors are often restricted in the amount of time they can dedicate to assessment. Thus it is important to have various methods of gaining reliable and valid information about a client's presenting problems in a relatively short time. Self-report and informant-report behavioral checklists and rating scales are practical assessment tools to identify problem behaviors and to obtain multidimensional information from clients and their significant others. When selected thoughtfully, respondents to checklists and rating scales provide valuable, accurate, cost-effective, and time-effective insight into client behaviors from the naturalistic settings.

> **Think About It 9.2**   Why would it be beneficial for a professional counselor to use both direct and indirect assessment approaches when evaluating a client?

BEHAVIORAL RATING SCALES AND INVENTORIES USED IN COUNSELING

The lines between clinical, behavioral, and personality assessments are quite blurred, the overlap in functions is sometimes pronounced. While there are innumerable assessment tools available for use by professional counselors, the tests and inventories that follow in this chapter are among the most commonly used for *indirect assessment* of behaviors. An overview of the format and psychometric properties of each instrument is provided. Hopefully, these reviews will help in the selection process of other instruments as well. It is important to note that only a few of the hundreds of available rating scales are reviewed below, but the skills in understanding and using tests garnered from this text will help the reader evaluate, select, and use other instruments.

Conners' Rating Scales—Revised (CRS-R)

The *Conners' Rating Scales—Revised* (*CRS-R*) (Conners, 1997) is a multi-informant inventory designed to assess psychopathology and problem behavior in children and adolescents ages 3 to 17 years. It can be completed by parents and teachers, and can also be self-reported by adolescents. The *CRS-R* is available in four primary formats based on length and respondent: (1) a short form (27 items) of the *Conners' Parent Rating Scales—Revised* (*CPRS-R:S*); (2) a short form (28 items) of the *Conners' Teacher Rating Scale—Revised* (*CTRS-R:S*); (3) a long form of 80 items for parents (*CPRS-R:L*); and (4) a long form of 59 items for teachers (*CTRS-R:L*). An adolescent self-report form, the *Conners-Wells Adolescent Self-Report Scale (CASS),* is available in long (*CASS-L*) and short (*CASS-S*) forms (Conners & Wells, 1997), and an adult form, the *Conners' Adult ADHD Rating Scales* (*CAARS*) (Conners, Erhardt, &

Sparrow, 1999), is also available. Items measure such facets as Oppositional, Social Problems, Cognitive Problems/Inattention, Psychosomatic, Hyperactivity, Symptom Subscales, Anxious-Shy, ADHD Index, Perfectionism, and a Conners' Global Index (Conners, 1997). In addition, the long forms provide two *DSM-IV* subscales (Inattention, Hyperactive-Impulsive), scored in a straight symptom count or in comparison to norms. Sample items from the *CPRS-R:S* include "Argues with adults," "Irritable," and "Deliberately does things that annoy other people." The *CRS-R* can be completed using pencil and paper in 5 to 10 minutes for the short version and 10 to 20 minutes for the long version. This inventory can be completed by computer, remotely, or over the telephone, and is available in English, Spanish, and French-Canadian languages.

The normative sample for the *CRS-R* consisted of over 8,000 cases in a large database compiled from over 200 collection sites throughout North America (Conners, 1997). This inventory requires Level B instrument qualifications and is written at the 10th-grade reading level for the parent and teacher forms, and at the 6th-grade level for the long-form adolescent self-report (*CASS:L*). Subscale internal consistency coefficients are satisfactory, ranging from 0.73 to 0.94 for the *CPRS-R:L*; 0.86 to 0.94 for the *CPRS-R:S*; 0.77 to 0.96 for the *CTRS-R:L*; 0.88 to 0.95 for the *CTRS-R:S*; and 0.75 to 0.92 for the *CASS:L* (Conners, 1997). Raw scores are converted into T scores and percentiles. The various versions of the *CRS-R* are helpful because they display AD/HD-type behaviors and track therapeutic progress (Giarnarris, Golden, & Greene, 2001; Townsend, Baylot, & Erford, 2006). Hand scoring of the protocols is easy using pressure-sensitive carbonless paper, but computer scoring and mail or fax scoring are also available. Clinicians need to be cautious when using this inventory for African American clients, because this group was underrepresented in the parent sample. It is an excellent screening device for AD/HD and general childhood psychopathology.

Attention Deficit Disorders Evaluation Scale—Third Edition (ADDES-3)

The *Attention Deficit Disorders Evaluation Scale—Third Edition* (*ADDES-3*) (McCarney & Arthaud, 2004a, 2004b) was designed to assess symptoms of AD/HD (inattentiveness, hyperactivity, impulsivity) in children and adolescents ages 4 to 18 years. It is available in two versions: a *Home Version* of 46 items for parent report (*ADDES-3-HV*) and a *School Version* of 60 items for teacher report (*ADDES-3-SV*). Each version consists of two subscales: Inattentive and Hyperactive-Impulsive. A child's demonstration of a given behavior is rated on a 6-point scale: 0—Not Developmentally Appropriate for Age; 1—Not Observed; 2—One to Several Times per Month; 3—One to Several Times per Week; 4—One to Several Times per Day; 5—One to Several Times per Hour. Such a rating system allows for substantial specificity in determining the frequency of display of a given behavior (Demaray & Elting, 2003). The *ADDES-3* is a Level B test and generally requires 15 to 20 minutes to administer and score. Scoring can be accomplished by hand or computer.

Raw scores can be converted to scaled scores ($M = 10$; $SD = 3$) and percentile ranks. Lower scaled scores or percentile ranks indicate higher levels of inattentiveness or hyperactivity of the client (Erford, 2006).

The standardization sample generally conformed to the 2000 U.S. Census population demographics. However, the *School Version* had a lower percentage of White participants (62.42%) than the national sample (71.89%), and both the *School Version* and the *Home Version* contained higher numbers of Black participants (24.64% and 15.13%, respectively) versus the national sample (12.14%). The *ADDES-3-SV* age category coefficient *alpha*s for the Inattentive subscale ranged from $r = 0.89$ to $r = 0.98$ (median = 0.98); the Hyperactive-Impulsive subscale ranged from $r = 0.89$ to $r = 0.99$ (median = 0.98); and the overall quotients ranged from $r = 0.98$ to $r = 0.99$ (median = 0.99). The *ADDES-3-HV* coefficient *alpha*s for the age categories of the Inattentive subscale ranged from $r = 0.90$ to $r = 0.97$ (median = 0.96); the Hyperactive-Impulsive subscale ranged from $r = 0.95$ to $r = 0.97$ (median = 0.96); and the overall quotient ranged from $r = 0.96$ to $r = 0.98$ (median = 0.98). However, it is not stated whether coefficients were derived from raw scores or standard scores. If raw scores served as the basis for reliability coefficients, the estimates would be inflated (Erford, 2006). Therefore, further analysis using standard scores should be conducted.

Criterion-related validity studies provided in the manual used the *ADDES-2,* which contained very similar items in most regards. Bussing, Schuhmann, and Belin (1998) found the *ADDES-2* produced a significant number of false positives and false negatives and that the results for girls were more accurate than those for boys. Overall, the psychometric characteristics of the *ADDES-3* appear adequate for screening symptoms of AD/HD. Ancillary publications have been developed, including *The Parents' Guide to Attention Deficit Disorders—Second Edition* (McCarney & Baker, 1995) and the *Attention Deficit Disorders Intervention Manual—Second Edition* (McCarney, 1994). Klecker (2001, p. 91) was quite critical of these supplements, however, stating that the materials were "too fragmented to be either readable or helpful. The supplements would be more useful with age-specific scenarios and practical examples."

Behavior Assessment System for Children (BASC)

The *Behavior Assessment System for Children* (*BASC*) (Reynolds & Kamphaus, 1992; 1998) was designed to aid in the identification and diagnosis of emotional and behavior disorders in children and adolescents ages 2.5 to 18 years. It is a multi-informant, multi-assessment battery composed of five components: (1) Teacher Rating Scales (TRS); (2) Parent Rating Scales (PRS); (3) Self-Report of Personality (SRP); (4) Structured Developmental History (SDH); and (5) Student Observation System (SOS). Items on the TRS and PRS utilize a 4-point frequency rating ranging from Never to Almost Always. These components yield 4 composite scores (Internalizing Problems, Externalizing Problems, Adaptive Skills, and the Behavioral Symptoms Index) as well as 10 scale scores (Aggression, Hyperactivity,

Anxiety, Depression, Somatization, Attention Problems, Atypicality, Withdrawal, Adaptability, and Social Skills). For each component, administration and scoring range from 10 to 30 minutes. The standardization samples generally conformed to the U.S. population demographics.

The internal consistency coefficients for the TRS composites are generally high, ranging from $r = 0.88$ to $r = 0.95$ for the younger preschool age group, and from $r = 0.90$ to $r = 0.96$ for the older preschool age group. Somewhat lower were the coefficients of the scales for both the younger ($r = 0.71–0.92$) and the older preschool age groups ($r = 0.78–0.90$). Test-retest studies, with a maximum of 2 months between administrations, yielded correlations ranging from $r = 0.90$ to $r = 0.95$ (composites) and from $r = 0.82$ to $r = 0.95$ (scales) (Erford, 2006). Validity evidence for the *BASC* is based on factor analysis of its theoretical model, correlations with similar tests, and correlation matrices between the TRS and PRS. The *BASC* psychometric characteristics are quite sound, and it appears a robust measure for screening emotional and behavior symptoms (Witt & Jones, 1998), but Erford (2006) urged the use of subscale results only for hypothesis generation and validation, not diagnosis, due to lower technical adequacy. Sandoval (1998) also indicated that the standardization sample overrepresented children from Catholic and university-affiliated schools. Finally, Wilder & Sudweeks (2003) indicated that a lack of specific psychometric data on culturally diverse subpopulations indicates the need for caution when assessing and making decisions about culturally diverse youth.

Disruptive Behavior Rating Scale (DBRS)

The *Disruptive Behavior Rating Scale* (*DBRS*) (Erford, 1993) was designed to provide quick, meaningful information regarding disruptive behaviors displayed by children ages 5–10 years. It assesses symptoms associated with distractibility, impulsive-hyperactivity, oppositional behavior, and antisocial conduct. The *DBRS* can be used as a preliminary screening tool, as part of a medical, psychological, or psychoeducational evaluation, to target specific behaviors, or as a pretest-posttest measure of intervention effectiveness (Erford, 1993). It is available in two versions (teacher and parent), and separate norms are provided for teachers, mothers, and fathers. To eliminate cross-respondent confounds, each version of the *DBRS* contains 50 items with identical wording. All items are answered based on a 4-point frequency scale: 0—Rarely/Hardly Ever; 1—Occasionally; 2—Frequently; and 3—Most of the Time. The *DBRS* generally requires 5 to 10 minutes for administration and is easily scored by hand or by computer (McKechnie, 2006). Raw scores are transformed into T scores, percentile ranks, and three interpretive ranges: Abnormal (T > 66); Borderline ($60 \leq T \leq 66$); and Normal (T < 60). The standardization sample underrepresented minorities, rural residents, and individuals whose parents had lower levels of education (Erford, 1993).

Cronbach's *alpha* reliability coefficients for the *DBRS* subscales were well above the minimum acceptable level ($r \geq 0.80$, discussed in Chapter 3) for the Distractible ($r = 0.92–0.95$; median = 0.92); Oppositional ($r = 0.86–0.96$; median = 0.88); and Impulsive-Hyperactivity ($r = 0.88–0.96$; median = 0.92) subscales. However, the

Antisocial Conduct subscale coefficients were substantially lower ($r = 0.67$–0.77; median = 0.73), most likely because it contains only four heterogeneous items. Similar results were found for 30-day test-retest studies. The *DBRS*'s content, construct, and criterion-related validity when compared to factors in other tests were moderate to high (Erford, 1996, 1997a, 1998; McKechnie, 2006). Table 9.3 provides a sample of output from the *DBRS* computerized scoring and interpretation system.

Coping Inventory for Stressful Situations (CISS)

The *Coping Inventory for Stressful Situations* (*CISS*) is a 48-item self-report inventory used to assess three major coping styles: (1) task-oriented, (2) emotion-oriented, and (3) avoidance-oriented. Each coping style is assessed through 16 items. The *CISS* is based on Endler's (one of the authors of the *CISS*) multidimensional interaction model of stress, anxiety, and coping. According to Endler (1997), task-oriented coping contains efforts such as problem solving and situation changing, whereas emotion-oriented coping contains self-oriented responses such as emotional reactions, self-preoccupation, and fantasizing. Avoidance-oriented coping contains activities or cognitive changes to avoid stressful situations (for details of the multidimensional interaction model and the three coping styles, see Endler, 1997). There are two versions of the *CISS:* an Adolescent version (ages 13–18) and an Adult version (ages 18 and older). Paper-and-pencil record forms called "QuikScore™" are available. A 21-item brief format for adults (*CISS: Situation Specific Coping* [*CISS:SSC*]) is also available to assess coping style in situations involving social evaluation and interpersonal conflicts (Multi-Health Systems, Inc., 2003). Current cost information and online ordering information are available on the website of Multi-Health Systems (2003).

Each item of the *CISS* is formatted on a Likert scale ranging from 1 (Not at All) to 5 (Very Much). The *CISS* takes approximately 10 minutes to complete and has a Level A qualification for administration and interpretation. An examiner scores the *CISS* using a scoring grid and obtains a percentile rank and T score using a profile sheet on the back side of the scoring grid. Provided scales are Task, Emotion, and Avoidance. Avoidance consists of two subscales: Distraction and Social Diversion.

Norms are provided for adults and adolescents (Tirre, 2003). For adults, separate male and female norms are provided for general-population and psychiatric patients, respectively. For adolescents, separate norms are provided for individuals ages 13–15 years and 16–18 years. Separate college student norms are also available. Endler (1997) found sufficient internal consistency and test-retest reliability for the *CISS*. Endler (1997) also found the scores of the *CISS* to be valid. Through an examination of construct validity, Endler discovered that some *CISS* scales were significantly correlated with related measures, such as the *Beck Depression Inventory* (*BDI*) and the *Eysenck Personality Inventory* (*EPI*).

Professional counselors interested in using the *CISS* are encouraged to explore Endler's multidimensional interaction model prior to use. Endler (1997) insisted on the necessity of examining not only the interaction *between* person and situation

Table 9.3   Computerized *DBRS r*eport for a 7-year-old boy named Billy

Respondent's name: Mrs. Jones, his teacher

Summary Statistics and Critical Analysis Tables

Scale	Raw score	*SEM*	T score; Range	%ile Rank; Range	Range of significance
Distractible	21	4	67; 63–71	96; 91–98	Borderline to Abnormal
Oppositional	5	6	55; 49–61	69; 47–87	Normal to Borderline
Impulsive-Hyperactive	21	5	74; 69–79	99; 97–99.81	Abnormal
Antisocial conduct (Aux)	1	13	55; 42–68	69; 21–96	Normal to Abnormal

Critical Item Analysis

Scale	Item	Statements
Distractible	8	Doesn't seem to remember what is said.
	22	Has difficulty following simple instructions.
	31	Does not finish activities undertaken.
Oppositional	None	
Impulsive- Hyperactive	3	Calls out unexpectedly.
	6	Fidgety.
	10	Finds it hard to await turn in group situations.
	13	Restless, squirmy.
	21	Interrupts.
	34	Has difficulty sitting still.
	42	Finds it hard to play quietly.
Antisocial conduct (Aux)	None	

Interpretation

The *Disruptive Behavior Rating Scale—Teacher Version* (*DBRS-T*) is a 50-item inventory of common childhood behaviors associated with distractible, impulsive-hyperactive, oppositional, and antisocial behavior. Mrs. Jones's responses to the *DBRS-T* indicate that Billy is observed to perform in the Borderline to Abnormal range of distractible behavior. Billy is more distractible than approximately 96% of boys his age. Billy is having particular difficulty remembering what is said, following simple instructions, and finishing activities undertaken.

Billy is observed as performing in the Abnormal range of impulsive-hyperactive behavior. Billy is more impulsive-hyperactive than approximately 99% of boys his age. Billy displays a significant inclination toward calling out unexpectedly, fidgeting, not awaiting turns in group activities, restless squirming, interrupting, difficulty in sitting still, and difficulty in playing quietly.

Additionally, Billy performs in the Normal to Borderline range of oppositional behavior. Billy is more oppositional than approximately 69% of boys his age. No critical items were determined for this factor.

Finally, Billy is rated to perform in the Normal to Abnormal range of antisocial conduct. Billy is more antisocial than approximately 69 percent of boys his age. No critical items were determined for this factor.

A diagnosis of Attention-Deficit Hyperactivity Disorder (AD/HD) should be considered. Validation of these findings through multiple methods of evaluation and multiple informants is recommended.

variables, but also the interaction *within* person variables (e.g., cognitive style, biological variables) and situation variables (e.g., stressful events, physical environments), given that "stress, anxiety, and coping all involve complex processes and all interact with one another" (Endler, 1997, p. 149).

SUMMARY/CONCLUSION

Professional counselors should remember that the referral question should always drive the assessment process. All too often, assessment reports are driven by a one-size-fits-all approach. It is important to gather data from multiple methods and multiple informants to evaluate how the identified individual differs from other individuals in the population (nomothetic comparisons) and to identify specific targets for remediation or therapy. Professional counselors should use a combination of behavioral interviews, rating scales, inventories, and direct observations to obtain a comprehensive picture of the client and the specific referral concerns. Doing so not only provides appropriate services but constitutes best practices for ethical and legal obligations of service provision in the area of assessment.

KEY TERMS

behavioral assessment
behavioral interview
direct assessment
functional behavioral assessment
  (FBA)

indirect assessment
interval recording
narrative recording
operational definition
self-monitoring

CHAPTER 10

Assessment of Intelligence

by Bradley T. Erford, Lauren Klein, and Kathleen McNinch

Intelligence is an important human characteristic with robust applications to the areas of academic achievement, career development, and psychopathology. There is no commonly accepted definition of intelligence, and numerous models have been offered to explain and measure this construct. This chapter explores these models and reviews many of the individual and group-administered tests designed to measure intelligence. In addition, important societal and educational issues and implications are discussed.

WHAT IS INTELLIGENCE?

"She's really smart." "He's about as bright as a burned-out light bulb." "She should aspire to raise her IQ to room temperature." "He's brilliant, simply brilliant!" At some time, most people have overheard (or perhaps made) a judgment about their own or someone else's probable level of **intelligence**. For more than a century, theorists and test developers have attempted to define and operationalize "intelligence."

In 1921, 17 experts responded to an invitation by the editor of the *Journal of Educational Psychology* to define and describe their perspectives on intelligence. In 1986, Sternberg and Detterman similarly consulted leading experts in the field. The result in both cases: The experts revealed great diversity and little commonality in their conceptions of what intelligence entails. Charles Spearman (1927, p. 14), a famous theoretician and researcher in the field of intelligence, pessimistically concluded, "In truth, intelligence has become . . . a word with so many meanings that finally it has none."

Various definitions of intelligence emphasized at least one of the following components (Sax, 1997): (1) *origin*—whether intelligence is inherited, learned, or both; (2) *structure*—its traits, facets, or components; and (3) *function*—its purpose, usually to aid in adjustment or survival. In a broad sense, intelligence is a human-contrived construct used to explain one's (genetic and/or learned) abilities to reason through and solve problems or dilemmas of importance to human adaptation. And as if defining intelligence isn't challenging enough, measuring it is even harder! The premier challenge confronting researchers and test developers in the field of intellectual assessment is to operationally define the construct of intelligence from often-divergent theoretical perspectives. Therefore, nearly all tests of intelligence available for use today measure some conception of cognitive capability, but each does so from a somewhat different perspective.

The term **intelligence testing** is virtually synonymous with the terms *cognitive ability testing* and *mental ability testing*. However, the term **aptitude**, while overlapping in many ways with intelligence, is a concept that implies a more specialized use of intellectual, perceptual, and motor abilities—usually with vocational or educational applications. The area of aptitude assessment will be covered in further detail in Chapter 11. Intelligence testing is undertaken to estimate a client's ability to comprehend and express verbal information; to solve problems through verbal or nonverbal means (i.e., spatial, figural, visual); to learn and remember information (i.e., short-term, long-term); and to assess information processing efficiency. In short, intelligence is a useful and robust concept with widespread clinical applications.

While professional counselors may not frequently be the professional administering a given intelligence test, it is essential that professional counselors understand the nature of intelligence, the practical features of intelligence tests, and how these tests are used for clinical and educational decision making and for treatment and remedial planning. For example, professional school counselors and other educational personnel use intelligence tests to help determine a student's eligibility for special education services under the Individuals With Disabilities Education Improvement Act (IDEIA), and often for educational accommodations under Section 504 of the U.S. Rehabilitation Act of 1973. Mental health and community counselors use intelligence test information to establish effective treatment plans and to advocate on behalf of clients with special needs. Career and professional school counselors use intelligence test information to help students and clients with educational planning and career choices. Intelligence test results are helpful decision-making tools applicable across a wide gamut of life decisions.

Think About It 10.1   How could intelligence testing be beneficial in working with students?

Unfortunately, there is no widespread consensus over the definition of intelligence. Various researchers and test developers have conceived of very diverse theories of, and perspectives on, intelligence. Indeed, one could support the assertion that each intelligence test published and available today has a somewhat different theoretical underpinning. The differences are frequently slight, at other times vast. But keep in mind, all purport to measure this concept referred to as "intelligence."

NATURE AND THEORIES OF INTELLIGENCE

For more than a century, numerous researchers and test developers have attempted to define the construct of intelligence. While there is great diversity in these conceptions of intelligence, typically intelligence tests measure, to a greater extent, verbal abilities and, to a lesser extent, abstract visual reasoning and quantitative skills. There is also general agreement that speed and efficiency of problem-solving capacities are characteristic of individuals with higher levels of intelligence (Jensen, 1985). Snyderman and Rothman (1986) surveyed 661 testing authorities, virtually all of whom agreed that intelligence involves, at a minimum, capacity to acquire knowledge, abstract reasoning, and general problem-solving capabilities. Some (e.g., Gardner, 1983) even integrate personality variables into their definition. What follows is a brief exploration of some conceptualizations, theories, and models of intelligence developed over the past century. Note how the construct of intelligence has at times evolved from simpler to more complex explanations, while at other times divergent pathways have led to new theoretical models and orientations.

Historical Conceptualizations of Intelligence

In the late 19th century, Sir Francis Galton and James McKeen Cattell believed in the importance of sensory acuities and capabilities as indications of intellectual prowess, because all information about the external world (and thus all potential learning) entered through the senses. To their way of thinking, the more highly developed and attuned one's senses, the more intelligent one could become. While plausible on its surface, such a perspective fails to account for thinking or reasoning processes. In 1890, Cattell coined the term *mental test,* giving rise to the field of study now known as *intellectual assessment.* Unfortunately, from early on, other researchers (Wissler, 1901) demonstrated that the type of "intelligence" Cattell and others were proposing had little relationship to academic performance, failing to explain why some students, particularly at the university level, do better or more poorly than others. Interestingly, Wissler's results later were criticized for using a sample with a restricted range of ability—a flaw that suppresses the magnitude of a correlation coefficient—as is discussed on the companion website.

From the early reliance on sensory processing, definitions of intelligence evolved with a heavier focus on internal thinking and reasoning processes. At the same time, however, the concept of intelligence was also discussed primarily as a general, unidimensional construct.

Alfred Binet

Alfred Binet defined intelligence as the "tendency to take and maintain a definite direction; the capacity to make adaptations for the purpose of attaining a desired end" (as cited in Terman, 1916a, p. 45). Binet and Henri (1895a, 1895b, 1895c) studied facets of human intelligence that were far more complex and less easily measured than the simple sensory functions observed by Galton, including tasks of reasoning, comprehension, memory, judgment, and abstraction (Varon, 1936). Binet believed distinct thinking abilities were integrated into a general ability that was called on when solving problems. Thus, when one is solving a problem such as, "What should you do if your boat begins to sink in the middle of a large lake?" Binet believed that it was difficult to sort out the influence of, say, practical experience, memory, reasoning, and verbal facility in the construction of an acceptable answer. This preliminary research led to the development of the first functional individual intelligence test by Binet and Simon (1905).

David Wechsler

Wechsler (1955, p. 7) once wrote:

> Intelligence, operationally defined, is the aggregate or global capacity of the individual to act purposively, to think rationally, and to deal effectively with his environment. It is aggregate or global because it is composed of elements or abilities which, though not entirely independent, are qualitatively differentiable. . . . The only way we can evaluate it quantitatively is by the measurement of the various aspects of these abilities.

In 1939, Wechsler developed a test to measure the intelligence of individual adults. His test was composed of a collection of subtests adapted from the Army *Alpha* and *Beta* tests from World War I. His verbal subtests were modeled from items off the Army *Alpha*, and his performance subtests were modeled after items off the *Army Beta*. Combining the scores from the verbal and performance subtests yielded a full-scale intelligence estimate that Wechsler believed a good representation of *g*. However, the development of the original test and its various revised editions were driven more by clinical practice and implications than by theoretical considerations.

Wechsler clearly acknowledged a general factor (*g*) composed of multiple components, and his intelligence tests, which will be discussed later in this chapter, have become the most commonly used in history. However, it is important to remember that while Wechsler stressed the essential role of cognitive capabilities in intellectual capabilities, he also recognized that a comprehensive understanding of intelligence involved noncognitive capacities, including "capabilities more of the nature of connative, affective, or personality traits . . . such as drive, persistence, and goal awareness . . . [and] . . . an individual's potential to perceive and respond to social, moral, and aesthetic values" (Wechsler, 1975, p. 136).

Piaget's developmental model

Swiss developmental psychologist Jean Piaget has made important theoretical contributions to the understanding of childhood intelligence (1954, 1971). Piaget believed that the function of intelligence was to help humans to adapt to the environment. As individuals become more intelligent, they progress through more advanced levels of symbolic representation. Eventually, physical trial and error is replaced by mental trial and error. To Piaget, learning was a consequence of an individual's interacting with the environment and encountering dilemmas that required mastery through a reorganization of thought. These organized structures were called **schemata**. Infants are born with some schemata (i.e., sucking, grasping) and learn about the environment by coordinating these schemata to take in new information (Cohen & Swerdlik, 1999). Thus infants may grasp objects and place them into their mouths to more fully appreciate the object. Eventually, schemata of greater and greater complexity develop, departing from sole reliance on the physical realm and leading to cognitive transformations. As the individual interacts with the environment, existing schemata are constantly being refined, and new schemata are formed.

Piaget proposed two methods by which humans organize their cognitive structures and adapt to new contexts. **Assimilation** is the process by which individuals make sense of new information in terms of a structure or process that already exists. For example, small children generally know what a dog is and know a dog when they encounter it or see a picture of it. Every time they see a dog and recognize it as a dog, they are assimilating this information—making sense of it in terms of an existing structure. New information is related to old structures. **Accommodation** is the process by which individuals make sense of new information by changing the existing structure or process, thus creating an adapted schema. For example, eventually children recognize that there are different types of dogs (i.e., golden retrievers, beagles, miniature poodles) and restructure the previously existing category (e.g., they're all dogs) into new, more meaningful categories designated by using diverse dog breed names. Thus new information is reorganized into new ways of thinking.

Piaget was also instrumental in developing the now common assumption that there are qualitative differences in the way children think at various ages. His theory proposes four stages of development. The *sensorimotor stage* occurs during the first several years of life, and cognitions of the infant and toddler are basically limited to the sensory processes in the immediate environment (i.e., touch, taste, smell, sight, hearing). The *preoperational stage* generally occurs between ages 2 and 7 years and evolves from the child's emerging ability to reason symbolically (i.e., to use words to symbolize objects). The *concrete operational stage* involves the beginnings of logical, systematic thinking and generally develops between ages 7 and 12 years. Concepts such as conservation and reversibility of operations are important, but problem solving is still predominated by direct, immediate experiences. Piaget's highest level of reasoning was called the *formal operational stage*. Generally emerging around age 12 years, this period is marked by problem-solving strategies that rely on increasing levels of abstract, systematic, hypothetical thinking. Individuals can evaluate their own thought processes (metacognition) and more easily see how several variables relate, interact, and can be used to learn from and predict. Piaget's theory has been very influential in education, influencing curricular activities, materials, and programs.

Think About It 10.2   How would being aware of Piaget's stages of development be useful when working with children?

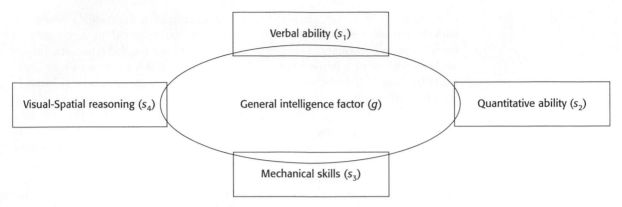

Figure 10.1   Spearman's two-factor theory of intelligence

Spearman's general-factor theory (g)

A British statistician and psychologist named Charles Spearman, the innovator of a useful statistical technique now known as factor analysis, proposed a theory of intelligence that is referred to as both a "two-factor theory" and a "general factor theory" of intelligence. His theory proposed that a **general factor** (g) stands at the center of one's cognitive capacity, and that (perhaps numerous) specific factors ($s_1, s_2, s_3, \ldots s_n$) are related to the general factor and help explain nuances and specialized characteristics observed in individuals. Spearman noticed that all measures of intelligence were positively correlated with academic performance, leading him to think that a common construct (the general ability factor [g]) underlay these measures and created the positive associations. Figure 10.1 provides a pictorial representation of Spearman's theory.

Spearman also noticed that as he began to aggregate (i.e., add together) scores obtained on the simple sensory tasks and the reasoning and comprehension tasks commonly associated with intelligence at that time, the measures correlated in the 0.30s with academic performance (Francher, 1985), substantially enhancing the predictive usefulness of these tasks. Spearman became convinced that all measures of intelligence were simply facets related to the general intelligence factor (g). Thus two tests measuring different facets of intelligence would overlap to some extent, depending on the strength of their relationship to g. He reasoned that if all intelligence tests measured only general mental ability, the correlations between these tests would approach $r = 1.00$. However, because these correlations were significantly less than $r = 1.00$, he assumed that a diverse set of specific factor elements (s_1, s_2, etc.) were what prevented the perfect correlations. "Spearman referred to g as the total mental energy available to a person while the s factors were the engines through which this energy was applied" (Janda, 1998, p. 209). Some cognitive tasks required more general ability (g) than others, but all cognitive tasks required at least some. Spearman's two-factor theory of intelligence was an important advance but was far from universally accepted.

Multiple-Factor Models

Multiple-factor theories propose that one's intellectual makeup is composed of many components that are more or less independent of each other. For example, while most people have normal or average verbal and visual-spatial reasoning abilities, others may be weak in both areas, and still others may be strong in both areas. Notice that, so far, this is in keeping with Spearman's general-factor theory. However, many people are normal or strong in verbal reasoning, but weak in visual-spatial reasoning, and vice versa. The intellectual structure of these individuals is not explained by a single, general factor but is better explained by a theory that suggests that these two factors are independent and *should* vary according to individual cognitive strengths and weaknesses. Of course, the more factors that are included in the theory, the more complex the scenarios can become.

Thurstone's Primary Mental Abilities

An American psychologist, Louis L. Thurstone, from the University of Chicago, proposed that a collection of mostly independent primary abilities underlay intelligence, rather than the global general factor and multitude of specific factors proposed by Spearman. Interestingly, one of the things we know today about factor analysis that wasn't widely known 75 years ago is that the number of factors derived is in large part due to the number and diversity of the input (i.e., items, subtests, tests). Using the statistical technique multiple-factor analysis, Thurstone analyzed responses of more than 200 college students to 56 ability tests and derived 13 mental factors. He eventually settled on seven *primary mental abilities,* described in Table 10.1. It is important to understand that even Thurstone admitted that these factors were not

Table 10.1 Thurstone's seven primary mental abilities

Ability	Description
Verbal Comprehension (V)	Assesses understanding and expression of ideas using language. (V) is measured by tasks involving vocabulary, analogies, and reading comprehension.
Number (N)	Assesses ability to solve numeric problems using basic math processes. (N) is measured by tasks involving rapid, accurate computation of simple math problems, story problems, and math calculation.
Word Fluency (W)	Assesses fluency of speech and writing. (W) is measured by tasks such as anagrams and word naming (e.g. words ending in-*ing*).
Spatial (S)	Assesses ability to visualize patterns and rotate objects in space. (S) is measured by tasks involving three-dimensional visualization, matrices, and block designs.
Reasoning (R)	Assesses inductive thinking and problem solving. (R) is measured by tasks involving logic, discerning a rule of operation or pattern, and number sequence patterns.
Memory (M)	Assesses rote memorization of information. (M) is measured by tasks involving recall of sentences, letters, digits, words, etc.
Perceptual Speed (P)	Assesses ability to quickly note and discriminate visual details. (P) is measured by tasks involving identification of similarities and differences in pictures or geometric objects.

Table 10.2   Factors of the Horn-Cattell model

Designation	Name	Description
Gf	Fluid intelligence	Nonverbal reasoning, novel circumstances
Gc	Crystallized intelligence	General knowledge, verbal comprehension and reasoning
Gq	Quantitative ability	Understanding and problem solving using mathematical concepts and symbols
Gv	Visual processing	Receiving and making decisions using visual and spatial stimuli
Ga	Auditory processing	Receiving and making decisions using auditory stimuli
Gs	Processing speed	Ability to maintain attention and make quick, accurate decisions
Gsm	Short-term memory	Ability to maintain and use information over a short time period (seconds to minutes)
Glr	Long-term retrieval	Ability to encode and store information for retrieval and use over a long time period (hours to years)

totally independent, and that any given intelligence test could measure one, several, or even all of these dimensions. In fact, Thurstone developed the *Primary Mental Abilities* intelligence test in 1938 to do just that. Unfortunately, Thurstone's own test showed that several of the factors were highly correlated (e.g., the Verbal and Reasoning factors correlated nearly $r = 0.60$), calling into question the independence of these components of intelligence. Of course, critics of multiple-factor models were quick to explain this observation by using Spearman's general-factor model. Perhaps the most damaging contradiction of Thurstone's model is the inclusion of a total-scale score for the *Primary Abilities Test*; an admission, although perhaps inadvertent, that a general global factor has some interpretable meaning or predictive usefulness.

Horn-Cattell Gc/Gf model

Raymond Cattell (1943, 1963, 1971, 1979) proposed that intellectual abilities could be divided into two broad categories or second-order factors. **Fluid abilities** (Gf) were primarily inherited, perceptual capabilities thought to be mostly free of potential **sociocultural bias.** Tests measuring visualization, nonverbal, and spatial reasoning capabilities are direct assessments of fluid ability. **Crystallized abilities** (Gc) were primarily learned, acquired knowledge and skills that were socioculturally laden and heavily influenced by formal and informal educational experiences. Tests measuring vocabulary, general information, verbal abstract reasoning, and social comprehension directly assess crystallized ability. Importantly, Cattell proposed that fluid and crystallized abilities are significantly correlated, especially among those who share a common cultural and educational background. Thus no pretense of factor independence was offered.

In 1966, Cattell and John Horn became the major proponents of this model, and the model was expanded by Horn and his colleagues in subsequent years to add on additional factors derived through rational and factor analytic studies of multiple test batteries. Currently, the Horn-Cattell model espouses eight components (see Table 10.2), many of which have more or less provided the theoretical underpin-

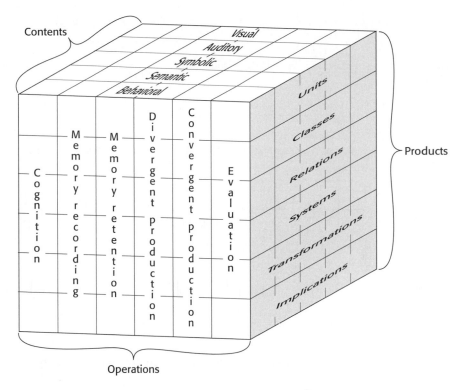

Figure 10.2   Guilford's structure-of-intellect model

nings of the *Stanford-Binet Intelligence Scales,* now in its fifth edition (*SB-5*) (Roid, 2003), and to a greater extent, the *Woodcock-Johnson Tests of Cognitive Abilities—Third Edition* (*WJ-III COG*) (Woodcock, Mather, & McGrew, 2001).

Guilford's Structure-of-Intellect Model

Guilford (1967, 1988; Guilford & Hoepfner, 1971) also used factor analysis to discern a model of intellect but arrived at quite different conclusions than Spearman or Vernon about the existence of *g,* and he rejected Thurstone's argument of the existence of a number of independent primary mental abilities. Instead, Guilford proposed a theory in which 3 dimensions gave rise to approximately 180 unique specific factors (see Figure 10.2), as expressed within a $6 \times 5 \times 6$ boxlike matrix. The first dimension, *mental operations,* indicates what an individual does and includes 6 components: cognition, memory recording, memory retention, divergent production, convergent production, and evaluation. The second dimension, *contents,* indicates the materials upon which the individual performs various operations and includes 5 components: visual, auditory, symbolic, semantic, and behavioral. The final dimension, *products,* indicates the format into which individuals store and process information and includes 6 facets: units, classes, relations, systems, transformations, and

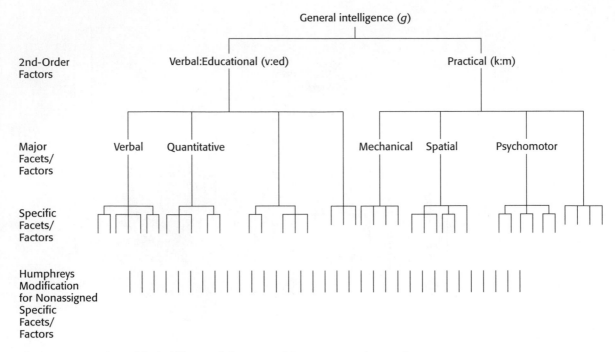

Figure 10.3   Hierarchical ability model proposed by Vernon and Humphrey

implications. Each of the resulting 180 cells may contain a specific factor or a combination of specific factors, but each factor can be described in terms of its 3 components. Guilford's model has had little impact on the standardized measurement of intelligence, but nonetheless is a helpful model for understanding intelligence, particularly as applied to education.

Hierarchical Models

Vernon (1960, 1965) suggested a model of intelligence that in some ways is a compromise between the divergent theories proposed by Spearman and Thurstone. Vernon agreed that *g* underlay all facets of intelligence but noticed that certain clusters of various types of intelligence tests or subtests were too high to conclude that *g* was the only factor accounting for the relationship. He proposed that two second-order factors comprised *g,* namely Verbal:Educational (v:ed) and Practical (k:m) aptitudes. From these second-order factors, various skill areas branch off, which may be broken down into even lower-level facets (see Figure 10.3). For example, the Verbal: Educational factor may be assessed using tests measuring verbal comprehension and quantitative skill. Verbal comprehension skills may be further delineated and assessed by tests measuring vocabulary development, social comprehension, general information, and verbal abstract reasoning. These latter tests are more similar to the *s* factors proposed by Spearman or the individual cells proposed by Guilford.

Other **hierarchical models**, such as the one proposed by Humphreys (1962, 1970), argued for more flexibility in accounting for or assigning specific factors to higher-level factors. For example, it can be argued that in testing one's ability to solve analogies, it is helpful to use spatial, verbal, and numerical cues, each of which is represented by specific factors. While the practical and theoretical applications of hierarchical models have allowed them to grow in popularity (Anastasi & Urbina, 1997), a primary limitation remains the lack of empirical validation of the model (Sax, 1997).

Sternberg's Triarchic Theory: An Information Processing Approach

Sternberg (1988), using an information processing perspective, described a triarchic model, so named because it was composed of three aspects (subtheoretical components) of intelligence: *componential* (the person's internal world), *experiential* (the person's external world and adaptation to novelty), and *contextual* (the person's external world and environmental adaptation or creation). This theory arose from Sternberg's (1986, p. 33) belief that intelligence involved "purposive adaptation to, shaping of, and selection of real-world environments relevant to one's life." Sternberg stated that available tests of intelligence failed to measure the complex processes proposed in his theory. Sternberg's primary criticism of currently available intelligence tests is that they measure primarily memory and analytical reasoning skills that are useful in predicting school performance, predominantly because they are contextualized to school and learning problems, are short, and have a single correct answer. He believes these tests have little usefulness in predicting "real-world" performances people encounter in the world of work; what some call practical intelligence.

In the *componential subtheory,* Sternberg identified three facets as being critical to the efficiency with which individuals process information. *Metacomponents* allow people to plan purposeful activities, self-monitor the implementation of these plans, and self-evaluate the effectiveness of the implementation. These are higher-level cognitive processes, sometimes called executive functioning, that help explain why some very bright and talented people accomplish a lot and others accomplish very little. According to Sternberg, the very intelligent person focuses on important tasks and issues—what some refer to as the "big picture"—plans them out, and accomplishes them. Less intelligent people focus on issues and situations that are less important— what some call the "little picture." *Performance components* allow individuals to process diverse information with varying degrees of efficiency by using mental skills such as information retrieval, encoding, or comparing. *Knowledge acquisition* involves an individual's capacity to select information relevant to a given problem context and then to compare and combine it with other relevant information, leading to insights, connections, and, eventually, new learning. Obviously, the more efficient one is at making relevant connections and gaining necessary insights, the greater one's capacity for learning (i.e., intelligence).

The *experiential subtheory* views intelligence as an interplay of experience and information processing. Thus, experienced individuals often appear more intelligent but only because they have encountered a problem in the past and recall how to resolve it appropriately. According to Sternberg, novel situations present a level playing field to determine adaptability and problem solving, because such circumstances favor those who process information more quickly and efficiently. In this way, Sternberg valued "automaticity," the ability to quickly learn information, processes, and procedures, thus freeing up the resources necessary for adaptation to novel situations.

Finally, Sternberg's *contextual subtheory* involves adaptability in the external world, the context for practical, pragmatic decision making that allows humans to shape, adapt, and select environments in which to thrive. For example, we have all known individuals who did not do well in school but had a knack for adapting to new situations (contexts) and who do quite well for themselves. These individuals read and adapt to the environmental context.

In 1994, Sternberg refined his theory by altering his terminology to include the terms *memory-analytic, synthetic-creative,* and *practical-contextual* abilities. Sternberg viewed memory-analytic functions as commonplace in education and science today, where people construct defined and delimited problems with predictable and "correct" solutions. Synthetic-creative problems are those that are not entrenched in common assumptions, such as when an illogical assumption is given and the examinee is required to follow the assumption to its inevitable conclusion. Such out-of-the-box thinking requires flexible cognitive and reasoning processes that are difficult to teach, but which are nonetheless critical to creative problem solving. Practical-contextual abilities, also termed *tacit knowledge* or *practical intelligence,* was defined as "action-oriented knowledge, acquired without direct help from others, that allows individuals to achieve goals they personally value" (Sternberg, Wagner, Williams, & Horvath, 1995, p. 916). Practical-contextual tasks help explain why some individuals who score low on traditional tests of intelligence are able to solve sometimes complex everyday situations with more ease than their "more intelligent" counterparts. As an application of Sternberg's theory, Table 10.3 contains the types of items derived from a triarchic model.

Fundamental to Sternberg's theory is that intelligence is not set; it is malleable and continually developing. Moreover, the display of an individual's intelligence can vary from one context to another; that is, people may be absolutely brilliant when in their "element" (i.e., the board room or chemistry lab), but substantially less so when not (i.e., the kitchen or nursery).

Gardner's Multiple Intelligences

Howard Gardner (1983, 1993) rejected the existence of *g* and identified eight distinct intelligences that aid in an individual's adaptation to the environment. He defined intelligence as the ability "to resolve general problems or difficulties as they are encountered" (Gardner, 1983, p. 60) and identified the following eight intelligences: (1) verbal-linguistic, (2) logical-mathematical, (3) spatial, (4) musical, (5) bodily-kinesthetic, (6) interpersonal, (7) intrapersonal, and (8) naturalist (see Table 10.4). Gardner criticized current tests of intelligence for being primarily measures of verbal, spatial, and logical reasoning while ignoring other abilities that are, in some ways, so

Table 10.3   Item types derived from Sternberg's triarchic model

Item type	Description
Componential: Verbal	Assesses a student's verbal ability when learning from relevant contexts, such as when a word is used in the context of a sentence and a student is asked to infer the word's meaning from context.
Componential: Quantitative	Assesses numerically based inductive reasoning abilities by extrapolating from sequences of numbers. For example: When given the following sequence of numbers: 2, 4, 8, 16, __?__; the student would choose *32* from a list of possible answers.
Componential: Figural	Assesses inductive reasoning abilities through figure classifications and analogies. For example:

Coping With Novelty: Verbal	Assesses the ability to think in relatively novel ways using hypothetical thinking or novel verbal analogies requiring counterfactual reasoning. For example: Assume snowflakes are made of sand. Which solution is now correct, given the assumption? Water is to drop as snow is to: (a) storm, (b) beach, (c) grain, (d) ice.
Coping With Novelty: Quantitative	Assesses quantitative coping with novelty skills by using number matrix items, but with an element of novelty. Usually, items involve symbols used in place of certain numbers and require the examinee to make a number substitution. For example:

$$\begin{array}{ccc} * & 2 & 7 \\ 12 & * & ? \\ * & = & 5 \end{array}$$

(a) 14, (b) 4, (c) 17, (d) 8.

| Coping with novelty: Figural | Assesses a student's ability to complete a pictorial series in a "newly mapped domain," (not the domain in which the student has constructed or inferred the rule). For example, |

continued

Table 10.3   continued

Item type	Description

Item type	Description
Automatization: Verbal	Assesses rapid decisions of a verbal nature. For example, are the following letters from the "same" category (both vowels, both consonants) or "different" categories (vowel or consonant): "b, n" (same); "e, m" (different); "u, o" (same); "g, i" (different).
Automatization: Quantitative	Assesses rapid decisions of a quantitative nature. For example, are the following numbers from the "same" category (both odd, both even) or "different" categories (odd or even): "2, 4" (same); "9, 6" (different); "7, 3" (same); "8, 5" (different).
Automatization: Figural	Assesses rapid decisions of a figural nature. For example, do the following figures have the "same" or "different" numbers of sides?

Item type	Description
Practical: Verbal	Assesses practical, everyday problem-solving abilities requiring verbal inferential reasoning. For example: The sign at Bill's Market reads, "The lowest meat prices in town." If the ad is for real, which of the following is most likely true? (a) Bill's Market charges more than Sam's. (b) No other market charges less than Bill's. (c) Bill is a successful businessman. (d) Bill's is the busiest market in town.
Practical: Quantitative	Assesses practical, everyday problem-solving abilities requiring quantitative reasoning. For example: Given a recipe for making two dozen cookies and an inventory of ingredients currently in the house, the examinee may be asked, "How many dozen cookies could be baked without having to go to the store for more supplies?"
Practical: Figural	Assesses practical, everyday problem-solving abilities requiring figural reasoning. For example: A student may be shown a town map and be asked to chart the shortest route from one place in the town to another.

much more important in adapting to the environment and solving real-world problems. For example, intelligence tests rarely identify outstanding musical, athletic, or intrinsic motivation potential. Gardner's relatively independent intelligences were

Table 10.4   Howard Gardner's multiple intelligences

Intelligence	Description
Linguistic	The ability to use language to express ideas and understand others. Linguistic intelligence is displayed by lawyers, teachers, orators, writers, and linguists.
Logical-Mathematical	The ability to understand underlying causal systems, inductive and deductive logic, scientific reasoning, numerical reasoning, and numerical operations. Logical-mathematical intelligence is displayed by mathematicians, logicians, scientists, and engineers.
Spatial	The ability to understand, visualize, and manipulate mental images, graphic representations, or objects in space. Spatial intelligence is displayed by sculptors, painters, surgeons, architects, and navigators.
Musical	The ability to think musically and rhythmically by hearing, remembering, and manipulating patterns. Musical intelligence is displayed by musicians of any kind.
Bodily-Kinesthetic	The ability to use one's body to solve complex motor problems through awareness and control of motor functions. Bodily-kinesthetic intelligence is displayed by athletes, dancers, actors, and seamstresses.
Interpersonal	The ability to understand and work with other people, read their verbal and nonverbal communication, be sensitive to the feelings of others, and solve problems of an interpersonal nature. Interpersonal intelligence is displayed by professional counselors, salespeople, managers, politicians, and just about anyone else who has to deal with people problems.
Intrapersonal	The ability to understand oneself; what one can do, can't do, self-motivations, propensities, and aversions. Intrapersonal intelligence involves metacognition, self-awareness, and abstract thinking. It relies on self-awareness and is important in virtually any endeavor.
Naturalist	The ability to discriminate among and classify objects. Naturalist intelligence is displayed by farmers, botanists, hunters, and chefs.

identified through a process that involved several criteria, including occurrence across cultures, the effects of localized brain damage, and the distinct history of exceptional ability.

While Gardner does not dispute the importance of genetics, he clearly points out that intelligence stems from an interaction between heredity and environment. For example, consider a case in which two children of equal musical talent are born into two separate families. The first family values musical talent and expends great time and effort to cultivate Johnny's burgeoning skills. The second family not only doesn't value musical talent, but actively punishes its expression whenever possible, frequently telling the child, "Stop playing with violins and cellos, Jimmy. You'll have no need of them in your career as a professional counselor!" Certainly, the odds of developing substantial musical intelligence are in Johnny's favor. Gardner's theory is thought provoking and has received much attention in classrooms and schools around the United States. Unfortunately, there are numerous problems when trying to measure several of the intelligences, and the empirical support behind the theory is less than robust.

Some Final Thoughts on the (Practical) Nature of Intelligence

Richard Hernstein and Charles Murray (1994), in their very controversial book *The Bell Curve: Intelligence and Class Structure in American Life,* categorized the theories proposed by Spearman, Binet, and their contemporaries as *classicist.* The common thread to classicist models was the adherence to a unifying factor, *g,* at the center of intellectual being. Another broad category proposed by Hernstein and Murray was the *revisionist* models. Revisionist theories proposed that there was indeed a unifying factor, *g,* at the center of cognitive structure, but *g* was composed of several secondary factors (i.e., verbal reasoning, nonverbal reasoning, working memory, processing speed), each of which contributes to one's total cognitive makeup. Furthermore, revisionist models assert that individual clients can have strengths and weaknesses in each of these processing categories. In the end, it is the combination of these strengths, weaknesses, or normal capacities that make up one's total cognitive function (*g*). However, various patterns or combinations of cognitive skills, while perhaps resulting in the same estimate of overall intelligence (*g*), may lead to very different results in terms of *how* problems are solved. For example, when required to write an extensive report about some social phenomenon, a client with excellent verbal reasoning skills and poor nonverbal reasoning skills may be able to excel at the task, while a client with the identical overall IQ (*g*), but with low verbal reasoning skills and outstanding nonverbal reasoning skills, may struggle mightily. Some well-known revisionist models include those of Vernon, Horn-Cattell, and Guilford. To this day, psychometricians and statisticians continue to debate whether intelligence can be meaningfully represented by a single global score (the classicist position) or is global with multidimensional refinements (the revisionist position).

Hernstein and Murray (1994) referred to a third movement within the field of intellectual assessment as the *radicals,* and pointed to Gardner's theory of multiple intelligences as a prime example. Gardner rejects the existence of *g* and lauds the independence of the intelligences he has identified. While appealing in its own right and widely used in education, little empirical support for the independent nature of the identified intelligences exists.

While development, classification, and description of intelligence tests is certainly important, perhaps it speaks volumes that the most commonly used tests of intelligence, the various versions of the *Wechsler* scales, put less emphasis on theoretical considerations and focus more attention on clinical usefulness and applications. After all, what guarantee is there that a well-constructed, theoretically pure measure of intelligence will help make better decisions or predictions about the clients and students to whom they are administered? It is this pragmatism that has lead some to urge that the assessment of intelligence consider not only the comprehensive measures of ability that predict one's learning potential, but also the wide-ranging cognitive processes that help diagnose individual strengths and weaknesses. For example, Salvia and Ysseldyke (2004, p. 317) suggested that intelligence tests sample the following domains of behavior: "discrimination, generalization, motor behavior, general knowledge, vocabulary, induction, comprehension, sequencing, detail recognition, analogical reasoning, pattern completion, abstract reasoning, and memory." No matter the theory of intelligence or intelligence test used, the key consideration rests in the practical clinical value of the results—how will this theory or test help professional counselors make better decisions about clients and students?

COMMONLY USED TESTS OF INTELLIGENCE

Tests of intelligence, cognition, or school abilities are available in group and individually administered formats and can be administered for screening or diagnostic purposes. Some of the most commonly used and currently available tests will be reviewed in the following sections.

Group-Administered Tests of Intelligence and School Ability

Group-administered intelligence tests are frequently used in schools, the military, or other venues in which large numbers of persons need to be assessed quickly and efficiently. Large-scale testing of this sort relies on objective administration and scoring formats, easy examiner instructions, and lower costs per administration. Because these tests are administered to large numbers of examinees at a time, **group-administered tests** often have well-developed item pools, norms, and technical estimates of score reliability and validity. Disadvantages of group testing include the examiner's inability to observe the specific test-related behaviors of all examinees and the lack of examiner flexibility to follow up on examinee responses. Often these tests present items in a multiple-choice format, and a variety of item types are mixed together (i.e., vocabulary, analogies, figural reasoning, matrix analogies) in some order of increasing difficulty. Generally, these tests are designed to be power tests but are administered under time limits that allow the vast majority of clients to complete all items.

Otis-Lennon School Ability Test (OLSAT)

The *OLSAT-8* (Otis & Lennon, 2004) measures a student's ability to solve school learning tasks and also serves as a screen for placement decisions (Salvia & Ysseldyke, 2004). It is frequently administered to students early in elementary school as a cognitive screening measure and has been used as a screening measure for identifying gifted students. The *OLSAT-8* has seven levels (A–G) and is administered to students in grades K–12. Administration times vary by level and run between 30 and 75 minutes. Items were developed to measure five clusters of cognitive skills: verbal comprehension, verbal reasoning, pictorial reasoning, figural reasoning, and quantitative reasoning (see Figure 10.4). According to Salvia and Ysseldyke (2004), standardization generally conformed to the U.S. population demographics.

The *OLSAT-8* is a quick, group-administered test of intelligence, but researchers debate the adequacy of test score validity. Raw scores can be converted into scaled scores, school ability indexes ($M = 100$; $SD = 16$), percentile ranks, stanines, and normal-curve equivalents (Salvia & Ysseldyke, 2004). At each level, most reliability

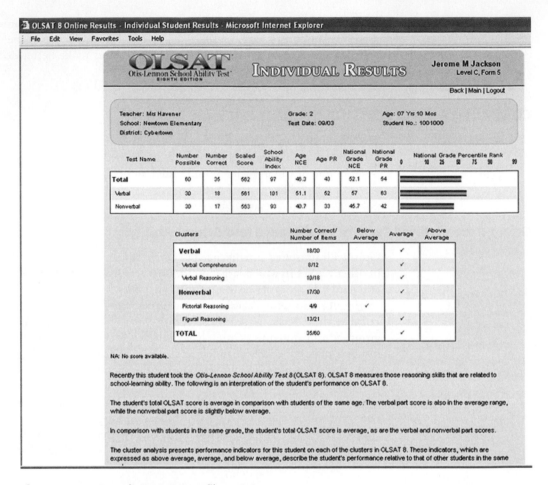

Figure 10.4   Sample *OLSAT-8* profile report

Source: © 2004 by Harcourt Assessment, Inc. Reproduced with permission.

coefficients ranged from 0.80 to 0.89, but some were as low as 0.63. No data on test stability were provided. Validity studies conducted yielded high correlations between the *OLSAT* and the *Stanford-Binet Intelligence Test*. Previous versions of the *OLSAT* were shown to underestimate the intellectual abilities of learning-disabled children, an important problem if using this information to generate referrals for special services. The authors also provided scant evidence of the relationship between *OLSAT* scores and school achievement (DeStephano, 2001).

Cognitive Abilities Test (CogAT)

The *Cognitive Abilities Test* (*CogAT*) (Lohman & Hagen, 2001) provides a measurement of level and pattern of cognitive development. The test can be administered to students K–12 and has 11 different levels. Both the primary battery (Levels K, 1,

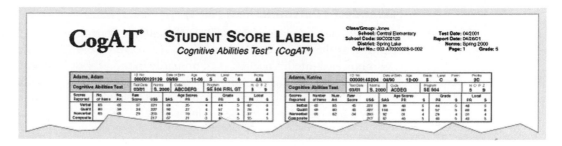

Figure 10.5   Sample *CogAT* score report

and 2) and the multilevel battery (Levels A–H) are broken into three batteries of skills: Verbal, Quantitative, and Nonverbal. The primary battery takes three sessions of 35 to 40 minutes each; the multilevel battery takes three sessions of 45 to 50 minutes each. Levels K, 1, and 2 have six subtests: Oral Vocabulary, Verbal Reasoning, Relational Concepts, Quantitative Concepts, Figure Classification, and Matrices. Levels A–H (used for 3rd- through 12th-graders) have nine subtests: Sentence Completion, Verbal Classification, Verbal Analogies, Quantitative Relations, Number Series, Equation Building, Figure Classification, Figure Analogies, and Figure Analysis. The number of items varies by level and subtest. Four scores— Verbal, Quantitative, Nonverbal, and Total—are given at each level, but subtest scores are not reported individually (see Figure 10.5 for a sample score report). The *CogAT* was standardized at the same time as the *Iowa Tests of Educational Development* (ITBD) and the *Iowa Test of Basic Skills* (ITBS) and conforms to U.S. population demographics (Salvia & Ysseldyke, 2004).

The *CogAT* offers a wide range of test levels for different-aged students. Standard age scores (M = 100; SD =15), national grade equivalents, age-based percentile ranks, and grade- and age-based stanines are available for the *CogAT.* Total battery score reliability coefficients for Level K range from $r = 0.85$ to $r = 0.89$; for Level 1, from $r = 0.87$ to $r = 0.93$; for Level 2, from $r = 0.86$ to $r = 0.92$; and for Levels A–H, from $r = 0.93$ to $r = 0.95$. The total-battery range is very high, from $r = 0.94$ to $r = 0.98$. Minimal validity data are provided in the manual (Salvia & Ysseldyke, 2004).

Multidimensional Aptitude Battery–II (MAB-II)

The *Multidimensional Aptitude Battery—II* (*MAB-II*) (Jackson, 1998) was designed as a group-administered alternative to the *Wechsler Adult Intelligence Scale—Revised* (*WAIS-R*—now *WAIS-III*), for administration to older adolescents and adults. Like the *Wechsler* adult version, the *MAB-II* yields a Verbal IQ score, Performance IQ score, and Full Scale IQ score. The Verbal and Performance scales are each composed of five subtests and each subtest has a time limit of 7 minutes.

Wonderlic Personnel Test (WPT)

The *Wonderlic Personnel Test* (*WPT*) (Wonderlic Personnel Test, 1998), formerly known as the *Wonderlic Personnel Test and Scholastic Level Exam,* is another group-administered intelligence test used primarily in industry or business. The *WPT* is a speeded test requiring the completion of 50 items within a 12-minute time limit. The *WPT* has several alternate forms and can be administered online, by computer, or by traditional paper-and-pencil format.

Individual Screening Tests of Intelligence

This section reviews several commonly used individualized tests of intelligence used primarily for screening purposes. Recall that screening tests are used to identify students or clients in need of deeper-level diagnostic testing to identify cognitive or learning strengths and weaknesses or to make placement decisions. It is inappropriate to use screening-level tests as the primary instruments for diagnostic or placement decisions, although they can be helpful in an ancillary capacity to validate those decisions.

Slosson Intelligence Test–Revised (SIT-R3)

The *SIT-R3* (Nicholson & Hipshman, 1997) is a 187-item screening test for verbal ability. It usually requires about 15 to 30 minutes to administer and score. Although the items measure diverse verbal subconstructs, including vocabulary, similarities and differences, comprehension, general information, quantitative, and auditory memory abilities, the total score is interpreted as a unidimensional construct called Total Standard Score (M = 100; SD = 16). The *SIT-R3* is a quick, cost-efficient, untimed test useful with clients ages 4 years through adulthood (Campbell & Ashmore, 1995; McKechnie & Erford, 2001). Items are scored correct (1 point) or incorrect (0 points), and age-related starting points are provided. Ten consecutive items are required to establish basal and ceiling levels. The *SIT-R3* standardization sample over-samples White participants but generally conforms to U.S. population estimates. Undersampling of minorities was noted (Watson, 1994), as was rural and urban sampling.

Raw scores are converted to standard scores, percentile ranks, and age and grade equivalents (see Figure 1.3 for a sample *SIT-R3* protocol). Because the *SIT-R3* measures only verbal abilities (e.g., crystallized intelligence), it is not a comprehensive indicator of intelligence in the same way as the *Wechsler Intelligence Scales for Children—Fourth Edition* (*WISC-IV*) or *SB-5*. In fact, the *SIT-R3* correlates substantially higher with Verbal IQ than Performance IQ (Nicholson & Hipshman, 1997). Substantial correlations with other verbal ability tests were reported. KR-20 estimates ranged from r = 0.88 to r = 0.97 (*Mdn* = 0.925), which appear more than adequate (Kamphaus, 1994). One study of test-retest reliability (n = 41) reported r = 0.96. This was a small sample for confidence in results (McKechnie & Erford, 2001), and no descriptions of these 41 subjects were provided (Johns & Van Leirsburg, 1994). The *SIT-R3* has been deemed useful as a screening test for mental retardation (Kunen, Overstreet, & Salles, 1996). With the gifted population, the *SIT-R3* has a tendency to inflate scores (Clark, McCallum, Edwards, & Hildman, 1987; Smith, Klass, & Stovall, 1992). Unfortunately, no age differentiation in norms is provided over age 18 years (Watson, 1994), as all adults 18 and older are lumped into this final age group.

Slosson Intelligence Test–Primary (SIT-P)

The *SIT-P* (Erford, Vitali, & Slosson, 1999) is a brief, 121-item screening-level test of typical developmental skills of early childhood that is used for children ages 2–7 years. It usually requires about 30 minutes to administer. A basal level is established when a child correctly answers seven consecutive questions; a ceiling is determined when the child is unable to answer seven consecutive items (Erford et al., 1999). Various theoretical models of intelligence were incorporated into the development of the test. Verbal and nonverbal items are used, drawing from many of the domains used in the *WISC-III* or the *SBIS-4*. Items are scored correct (1 point) or incorrect (0 points), and are simply totaled to reach the Verbal Scale Total Score, Nonverbal Scale Total Score, and Total Score. Conversion tables in the manual convert the scores to percentile ranks, age equivalencies, and standard scores ($M = 100$; $SD = 15$) (Erford et al., 1999).

The standardization sample was made up of children from Virginia and Maryland ages 2–7 years. The sample generally conformed to the 1990 U.S. Census statistics, though the socioeconomic level of the sample was slightly higher than average, and there were slightly more White and slightly fewer Hispanic children in the sample. KR-20 coefficients ranged from $r = 0.72$ to $r = 0.97$, and internal consistency coefficients for the Verbal, Nonverbal, and Total scales for the entire standardization sample were $r = 0.95$, 0.97, and 0.98, respectively (Erford, Vitali, & Slosson, 1999). The *SIT-P* was correlated with scores on similar tests (*SBIS-4, WISC-III, SIT-R TSS, PPVT-R,* and *EOWPVT-R*), and the total-scale score correlation ranged from 0.46 to 0.74. Several techniques were used to demonstrate the construct validity of the *SIT-P,* and all highly asserted construct validity.

Wechsler Abbreviated Scale of Intelligence (WASI)

The *Wechsler Abbreviated Scale of Intelligence* (*WASI*) (Wechsler, 1999) is an individually administered brief measure of intelligence for clients ages 6–89 years. It is most often used for screening purposes, when time or resources are limited, for quickly estimating full-scale IQ, or for reevaluations. The test is made up of the four subtests yielding the most reliable and valid scores from the Verbal Comprehension and Perceptual Reasoning Indexes of the *Wechsler* series of IQ tests (i.e., Block Design, Matrix Reasoning, Vocabulary, and Similarities). All four subtests can be administered in about 30 minutes, or two subtests can be administered in about 15 minutes. The test's norm sample had 2,245 cases and generally conformed to U.S. population demographics. Raw scores can be converted to standard scores, T scores, percentile ranks, Verbal IQ, Performance IQ, and Full Composite IQ scores ($M = 100$; $SD = 15$) (The Psychological Corporation, 2005a). *WASI* scores correlate to a very high degree with complementary subtests and Index scores on the diagnostic *Wechsler* series, but like other *Wechsler* scales, *WASI* scores rarely connect to anything beyond the *Wechsler* terminology. Split-half reliabilities for all tests and all age levels are in an acceptable 0.81 to 0.98 range for subtests and 0.92 to 0.98 for IQs. Test-retest coefficients (2- to 12-week intervals) range from 0.83 to 0.95. Validity information supports the use of the *WASI* but could be more complete (Keith, 2001).

Kaufman Brief Intelligence Test–Second Edition (KBIT-2)

The *Kaufman Brief Intelligence Test—Second Edition* (*KBIT-2*) (Kaufman & Kaufman, 2004b) is a quick (15- to 30-minute) estimate of intelligence and can be used to screen students for potential educational problems and gifted programs. It can be used with clients ages 4–90 years. The *KBIT-2* consists of an IQ composite score with two subtests: Vocabulary (verbal, crystallized) and Matrices (nonverbal, fluid). Items are scored right (1 point) or wrong (0 points). During the standardization process, adequate consideration was given to U.S. population demographics based on the U.S. Census (Overton, 1996). Raw scores can be converted to standard scores and national percentile ranks by age. Split-half reliability and test-retest coefficients are satisfactory, ranging between 0.80 and 0.90. Criterion-related validity studies were conducted with the original *K-BIT,* the *WISC-R,* the *K-ABC,* and the *WAIS-R*, yielding satisfactory validity coefficients (Overton, 1996). Hayes (1999) reported the original *KBIT* appeared culture-fair and relatively free of gender or ethnic bias. Overall, the *KBIT-2* is a brief, efficient, and technically adequate screening measure for a balanced estimate of intellectual ability.

Individual Diagnostic Tests of Intelligence

When making diagnostic or placement decisions for students or clients, individualized tests of intelligence are frequently used. To belong to this category, intelligence tests must demonstrate a high degree of score reliability and validity, and be helpful in determining learning or cognitive strengths and weaknesses. These tests are frequently used in education to determine whether a child has a learning disability or mental retardation, and are part of comprehensive psychological and neuropsychological assessments for adult clients. Following are a number of the most popular individual diagnostic tests of intelligence used in education and clinical practice.

The various *Wechsler* tests (*WAIS-III, WISC-IV, WPPSI-III*)

- *Wechsler Preschool and Primary Scale of Intelligence—Third Edition* (*WPPSI-III*) (Wechsler, 2002): ages 2 years, 6 months–7 years, 3 months
- *Wechsler Intelligence Scale for Children—Fourth Edition* (*WISC-IV*) (Wechsler, 2001a, 2001b): ages 6–16 years
- *Wechsler Adult Intelligence Scale—Third Edition* (*WAIS-III*) (Wechsler, 1997): ages 16 years through adult

Each of the *Wechsler* tests is designed to measure intellectual ability of students or clients at various age levels ranging from 2 years, 6 months through adult. Table

Table 10.5   Index and subtest composition of the *WPPSI-III*, *WISC-IV*, and *WAIS-III*

WPPSI-III	*WISC-IV*	*WAIS-III*
Verbal	**Verbal comprehension**	**Verbal comprehension**
Similarities	Similarities	Similarities
Vocabulary	Vocabulary	Vocabulary
Comprehension	Comprehension	Comprehension
Information	Information	Information
Word Reasoning	Word Reasoning	
Picture Naming		
Receptive Vocabulary		
Performance	**Perceptual reasoning**	**Perceptual organization factor**
Block Design	Block Design	Block Design
Picture Concepts	Picture Concepts	Picture Arrangement
Matrix Reasoning	Matrix Reasoning	Matrix Reasoning
Picture Completion	Picture Completion	Picture Completion
Object Assembly		Object Assembly
	Working memory	**Working memory**
	Digit Span	Digit Span
	Letter-Number Sequencing	Letter-Number Sequencing
	Arithmetic	Arithmetic
Processing speed	**Processing speed**	**Processing speed**
Coding	Coding	Digit Symbol–Coding
Symbol Search	Symbol Search	Symbol Search
	Cancellation	

10.5 indicates subtest components of the various index scores, and Table 10.6 provides brief descriptions of various *WPPSI-III, WISC-IV,* and *WAIS-III* subtests. The Full Scale IQ composite score is composed of different subtest configurations, depending on the *Wechsler* level used. All *Wechsler* versions require Level C qualifications. Administration time varies by version, as does the number of subtests given. Generally, the *WPPSI-III* takes between 45 and 75 minutes, while the *WISC-IV* and *WAIS-III* may take from 60 to 90 minutes. Scoring for most subtests is completed using a 0 (wrong) and 1 (correct) point scale. However, several verbal comprehension subtests use a 0 to 2 scale, dependent on answer quality, and scoring can become quite difficult (Slate & Hunnicutt, 1988). Scoring criteria are thoroughly described in the various *Wechsler* administration and scoring manuals. Starting points for each subtest are designated, but if clients miss one of the first several items, the test administrator reverses the administration sequence to determine the basal level; ceiling levels are designated for most subtests. According to Sattler and Dumont (2004), the stratified sampling methods used for the *WISC-IV* and *WPPSI-III* were

Table 10.6 *WISC-IV* subtests

Similarities	Measures verbal abstract reasoning, verbal concept formation. Two objects or concepts are presented verbally, and the client tells how the concepts are alike or the same.
Vocabulary	Measures word knowledge, word usage, and verbal fluency. Clients define words.
Comprehension	Measures social knowledge, common sense, level of social maturation, and moral judgment. Clients respond to questions about what to do in social situations requiring problem solving.
Information	Measures general cultural knowledge, long-term memory, and acquired facts. Clients are asked a wide range of questions covering general information that is taught in school.
Word Reasoning	Measures verbal abstract reasoning, concept formation, and expression. Clients are presented with one-word descriptive clues and are asked to identify an object or concept.
Block Design	Measures the spatial reasoning and visual analysis. Clients are asked to reproduce increasingly abstract designs using red and white plastic blocks. This task is timed.
Picture Concepts	Measures categorical, abstract reasoning. Clients compare rows of pictures and choose one picture from each row that is conceptually similar to a picture in another row.
Matrix Reasoning	Measures nonverbal, analogical reasoning, and simultaneous processing. The child chooses the pattern that best completes the visual matrix set from among several possible pattern choices.
Picture Completion	Measures recognition of familiar items and identification of missing parts. The client is asked to identify missing parts within a whole object or picture.
Digit Span	Measures short-term auditory memory and attention span. The examiner presents a set of random digits, and the client is asked to remember and recite the numbers. On the second part, the client recites the digits in reverse order.
Letter-Number Sequencing	Measures attention span, short-term auditory memory, and organizational and sequencing abilities. The client listens to a set of random digits and letters and then must recite the numbers in chronological order and the letters in alphabetical order.
Arithmetic	Measures numerical accuracy and reasoning, and attention/distractibility. The test consists of basic mathematical story problems, which are presented orally to the client. Without using pencil and paper, the client must determine the correct answers. This task is timed.
Coding	Measures processing speed, associative nonverbal learning, and short-term visual memory. The client must quickly write in symbols paired with digits. The quicker a client processes information and visually memorizes the digit-symbol pair, the faster the performance. This task is timed.
Symbol Search	Measures speed in recognizing symbols. The client is presented with a stimulus symbol and asked to find this symbol quickly in another set of symbols. This task is timed.
Cancellation	Measures speed in processing visual information, visual vigilance or neglect, and selective attention. The examinee is presented with a target stimulus (i.e., animals). The client is then presented with a group of items and asked to draw a line through all those that do not have the same characteristics as the target stimulus. This task is timed.

outstanding. Standardization of the *WAIS-III* was adequate, and the norm sample was stratified according to U.S. population demographics based on the 1990 census (Drummond, 2000).

The *WPPSI-III, WISC-IV,* and *WAIS-III* all report deviation IQs (M = 100; SD = 15) for the Full Scale IQ and Index scores, and scaled scores (M = 10; SD = 3) for the individual subtests (see Figure 10.6). Norm tables provided in the administration and scoring manuals are well designed and allow standard scores to be converted to percentile ranks, age equivalents, and qualitative descriptors. Convenient norm tables present 90% and 95% confidence intervals for standard

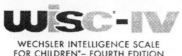

WECHSLER INTELLIGENCE SCALE FOR CHILDREN® – FOURTH EDITION

Child's Name ___SARAH___

Examiner's Name _____

Calculation of Child's Age

	Year	Month	Day
Date of Testing	2006	8	21
Date of Birth	1993	3	5
Age at Testing	13	5	16

Total Raw Score to Scaled Score Conversions

Subtest	Raw Score	Scaled Scores				
Block Design	9		9			9
Similarities	17	17				17
Digit Span	9			9		9
Picture Concepts	10		10			10
Coding	11				11	11
Vocabulary	10	10				10
Letter–Number Seq.	8			8		8
Matrix Reasoning	12		12			12
Comprehension	13	13				13
Symbol Search	16				16	16
(Picture Completion)	11		(11)			(11)
(Cancellation)	12				(12)	(12)
(Information)	10	(10)				(10)
(Arithmetic)	10			(10)		(10)
(Word Reasoning)	11	(11)				(11)
Sums of Scaled Scores		40	31	17	27	115
		Verbal Comp.	Perc. Rsng.	Work. Mem.	Proc. Speed	Full Scale

Sum of Scaled Scores to Composite Score Conversions

Scale	Sum of Scaled Scores	Composite Score	Percentile Rank	___% Confidence Interval
Verbal Comprehension	40	VCI 119	90	111-125
Perceptual Reasoning	31	PRI 102	55	94-109
Working Memory	17	WMI 91	27	84-99
Processing Speed	27	PSI 121	92	110-127
Full Scale	115	FSIQ 111	77	106-116

Ⓨ**PsychCorp**™

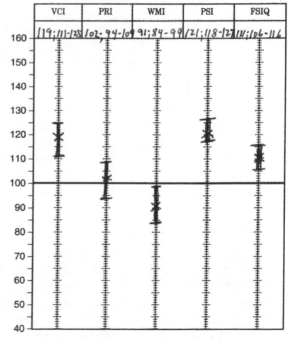

Figure 10.6 *WISC-IV* protocol cover sheet for Sarah

Source: Copyright 2003 by The Psychological Corporation, a Harcourt Assessment, Inc. Company. Reproduced with permission.

scores. All index scores have high enough reliability to allow for confident diagnostic interpretation; however, subtest reliability coefficients vary substantially across age levels, and most do not reach the level of confidence required for diagnostic purposes. Thus subtest interpretation must be undertaken with caution and validated through other measures. The best use of subtest scores is for hypothesis generation or validation.

Overall, internal consistency reliability coefficients for the *WISC-IV* scores ranged from $r = 0.91$ to $r = 0.95$ on the Verbal Comprehension Index; from $r = 0.91$ to $r = 0.93$ on the Perceptual Reasoning Index; from $r = 0.90$ to $r = 0.93$ on the Working Memory Index; from $r = 0.81$ to $r = 0.90$ on the Processing Speed Index; and from $r = 0.96$ to $r = 0.97$ for the full-scale IQ. Overall, internal consistency reliability for the *WPPSI-III* ranged from $r = 0.94$ to $r = 0.96$ on the Verbal IQ; from $r = 0.89$ to $r = 0.95$ on the Performance IQ; and from $r = 0.95$ to $r = 0.97$ for the Full Scale IQ (Sattler & Dumont, 2004). The *WAIS-III* also had good overall reliability coefficients, with split-half reliability coefficients of $r = 0.98$ for the Full Scale IQ; $r = 0.97$ for the Verbal IQ; and $r = 0.94$ for the Performance IQ. Test-retest reliability coefficients were lower, ranging from the high 0.80s to mid-0.90s (Drummond, 2000). The *WISC-III* was shown to yield stable scores over 2–3 years with a sample of disabled students (Canivez & Watkins, 1998).

Validity studies reported in the manuals conducted on the *Wechsler* tests are adequate. Most of the validity study participants tested yielded average intelligence; therefore, it may be argued that little is known about how the test performs in the extreme ranges of intellectual ability (Sattler & Dumont, 2004). Sattler (2001) raised potential concerns over cultural bias of some *WAIS-III* items, particularly on the Picture Arrangement and Comprehension subtests. Kwate (2001) went so far as to call the *WISC-III* "Euro-centrist" and not appropriate for assessing racial and ethnic minorities in the United States. Some concern has also been raised about the scales' score sensitivity and differential capabilities for use with individuals who are extremely gifted or severely mentally retarded. Also, gifted students with uneven profiles may not be identified using the *WISC Full Scale IQ* (Fishkin & Kampsnider, 1996). Several of the less technically adequate subtests were eliminated on the *WISC-IV,* perhaps presaging their eventual elimination from the next edition of the *WAIS* (e.g., Object Assembly, Picture Arrangement). A strength of the *Wechsler* scales continues to be the latitude given to examiners to actively probe and clearly evaluate examinee understanding (Sattler & Dumont, 2004). The materials are colorful, attractive, and engaging. The game-like features of subtests hold the interest of even young children.

The conorming of the *WISC* and *WIAT* allows examiners to minimize the effects of statistical regression when comparing discrepancies between intellectual ability and academic achievement (Kaufman & Lichtenberger, 2000). Criticisms of the use of the bonus points for speed on subtests of previous versions (Branden, 1995) were addressed on the *WISC-IV* by elimination of most bonus elements. Such practices were suspected of suppressing the scores of bright, yet reflective, children.

Because the correlations between previous versions of the *Wechsler* tests correlate so highly with the most recent editions ($r = 0.85$–0.95, usually), much of the technical adequacy demonstrated by previous versions (and interpretive strategies) should also be applicable to the revised editions. Previous versions of the *Wechsler* scales were among the most frequently studied intelligence tests (Sandoval, 1995). The technical characteristics have traditionally been outstanding and by all appearances, the most recent editions have improved on these traditions. Thus the *Wechsler* series of intelligence tests continue to set the standard for measurement of intelligence.

Stanford-Binet Intelligence Scales—Fifth Edition (SB-5)

The *SB-5* (Roid, 2003) is used to measure intelligence and cognitive abilities for clients ages 2–85 years. The *SB-5* has two routing tests, one each for the verbal and the nonverbal domains, and a total of five subscales under each: Fluid Reasoning, Knowledge, Quantitative Reasoning, Visual-Spatial Processing, and Working Memory (see Figure 10.7). The test is untimed, with an average testing time of about 5 minutes per facet. The examiner determines the basal (4 items/points passed) and ceiling levels (2 or fewer items/points correct).

Standardization was stratified according to U.S. population demographics, based on the U.S. Census.

The *SB-5* is helpful in assessing clients with minimal English abilities, deafness, and communication disorders. Raw scores can be transformed into scaled scores ($M = 10$; $SD = 3$) and combined to yield standard scores ($M = 100$; $SD = 15$), percentile ranks, age equivalents, and change-sensitive scores. Reliability for *SB-5* scores appears adequate, and criterion-related validity coefficients were moderate to strong with other measures. The previous version, *SBIS-4* (Thorndike, Hagen, & Sattler, 1986a, 1986b), was reportedly a useful test for making decisions about students with learning disabilities and short-term memory deficiencies (Laurent, Swerdlik, & Ryburn, 1992), but of questionable value when used to assess individuals with mental retardation or the gifted at certain ages (Bracey, 1994; Laurent et al., 1992; Silverman, 1986; Silverman & Kearney, 1992). Robinson (1992) found even the most difficult items on many subtests to be easy for gifted students above 11 years of age. Whether these deficiencies have been corrected in the *SB-5* remains in question.

Kaufman Assessment Battery for Children—Second Edition (KABC-II)

The *KABC-II* (Kaufman & Kaufman, 2004a) is an individually administered test used to assess cognitive ability. The test is based on two theoretical models, the Luria neuropsychological model (which excludes verbal ability) and the Cattell-Horn-Carroll model (CHC). The test administrator can choose which form, the Luria or the CHC, to use based on the client's cultural and/or language background. The Luria format takes 25 to 55 minutes to administer, while the CHC format requires 35 to 70 minutes. The *KABC-II* can be used with clients ages 3–18 years, with applicable subtests varying by age. The five scales (and related subtests) on the *KABC-II* include Simultaneous (Triangles, Face Recognition, Pattern Reasoning, Block Counting, Story Completion, Conceptual Thinking, Rover, Gestalt Closure);

Name THOMAS Sex: F M
Last   First   MI

ID # _____ **Examiner** _____

School/Agency _____ **Grade** _____

Stanford BINET Intelligence Scales Fifth Edition
Record Form

	Year	Month	Day
Testing Date	2006	6	12
Birth Date	1984	2	8
Age	22	4	4

Nonverbal (NV) Domain

	FR	KN	QR	VS	WM	
Raw Scores: Level 1	(ROUTING)			4	4	
Level 2	6	6	6	6		
Level 3	6	6	6	6		
Level 4	6	6	5	4		
Level 5	5	3	1	0		
Level 6	1	0	0	0		
Raw Score Total	28	24	21	22	20	Nonverbal Sum of Scaled Scores
NV Scaled Score Appendix A	10+	11+	8+	9+	7 =	45

Verbal (V) Domain

	FR	KN	QR	VS	WM	
Raw Scores: Level 2	6	(ROUTING)	6	6	6	
Level 3	6		6	6	6	
Level 4	6		5	6	6	
Level 5	3		2	6	7	
Level 6	0		0	2	0	Verbal Sum of Scaled Scores
Raw Score Total	21	45	19	26	20	
V Scaled Score Appendix A	11+	11+	9+	13+	8 =	52

	FR	KN	QR	VS	WM
Sum of NV and V Scaled Scores	21	22	17	22	15

Appendix B

	Sum of Scaled Scores	Standard Score	Percentile Rank	____% Confidence Interval
NVIQ +	45	93	32	87 to 99
VIQ =	52	102	55	96 to 108
FSIQ	97	98	45	94 to 102
FR	21	103	58	95 to 111
KN	22	106	66	98 to 114
QR	17	92	30	85 to 101
VS	22	106	66	98 to 114
WM	15	86	18	79 to 95

Composite Profile-Standard Scores

NVIQ	VIQ	FSIQ	FR	KN	QR	VS	WM
93	102	98	103	106	92	106	86

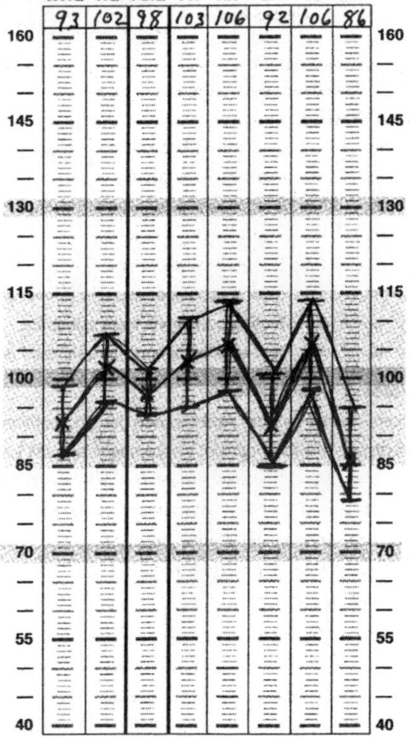

Subtest Profile-Scaled Scores

	Nonverbal (NV)					Verbal (V)				
	FR	KN	QR	VS	WM	FR	KN	QR	VS	WM
	10	11	8	9	7	11	11	9	13	8

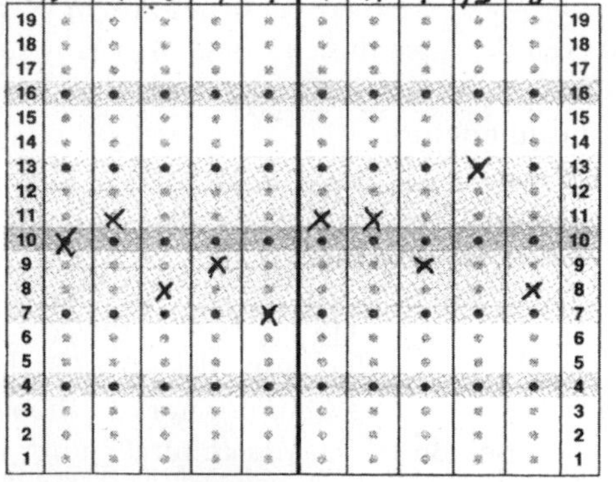

Riverside Publishing

Figure 10.7 *SB-5* cover sheet for Thomas

Sequential (Word Order, Number Recall, Hand Movements); Planning (Pattern Reasoning, Story Completion); Learning (Atlantis, Atlantis Delayed, Rebus, Rebus Delayed); and Knowledge (*CHC* model only) (Riddles, Expression Vocabulary, Verbal Knowledge). The standardization sample of 3,025 individuals generally conformed to U.S. population demographics in terms of ethnicity and was generally equally divided by sex (Kaufman & Kaufman, 2004a).

The *KABC-II* is a culturally sensitive measure of cognitive ability. Raw scores can be transformed into age-based scaled scores, standard scores ($M = 100$; $SD = 15$), age equivalents, and percentile ranks. Test scale scores had mean reliability coefficients ranging from 0.87 to 0.96. Subtest score mean reliability coefficients were more variable, ranging from 0.74 to 0.92. The validity of the original *KABC* has been widely disputed; however, the validity of the revised *KABC-II* seems adequate according to the technical manual (Kaufman & Kaufman, 2004a).

Woodcock-Johnson Tests of Cognitive Ability—Third Edition (WJ-III-COG)

The *WJ-III COG* (McGrew & Woodcock, 2001; Woodcock, Mather, & McGrew 2001) is a comprehensive assessment of intelligence and general ability based on the Cattell-Horn-Carroll (CHC) model of cognitive abilities, one of the best and most theoretically sound descriptions of the structure of intelligence (Keith, Kransler, & Flanagan, 2001). It is designed to help with diagnosis of learning disabilities, determine educational discrepancies, develop educational plans for individuals, assess growth, and offer guidance in educational and clinical settings for anyone over 24 months of age. A total of 20 subtests (see Table 10.7) can be administered individually (some can be adapted for group administration). Depending on examiner or examinee needs, different combinations of the tests can be used. For example, by using the Verbal Comprehension, Concept Formation, and Visual Matching subtests, a Brief Intelligence Ability score can be derived that is helpful for screenings or reevaluations without a comprehensive assessment. Likewise, a General Intellectual Ability score can also be found using multiple subtests from the battery. Each subtest is easy to administer and takes about 5 minutes to complete. Scoring must be accomplished using the accompanying Compuscore software. There is a standard and an extended version of the battery. The standard version of the test is made up of the first 10 subtests, and the extended version includes the last 10 subtests. The subtests were designed to measure the seven factors of the Cattell-Horn-Carroll model: Comprehension-Knowledge (Gc); Long-Term Retrieval (Glr); Visual-Spatial (Gv); Reasoning (Gf); Processing Speed (Gs); and Short-Term Memory (Gsm).

This norm-referenced test is very useful for developing a wide range of derived scores, including standard scores ($M = 100$; $SD = 15$), age and grade equivalents, percentile ranks, discrepancy scores, and many scores reported using the scales developed for this specific test (Cizek, 2003). The reliability and validity results are impressive, and the test's normative data are sufficient to be able to use the test as an accurate diagnostic tool. Cizek commented that some diagnostic examples and intervention strategies would be useful, in addition to some Compuscore reports and interpretations. Sandoval (2003) commented that all of the materials are very well done and

Table 10.7 *WJ-III COG* subtests

Subtest and factor association	Description
1. Verbal Comprehension (Gc)	Measures lexical knowledge and language development. Examinees are asked to identify pictures of familiar and unfamiliar objects and to respond to antonyms, synonyms, and verbal analogies.
2. Visual-Auditory Learning (Glr)	Measures visual-auditory association. Examinees must associate new visual symbols with familiar words and translate a series of symbols into verbal sentences.
3. Spatial Relations (Gv)	Measures visual processing. Examinees select from a visual list the component parts needed to complete the whole shape.
4. Sound Blending (Ga)	Measures auditory phonics coding. Examinees must integrate and say whole words after hearing parts of them.
5. Concept Formation (Gf)	Measures ability to deduce relations. Examinees identify the rules for concepts when shown illustrations of both instances and noninstances of the concepts.
6. Visual Matching (Gs)	Measures speed in visual discrimination. Examinees visually identify two numerals that are alike in a row of six numbers. As the items progress, the task becomes increasingly difficult.
7. Numbers Reversed (Gsm)	Measures short-term auditory memory. Examinees repeat a series of random numbers backward.
8. Incomplete Words (Ga)	Measures auditory closure. Examinees must state a complete word after listening to a word missing one or more phonemes.
9. Auditory Working Memory (Gsm)	Measures working memory. Examinees are first asked to listen to a mixed set of numbers and words, then put this series in sequential order, words first, then numbers.
10. Visual-Auditory Learning-Delayed (Glr)	Measures delayed recollection after 1 to 8 days. Examinees are presented with symbols from Visual-Auditory Learning, state the name of each, and are retested later, without knowing the retest will occur.
11. General Information (Gc)	Measures general verbal information and contains two subtests. In the first subtest, examinees are asked where one would find a certain object. In the second subtest, examinees are asked what one would do with this object.
12. Retrieval Fluency (Glr)	Measures ideation fluency. Examinees are given a category and asked to name as many examples from that category as possible in 1 minute.
13. Picture Recognition (Gv)	Measures visual memory. Examinees must recognize a subset of previously presented pictures within a field of distracting pictures.
14. Auditory Attention (Ga)	Measures speech-sound discrimination and resistance to auditory stimulus distortion. Examinees are presented with four pictures and are asked to listen to a word that is audiotaped and superimposed over background noise. Examinees are then asked to point to the correct picture for that word..
15. Analysis-Synthesis (Gf)	Measures analysis of deductive reasoning. Examinees must analyze a puzzle composed of colored squares.
16. Decision Speed (Gs)	Measures semantic processing speed. Examinees are presented with a row of pictures and are asked to identify the two pictures that are most similar.
17. Memory for Words (Gsm)	Measures serial auditory memory. Examinees repeat lists of unrelated words in correct sequences.
18. Rapid Picture Naming (Gs)	Measures naming facility and speed. Examinees are presented with a series of pictures and are asked to name them within a 2-minute time limit.
19. Planning (Gv)/(Gf)	Measures executive processing, spatial scanning, and general sequential reasoning. Examinees are asked to trace an outline without picking up their pencil or retracing lines.
20. Pair Cancellation (Gs)	Measures attention and concentration. Examinees are asked to identify and circle a repeated pattern in a 3-minute time limit.

useful, and the manual is very comprehensive. Rizza, McIntosh, & McGunn (2001) indicated the cognitive battery provides multiple means for analyzing specific strengths and weaknesses of gifted students. Proctor and Prevatt (2003) reported that the six different types of discrepancies scores derived can be very helpful in the diagnosis of learning disabilities.

Das-Naglieri Cognitive Assessment System (CAS)

The *CAS* (Naglieri & Das, 1996) is a measure of cognitive processing that uses a battery of tasks. It is very well researched, uses nontraditional approaches for assessing differences in intelligence (Meikamp, 2001), and, in general, reduces the emphasis on client verbal and language skills compared with other prominent intelligence tests. It has two formats, basic and standard. The Basic Battery has 8 subtests and can be administered in 40 minutes. The Standard Battery has 12 subtests and can be administered in 60 minutes. The *CAS* is individually administered and is appropriate for clients ages 5 to 17 years. The test is based on the PASS approach, developed by its authors, which is supported by the basic cognitive functions of Planning, Attention, and Simultaneous and Successive processing (Anastasi & Urbina, 1997). The Planning function includes the Matching Numbers, Planned Codes, and Planned Connections subtests. The Attention function includes the Expressive Attention, Number Detection, and Receptive Attention subtests. The Simultaneous Processing function includes the Nonverbal Matrices, Verbal-Spatial Relations, and Figure Memory subtests. The Successive Processing function includes the Word Series, Sentence Repetition, Speech Rates (ages 5 to 7 years), and Sentence Questions (ages 8 to 17 years) subtests. The inclusion of the Planning and Attention scales make this test unique compared with other traditional methods of intelligence assessment (Meikamp). Thompson (2001) reported that the directions for administration are straightforward, and it is easy to learn to administer. According to the test publisher (Riverside Publishing, 2005a), stratified standardization samples (*n* = 2,200) conformed to U.S. population demographics.

Raw scores for the *CAS* can be converted into scaled scores, standard scores (*M* = 100; *SD* = 15 for the Full Scale score), percentile ranks, and age equivalents. According to the *Interpretive Handbook,* score reliability is reportedly excellent, as the full-scale internal consistency coefficient was 0.96, and PASS scale reliabilities ranged between 0.83 and 0.93. The test-retest reliability coefficients ranged from *r* = 0.64 to *r* = 0.92, with an average interval of 21 days (Meikamp, 2001). Discriminant validity was supported in the *Interpretive Manual,* and other reliability and validity studies were reviewed (Riverside Publishing, 2005a). Meikamp warned that even though the *CAS* can help to gain a broader understanding of individual differences, comparisons of PASS scales and subtest scores may be easily misinterpreted, and further empirical research is necessary. Thompson (2001) concluded that he found the *CAS* to be a more superior measure of intelligence than the *Stanford-Binet (Fourth Edition)*, but because of easier use and scoring interpretation, he preferred the *Wechsler* scales.

ASSESSING MENTAL RETARDATION

The assessment of **mental retardation** involves obtaining information in three primary areas: (1) sociocultural history (2) intellectual functioning, and (3) adaptive functioning. Both the *DSM-IV-TR* (APA, 2000) and the Individuals With Disabilities Education Improvement Act (IDEIA) indicated that the essential features of mental retardation are significant subaverage intellectual and adaptive functioning. However, it is critical that a comprehensive assessment of social and cultural factors be undertaken. Evaluators must ensure that any noted cognitive deficiency does not result primarily from social, language, or cultural deprivation or from other factors that may create an unfair bias in test scores and hold the child at a disadvantage. The legal history of intelligence assessment is replete with instances in which poor practice decisions led to inaccurate diagnoses.

Importantly, **significant subaverage** has traditionally been defined as a performance falling at least two standard deviations below the mean on an individualized, standardized diagnostic test. Thus, on a norm-referenced test with $M = 100$ and $SD = 15$, significant subaverage performance would be any standard score of 70 or lower, effectively identifying approximately 2.27% of the population. Of course, some school systems set a more lenient criterion for identification. For example, it is not unusual for some local education agencies (LEAs, or school system) to allow identification of children with an IDEIA handicapping condition of Mental Retardation if their IQ test score goes as high as 75. Caution is warranted when making decisions using this more lenient criterion. Recall that using a standard score of 75 will identify approximately 5% of a normal school-aged population, effectively doubling the number of students eligible for special educational services with a handicapping condition of Mental Retardation.

Intellectual functioning is typically assessed using individualized, diagnostic intelligence tests, such as the *Wechsler Intelligence Scale for Children—Fourth Edition* (*WISC-IV*) (Wechsler, 2001a), *Stanford-Binet Intelligence Scales—Fifth Edition* (*SB-5*) (Roid, 2003), or the *Kaufman Assessment Battery for Children—Second Edition* (*KABC-II*) (Kaufman & Kaufman, 1983a, 1983b). Generally, in the identification of mental retardation, the test's Total Standard Score is used as the representative deviation IQ score, and examiners should ensure that very little index or subtest scatter is apparent.

Adaptive functioning is typically assessed using individual tests of adaptive behavior, such as the *Vineland Adaptive Behavior Scales* (*VABS*) (Harrison, 1985; Sparrow, Balla, & Cicchetti, 1984a, 1984b), or the American Association on Mental Retardation's *AAMR Adaptive Behavior Scale* (Lambert, Nihira, & Leland, 1993) These scales measure self-care, motor, social, and functional communication skills to determine an individual's ability to achieve independent living skills across wide areas of functioning. Again, standard scores in the Deficient to Low Borderline ranges (standard scores of about 75 and below; $M = 100$; $SD = 15$) generally are required to demonstrate significant subaverage adaptive functioning.

As examples, *WISC-IV* index and subtest profiles and *Vineland Adaptive Behavior Scales* profiles for Julie, Juan, and Latoya are given in Table 10.8. Even

Table 10.8   Comparison of *Wechsler Intelligence Scale for Children—Fourth Edition (WISC-IV)* and *Vineland Adaptive Behavior Scales—Classroom Edition (VABS-CE)* standard score profiles for three students being evaluated for possible mental retardation

	Julie	Juan	Latoya
WISC-IV Indices and Subtests			
Full Scale IQ (FSIQ)	69	69	69
Verbal Comprehension Index (VCI)	67	63	69
Similarities	4	3	4
Vocabulary	4	4	4
Comprehension	5	4	5
Perceptual Reasoning Index (PCI)	71	82	71
Block Design	5	7	5
Picture Concepts	6	6	6
Matrix Reasoning	5	8	5
Working Memory Index (WMI)	77	71	77
Digit Span	7	5	7
Letter-Number Sequencing	5	5	6
Processing Speed Index (PSI)	83	83	83
Coding	7	7	7
Symbol Search	7	7	7
Vineland Adaptive Behavior Scales—Classroom Edition (VABS-CE)			
Communication Domain	65	69	83
Daily Living Skills Domain	71	83	87
Socialization Domain	62	84	83
Adaptive Behavior Composite	63	75	82

though they have the identical Full Scale IQ score (FSIQ = 69), it is likely that Julie will be identified with Mental Retardation, while Juan and Latoya will not. Julie's cognitive profile is evenly developed, with no significant differences between the *WISC-IV* index scores or subtests. This means that her cognitive skills are evenly developed and fall in the Mildly Deficient to Borderline range. The same is true for her adaptive behavior as measured by the *VABS*—evenly developed and falling consistently in the Mildly Deficient to Low Average range. In contrast, Juan's *WISC-IV* Verbal Comprehension Index (VCI)—Perceptual Reasoning Index (PRI) split is too large, and the subtest profile is too scattered to have confidence that the low overall intellectual performance is not better explained by another cognitive or learning problem. Juan's adaptive behavior is also a bit too high and varied to conclude that he displays significant subaverage adaptive functioning. Juan's Daily Living Skills and Socialization Domains both fall in the Borderline to Low Average range, while his

Communication Domain standard score was a 69—tracking nicely with his demonstrated verbal skills on the *WISC-IV*. In Latoya's case, even though her *WISC-IV* scores are identical to Julie's, her adaptive behavior is clearly too high (i.e., consistently Low Average) to qualify for a handicapping condition of mentally retarded. Further exploration of developmental and socioeconomic factors should be conducted in her case.

Various degrees of severity are generally associated with Mental Retardation (MR). In general, examinees with deviation IQ scores ranging from 50–55 through 70 are identified with mild Mental Retardation, and these individuals are able to master some basic academic skills. Individuals with mild MR are frequently able to function independently for periods of time but generally require periodic supervision. Individuals with scores ranging from 35–40 through 50–55 are identified with moderate Mental Retardation and are generally unable to learn even basic academic skills, but they can be trained to perform manual tasks. Individuals with moderate MR require frequent supervision and are generally unable to maintain an independent lifestyle. Individuals with scores ranging below 35–40 are identified with severe and profound Mental Retardation, require constant supervision, and are frequently placed in residential treatment facilities during their adult years. Individuals with severe and profound MR often present with multiple handicapping conditions (i.e., orthopedic, visual, hearing).

ASSESSING GIFTEDNESS

Tests of intelligence measure wide-ranging intellectual capabilities and are helpful in identifying individuals performing at both ends of the intellectual continuum. The previous section dealt the identification of those in the significant subaverage range of ability—mental retardation. The other end of the continuum is the significant superaverage range—intellectual **giftedness**.

Terman (et al., 1925) was the first to systematically explore giftedness by administering his 1916 edition of the *Stanford-Binet* and identifying 1,528 children with an IQ of 140 or higher. His longitudinal study of these children over many years led him to conclude that they continued to perform in a very superior manner, intellectually, committed fewer than average crimes, held moderate social and political views, were in better-than-average physical condition, had lower-than-average mortality rates, and were educationally and vocationally successful. But the defining characteristics of giftedness have remained somewhat elusive even today, perhaps because of the wide-ranging abilities that truly gifted and talented individuals possess. Public Law 95-561 was one of the first federal attempts to help identify and serve the needs of gifted children. This law described gifted children as displaying consistently superior intellectual, leadership, mechanical, figural and visual, or creative abilities. Most of the impetus on identifying gifted individuals has fallen on to school systems.

Early on, most schools relied exclusively on intelligence tests to identify this population. Several problems arose from strict adherence to the sole use of IQ tests. First, most used the global ability score from these tests (i.e., the Full Scale IQ score on the *WISC-IV* or *SB-5*), which is a combination of all subtest scores. Generally, schools used a deviation IQ score of about 130 (two standard deviations above the mean) as a criterion for superior cognitive performance. As mentioned earlier, many brilliant people have strengths and weaknesses in their cognitive profile and these do not always average out to a Full Scale IQ of 130. Indeed, most IQ tests weight all subtests equally, even though each has a different relationship to *g*. Thus a brilliant, albeit anxious-perfectionistic individual may receive Very Superior scores on all subtests of the *WISC-IV* except for average performances on the two processing speed subtests and not reach the 130 IQ criterion. Second, it stands to reason that the purpose or goal of the program for gifted students should be taken into consideration in the selection process. Many school system programs for gifted students are little more than (or the equivalent of) honors or advanced placement courses found in numerous high schools today. Thus it makes sense to many jurisdictions that academic criteria should be in place to ensure that individuals with high IQs can also benefit from and be competitive in these advanced classes. That is, identification of an incredibly bright child should, in itself, not be the goal of a program for the gifted, if that child will not benefit from the services that school system affords a gifted child. For this reason, school systems often put an additional criterion in place related to academic performance. For example, a child may be required to score at the 95th or 98th percentile on a group- or individually administered test of achievement in one or more academic areas to be identified as a gifted student. In this way, the school system requires Superior to Very Superior intellectual abilities and academic skills of students being considered for gifted programming.

A third criterion is sometimes also added: ratings of gifted characteristics. Some researchers have identified behavioral characteristics of gifted students (e.g., enter into activities with eagerness, behavior dictated by personal values, receptive to new experiences), and some (Clark, 1979; Renzulli et al., 2002) have even developed rating scales of these characteristics for teachers to complete. While these rating scales can provide an additional helpful layer of identification, they can sometimes complicate the process and restrict program access for students who are something less than a model student. For example, an intellectually and academically superior student with a learning disability or AD/HD may be rated less worthy than a well-behaved but less intellectually and academically capable student. Any decision-making model will have its strengths and weaknesses. The important point here is that flexibility should be built into any decision-making system, and any placement decision should always be based on more than one test score. For this reason, great flexibility has been afforded school systems in identifying students for gifted services.

Importantly, some thought should be given to how students will be screened for placement consideration. Many school systems use a teacher nomination process, even though such systems have been shown unreliable at best (Jacobs, 1970; Tuttle & Becker, 1980) and biased at worst (i.e., girls nominated in far higher percentages than boys). As a result, many school systems use their already-existing group-administered standardized testing process to aid in screening. For example, by 2nd or 3rd grade, many schools have administered the *Otis-Lennon*

School Ability Test (*OLSAT*) or *Cognitive Abilities Test* (*CogAT*), as well as an achievement series such as the *TerraNova 2* or *Iowa Test of Basic Skills* (*ITBS*). Student scores on these tests can be used to make referrals for individualized diagnostic assessment and eventual placement decisions. Interestingly, these placement decisions are often made using the three decision-making methods discussed in Chapter 4, "Validity" (i.e., clinical judgment, multiple cutoff, and [modified] multiple regression).

SUMMARY/CONCLUSION

This chapter has provided insights into how various scholars have defined and conceptualized intelligence and how professional counselors can use intelligence tests and results to make decisions about, and advocate for, students and clients. The term *intelligence* is virtually synonymous with the terms *cognitive, mental, and school ability* but differs from the term *aptitude,* which predicts more proscribed vocational or educational abilities.

The early perspectives of Galton and Cattell relied on sensory information as determinants of intelligence. Spearman developed the single-global-factor (*g*) theory, and subsequent attempts to construct a theory of intelligence have basically been reactions to Spearman's model, including Thurstone's theory of primary mental abilities, the Horn-Cattell Gc/Gf model, Guilford's structure-of-intellect model, Vernon's hierarchical model, Sternberg's triarchic theory, and Gardner's theory of multiple intelligences.

Several controversial IQ issues were discussed: (1) IQ scores predict school performance and occupational success fairly well; (2) beyond early childhood, IQ scores tend to be stable throughout the lifespan; and (3) while racial and gender differences are observed from time to time, these differences are either relatively small or can be accounted for by various mediating variables (e.g., socioeconomic status, culture, environment experiences).

Numerous commonly used tests of intellectual ability were presented and reviewed. Some of these tests are group administered, others individually administered; some are screening-level instruments, others diagnostic tools. Their uses were sometimes explored in the context within which decisions may be made, including when diagnosing mental retardation or giftedness, or when assessing clients from different cultures or with low-incidence handicaps.

Whether professional counselors are administering, interpreting, or reading the results of intelligence tests to better understand client needs and concerns, understanding the theory and applications of intellectual assessment information is critical to effective advocacy, diagnosis, and treatment of clients and students.

KEY TERMS

accommodation	assimilation
adaptive functioning	crystallized abilities
aptitude	fluid abilities

general factor (*g*)
giftedness
group-administered test
hierarchical model
intelligence
intelligence testing

mental retardation
multiple-factor theories
schemata
significant subaverage
sociocultural bias

CHAPTER 11

Assessment of Other Aptitudes

by Bradley T. Erford and Kathleen McNinch

While intelligence tests are a type of aptitude measure, this chapter deals with more widely construed measures of scholastic and general aptitude, as well as measures of specific aptitudes. Scholastic aptitude tests such as the *Scholastic Assessment Test* (*SAT*) and the *American College Testing Assessment* (*ACT*) will be reviewed, as well as more generalized aptitude measures, such as the *Differential Aptitude Test* (*DAT*) and the *Armed Services Vocational Aptitude Battery* (*ASVAB*).

Tests that measure aptitudes, intelligence, and achievement overlap in some very important ways. For example, all three types of tests assess verbal abilities, numerical and quantitative skills, and reasoning (problem solving). However, the primary difference among these three categories of assessment involves the purpose for which each is used. *Aptitude* and *intelligence tests* are used primarily to predict future performance, while *achievement tests* are designed to measure what a student or client has already learned, usually through some sort of structured curricular activity. In this way, achievement tests describe current academic skills that are emerging or have been mastered. Performance on tests measuring aptitudes is influenced not by previously learned content or instruction in an academic domain, but rather by previous, less formalized learning experiences. Some make absolutely no distinction between aptitude and intelligence or propose that intelligence tests are a subcategory of aptitude measures.

Aptitude and intelligence tests are similar to the extent that both are cognitive or psychomotor in orientation and stem from unstructured, less formal life experiences; learning, motivation, and psychological factors; and, to some degree, innate potential or ability. (Note: Although some view a characteristic of aptitude as an absence of innate ability, separation of innate from environmental ability on tests of this nature is virtually impossible). However, aptitude and intelligence tests also differ in purpose, although sometimes the distinctions are minor. Both serve to predict future performance, but intelligence tests tend to have more global predictive applications. An intelligence test can be used to predict overall achievement across broad academic domains (i.e., reading, writing, mathematics, science, history) and therefore is useful in identifying children with learning disabilities as well as the intellectually and academically gifted. Intelligence tests are also helpful in identifying intrapersonal strengths and weaknesses in cognitive or learning styles. In addition, intelligence tests can be helpful in determining neurological dysfunction and brain damage when used as part of a comprehensive evaluation system.

Aptitude tests, on the other hand, generally are developed with the intention of predicting a narrow range of skills and abilities, although this is not always the case. Recall that the global-factor (or two-factor) theory of intelligence proposed that a global intelligence factor predominates, but that other more specific factors may exist. If a single global score (g) were the best predictor of all specific job or academic performances, there would be no need to develop more specific aptitude measures. If IQ predicted everything better than anything else, why bother developing tests that measured other abilities? The simple truth is that intelligence tests predict many things very well, but certainly not everything equally well. This is where more generalized aptitude batteries or specific ability tests can become very helpful to professional counselors. Aptitude tests are frequently used to help make college or postgraduate admission decisions, various course placements, occupational or workplace decisions, and placement decisions in the armed services, vocational rehabilitation, or government employment agencies. Such tests can be powerful predictors of future success in attaining the proficiency desired by those making these important decisions. At the classroom level, aptitude tests can be used with school-aged youth to diagnose learning problems, assess learner readiness, identify underachieving students, and individualize instruction. The applications for aptitude tests by professional counselors are quite broad.

By now you may have realized that the term *prediction* has been used frequently in the preceding paragraphs. Recall from Chapter 4 that the term *predictive criterion-related validity* was defined as the degree to which a test score predicts some criterion performance at some point in the future. In a nutshell, this is the key reason that aptitude tests are used; aptitude tests help professional counselors, students, and clients make decisions based on likely future performances. The more accurate the aptitude test is, the more accurate the decision about likely future performance. But not all tests that predict are aptitude tests. Personality, attitude, and interest inventories predict human characteristics and likely future behaviors but are not tests of aptitude. Aptitude tests are basically limited to cognitive and psychomotor facets. Three major types of aptitude tests are covered in this chapter: aptitude tests designed for scholastic admission decisions, multiaptitude batteries, and measures of special abilities.

APTITUDE TESTS DESIGNED FOR ADMISSION DECISIONS

There is little agreement on the differences between the terms *intelligence* and *scholastic aptitude*. Are they the same or different, and if different, how? In this book, the terms will be viewed with a great deal of similarity, so long as the purpose of the test's administration is to predict academic achievement. The reader may recall from the previous chapter that intelligence tests are frequently administered to school-aged youth to predict their academic performance. In this way, the intelligence test is being used as a measure of scholastic aptitude—and, in general, diagnostic intelligence tests are well suited for this purpose, particularly with learning-disabled youth.

Aptitude tests assess a student's potential for learning. An important niche for aptitude assessment has developed in the area of **scholastic aptitude** over the past 50 years or so, driven by the need to efficiently identify college-bound youth who have the "aptitude" to be successful at the college level and beyond. Admittedly, college admission officials could (and sometimes do) use numerous indicators to predict whether a student will successfully complete college: high school grade-point average (GPA), class rank, reference letters from teachers, even parents' income. While each of these indicators may provide a level of predictability, unfortunately, each possesses a good deal of error due to lack of comparability. For example, a GPA of 3.50 at School A may represent an entirely different degree of achievement than the same GPA at School B. This difference could be due to anything from grade inflation to the rigor of a curriculum or the variability of courses taken. Even though parent income was mentioned partially in jest, even standard of living differs from state to state or from rural to urban residence. The important point is that these indicators are variable, offering admissions officers an apples-to-oranges comparison, rather than the desired apples-to-apples comparison. Here is where scholastic aptitude examinations play an important role.

Scholastic aptitude assessments such as the *SAT-I* or *ACT* allow direct comparability across students in a manner that levels the playing field. Because the tests are equated, admissions officers can be reasonably assured that one student who scores higher than another has a higher likelihood of being more successful in college. A student who scores incredibly high on a music or foreign language aptitude test can be reasonably identified for advanced instruction. In the same manner, students with low scores can be identified in need of remedial instruction. This standardized approach allows comparisons to be made on a student-by-student basis and—when considered in the context of grades, rank, and character references—helps to provide multiple sources of information useful in arriving at an accurate admission decision. Of course, no system offers perfect predictability. But the reason scholastic aptitude tests are used is that they help admissions officers to make decisions more accurately than would a more subjective decision-making system.

Commonly Used Admission Tests

Scholastic Assessment Test (SAT)

The *SAT* (College Board, 2005c) is one of the most commonly used nationally administered college entrance exams. Originally called the *Scholastic Aptitude Test,* the *SAT* has been in existence since 1926 and has been revised periodically. The term *aptitude* was changed to the current term *assessment* to avoid prevalent misconceptions that the *SAT* measured "innate ability." The *SAT* helps colleges, scholarship committees, and students with educational decision making and planning. It provides college admission personnel with a common standard of comparison and is often used in conjunction with other sources of information (e.g., grades, letters of recommendation) in college admission decisions. Currently, the *Scholastic Assessment Test* consists of the *SAT-I,* a 3-hour reasoning test, and the *SAT-II,* subject content tests (e.g., biology, French). Typically, college-bound students take the *SAT* during the latter half of their junior year or the early part of their senior year of high school.

In early 2005, the College Board announced major changes in the *SAT,* and the new exam was first administered in March 2005. The original timed *SAT* exam had two components, Math and Verbal. The new *Sat-I* exam has three components, Writing, Critical Reading, and Math. The new Writing component has four subtests: Identifying Sentence Errors, Improving Sentences, Improving Paragraphs, and an Essay, all of which are combined and reported on a scale of 200 to 800 points. Students are allotted a maximum of 60 minutes to complete the Writing component. The Critical Reading component has three subtests: Reading Comprehension, Sentence Completion, and Paragraph-Length Critical Reading. The analogy subtest has been eliminated. Students are allotted a maximum of 70 minutes to complete the Critical Reading component, which is three subtests combined and reported on a scale of 200 to 800 points. The Mathematics component has four subtests: Number and Operations; Algebra I and II and Functions; Geometry; and Statistics, Probability, and Data Analysis. Students are allotted a maximum of 70 minutes to complete the Mathematics component, whose four subtests are combined and reported on a scale of 200 to 800 points. A minimum of 600 and maximum of 2,400 points can be attained on the new version of the *SAT-I* for the three components combined.

Reliability and validity studies are currently underway for the new version of the *SAT,* and past reviews for old editions generally yielded satisfactory results. Studies show that changes in the exam likely will increase predictive validity and will provide colleges with a better overview of a student's ability. The College Board scores all *SAT* tests electronically. A student gets 1 full point for each correct answer, 0 points for each unanswered or incorrect student-produced response question, and loses ¼ point for each incorrect multiple-choice question.

Raw scores are converted into standard scores and percentile ranks. Mean standard scores for the old versions of the *SAT* were 500 (*SD* = 100) on both the Verbal and Math components (College Board, 2005c). Mean scores on the *SAT* declined substantially between 1950 and 1995, primarily due to the increased opportunity for diverse groups of students to attend college in the United States and the fixed-reference-group norming procedures used since the 1940s. In 1995, the mean for both the Verbal and Mathematical reasoning scales was recentered from means in the low- to mid-400s closer to a new mean of 500. Educational Testing Service (ETS) supplies personal and college profiles to individual students and the high schools administering the exams to help identify strengths and limitations. Information on the *SAT,* including test preparation materials, sample test questions, scoring information, and resources for professional school counselors can be found at www.collegeboard.org.

The *SAT-II: Subject Tests* are specifically designed to measure a student's proficiency in a particular subject. Tests are given in a 1-hour time frame and are primarily multiple-choice tests. Subject tests are given in foreign languages, mathematics, sciences, literature, and history and reflect current trends in high school curricular content. Scores on the *SAT-II* are also reported on a scale of 200 to 800 except in the case of the English Language Proficiency Test, for which scores are reported on a scale of 901 to 999. Raw scores are converted to standard scores, and percentile ranks and scores are presented in a user-friendly personal report profile.

Preliminary Scholastic Assessment Test/National Merit Scholarship Qualifying Test (PSAT/NMSQT)

The *Preliminary Scholastic Assessment Test / National Merit Scholarship Qualifying Test* (*PSAT/NMSQT*), known as the *PSAT* (College Board, 2005b), is a practice assessment for the *SAT* and is also a qualifying exam for National Merit Scholarship opportunities. This test is typically given to students in their sophomore and/or junior years of high school. Like the *SAT,* the *PSAT* measures Mathematics, Critical Reading, and Writing abilities. Scoring is similar to that of the *SAT-I* and *SAT-II*, although each scale ranges from 20 to 80, rather than from 200 to 800. The mean for each scale is 50 ($SD = 10$). Thus a score of 65 on the *PSAT* mathematics scale would indicate a likely score of approximately 650 on the *SAT-I* mathematics scale. Scores from the *PSAT* allow students to assess their strengths and weaknesses and to begin studying accordingly. In addition, professional counselors can use *PSAT* performance to help students with educational planning and decision making. Professional counselors, particularly those working in schools, will find the publication *Guidelines and Uses of College Board Test Scores and Related Data* very helpful in understanding interpretation of test scores and decision-making strategies (College Entrance Examination Board, 2002).

American College Testing Assessment (ACT)

Another commonly used scholastic aptitude test, the *American College Testing Assessment* (*ACT*) (American College Testing, 2005), is used to measure high school students' ability in four core areas and to predict students' ability to complete college-level work. The four core areas of the *ACT* are English (45 minutes), Mathematics (60 minutes), Reading (35 minutes), and Science (35 minutes). A new, optional 30-minute Writing component is now available. Each core component is scored on a scale of 1 to 36, and all components are then averaged and rounded to the nearest whole number to attain a full composite score. The English, Mathematics, and Reading components are each composed of two subscore areas ranging from 1 to 18. The average composite score for the *ACT* in 2004 was 20.9. Importantly, the mean and standard deviation vary from year to year. Percentile ranks are also provided. Standard error of measurement varies by component but is generally equal to 2 points for component scores and 1 point for the composite score.

The *ACT* was first administered in 1959 and became available in all 50 states in 1960. Internal consistency coefficients are in 0.90s for the composite and range from the high 0.70s to the high 0.80s for each of the four subdomains. The *ACT* compares strongly with the *SAT* in predicting college GPA and in correlation with high school GPA, usually in the high 0.80s. Noble and Camera (2003) reported the *ACT* composite had a correlation of $r = 0.92$ with the *SAT*. The *ACT* had a correlation of $r = 0.43$ with first-year college GPAs, and when high school GPAs were factored in, the correlation increased to $r = 0.53$. Woodruff (2003) indicated that the *ACT* composite's correlation of $r = 0.52$ with high school GPA is substantial evidence of construct validity. The holistically scored writing essay recently added to the *ACT* likely will increase the accuracy of freshman composition placement (Matzen & Hoyt, 2004). Information on the *ACT*, including test preparation materials, sample test questions, scoring information, and resources for professional school counselors, can be found at www.act.org.

In addition to the results of the four academic areas and high school course and grade information, professional counselors will also find the *ACT Interest Inventory* and *Student Profile Section* quite helpful. Both of these sections provide the professional counselor with summaries of a student's academic needs, interests, and career planning. The *ACT Interest Inventory* parallels Holland's (1997) six areas of career interest, is compared to the interests of the national sample, and is interpreted as percentile ranks with standard error of measure bands. Ancillary to the *ACT Interest Inventory* is the World-of-Work Map on the reverse side, which helps identify preferences for Data, People, Ideas, and Things, even providing comparisons with occupational categories corresponding to the interests identified by the student. Figure 11.1 shows a sample *ACT* score report.

Miller Analogies Test (MAT)

The *Miller Analogies Test* (*MAT*) (Harcourt Assessment, Inc., 2005; Miller, 1992) is a graduate entrance exam that assesses ability in analytical thinking using only verbal measures; it is often used in place of, or supplementary to, the *Graduate Record Exam* (*GRE*). Originally developed in 1926, the test continues to differentiate among top-ranked, high-ability graduate students (Ivens, 1995). The test has 100 multiple-choice analogy items and has a 50-minute time limit. In addition, seven forms are available, which allows for retesting, and the test can be scored on-site, which saves time and expedites the admissions decision-making process (Frary, 1995). Although knowledge of vocabulary is a factor, understanding of analogous relationships and analytical thinking play a more important role when answering questions. Since the test covers a variety of nine subjects (language usage, biological sciences, social sciences, history, literature-philosophy, fine arts, mathematics, physical sciences, and general information), it is a good measure of educational background and problem-solving ability (Frary, 1995). Scores are computed by Harcourt Assessment, Inc. and are reported in scaled scores, percentiles based on intended major, and percentiles based on a normative population of *MAT* examinees who took the test for the first time between 1990 and 1992 (Frary). The manual addresses issues of possible race, ethnic, and/or gender bias, but only in uninterpreted tables (Ivens, 1995).

Split-half reliability coefficients are reported in the high 0.80s. The KR-20 reliability coefficients are reported as being between 0.90 and 0.94 for all of the forms, but little evidence of equivalence across the seven forms is available, a potential problem when it comes to actual comparability of scores across forms. Validity coefficients of scores vary depending on the sample (median to high 0.30s), but there is a high correlation with the *GRE* (low 0.80s). No content validity is presented. There is some discrepancy in prediction of GPA in certain samples, such as overestimation in men and underestimation in women. It is also important to remember that the *MAT* assesses only verbal analytical thinking and leaves out other domains important to graduate school performance and intellectual ability (Kaplan & Saccuzzo, 2001).

Graduate Record Examination (GRE)

The *Graduate Record Examination* (*GRE*) (College Board, 2005a) is a widely used graduate school entrance exam that measures graduate student scholastic ability as opposed to the *SAT-I* and *ACT,* which are commonly used for admission at the undergraduate level. Importantly, the *GRE* is a general aptitude test for graduate study. There are a number of more specific graduate school admissions tests, including the *Medical College Admissions Test* (*MCAT*), *Law School Admission Test* (*LSAT*), *Graduate Management Admission Test* (*GMAT*), and *Dental Admission Test* (*DAT*). The *GRE* assessed three core sections: Analytical Writing (75 minutes); Verbal (30 minutes); and Quantitative (45 minutes). The Verbal section measures ability to recognize relationships between words and concepts, synthesize information, analyze and evaluate written material, and analyze sentences. The Quantitative section assesses understanding of algebra, geometry, data analysis, math reasoning, and problem solving. Verbal and Math components are scored on a scale of 200 to 800, and Writing is scored on a scale of 0 to 6. The Writing section measures articulation of complex ideas, evaluation of evidence, appropriate support of ideas, coherence, and use of standard written English. Raw scores are converted to standard scores (M =500; SD = 100) and percentile ranks. On any given test, there may be an added research or pretest section that is experimental and which does not count.

A complete guide to understanding *GRE* scores is available at www.gre.org. According to Kaplan and Saccuzzo (2001), the normative sample for the *GRE* is smaller than that of the *SAT* and other scholastic abilities tests, and the psychometric measures are less impressive. They indicate that the split-half reliability appears adequate, but not the predictive validity of scores. Many researchers debate whether the *GRE* is an adequate predictor of GPA and academic success, but the *GRE* continues to be an accepted standard for entry into many graduate school programs (Kaplan & Saccuzzo, 2001).

The *GRE* was among the first scholastic tests to explore the use of computer-adaptive assessment, and the evidence concludes that this method is equivalent to paper-and-pencil formats (GRE Board, 1997). Numerous computerized testing sites are available across the country, so students can simply make a test appointment, rather than wait for a scheduled testing date. As explained in Chapter 1, computer-adaptive testing allows the computer software to select more or less difficult questions based on student responses, usually leading to less time being required to administer the exam. Also, results are scored immediately and are available to the student on completion of the exam.

TRACY ARTHUR C
7852 W 46TH ST
WHEAT RIDGE CO 80033

392-11-2004
HSC 067-890
90210-000003456S

YOUR ACT TEST SCORES Your 04/05 ACT scores, listed below, provide one way to estimate your level of educational development. The ranks show how your scores compare with those of recent high school graduates who took the ACT while in high school. For instance, your READING score (25) has a rank of 75. This means that 75% of the ACT-tested students scored at or below your READING score. The rank of your Composite (average) score indicates that your overall educational development is likely in the middle half of ACT-tested students.

To emphasize that test scores are only estimates, bands are drawn around your ranks. Check the bands for the four tests (English, Math, Reading, Science). If bands for two tests do **not** overlap, your ranks probably differ. For three of the tests, additional scores (subscores) are provided. Check the subscore bands for English, then Math, then Reading. If the subscore bands for a test do **not** overlap, your ranks probably differ. Use the bands to identify knowledge and skill areas you may want to work on. The areas are described in *Using Your ACT Assessment Results*.

KNOWLEDGE AND SKILL AREAS	SCORES (1-36) (1-18)	RANK: PERCENT OF ACT-TESTED STUDENTS AT OR BELOW YOUR SCORES
ENGLISH	24	76
Usage/Mechanics	13	79
Rhetorical Skills	12	75
MATHEMATICS	17	34
Pre-Algebra/Elem. Alg.	09	41
Alg./Coord. Geometry	10	55
Plane Geometry/Trig.	08	25
READING	25	75
Soc. Studies/Sciences	10	51
Arts/Literature	14	79
SCIENCE	18	30
COMPOSITE (Average)	21	**57**

(Rank scale: 1, 10, 25, 50, 75, 90, 99)

PLUS WRITING SCORES

	(1-36)	(2-12)	% at or below
English/Writing	25		81
Writing		10	96

(See Comments on Your Essay, below.)

TRACY ARTHUR C
7852 W 46TH ST
WHEAT RIDGE CO 80033

000000001

H.S. GPA computed from grades you reported in English, Math,
Natural Sciences, & Social Studies courses (4.0 scale) = 3.29

YOUR COLLEGE PLANNING Admissions standards differ among colleges and, sometimes, among programs of study within a college. A list of typical class ranks and ACT composite scores at colleges with different admissions policies is provided on the back of this report. Check with the admissions office at the college of your choice if you have any questions.

The table below gives information about the colleges you listed when you registered for the ACT. For example, UNIVERSITY OF OMEGA has a traditional admissions policy. Your ACT Composite score is estimated to rank in the middle half of entering students. The average high school GPA for freshmen is 2.76—lower than the 3.29 for the grades you reported. Students with ACT scores and grades like yours, if admitted to this college, would have about 6 chances in 10 of earning a "C" average or higher during the freshman year. The program of study you listed at ACT registration (POLITICAL SCI/GOVERNMENT) is available. The approximate cost of tuition/fees is $1,700/year, which does not include housing, meals, books, transportation, etc. About 67% of the current freshman class receives student aid based on financial need.

COLLEGE CODE AND NAME	ADMISSIONS POLICY	ESTIMATED RANK OF YOUR ACT COMPOSITE SCORE (ENROLLED FRESHMEN)	H.S. AVERAGE (ENROLLED FRESHMEN)	CHANCES IN 10 OF "C" OR HIGHER	YOUR PROGRAM OF STUDY AVAILABLE	APPROX. YEARLY TUITION & FEES (minus room/board)	PERCENT FRESHMAN CLASS RECEIVING FINANCIAL AID BASED ON NEED
9521 UNIVERSITY OF OMEGA	TRAD	MIDDLE HALF	2.76	6	YES: 4-YR DEGREE	1700	67
9059 ALPHA UNIVERSITY	SEL	MIDDLE HALF	3.12	5	YES: 4-YR DEGREE	4500	85
8866 BETA COMMUNITY COLL	OPEN	UPPER QUARTER	2.49	9	YES: 2-YR DEGREE	1200	58
8905 MAGNA COLLEGE	TRAD	MIDDLE HALF	2.71	6	YES: 4-YR DEGREE	8500	90

A dash (—) means ACT™ has no information available. See *Using Your ACT Assessment Results* for an explanation of program of study and tuition/fees categories.

Remember that test scores and past grades do not guarantee success or failure in college. Other factors, such as program of study and motivation, count too. Most colleges have special programs for students wanting help in particular areas. You reported that you would like help with educational or vocational plans and mathematics. Check with your high school counselor, the college catalog, or the college admissions office to learn whether this special help is available at the college of your choice.

Section 2 of *Using Your ACT Assessment Results* provides more information about choosing a college.

YOUR EDUCATIONAL/OCCUPATIONAL PLANNING Since many people consider several possibilities before making definite career plans, ACT has grouped similar occupations and programs of study into "areas" as a career exploration aid. For example, the program of study you indicated (POLITICAL SCI/GOVERNMENT) best fits Career Area S (SOCIAL SCIENCE); the occupational choice you indicated (LAW) best fits Career Area Y (COMMUNITY SERVICES). If you would like to identify other careers in these areas, check the Career Area List on the back of this report.

Occupations differ in how much they involve working with data (facts, records); ideas (theories, insights); people (care, services); and things (machines, materials, lab equipment). Your responses to the ACT Interest Inventory indicate that you might enjoy opportunities to work with PEOPLE and ideas. Career Areas V, W, and X include many occupations and programs of study which emphasize these "work tasks." If you scan these areas, you may find additional career possibilities that you would like to explore. You can identify other Career Areas emphasizing people and ideas "work tasks" by using the World-of-Work Map (Found in Section 3 of *Using Your ACT Assessment Results*). See, especially, Map Regions 11 and 12. Remember, however:

*Occupations within each area differ in the proportion of time spent with each of the work tasks.

*Interest scores, like other test scores, are estimates; also, interests may change with experience.

*Interests and abilities may differ; consider both in your educational/occupational planning.

If you will now turn to Section 3 of *Using Your ACT Assessment Results*, you will find a list of activities which can help you identify and explore career options.

COMMENTS ON YOUR ESSAY Your essay showed recognition of the complexity of the issue by partially evaluating its implications. The general statements in your essay were well supported with reasons, examples, and details. Some varied sentence structure and precise word choice added clarity and interest to your writing.

Figure 11.1 Sample *ACT* score report

Source: Reprinted by permission of ACT, Inc.

COLLEGE ADMISSION POLICIES

College admission policies may be characterized as follows:

	Typical ACT Composite Scores		Typical ACT Composite Scores
Highly Selective: Majority of accepted freshmen in top 10 percent of high school graduating class	27–31	**Liberal:** Some freshmen from lower half of high school graduating class	18–21
Selective: Majority of accepted freshmen in top 25 percent of high school graduating class	22–27	**Open:** All high school graduates accepted, to limit of capacity	17–20
Traditional: Majority of accepted freshmen in top 50 percent of high school graduating class	20–23		

CAREER AREA LIST (3rd Edition)

Typical occupations and college programs of study associated with each ACT Career Area are listed below. Page numbers for each area refer to pages in the Occupational Outlook Handbook (OOH), 2002–03 edition, published by the U.S. Department of Labor. The OOH includes more occupations than can be given here, and also provides descriptions of the occupations, what the work is like, characteristics of workers, training required, earnings, and employment prospects. The OOH is available in most libraries and online at http://www.bls.gov/oco.

The Bureau of Labor Statistics (BLS) provides employment projections every two years in a variety of publications such as the Occupational Outlook Quarterly and Employment Outlook: 1996–2006. The data and information in these publications are also accessible via the Office of Employment

Projections home page: http://www.bls.gov/emp. This important information is useful for long-term career planning.

In the lists below, occupations that may require some training beyond high school are designated as (2) and those typically requiring 4 years or more of college as (4). When both numbers appear, 4 years is the recommended amount of training. However, the actual educational requirements for jobs will differ among employers.

Programs of study are designated (2) if they are usually offered by 2-year colleges and (4) if they are usually offered by 4-year colleges. Programs often offered by both are designated (2, 4).

ADMINISTRATION & SALES

EXAMPLE OCCUPATIONS	EXAMPLE PROGRAMS OF STUDY
A. Employment-Related Services (page 60)	
Employment Interviewer (2, 4), Employee Benefits Manager (4), Human Resources Manager (4), Human Resources Recruiter (4), Job Analyst (4)	Business Administration (2,4), Human Resources Management (2, 4), Economics (4), Psychology (4)
B. Marketing & Sales (pages 26, 80, 359-376)	
Insurance Agent (2, 4), Real Estate Agent (2, 4), Travel Agent (2, 4), Advertising Manager (4), Buyer (4), Financial Services Representative (4), Sales/Marketing Manager (4)	General Business (2,4), Insurance/Real Estate (2, 4), Retailing/Marketing (2, 4), Business Administration (2, 4), Specialized fields related to sales (2, 4)
C. Management (pages 52-58, 70-72, 77, 86, 417)	
Administrative Assistant (2), Hotel/Motel Manager (2, 4), Executive (4), Financial Manager (4), Foreign Service Officer (4), Management Consultant (4), Property Manager (4)	Administrative/Secretarial Services (2), Business Administration (2, 4), Hotel/Restaurant Management (2, 4), Office Management (2, 4), Business Economics (4)
D. Regulation & Protection (pages 344-350, 594)	
Police Officer (2), Park Ranger (2, 4), Detective (2, 4), Customs Inspector (4), Insurance Claim Representative (4), Security Manager (4)	Criminal Justice and Corrections (2, 4), Law Enforcement (2, 4), Parks and Recreation Studies (4)

BUSINESS OPERATIONS

EXAMPLE OCCUPATIONS	EXAMPLE PROGRAMS OF STUDY
E. Communications & Records (pages 206, 386-390, 394-401, 405-406, 419, 422)	
Billing Clerk (2), Health Information Technician (2), Interviewing/New Account Clerk (2), Hotel Clerk (2), Medical Transcriptionist (2), Secretary (2), Court Reporter (2, 4)	Secretarial Services (2), and specialized (e.g., Executive, Legal, Medical) secretarial programs (2, 4), Accounting (2, 4), Health Administrative Services (2, 4)
F. Financial Transactions (pages 21, 29, 66, 353, 393, 594)	
Cashier (2), Budget/Credit Analyst (2, 4), Real Estate Appraiser (2, 4), Accountant/Auditor (4), Insurance Underwriter (4), Tax Accountant (4)	Taxation (2), Accounting (2, 4), Business Administration (2, 4), Financial Management (2, 4)
G. Distribution & Dispatching (pages 407, 412, 414, 565)	
Shipping/Receiving Clerk (2), Warehouse Supervisor (2, 4), Air Traffic Controller (4), Flight Dispatcher (4)	Administrative/Secretarial Services (2), Air Transportation (2, 4), Retailing/Distribution (2, 4), On-the-Job Training, Apprenticeship

TECHNICAL

EXAMPLE OCCUPATIONS	EXAMPLE PROGRAMS OF STUDY
H. Transport Operation & Related (pages 562, 570, 576, 582)	
Bus Driver (2), Sailor (2), Truck Driver (2), Aircraft Pilot (2, 4), Ship Captain (4)	Vehicle and Equipment Operating (2), Aerospace/Aeronautical Engineering (4), On-the-Job Training
I. Agriculture, Forestry & Related (pages 47, 222, 302, 324, 598)	
Animal Caretaker (2), Arborist (2, 4), Farmer (2, 4), Greenhouse Manager (2, 4), Forester (4)	Agricultural Business and Management (2, 4), Agriculture (4), Animal/Plant Sciences (4), On-the-Job Training, Apprenticeship
J. Computer & Information Specialties (pages 163, 166-171, 180, 190)	
Library Technician (2), Web Site Developer (2, 4), Actuary (4), Computer Programmer (4), Computer Systems Analyst (4)	Data Processing Technology (2), Computer and Information Sciences (2, 4), Computer Programming (2, 4), Mathematics (4)
K. Construction & Maintenance (pages 341, 435-469)	
Building/Construction Inspector (2), Carpenter (2), Electrician (2), Firefighter (2), Plumber (2), Security System Installer (2)	Carpentry (2), Drafting (2), Electrical Equipment Installation and Repair (2), On-the-Job Training, Apprenticeship
L. Crafts & Related (pages 306, 542, 552)	
Jeweler (2), Tailor/Dressmaker (2), Baker (2, 4), Chef/Cook (2, 4)	Culinary Arts/Chef Training (2), Design and Applied Arts (2, 4), Clothing and Textile Studies (4), Apprenticeship
M. Manufacturing & Processing (pages 470, 514, 526-530, 535)	
Bookbinder (2), Sheet Metal Worker (2), Tool and Die Maker (2), Water Plant Operator (2), Welder (2)	Graphic and Printing Equipment Operation (2), Industrial Equipment Operation and Repair (2), Precision Metal Work (2), On-the-Job Training, Apprenticeship
N. Mechanical & Electrical Specialties (pages 475-511)	
Line Installer/Cable Splicer (2), Millwright (2), Specialized (e.g. Aircraft, Heating and Air Conditioning, Communications Equipment), Mechanics and Technicians (2, 4)	Electrical Equipment Installation and Repair (2), Precision Metal Work (2), Vehicle Equipment Mechanics (2), Apprenticeship

SCIENCE & TECHNOLOGY

EXAMPLE OCCUPATIONS	EXAMPLE PROGRAMS OF STUDY
O. Engineering & Technologies (pages 90, 95, 103-117)	
Engineers (e.g. Aerospace, Computer, Mechanical) and Technicians (e.g., Energy, Laser, Quality Control) in various fields (2, 4), Architect (4), Surveyor (4)	Drafting (2), Computer and Information Sciences (2, 4), General Engineering (2, 4), Architecture (4), Specialized engineering fields (2, 4)
P. Natural Science & Technologies (pages 174, 178, 216-236)	
Science Technician (2), Astronomer (4), Biologist (4), Food Technologist (4), Geologist (4), Physicist (4), Statistician (4)	Biology (2, 4), Information Sciences and Systems (2, 4), Chemistry (4), Geology (4), Mathematics (4), Physics (4)
Q. Medical Technologies (pages 252, 257, 277-279, 289-298)	
Optician (2), Radiographer (2, 4), Pharmacist (4), Technologists (e.g., Medical, Surgical) in various fields (2, 4)	Medical Diagnostic/Treatment Services (2), Medical Lab Technologies (2, 4), Chemistry (4), Microbiology (4)
R. Medical Diagnosis & Treatment (pages 248-264, 274, 284)	
Emergency Medical Technician (2), Dentist (4), Nurse Anesthetist (4), Optometrist (4), Physical Therapist (4), Physician (4), Physician Assistant (4), Veterinarian (4)	Medical Diagnostic/Treatment Services (2), Biology (4), Chemistry (4), Rehabilitation/Therapeutic Services (4), Pre-medicine (4)
S. Social Science (pages 239-246)	
Anthropologist (4), Experimental Psychologist (4), Political Scientist (4), Sociologist (4), Urban Planner (4)	Social Sciences (2, 4), Anthropology (4), History (4), Psychology (4), Sociology (4)

ARTS

EXAMPLE OCCUPATIONS	EXAMPLE PROGRAMS OF STUDY
T. Applied Arts (Visual) (pages 118-120, 139)	
Artist (2, 4), Fashion/Floral/Interior Designer (2, 4), Graphic Artist (2, 4), Photographer (2, 4)	Design and Applied Arts (2, 4), Film/Video and Photographic Arts (2, 4), Fine Arts and Art Studies (2, 4), Clothing/Textile Studies (4), Apprenticeship
U. Creative & Performing Arts (pages 124, 129-131, 145, 356)	
Fashion Model (2), Actor (2, 4), Dancer/Choreographer (2, 4), Musician (2, 4), Singer (2, 4), Writer/Author (2, 4)	Dance (4), Drama/Theatre Arts (4), Music (4), Visual and Performing Arts (4), Creative Writing (4)
V. Applied Arts (Written & Spoken) (pages 133-137, 141, 145, 188)	
Interpreter (2, 4), Advertising Copywriter (4), Editor (4), Librarian (4), Public Relations Specialist (4), Reporter/Journalist (4)	Advertising (4), English Language and Literature (4), Foreign Language (4), Journalism (4), Radio/Television Broadcasting (4)

SOCIAL SERVICE

EXAMPLE OCCUPATIONS	EXAMPLE PROGRAMS OF STUDY
W. Health Care (pages 74, 266-268, 281, 312-314, 595)	
Physical Therapist Assistant (2), Dental Assistant/Hygienist (2, 4), Nurse (2, 4), Athletic Trainer (4), Health Services Administrator (4) Recreational Therapist (4)	Dental/Medical Assisting (2), LPN/RN Nurse Training (2, 4), Medical Administrative Services (2, 4), Exercise Sciences (4), Rehabilitation/Therapeutic Services (4)
X. Education (pages 42, 126, 194-203)	
Athletic Coach (4), Educational Administrator (4), Elementary/Secondary Teacher (4), Teachers (Art, Music, Physical Education, Vocational, etc.) in various specialties (4)	Individual/Family Development Studies (2), General/Elementary/Secondary Teacher Education (4), Specialized fields (e.g., Music, Science) related to education (4)
Y. Community Services (pages 148-151, 158-160, 208-213)	
Legal Assistant (2, 4), Clergy (4), Counselors (Career, Mental Health, Rehabilitation, etc.) in various specialties (4), Home Economist (4), Lawyer (4), Social Service Director (4), Social Worker (4)	Individual/Family Development Studies (2), Criminal Justice and Corrections (2, 4), Social Work (2, 4), Psychology (4), Sociology (4), Theology (4)
Z. Personal Services (pages 317, 324-331, 335)	
Barber/Hairstylist (2), Home Health Aide (2), Travel Guide (2), Animal Trainer (2, 4), Flight Attendant (2, 4)	Child Care and Guidance (2), Cosmetic Services (2), Culinary Arts and Related Services (2), Tourism and Travel Services Marketing (2)

5278

Figure 11.1 continued

TESTS OF GENERAL AND SPECIFIC APTITUDE

Aptitude tests with educational and vocational applications are frequently categorized according to whether they include a battery of tests or measure a single, specific aptitude.

Multiaptitude Batteries

The increase in vocational counseling services has created a need for identifying student or client career-related skills and abilities. Knowing what a high school student is interested in and good at can provide a valuable impetus to further exploration of careers or jobs aligned with those interests and skills (see Chapter 13). **Multiaptitude batteries** have filled this need by providing professional counselors with the tools to identify student and client aptitudes. Knowledge of these aptitudes can help individuals make important career-based decisions. But how good are these multiaptitude tests at differentially predicting future performance?

Differential prediction relates to how well a group of people's test scores help indicate who will be more or less successful at certain academic or occupational tasks in the future. In general, aptitude batteries are not very good at achieving this very desirable result, not because the tests lack psychometric rigor, but more because of the nature of the criteria to be predicted. More succinctly, one's success at a given job is not simply a function of global intelligence or any specific ability (aptitude). While intelligence and aptitudes are important, job success also hinges on motivation to perform, person-environment fit, and social and personality characteristics. That is, an accountant's job success at a given accounting firm may not be due solely to how good the person is with numbers, but may be even more closely aligned with the individual's motivations and personality characteristics and how well these align with the internal environment of that specific accounting firm. It is not hard to imagine that the same individual could be perceived in two entirely different ways depending on the context of the work environment (i.e., a company may be nurturing or competitive, discouraging of social connectedness, and engaging in illegal or unethical activities).

However, career counselors frequently highlight the importance of describing client skills and abilities to bring the client to a greater level of awareness and depth of understanding. Such information often empowers clients to see possibilities in vocational opportunities where, previously, they may not have. Thus the lack of predictive efficiency of aptitude tests may become secondary to the descriptive usefulness of multiaptitude batteries.

A number of multiaptitude batteries have been developed. The *Armed Services Vocational Assessment Battery* (*ASVAB*) was specifically developed for use in assigning recruits to military occupational specialty areas. A tremendous amount of data has been generated through large-scale *ASVAB* administrations over the years, but, as is the case with most aptitude batteries, the *ASVAB* is much better at predicting recruit success in completing the training program than actual job success. Multiaptitude batteries such as the *Differential Aptitude Test* (*DAT*) and the Occupational Information Network's *O*NET Ability Profiler* (*O*NET*) were designed for civilian use in vocational counseling and job placement.

Differential Aptitude Test (DAT)

The *Differential Aptitude Test—Fifth Edition* (*DAT*) (Bennett, Seashore, & Wesman, 1990) is a vocational and educational guidance battery designed to help students plan for their future. There are three versions available: one for students in grades 7–9, one for students in grades 10–12, and one for adults. There are eight subtests: Verbal Reasoning, Numerical Reasoning, Abstract Reasoning, Perceptual Speed and Accuracy (two parts), Mechanical Reasoning, Space Relations, Spelling, and Language Usage. The total testing time is 235 minutes; 181 minutes are for testing, and the remaining 54 minutes are for giving administration directions and scoring of the test. The computer-adapted version requires only about 90 minutes to complete, and immediate score results are available with this version (Drummond, 2000). The test manual (Bennett et al., 1990), the *Guide to Careers Student Workbook,* the *Career Interest Inventory,* and several ancillary books are useful tools for professional counselors administering the test. The test can be computer- and hand-scored. The normative information has been improved from previous versions, and the score reliability and validity information supports the use of the test as a helpful aptitude assessment tool. Even though each revision has been an improvement over the previous versions, especially with regard to the normative information, there is still a lack of evidence for differential and incremental validity (Hattrup, 1995).

O*Net Ability Profiler

The *O*NET Ability Profiler* (U.S. Department of Labor, 2005) replaced the *General Aptitude Test Battery* (*GATB*) and is used in vocational guidance, usually by employment services or secondary schools to help individuals investigate and plan their work future. The *Ability Profiler* is one of three assessments from *O*Net* (the other two being the *Work Importance Profiler* and the *Interest Profiler* (see Figure 11.2 for the beginning Self-Report Skills Search Inventory). In addition, the *Occupational Information Network* replaced the *Dictionary of Occupational Titles* (*DOT*), and is one of the best sources of occupational information. The *Ability Profiler* is used with high school students and adults, ages 16 years and older. Eleven parts or exercises make up the test, and 5 of the exercises involve psychomotor assessment. Each part can be administered alone, but it is recommended that all 11 tasks be administered together, requiring about 2 ½ hours. Scores are in nine categories: Verbal Abilities, Arithmetic Reasoning, Computation, Spatial Ability, Form Perception, Clerical Perception, Motor Coordination, Finger Dexterity, and Manual Dexterity. Raw scores and percentile scores are reported.

Armed Services Vocational Aptitude Battery (ASVAB)

The *Armed Services Vocational Aptitude Battery* (*ASVAB*) (U.S. Military Entrance Processing Command, 2005) is a test given by the armed forces but can be used as an educational and vocational tool for counseling students in 10th grade and above in job and training opportunities in the armed services and in civilian careers. The test helps students to assess their abilities and interests, select career exploration activities, and examine potential career choices (Drummond, 2000). It is primarily used as a qualification test for entering the armed forces, but it can also be used for

Editor's comment: The *O*NET* begins with a self-report skills search inventory, included below:

Skills Search

Select **skills** from one or more of the six skill groups below. Start by selecting as many skills as you have or plan to acquire. (See <u>Skills Search</u> for more details.)

<u>Basic Skills</u> | <u>Complex Problem Solving Skills</u> | <u>Resource Management Skills</u> | <u>Social Skills</u> | <u>Systems Skills</u> | <u>Technical Skills</u>

Basic Skills
Developed capacities that facilitate learning or the more rapid acquisition of knowledge

- ☑ **Active Learning** — Understanding the implications of new information for both current and future problem-solving and decision-making.

- ☑ **Active Listening** — Giving full attention to what other people are saying, taking time to understand the points being made, asking questions as appropriate, and not interrupting at inappropriate times.

- ☑ **Critical Thinking** — Using logic and reasoning to identify the strengths and weaknesses of alternative solutions, conclusions or approaches to problems.

- ☐ **Learning Strategies** — Selecting and using training/instructional methods and procedures appropriate for the situation when learning or teaching new things.

- ☑ **Mathematics** — Using mathematics to solve problems.

- ☐ **Monitoring** — Monitoring/Assessing performance of yourself, other individuals, or organizations to make improvements or take corrective action.

- ☑ **Reading Comprehension** — Understanding written sentences and paragraphs in work related documents.

- ☑ **Science** — Using scientific rules and methods to solve problems.

- ☑ **Speaking** — Talking to others to convey information effectively.

- ☑ **Writing** — Communicating effectively in writing as appropriate for the needs of the audience.

Complex Problem Solving Skills
Developed capacities used to solve novel, ill-defined problems in complex, real-world settings

- ☑ **Complex Problem Solving** — Identifying complex problems and reviewing related information to develop and evaluate options and implement solutions.

Resource Management Skills
Developed capacities used to allocate resources efficiently

- ☐ **Management of Financial Resources** — Determining how money will be spent to get the work done, and accounting for these expenditures.

- ☑ **Management of Material Resources** — Obtaining and seeing to the appropriate use of equipment, facilities, and materials needed to do certain work.

Figure 11.2 Sample *O*NET* output for an adolescent girl

☐ **Management of Personnel Resources** — Motivating, developing, and directing people as they work, identifying the best people for the job.

☑ **Time Management** — Managing one's own time and the time of others.

Social Skills
Developed capacities used to work with people to achieve goals

☑ **Coordination** — Adjusting actions in relation to others' actions.

☑ **Instructing** — Teaching others how to do something.

☐ **Negotiation** — Bringing others together and trying to reconcile differences.

☐ **Persuasion** — Persuading others to change their minds or behavior.

☐ **Service Orientation** — Actively looking for ways to help people.

☐ **Social Perceptiveness** — Being aware of others' reactions and understanding why they react as they do.

Systems Skills
Developed capacities used to understand, monitor, and improve socio-technical systems

☑ **Judgment and Decision Making** — Considering the relative costs and benefits of potential actions to choose the most appropriate one.

☐ **Systems Analysis** — Determining how a system should work and how changes in conditions, operations, and the environment will affect outcomes.

☐ **Systems Evaluation** — Identifying measures or indicators of system performance and the actions needed to improve or correct performance, relative to the goals of the system.

Technical Skills
Developed capacities used to design, set-up, operate, and correct malfunctions involving application of machines or technological systems

☐ **Equipment Maintenance** — Performing routine maintenance on equipment and determining when and what kind of maintenance is needed.

☐ **Equipment Selection** — Determining the kind of tools and equipment needed to do a job.

☐ **Installation** — Installing equipment, machines, wiring, or programs to meet specifications.

☐ **Operation and Control** — Controlling operations of equipment or systems.

☐ **Operation Monitoring** — Watching gauges, dials, or other indicators to make sure a machine is working properly.

☐ **Operations Analysis** — Analyzing needs and product requirements to create a design.

Figure 11.2   continued

☐   **Programming** — Writing computer programs for various purposes.

☑   **Quality Control Analysis** — Conducting tests and inspections of products, services, or processes to evaluate quality or performance.

☐   **Repairing** — Repairing machines or systems using the needed tools.

☐   **Technology Design** — Generating or adapting equipment and technology to serve user needs.

☐   **Troubleshooting** — Determining causes of operating errors and deciding what to do about it.

Go		Reset Selections

Editor's comment: Next, the *O*NET* program analyzes the self-reported skills and matches these skills with occupations. What follows is a list of matches for the same client.

Skills Search for:
Reading Comprehension, Active Listening, Writing, Speaking, Mathematics, Science, Critical Thinking, Active Learning, Coordination, Instructing, Complex Problem Solving, Quality Control Analysis, Judgment and Decision Making, Time Management, Management of Material Resources (40 matches)

Select from Skills Matched to view how your selected skills compare to all skills for that occupation.

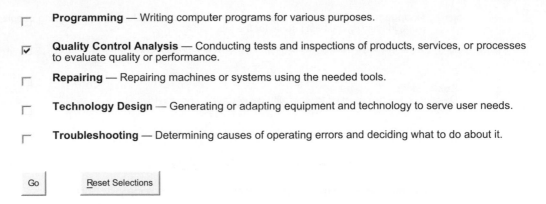

Skills Matched	Job Zone	Code	Occupation
14	3	29-2054.00	Respiratory Therapy Technicians
13	3	29-2061.00	Licensed Practical and Licensed Vocational Nurses
13	4	19-1022.00	Microbiologists
13	4	19-1041.00	Epidemiologists
13	4	19-1042.00	Medical Scientists, Except Epidemiologists
13	4	19-2031.00	Chemists
13	5	25-1054.00	Physics Teachers, Postsecondary
13	5	29-1131.00	Veterinarians
13	5	29-9091.00	Athletic Trainers
12	3	29-1124.00	Radiation Therapists
12	3	29-2033.00	Nuclear Medicine Technologists
12	3	47-2031.01	Construction Carpenters
12	4	11-2021.00	Marketing Managers
12	4	17-2141.00	Mechanical Engineers

Figure 11.2   continued

Editor's comment: The *O*NET* Skills Search usually provides about 40 matches for this function. Finally, clients can click on the occupation hotlinks and read information related to the matched occupations. What follows is truncated output from the first listed skills match occupation.

Summary Report for:
29-2054.00 - Respiratory Therapy Technicians

Provide specific, well defined respiratory care procedures under the direction of respiratory therapists and physicians.

This newly defined occupation contains data obtained through the O*NET data collection program and has not yet been rated for Interests and Work Values.

Sample of reported job titles: Respiratory Therapy Technician, Respiratory Technician, Certified Respiratory Therapy Technician, CRT (Certified Respiratory Therapist), CRTT (Certified Respiratory Therapy Technician)

View report:	Summary	Details	Custom

Tasks | Knowledge | Skills | Abilities | Work Activities | Work Context | Job Zone | Work Styles | Wages & Employment

Tasks

- Use ventilators and various oxygen devices and aerosol and breathing treatments in the provision of respiratory therapy.
- Work with patients in areas such as the emergency room, neonatal/pediatric intensive care, and surgical intensive care, treating conditions including emphysema, chronic bronchitis, asthma, cystic fibrosis, and pneumonia.
- Read and evaluate physicians' orders and patients' chart information to determine patients' condition and treatment protocols.
- Keep records of patients' therapy, completing all necessary forms.
- Set equipment controls to regulate the flow of oxygen, gases, mists, or aerosols.
- Provide respiratory care involving the application of well-defined therapeutic techniques under the supervision of a respiratory therapist and a physician.
- Assess patients' response to treatments and modify treatments according to protocol if necessary.
- Prepare and test devices such as mechanical ventilators, therapeutic gas administration apparatus, environmental control systems, aerosol generators and EKG machines.
- Monitor patients during treatment and report any unusual reactions to the respiratory therapist.
- Explain treatment procedures to patients.

Knowledge

Medicine and Dentistry — Knowledge of the information and techniques needed to diagnose and treat human injuries, diseases, and deformities. This includes symptoms, treatment alternatives, drug properties and interactions, and preventive health-care measures.

Customer and Personal Service — Knowledge of principles and processes for providing customer and personal services. This includes customer needs assessment, meeting quality standards for services, and evaluation of customer satisfaction.

Figure 11.2   continued

Chemistry — Knowledge of the chemical composition, structure, and properties of substances and of the chemical processes and transformations that they undergo. This includes uses of chemicals and their interactions, danger signs, production techniques, and disposal methods.

Psychology — Knowledge of human behavior and performance; individual differences in ability, personality, and interests; learning and motivation; psychological research methods; and the assessment and treatment of behavioral and affective disorders.

English Language — Knowledge of the structure and content of the English language including the meaning and spelling of words, rules of composition, and grammar.

Mathematics — Knowledge of arithmetic, algebra, geometry, calculus, statistics, and their applications.

Education and Training — Knowledge of principles and methods for curriculum and training design, teaching and instruction for individuals and groups, and the measurement of training effects.

Biology — Knowledge of plant and animal organisms, their tissues, cells, functions, interdependencies, and interactions with each other and the environment.

Public Safety and Security — Knowledge of relevant equipment, policies, procedures, and strategies to promote effective local, state, or national security operations for the protection of people, data, property, and institutions.

Physics — Knowledge and prediction of physical principles, laws, their interrelationships, and applications to understanding fluid, material, and atmospheric dynamics, and mechanical, electrical, atomic and sub- atomic structures and processes.

Skills

Time Management — Managing one's own time and the time of others.

Critical Thinking — Using logic and reasoning to identify the strengths and weaknesses of alternative solutions, conclusions or approaches to problems.

Reading Comprehension — Understanding written sentences and paragraphs in work related documents.

Troubleshooting — Determining causes of operating errors and deciding what to do about it.

Active Listening — Giving full attention to what other people are saying, taking time to understand the points being made, asking questions as appropriate, and not interrupting at inappropriate times.

Instructing — Teaching others how to do something.

Operation Monitoring — Watching gauges, dials, or other indicators to make sure a machine is working properly.

Judgment and Decision Making — Considering the relative costs and benefits of potential actions to choose the most appropriate one.

Service Orientation — Actively looking for ways to help people.

Speaking — Talking to others to convey information effectively.

Abilities

Oral Expression — The ability to communicate information and ideas in speaking so others will understand.

Problem Sensitivity — The ability to tell when something is wrong or is likely to go wrong. It does not involve solving the problem, only recognizing there is a problem.

Oral Comprehension — The ability to listen to and understand information and ideas presented through spoken words and sentences.

Figure 11.2   continued

Written Comprehension — The ability to read and understand information and ideas presented in writing.

Information Ordering — The ability to arrange things or actions in a certain order or pattern according to a specific rule or set of rules (e.g., patterns of numbers, letters, words, pictures, mathematical operations).

Near Vision — The ability to see details at close range (within a few feet of the observer).

Speech Clarity — The ability to speak clearly so others can understand you.

Speech Recognition — The ability to identify and understand the speech of another person.

Inductive Reasoning — The ability to combine pieces of information to form general rules or conclusions (includes finding a relationship among seemingly unrelated events).

Deductive Reasoning — The ability to apply general rules to specific problems to produce answers that make sense.

Work Activities

Assisting and Caring for Others — Providing personal assistance, medical attention, emotional support, or other personal care to others such as coworkers, customers, or patients.

Inspecting Equipment, Structures, or Material — Inspecting equipment, structures, or materials to identify the cause of errors or other problems or defects.

Performing for or Working Directly with the Public — Performing for people or dealing directly with the public. This includes serving customers in restaurants and stores, and receiving clients or guests.

Communicating with Supervisors, Peers, or Subordinates — Providing information to supervisors, co-workers, and subordinates by telephone, in written form, e-mail, or in person.

Identifying Objects, Actions, and Events — Identifying information by categorizing, estimating, recognizing differences or similarities, and detecting changes in circumstances or events.

Making Decisions and Solving Problems — Analyzing information and evaluating results to choose the best solution and solve problems.

Getting Information — Observing, receiving, and otherwise obtaining information from all relevant sources.

Updating and Using Relevant Knowledge — Keeping up-to-date technically and applying new knowledge to your job.

Establishing and Maintaining Interpersonal Relationships — Developing constructive and cooperative working relationships with others, and maintaining them over time.

Organizing, Planning, and Prioritizing Work — Developing specific goals and plans to prioritize, organize, and accomplish your work.

Work Context

Contact With Others — How much does this job require the worker to be in contact with others (face-to-face, by telephone, or otherwise) in order to perform it?

Face-to-Face Discussions — How often do you have to have face-to-face discussions with individuals or teams in this job?

Indoors, Environmentally Controlled — How often does this job require working indoors in environmentally controlled conditions?

Figure 11.2   continued

Exposed to Disease or Infections — How often does this job require exposure to disease/infections?

Telephone — How often do you have telephone conversations in this job?

Physical Proximity — To what extent does this job require the worker to perform job tasks in close physical proximity to other people?

Structured versus Unstructured Work — To what extent is this job structured for the worker, rather than allowing the worker to determine tasks, priorities, and goals?

Consequence of Error — How serious would the result usually be if the worker made a mistake that was not readily correctable?

Work With Work Group or Team — How important is it to work with others in a group or team in this job?

Frequency of Decision Making — How frequently is the worker required to make decisions that affect other people, the financial resources, and/or the image and reputation of the organization?

Job Zone

Title	Job Zone Three: Medium Preparation Needed
Overall Experience	Previous work-related skill, knowledge, or experience is required for these occupations. For example, an electrician must have completed three or four years of apprenticeship or several years of vocational training, and often must have passed a licensing exam, in order to perform the job.
Job Training	Employees in these occupations usually need one or two years of training involving both on-the-job experience and informal training with experienced workers.
Job Zone Examples	These occupations usually involve using communication and organizational skills to coordinate, supervise, manage, or train others to accomplish goals. Examples include electricians, fish and game wardens, legal secretaries, personnel recruiters, and recreation workers.
SVP Range	(6.0 to < 7.0)
Education	Most occupations in this zone require training in vocational schools, related on-the-job experience, or an associate's degree. Some may require a bachelor's degree.

Work Styles

Dependability — Job requires being reliable, responsible, and dependable, and fulfilling obligations.

Integrity — Job requires being honest and ethical.

Attention to Detail — Job requires being careful about detail and thorough in completing work tasks.

Concern for Others — Job requires being sensitive to others' needs and feelings and being understanding and helpful on the job.

Cooperation — Job requires being pleasant with others on the job and displaying a good-natured, cooperative attitude.

Self Control — Job requires maintaining composure, keeping emotions in check, controlling anger, and avoiding aggressive behavior, even in very difficult situations.

Stress Tolerance — Job requires accepting criticism and dealing calmly and effectively with high stress situations.

Figure 11.2   continued

Independence — Job requires developing one's own ways of doing things, guiding oneself with little or no supervision, and depending on oneself to get things done.

Adaptability/Flexibility — Job requires being open to change (positive or negative) and to considerable variety in the workplace.

Social Orientation — Job requires preferring to work with others rather than alone, and being personally connected with others on the job.

Figure 11.2   continued

students not interested in the military, simply as a career counseling tool. There are 334 questions divided among eight subtests, and three composite scores are derived after approximately 3 hours of testing. The eight subtests are General Science, Arithmetic Reasoning, Word Knowledge, Paragraph Comprehension, Auto and Shop, Mathematics Knowledge, Mechanical Comprehension, and Electronics Information. The composite scores derived are Science and Technical Skills, Verbal, and Math. The test battery was normed on a nationally representative sample, and the psychometric properties are appropriate for a battery of this type.

The composite score reliability estimates ranged from $r = 0.87$ to $r = 0.92$, and the individual tests range from $r = 0.66$ to $r = 0.88$. Criterion-related validity predicts job performance and success in civilian occupations, and construct validity shows a strong relationship between this test and similar achievement and ability tests (i.e. *SAT* and *ACT*). Few aptitude tests compare to the breadth and depth this test provides. Figure 11.3 provides a sample *ASVAB* report.

Measures of Special Abilities

A special aptitude is "a person's potential ability (or capacity to acquire proficiency) in a specified type of activity" (Mehrens & Lehmann, 1991, p. 335). Use of **special-ability aptitude tests** has a long history in workplace and vocational counseling settings and basically arose from the philosophy that an accurate match between employee ability and employment task demands would lead to greater productivity for the company and greater satisfaction for the employee. In this way, employees with certain abilities would be "matched" to the job most closely associated with their particular talents. Numerous special-ability tests commonly used in occupational settings have been developed over the years and are far too numerous to be expanded on in substantial detail here. Tables 11.1 through 11.6 provide a brief listing and description of some of these special-ability tests. In general, this type of test is probably most helpful in making placement decisions in the workplace, rather than for vocational or personal counseling.

Special-ability tests cover wide-ranging areas of interest, including mechanical, clerical, musical, and artistic aptitudes. The validity of scores on these tests varies widely depending on the individuals tested [i.e., sex, race, age, socioeconomic status (SES), values, motivation], situations, and criteria employed. Even though tests of special abilities have been specifically designed to predict job performance, many of

ASVAB SUMMARY RESULTS

PUBLIC, JANE Q
11th Gr Female (Form 23A)
SSN: XXX-XX-0534
Test Date: Mar 8, 2005
Any School H.S. ....
City......ST

Counselor Code: XXX

Prnt No. XXXXX

ASVAB Results

ASVAB Results	Percentile Scores				11th Grade Standard Score
	11th Grade Females	11th Grade Males	11th Grade Students		
Career Exploration Scores					
Verbal Skills	62	64	63		55
Math Skills	44	45	45		46
Science and Technical Skills	66	43	54		51
ASVAB Tests					
General Science	56	43	49		49
Arithmetic Reasoning	36	34	35		44
Word Knowledge	75	74	75		57
Paragraph Comprehension	44	56	50		51
Mathematics Knowledge	49	56	53		48
Electronics Information	77	52	65		53
Auto and Shop Information	68	35	51		48
Mechanical Comprehension	76	48	62		52

Military Entrance Score (AFQT)   39

11th Grade Female Standard Score Bands

EXPLANATION OF YOUR ASVAB PERCENTILE SCORES

Your ASVAB results are reported as percentile scores in the three highlighted columns to the left of the graph. Percentile scores show how you compare to other students - males and females, and for all students - in your grade. For example, a percentile score of 65 for an 11th grade female would mean she scored the same or better than 65 out of every 100 females in the 11th grade.

For purposes of career planning, knowing your relative standing in these comparison groups is important. Being male or female does not limit your career or educational choices. There are noticeable differences in how men and women score in some areas. Viewing your scores in light of your relative standing both to men and women may encourage you to explore areas that you might otherwise overlook.

You can use the **Career Exploration Scores** to evaluate your knowledge and skills in three general areas (Verbal, Math, and Science and Technical Skills). You can use the **ASVAB Test Scores** together with information on specific skill areas. *Together, these scores provide a snapshot of your current knowledge and skills.* This information will help you develop and review your career goals and plans.

EXPLANATION OF YOUR ASVAB STANDARD SCORES

Your ASVAB results are reported as standard scores in the above graph. Your score on each test is identified by the "X" in the corresponding bar graph. You should view these scores as *estimates* of your true skill level in that area. If you took the test again, you probably would receive a somewhat different score. Many things, such as how you were feeling during testing, contribute to this difference. This difference is shown with gray score bands in the graph of your results. Your standard scores are based on the ASVAB tests and composites based on your grade level.

The score bands provide a way to identify some of your strengths. Overlapping score bands mean your true skill level is similar in both areas, so the real difference between specific scores might not be meaningful. If the score bands do not overlap, you probably are stronger in the area that has the higher score band.

The ASVAB is an aptitude test. It is neither an absolute measure of your skills and abilities nor a perfect predictor of your success or failure. A high score does not guarantee success, and a low score does not guarantee failure, in a future educational program or occupation. For example, if you have never worked with shop equipment or cars, you may not be familiar with the terms and concepts assessed by the Auto and Shop Information test. Taking a course or obtaining a part-time job in this area would increase your knowledge and improve your score if you were to take it again.

USING ASVAB RESULTS IN CAREER EXPLORATION

Your career and educational plans may change over time as you gain more experience and learn more about your interests. *Exploring Careers: The ASVAB Career Exploration Guide* can help you learn more about yourself and the world of work, to identify and explore potential goals, and develop an effective strategy to realize your goals. The *Guide* will help you identify occupations in line with your interests and skills. As you explore potentially satisfying careers, you will develop your career exploration and planning skills.

Meanwhile, your ASVAB results can help you in making well-informed choices about future high school courses.

We encourage you to discuss your ASVAB results with a teacher, counselor, parent, family member or other interested adult. These individuals can help you to view your ASVAB results in light of other important information, such as your interests, school grades, motivation, and personal goals.

MILITARY ENTRANCE SCORES

The **Military Entrance Score** (also called AFQT, which stands for the Armed Forces Qualification Test) is the score used to determine your qualifications for entry into any branch of the United States Armed Forces or the Coast Guard. The **Military Entrance Score** predicts in a general way how well you might do in training and on the job in military occupations. Your score reflects your standing compared to American men and women 18 to 23 years of age.

USE OF INFORMATION

Personal identity information (name, social security number, street address, and telephone number) and test scores will not be released to any agency outside of the Department of Defense (DoD), the Armed Forces, the Coast Guard, and your school. Your school or local school system can determine any further release of information. The DoD will use your scores for recruiting and research purposes for up to two years. After that the information will be used by the DoD for research purposes only.

Use Access Code:

Access code expires:

Explore career possibilities by using your Access Code at

www.asvabprogram.com

SEE YOUR COUNSELOR FOR FURTHER INFORMATION

ASVAB SCORE AND TEST DESCRIPTIONS

Verbal Skills is a general measure of language and reading skills which combines the Word Knowledge and Paragraph Comprehension tests. People with high scores tend to do well in tasks that require good language or reading skills, while people with low scores have more difficulty with such tasks.

Math Skills is a general measure of mathematics skills which combines the Mathematics Knowledge and Arithmetic Reasoning tests. People with high scores tend to do well in tasks that require a knowledge of mathematics, while people with low scores have more difficulty with these kinds of tasks.

Science and Technical Skills is a general measure of science and technical skills which combines the General Science, Electronics Information, and Mechanical Comprehension tests. People with high scores tend to do well in tasks that require scientific thinking or technical skills, while people with low scores have more difficulty with such tasks.

General Science (GS) tests the ability to answer questions on a variety of science topics drawn from courses taught in most high schools. The life science items cover botany, zoology, anatomy and physiology, and ecology. The earth and space science items are based on astronomy, geology, meteorology, and oceanography. The physical science items measure force and motion mechanics, energy, fluids, atomic structure, and chemistry.

Arithmetic Reasoning (AR) tests the ability to solve basic arithmetic problems one encounters in everyday life. One-step and multi-step word problems require addition, subtraction, multiplication, and division, and choosing the correct order of operations when more than one step is necessary. The items include operations with whole numbers, operations with rational numbers, ratio and proportion, interest and percentage, and measurement. Arithmetic reasoning is one factor that helps characterize mathematics comprehension and it also assesses logical thinking.

Word Knowledge (WK) tests the ability to understand the meaning of words through synonyms - words having the same or nearly the same meaning as other words. The test is a measure of one component of reading comprehension since vocabulary is one of many factors that characterize reading comprehension.

Paragraph Comprehension (PC) tests the ability to obtain information from written material. Students read different types of passages of varying lengths and respond to questions based on information presented in each passage. Concepts include identifying stated and reworded facts, determining a sequence of events, drawing conclusions, identifying main ideas, determining the author's purpose and tone, and identifying style and technique.

Mathematics Knowledge (MK) tests the ability to solve problems by applying knowledge of mathematical concepts and applications. The problems focus on concepts and algorithms and involve number theory, numeration, algebraic operations and equations, geometry and measurement, and probability. Mathematics knowledge is one factor that characterizes mathematics comprehension; it also assesses logical thinking.

Electronics Information (EL) tests understanding of electrical current, circuits, devices, and systems. Electronics information topics include electrical circuits, electrical and electronic systems, electrical currents, electrical tools, symbols, devices, and materials.

Auto and Shop Information (AS) tests aptitude for automotive maintenance and repair and wood and metal shop practices. The test covers several areas commonly included in most high school auto and shop courses such as automotive components, automotive systems, automotive tools, troubleshooting and repair, shop tools, building materials, and building and construction procedures.

Mechanical Comprehension (MC) tests comprehension of the principles of mechanical devices and properties of materials. Mechanical comprehension topics include simple machines, compound machines, mechanical motion, fluid dynamics, properties of materials, and structural support.

Military Entrance Score (AFQT) is the score used if an individual decides to enter any of the armed services. See your local recruiter for details.

Figure 11.3   Sample *ASVAB* report

Source: Copyright 2005 by USMEPCOM. Reproduced with permission.

Table 11.1   Measures of clerical aptitude

Clerical Aptitude Test *(Kobal, Wrightstone, & Kunze, 1944)*

Publisher/Address:	Psychometric Affiliates, 118 Oakcrest Road, Huntsville, AL 35811
Purpose:	Measures abilities for clerical performance
Format/Subtests:	Three parts: Number Checking; Business Practice; Date, Name, Address Checking
Administration:	Pencil-and-paper

Curtis Verbal-Clerical Skills Test *(Curtis, n. d.)*

Publisher/Address:	Psychometric Affiliates, 118 Oakcrest Road, Huntsville, AL 35811
Format/Subtests:	Four subtests: Clerical and Verbal Abilities; Practical Arithmetic; Checking and Perceptual Speed and Accuracy; Reading Comprehension

General Clerical Test *(The Psychological Corporation, 1988)*

Publisher/Address:	The Psychological Corporation, 19500 Bulverde Road, San Antonio, TX 78259
Purpose:	Measures clerical speed and accuracy, numerical skills, language-related skills
Format/Subtests:	Nine parts, three subscores: Clerical Speed and Accuracy; Numerical Ability; Verbal Ability
Administration:	1 hour; clerical applicants and workers; individual and group administration; dichotomous scoring; hand scoring
Mental Measurement Yearbook (MMY)Review:	Newman (1995); Smith (1995)

Hay Aptitude Test Battery—Revised (HATB) *(Hay, 1999)*

Publisher/Address:	Wonderlic, Inc., 1795 N. Butterfield Rd., Libertyville, IL 60048
Purpose:	Measures speed and accuracy to identify individuals who can produce large amounts of work with few errors; predicts aptitude for accounting, keypunching, typing, filing, stockroom work, mail sorting positions
Format/Subtests:	One Warm-Up test, three subtests: Number Perception; Name Finding; Number Series Completion
Administration:	4 minutes per subtest (13 minutes total); cassette tapes available for (individual or group) administration and timing; speeded, paper-and-pencil, French, and Spanish versions available
Reliability/Validity:	Split-half reliability: Number Perception, 0.85; Name Finding, 0.94; Number Series Completion, 0.94; validity studies: 1972 and 1988 versions deemed equivalent
MMY Review:	Albanese (2001); Kane (2001)

Minnesota Clerical Test (MCT) *(Andrew, Paterson, & Longstaff, 1979)*

Publisher/Address:	The Psychological Corporation, 19500 Bulverde Road, San Antonio, TX 78259
Purpose:	Measures elements of perceptual speed and accuracy required for various clerical activities

Format/Subtests:	Two parts: Number and Name Comparison; 200 pairs of numbers, 200 pairs of names
Administration:	15 minutes (8 minutes for numbers; 7 minutes for names); grades 8 to adult; individual or group; speeded
Reliability/Validity:	Test-retest coefficients: 0.81–0.87; validity studies: correlated with measures of job performance, training outcome, scores from other similar tests
MMY Review:	Ryan (1985); Thomas (1985)

Office Skills Test (OST) *(Science Research Associates, 1977)*

Publisher/Address:	Reid London House, One North Dearborn, Suite 1600, Chicago, IL 60602
Purpose:	Measures aptitude for 12 on-the-job skills for entry-level employment
Format/Subtests:	Twelve subtests: Checking; Coding; Filing; Forms Completion; Grammar; Numerical Skills; Oral Directions; Punctuation; Reading Comprehension; Spelling; Typing; Vocabulary
Administration:	3–10 minutes per subtest; group or individual; alternate forms (A and B); paper-and pencil
Reliability/Validity:	Internal reliability coefficients: 0.72–0.99 (Form A); 0.56–0.96 (Form B)
MMY Review:	Shimberg (1985); Thayer (1985)

PSI Basic Skills Tests for Business, Industry, and Government *(Ruch, Shub, Moinat, & Dye, 1982)*

Publisher/Address:	Psychological Services Inc., 100 West Broadway, Suite 1100, Glendale, CA 91210
Purpose:	Measures abilities and skills important for clerical, administrative, and customer service positions
Format/Subtests:	Fifteen subtests: Classifying; Coding; Computation; Decision Making; Filing Names; Filing Numbers; Following Oral Directions; Forms Checking; Language Skills; Memory; Problem Solving; Reading Comprehension; Reasoning; Typing Practice Copy; Typing Revised Copy; Typing Straight Copy; Typing Tables; Visual Speed and Accuracy; Vocabulary
Administration:	5–15 minutes per test; group or individual; speeded
Reliability/Validity:	Reliability: none reported; overall validity relating to all job families together: 0.13–0.26
MMY Review:	Stahl (1985); Zedeck (1985)

SRA Clerical Aptitudes Test (CAT) *(Science Research Associates, 1947)*

Publisher/Address:	Science Research Associates, Inc., 155 N. Wacker Drive, Chicago, IL 60606
Purpose:	Measures general aptitude necessary for clerical work
Format/Subtests:	Three subtests: Office Vocabulary; Office Arithmetic; Office Checking
Administration:	Pencil-and-paper

Table 11.2   Measures of mechanical aptitude

Bennett Mechanical Comprehension Test (BMCT) *(Bennett, 1980)*

Publisher/Address:	The Psychological Corporation, 19500 Bulverde Road, San Antonio, TX 78259
Purpose:	Measures ability to apply physical and mechanical principles in practice; screens applicants for positions requiring complex machine operation and repair
Format/Subtests:	Total score only, alternate S and T forms; individual understanding of mechanical relationships; laws of physics in practical situations
Administration:	30 minutes; industrial employees, high school and above; individual or group; English and Spanish forms, tape version available
Reliability/Validity:	Split-half reliabilities above 0.80; validity coefficients of 0.30–0.60 in predicting success in engineering-type occupations
MMY Review:	(Sax, 1997) Wing (1992)

Mechanical Aptitude Test *(Kobal, Wrightstone, & Kunze, 1943)*

Publisher/Address:	Psychometric Affiliates, 118 Oakcrest Road, Huntsville, AL 35811
Purpose:	Measures interests and abilities associated with aptitudes for skilled trades; comprehension of mechanical tasks, use of tools and materials, matching tools with operations
Format/Subtests:	Three subtests: Mechanical Knowledge; Space Relations; Shop Arithmetic
Administration:	45 minutes; high school students and above

Revised Minnesota Paper Form Board—Revised (RMPFBT-R) *(Likert & Quasha, 1995)*

Publisher/Address:	The Psychological Corporation, 19500 Bulverde Road, San Antonio, TX 78259
Purpose:	Measures aspects of mechanical ability requiring the capacity to visualize and manipulate objects in space; assists in selection of employees for jobs or training programs that require capacity for spatial ability or visualization and manipulation of objects in space; prediction of performance in vocational-technical training settings
Format/Subtests:	Total score only, alternate A and B forms; mechanical aptitude
Administration:	20 minutes; 64 items; grade 9 and above; individual or group; speed and power test; hand- or machine-scored
Reliability/Validity:	Internal consistency coefficients: hand-scored A and B versions, split-half: 0.93 and 0.95; alternate forms: 0.86 and 0.91; test-retest on machine-scored version: 0.71 (delayed readministration [0–88 months]) to 0.85 (immediate readministration)
MMY Review:	Pearson (2001); Roszkowski (2001)

SRA Mechanical Aptitude Test *(Science Research Associates, n. d. a)*

Publisher/Address:	Science Research Associates, Inc., 155 N. Wacker Dr., Chicago, IL 60606

Purpose:	Measures ability to learn mechanical jobs
Format/Subtests:	Three subtests: Mechanical Knowledge; Space Relations; Shop Arithmetic
Administration:	35–40 minutes; high school and above

SRA Test of Mechanical Concepts *(Science Research Associates, n. d. b)*

Publisher/Address:	Science Research Associates, Inc., 155 N. Wacker Dr., Chicago, IL 60606
Purpose:	Measures ability to visualize and understand basic mechanical and spatial interrelationships
Format/Subtests:	Three subtests: Mechanical Interrelationships; Mechanical Tools and Devices; Spatial Relations
Administration:	35–40 minutes; high school and above
Reliability/Validity:	Criterion-related coefficients below 0.30
MMY Review:	(Sax, 1997)

Table 11.3   Measures of psychomotor ability

Bennett Hand-Tool Dexterity Test *(Bennett, 1985)*

Publisher/Address:	Harcourt Assessment, Inc., 19500 Bulverde Road, San Antonio, TX 78259
Purpose:	Measures manual dexterity independent of intellectual factors
Format/Subtest:	Take apart 12 assemblies of nuts, bolts, and washers from a wooden frame and reassemble with wrenches and screwdrivers
Administration:	5–10 minutes; individual; score determined by completion

Complete Minnesota Manual Dexterity Test (CMDT)
(Lafayette Instrument Company, n. d. a)

Publisher/Address:	Lafayette Instrument Company, PO Box 5729, 3700 Sagamore Parkway, North Lafayette, IN 47903
Purpose:	Measures capacity for simple but rapid eye-hand-finger coordination needed for semiskilled shop and clerical operations (i.e., wrapping, sorting, packing)
Format/Subtests:	Five subtests: Placing; Turning; Displacing; One-Hand Turning; Two-Hand Turning and Placing
Administration:	Approximately 15 minutes; ages 13–adult; individual or group
MMY Review:	Erickson (1995); Westman (1995)

Crawford Small Parts Dexterity Test (CSPD) *(Crawford & Crawford, 1985)*

Publisher/Address:	The Psychological Corporation, 19500 Bulverde Road, San Antonio, TX 78259
Purpose:	Measures eye-hand coordination, dexterity, and fine-motor skills; helps predict success in jobs requiring small parts
Format/Subtests:	Two parts: Part 1: using tweezers to assemble pin and collar assemblies; Part 2: screwing small screws into threaded holes in a plate
Administration:	8–15 minutes; individual or group

continued

Table 11.3   continued

Minnesota Rate of Manipulation Test *(American Guidance Services, 1969)*

Publisher/Address:	American Guidance Services, 4201 Woodland Rd., Circle Pines, MN 55014-1796
Purpose:	Measures finger-hand-arm dexterity; used to select employees for jobs requiring manual dexterity; used in vocational and rehabilitation training programs
Format/Subtests:	One single test
Administration:	Individual

O'Connor Tweezer Dexterity Test *(Lafayette Instrument Company, n. d. b)*

Publisher/Address:	Lafayette Instrument Company, 3700 Sagamore Parkway North, P. O. Box 5729, Lafayette, IN 47903
Purpose:	Measures speed in which an individual can pick up small objects and place them in holes
Format/Subtests:	Fine eye-hand coordination, ability to use small hand tools
Administration:	Individual

Stromberg Dexterity Test *(Stromberg, 1985)*

Publisher/Address:	Creative Organizational Design, 116 College Street, Kitchener, Ontario N2H 5A3
Purpose:	Measures manipulative skills (i.e., speed and accuracy of arm and hand movements)
Format/Subtests:	Manipulative skills in sorting by color and sequence
Administration:	5–10 minutes; individual

Table 11.4   Measures of artistic aptitude

Graves Design Judgment Test *(Graves, 1948)*

Publisher/Address:	The Psychological Corporation, 19500 Bulverde Road, San Antonio, TX 78259
Purpose:	Measure client ability to differentiate aesthetic quality within sets of geometric designs
Format/Subtests:	90 sets of two- or three-dimensional designs that vary in unity, balance, symmetry, or other aesthetic orders; individual selects best in each set

Meier Art Test: Aesthetic Perception *(Meier, 1940)*

Publisher/Address:	Bureau of Educational Research and Service, University of Iowa, Iowa City, IA 52242
Format/Subtests:	Four versions of same work presented, differing in proportion, unity, form, or design; individual ranks each set in order of merit

Table 11.5 Measures of musical aptitude

Musical Aptitude Profile—Fourth Edition *(Gordon, 1995)*

Publisher/Address:	GIA Publications, Inc., 7404 South Mason Avenue, Chicago, IL 60638
Purpose:	Evaluates music aptitude
Format/Subtests:	Three subtests: Tonal Imagery,(Melody and Harmony); Rhythm Imagery (tempo and meter); Musical Sensitivity (phrasing, balance, and style); pairs of selections are played on violin and cello, and examinee determines whether they are the same, or which of the two is a better performance
Administration:	3 ½ hours; 4th- to 12th-graders; individual or group; manual scoring
Reliability/Validity:	Reliability coefficients: individual subtests, 0.70s–0.80s; total battery, 0.90s
MMY Review:	Johnson (2005); Sherbon (2005)

Seashore Measures of Musical Talents—Revised *(Seashore, Lewis, & Saetveit, 1960)*

Publisher/Address:	The Psychological Corporation, 19500 Bulverde Road, San Antonio, TX 78259
Purpose:	Measures dimensions of auditory discrimination
Format/Subtests:	Six subtests: Pitch; Loudness; Time; Timbre; Rhythm; Tonal Memory
Administration:	1 hour; grade 4–adults; audiotape

Table 11.6 Measures of computer aptitude

Computer Operator Aptitude Battery (COAB)

Publisher/Address:	Creative Organizational Design, 116 College St., Kitchner, ON N214 5A3
Purpose:	Helps to predict performance of computer operators
Format/Subtests:	Three subtests: Sequence Recognition; Format Checking; Logical Thinking
Administration:	45 minutes; pencil-and-paper

Computer Programmer Aptitude Battery—Third Edition (CPAB-3)
(Palormo, Fisher, & Saville, 1985)

Publisher/Address:	Science Research Associates, Inc., 155 N. Wacker Dr., Chicago, IL 60606
Purpose:	Measures abilities related to success in computer programming and systems analysis fields
Format/Subtests:	Five subtests, 151 items: Verbal Meaning; Reasoning; Letter Series; Number Ability; Diagramming (problem analysis and logical solutions)
Administration:	75–90 minutes; pencil-and-paper; multiple-choice; adults; individual or group
Reliability/Validity:	Reliability coefficients: 0.67 (Letter Series) to 0.94 (Diagramming); Validity: training programs: 0.30–0.71 for total score, 0.09–0.69 for subtests; Job performance criteria: 0.02–0.61 for total score, 0.03–0.57 for subtests
MMY Review:	Mahurin (1992); Schafer (1992)

these scales yield scores with very low validity coefficients. In a review by Ghiselli (1973), validity coefficients for these measures were typically in the 0.20s. Importantly, correlations with on-the-job performance criteria were generally lower than training program success criteria. When special-ability tests are used for job placement purposes, it is recommended that the validity of candidate scores be validated using the test in the specific job-related context, using criteria appropriate to the actual job or task, and using participants with characteristics appropriate to the employees who will be hired.

> **Think About It 11.1**   Based on your experiences, discuss whether you believe aptitude test scores provide accurate predictions of future scholastic or vocational performance.

SUMMARY/CONCLUSION

Aptitude assessment is of critical importance in schools and career counseling because it helps clients and students understand strengths and limitations that may facilitate educational and vocational planning. Aptitude tests such as the *SAT-I* or the *ACT* are commonly used by universities to aid in admission decisions. General aptitude tests are frequently administered in schools and career counseling to help facilitate career and educational planning. The *ASVAB, O*Net,* and *Differential Aptitude Test* are three commonly used general aptitude batteries. Finally, employers and career counselors sometimes employ tests of specific aptitude (e.g., clerical, mechanical, musical, artistic). Aptitude tests help professional counselors and clients predict likely future performances in educational and vocational tasks.

KEY TERMS

aptitude test
differential prediction
multiaptitude battery

scholastic aptitude
special-ability aptitude test

CHAPTER 12

Assessment of Achievement

by Bradley T. Erford and Kathleen Hall

T his chapter covers the basic information necessary to understand the use of achievement testing in counseling so professional counselors can be prepared both to use achievement tests in practice and to advocate for individuals with special needs. Attention is paid to the Individuals With Disabilities Education Improvement Act (**IDEIA**) and **Section 504** of the U.S. Rehabilitation Act of 1973, two of the major laws applicable to the education of individuals with special needs. The various ways that tests can be categorized and basic elements assessed in the major subject areas are also discussed. Finally, commonly used group- and individually administered tests of achievement and language proficiency are reviewed.

WHY ASSESS ACHIEVEMENT?

Achievement tests are by far the most commonly used assessment devices in schools. Among all types of **achievement tests**, teacher-made, criterion-referenced tests are the most frequently administered, and are used mainly for the purpose of evaluating student performance and progress toward mastering educational standards. Seldom will professional school counselors be asked to consult with classroom teachers on the design and implementation of classroom tests. However, professional counselors, and professional school counselors specifically, should be aware of how standardized group- and individually administered tests of achievement are used in the school and clinical practice.

Achievement tests measure an individual's learning acquired through structured, education-based experiences. Usually, the assessment results are categorized according to how the academic instruction was implemented. For example, many achievement tests provide scores for reading (sight-word vocabulary, reading comprehension); written language (spelling, mechanics, written expression); mathematics (computation, problem solving); social studies; and science, among others. Such a score reporting system aligns with the implementation of educational instruction in many school systems and allows decision makers to make judgments about instructional effectiveness, as well as learning progress for individual students and groups of students when aggregated.

Achievement tests measure mastery of academic content. As such, the content or item composition of achievement tests is critical. Because achievement tests measure acquired knowledge, individuals who have not been exposed to information assessed by a test will be at a disadvantage. In such cases, a lower score reflects this lack of exposure to content, rather than a failure to master that content. In other words, until a student is taught something (exposure), it cannot be assumed the student is incapable of learning it (mastery). Thus great effort is expended to ensure that achievement test scores have **content validity**. Test items must align with classroom exposure and instruction to arrive at valid achievement scores. For example, if a "2nd-grade" math calculation test is administered to a group of 2nd-graders who have been taught only half of the concepts and procedures the test items measure, it is likely the students will do poorly. But these students may, on average, correctly answer 90% of the questions measuring content they have been taught. Thus their performance on content they have been exposed to may be excellent, but it may be dismal on content they have not been exposed to. To this way of thinking, achievement test scores reflect a combination of content exposure and mastery.

Achievement assessment has several purposes. Expanding on the four purposes of assessment outlined in Chapter 1—screening; diagnosis; treatment planning and goal identification; progress evaluation—educators use achievement tests for at least five specific purposes: (1) to make high-stakes decisions about students; (2) to assess the effectiveness of a school's curriculum; (3) to assess the progress or academic development of individual students; (4) to identify learning problems in individual students; and (5) to make placement or program eligibility decisions.

The first three purposes are currently addressed through large-scale and high-stakes assessments commonly administered in the schools. A test is considered **high stakes** if it carries with it serious consequences for students or educators. Some high-stakes tests have been used to determine if students will be promoted to the next grade level or receive a high school diploma. Student performance on some high-stakes tests also may lead to sanctions or rewards for schools or school systems. High-stakes testing has been on the rise in the United States and is widely attributed to the No Child Left Behind (NCLB) Act of 2001, which places a key emphasis on school accountability and the use of high-stakes testing to raise academic achievement for all students. Among other things, NCLB requires that all states administer reading and mathematics tests in grades 3–8 and 10–12, and that the content of these tests align with state educational standards. This is a function of the third purpose listed above: to assess the progress or academic development of individual students. It is up to local school systems to align their curricula with the state standards and to demonstrate that students are making adequate yearly progress toward the attainment of these state standards and learning targets. This is a function of the second purpose listed above: to assess the effectiveness of a school's curriculum. Curriculum effectiveness traditionally has been addressed through large-scale assessment and, more recently, high-stakes testing. The companion website for this text provides an in-depth analysis of the facets of high-stakes testing of which professional counselors must be aware. Some professional counselors make the mistake of thinking NCLB is applicable only to professional school counselors. NCLB has changed the landscape of education, and professional counselors, regardless of specialty area, will deal with its consequences, intended or otherwise.

The fourth and fifth purposes listed above involve identification of learning problems in individual students and subsequent placement or program eligibility decisions. While there are many funded and unfunded remedial programs in operation in any given school system, the two law-based processes most frequently encountered by professional school counselors employed within the school system, and professional counselors practicing in agencies or in private practice, are IDEIA (special education) and Section 504. Professional counselors are well advised to become very familiar with these laws and local implementation procedures to best advocate for students and clients.

USES OF ACHIEVEMENT TESTS IN COUNSELING

Professional school counselors, college counselors, and career counselors are probably the counseling specialty areas most intimately associated with achievement testing, but all professional counselors should have a basic understanding of this important assessment domain. In the schools, professional school counselors sometimes use achievement tests to screen children for potential learning problems, whether by administering individualized tests or by reviewing individual student results from a large-scale testing program. Either way, professional school counselors must be familiar with the specific tests used, what each measures, and how to administer, score, and interpret the tests. Sometimes, a professional school counselor serves as a school's testing coordinator and may be responsible for receiving, securing, distributing, administering, collecting, and shipping testing materials for a school's large-scale testing program. Frequently, the professional school counselor will also receive and distribute the school's results and parent report forms. Such responsibilities require outstanding organization, attention to detail, and follow-up.

Professional school, college, career, mental health, and community counselors are often advocates for students and clients with special needs and ensure that students receive appropriate services and learning accommodations. To be an effective **advocate**, professional counselors must understand educational and civil rights laws, psychometrics, the domain of behavior assessed by a test, and what scores on achievement and other tests may imply regarding student eligibility. Depending on state practice law and regulations, and the professional counselor's personal competence in assessment, professional counselors may be able to administer, score, and interpret achievement and other learning-related inventories to diagnose learning problems and provide advocacy for those already diagnosed.

Think About It 12.1   In what ways can a professional counselor be an advocate for a client? Why is this an important aspect of the counseling profession? What role can a professional counselor skilled in assessment play as an advocate?

Achievement test information can also be incredibly helpful in career and educational planning and decision making. Often clients and students know where their interests lie but are unsure whether they have the skills and knowledge to handle the college-level or technical coursework required to access the desired occupation. This is a primary reason why intelligence, aptitude, and achievement tests are so important to the practice of professional counselors and the clients they serve. One of the unwritten laws of behavior is that the best indicator of future performance is past performance. For example, if a student's field of interest is math-intensive, assessing the student's past and current mathematics achievement level may provide insight into the likelihood the student might perform adequately in higher-level mathematics courses.

ACHIEVEMENT TESTING AND INDIVIDUALS WITH SPECIAL NEEDS

One of the most important applications of achievement testing is in the public school realm of special education. Professional counselors in general, and professional school counselors specifically, who are not aware of the applicable laws, policies, and procedures governing the administration of special education services can not effectively advocate for students with special needs. The two laws that apply most directly to individuals with special educational needs are the Individuals With Disabilities Education Improvement Act and Section 504 of the U.S. Rehabilitation Act of 1973.

The Individuals With Disabilities Education Improvement Act (IDEIA)

IDEIA defines the following categories of handicapping conditions: autism; deaf-blindness; deafness; developmental delay; emotional disturbance; hearing impairment; mental retardation; orthopedic or other health impairment; specific learning disability; speech or language impairment; traumatic brain injury; visual impairment, including blindness; and multiple disabilities. Achievement testing may be a component of a comprehensive assessment in any of these categories. IDEIA guarantees the right of special education services to qualified students from birth to age 21 years, an individualized education program (IEP), education in the least restrictive environment (LRE), protection in evaluation procedures, and due process. While beyond the scope of this text, a comprehensive discussion of these provisions and the role of the professional school counselor can be found in Lockhart (2003).

The handicapping condition of **specific learning disability** (LD) perhaps is of greatest interest to the discussion of achievement testing. A specific learning disability was defined in Section 5(b)(4) of the Education for All Handicapped Children Act of 1975 (Public Law 94-142) as

> a disorder in one or more of the basic psychological processes involved in understanding or in using language, spoken or written, which may manifest itself in an imperfect ability to listen, think, speak, read, write, spell, or do mathematical calculations. The term includes such conditions as perceptual handicaps, brain injury, minimal brain dysfunction, dyslexia, and developmental aphasia. The term does not include children who have learning problems which are primarily the result of visual, hearing, or motor handicaps, or mental retardation, or of environmental, cultural, or economic disadvantages.

The diagnosis of LD requires documentation of three elements: (1) the absence of other primary handicapping conditions and environmental, cultural, and economic disadvantage as the primary cause; (2) a specific processing disorder (e.g., short-term memory, visual processing, auditory processing, processing speed, visual-motor integration); and (3) an educational deficiency in a qualifying academic content area so serious that it is significantly discrepant from ability. Specifically, a diagnosis of LD can be made if the student demonstrates a significant discrepancy between **ability** (normally assessed using individualized intelligence tests) and **achievement** (normally assessed using individualized achievement tests) in one or more of the following seven academic areas: oral expression, listening comprehension, basic reading skill, reading comprehension, written expression, mathematics calculation, and mathematics reasoning. Fortunately or unfortunately, the federal government never defined what a significant discrepancy between ability and achievement consisted of, so states and local school systems have been left to their own devices. On the other hand, the *Diagnostic and Statistical Manual of Mental Disorders—Fourth Edition—Text Revision* (*DSM-IV-TR*) defines a significant discrepancy as two standard deviations (i.e., 30 deviation IQ points). This can lead to substantial differences in eligibility requirements from state to state, and even from local school system to school system within the same state. For this and other reasons, many have criticized the efficiency and fairness of using discrepancy formulas (Fletcher et al., 1994; Kavale, 1995). Telzrow (1985) provided a well-written account of problems related to the use of discrepancy formulas.

To resolve the controversy over the lack of a clear definition of ability-achievement discrepancy, most states or localities have settled on one of three decision-making models for determining a significant discrepancy between ability and achievement: (1) the grade-equivalent discrepancy model, (2) the standard score point discrepancy model, and (3) the standard score point discrepancy with statistical regression model. Determining **grade-equivalent discrepancies** was somewhat popular in the 1970s but was largely abandoned as decision makers became more aware of the dangers of making decisions using grade and age equivalents. This model basically involved determining how many grade levels below current grade placement (or estimated expected grade placement based on an ability test score) a student needed to fall before a significant discrepancy could be claimed. For example, if the student was of average ability and in grade 5.2 (i.e., the 2nd month of the 5th-grade year), and it was determined that a significant discrepancy was 2.0 grade equivalents, the student would have to have one or more qualifying achievement area grade-equivalent scores of 3.2 (2nd month of 3rd grade) or lower to qualify for services. This method appears simple on the surface, but recall from Chapter 5 that grade and age equivalents *cannot* be manipulated mathematically (e.g., added, subtracted) because they are not transformed using an equal interval procedure the same way that standard scores are. Thus grade-equivalent discrepancies lead to inaccurate results.

The second model, the **standard score point discrepancy**, is very commonly used within the United States. In this model, the student's achievement test standard score is subtracted from the deviation IQ score (both with an $M = 100$; $SD = 15$). For example, a student with an IQ score of 115 and math calculation standard score of 85 would have a discrepancy score of 30 standard score points. If the discrepancy score exceeds the standard agreed to within the state or local education agency, the student may qualify for special education services. The cutoff criterion score varies by locale but usually falls between one and two standard deviations (a 15- to 30-point discrepancy). As discussed in Chapter 4, where the criterion (cutoff score) is set has important consequences, both for individual students and for the percentage of the population that will eventually qualify for services. In the example given above, if the student's discrepancy was 30 standard score points and the school system's criterion was 25 standard score points, the student might qualify for services.

The third model, the standard score point discrepancy with **statistical regression**, is becoming more commonly used within the United States This procedure is somewhat complicated, and states and school systems often produce regression and discrepancy tables to minimize errors of computation. Recall from Chapter 4 that the term *regression* has to do with prediction (i.e., what may be expected). Statistical regression in this context involves the prediction of a student's expected achievement level given a known (observed) intelligence ability score. While the regression values rely on test reliabilities and correlation coefficients between the tests, normally there are about six standard score points of regression for each standard deviation. In the example given above, an IQ score of 115 would lead to a predicted achievement score of 109 (i.e., 115 is exactly one standard deviation above the mean [6 points of regression] so $115 - 6 = 109$). If the school system uses the discrepancy criterion of 25 standard score points, any student with an IQ of 115 would need to have an achievement test standard score of 84 ($109 - 25 = 84$) to qualify for special education services. As you can see, using an eligibility criterion of 25 standard score points with statistical regression led to a net required discrepancy of 31 standard score points (i.e., $115 - 84 = 31$).

Table 12.1 provides ability (IQ scores) and expected educational achievements for various points in the standard score distribution, as well as commonly used dis-

Table 12.1 Ability and expected achievement calculations using a statistical regression model

IQ score	Regression points	Expected achievement	Minus 20 SS points	Minus 25 SS points	Minus 30 SS points
145	−18	127	107	102	97
140	−16	124	104	99	94
135	−14	121	101	96	91
130	−12	118	98	93	88
125	−10	115	95	90	85
120	−8	112	92	87	82
115	−6	109	89	84	79
110	−4	106	86	81	76
105	−2	103	83	78	73
100	0	100	80	75	70
95	+2	97	77	72	67
90	+4	94	74	69	64
85	+6	91	71	66	61
80	+8	88	68	63	58
75	+10	85	65	60	55
70	+12	82	62	57	52

Note: SS = standard score.

crepancy cutoffs. Of course, the concept of regression to the mean applies to ability scores that fall below the mean, but in the opposite direction to scores that fall above the mean. For example, in the 25-point-discrepancy decision-making system described above, an IQ score of 85 would also regress about 6 points toward the mean, resulting in an expected achievement level of 91. Subtracting the 25-point criterion from 91 yields a discrepancy cutoff of 66 (91 − 25 = 66). This is a net discrepancy standard score difference of only 19 points (IQ of 85 − 66 = 19). Of course, if the student's IQ score is at the mean (IQ = 100), regression is zero. Several publishers have conormed intelligence and achievement batteries to provide accurate regression models that generate expected difference scores. These include the *Wechsler Intelligence Scale for Children—Fourth Edition (WISC-IV)*, the *Wechsler Individual Achievement Test—Second Edition (WIAT-II)*, and the *Woodcock-Johnson Tests of Achievement—Third Edition (WJ-III-ACH)*.

Each of these three discrepancy models and various criterion cutoffs frequently will yield different results in terms of student eligibility for learning disability services. Table 12.2 contains a comparison of potential decision outcomes for one child based on the same test score performance. It is essential to understand that such variations in decision-making models have implications not only for an individual student, but also for the percentage of a school-aged population that will actually qualify for special education services. As advocates for students with special needs, the more professional counselors know about these decision-making models and special education policies and procedures, the better prepared they will be for providing effective advocacy.

Table 12.2 Comparison of various discrepancy models for a 10-year-old, 4th-grade student with an IQ of 120 (mental grade equivalent = 7.0) and a basic reading skills standard score of 93 (achievement grade equivalent = 3.7)

Model	Expected achievement score/equivalent	Actual achievement score/equivalent	Actual discrepancy	Cutoff criterion	Discrepancy decision
2.0 Grade equivalents	7.0	3.7	3.3 GE	2.0 GE	Eligible
2.5 Grade eequivalents	7.0	3.7	3.3 GE	2.5 GE	Eligible
3.0 Grade equivalents	7.0	3.7	3.3 GE	3.0 GE	Eligible
20 Standard score points	120	93	27 SS	20 SS	Eligible
25 Standard score points	120	93	27 SS	25 SS	Eligible
30 Standard Score points	120	93	27 SS	30 SS	Not eligible
20 Regressed stan. score	112	93	19 SS	20 SS	Not eligible
25 Regressed stan. score	112	93	19 SS	25 SS	Not eligible
30 Regressed stan. score	112	93	19 SS	30 SS	Not eligible

Note: SS means standard score points ($M = 100$, $SD = 15$); GE means grade equivalents in years (e.g., a GE of 3.3 means three whole grade levels plus three-tenths of a whole grade level).

Section 504 of the U.S. Rehabilitation Act of 1973

A second major piece of legislation that relates to services for individuals with special needs is known as "Section 504" (Public Law 93-112). Section 504 is civil rights legislation that protects persons with disabilities from discrimination. It was follow-up legislation to the Civil Rights Act of 1964, and the predecessor to the 1991 Americans With Disabilities Act (ADA; Public Law 101-336). Section 504, administered by the federal Office of Civil Rights (OCR), can result in the withholding of federal funds from institutions (e.g., state departments of education, local education agencies, universities) that discriminate against individuals with disabilities, fail to comply with the act, or choose not to correct noncompliance with the act. The act [104.3(j)] provides several important definitions:

Handicapped persons means any person who (i) has a physical or mental impairment which substantially limits one or more major life activities, (ii) has a record of such an impairment, or (iii) is regarded as having such an impairment. . . .

Physical or mental impairment means (A) any physiological disorder or condition, cosmetic disfigurement, or anatomical loss affecting one or more of the following body systems: neurological; musculoskeletal; special sense organs; respiratory, including speech organs; cardiovascular; reproductive, digestive, genitourinary; hemic and lymphatic; skin; and endocrine; or (B) any mental or psychological disorder, such as mental retardation, organic brain syndrome, emotional or mental illness, and specific learning disabilities. . . .

Major life activities means functions such as caring for one's self, performing manual tasks, walking, seeing, hearing, speaking, breathing, learning, and working.

Section 504 is often used to secure educational services or accommodations for individuals with Attention-Deficit/Hyperactivity Disorder (AD/HD) or other mental disorders whose learning is affected, but who are not eligible for services under IDEIA. Section 504 provides no federal funding to schools for these services or accommodations as IDEIA does. Also, while disagreements and appeals over IDEIA services are generally handled through internal school system procedures and rarely at the state education department level, Section 504 is civil rights legislation and can be submitted to the courts at any juncture. Knowledge of Section 504, ADA, and other civil rights legislation is critical to effective advocacy for school- and college-aged clients by professional counselors.

CATEGORIZING ACHIEVEMENT TESTS

Many ways exist for measuring and categorizing achievement tests. Whiston (2005) proposed categories of (1) survey achievement batteries, (2) individual diagnostic achievement tests, (3) criterion-referenced and minimum-level skills tests, and (4) subject area tests. Drummond (2004) proposed similar categories but split out individual achievement and diagnostic achievement, as well as criterion-referenced and minimum-level skills tests. **Survey batteries** measure wide-ranging subject areas (e.g., reading, written expression, mathematics, science, social studies) and are usually group administered. Many large-scale testing programs use survey achievement batteries, such as the *TerraNova-2* or *Iowa Test of Basic Skills-Sixth Edition* (*ITBS*). **Individual diagnostic achievement tests** are individually administered and used to diagnose learning problems or to provide a reliable estimate of current academic performance. These tests are often used in psychoeducational or educational assessments related to eligibility for special education services. Some **criterion-referenced** and **minimum-level skills tests** may be individually administered, while some may be group administered. They measure knowledge and skills and compare a student's performance to some standard of competence. Many group-administered high-stakes tests used by state departments of education fall into this category. An example of an individually administered criterion-referenced test is the *Brigance Inventory of Basic Skills*. *Single-subject tests* are usually developed by teachers and used in individual classrooms to determine mastery of a particular subject area.

There are, of course, many other ways to categorize tests, most of which are subcategories of those listed above. Nitko (2001) discussed single-level and multilevel tests. **Single-level tests** measure a single subject in a single time period (e.g., 2nd grade, freshman year of college). Such tests are a snapshot of achievement at one point in time and do not allow the evaluation of growth over time. Examples of single-level tests would be an Algebra I exam or the final evaluation in a graduate-level assessment course. **Multilevel batteries** do allow the monitoring of skill development over time. This type of test can be used to assess a single subject or survey several subjects over the course of several to many years. The *TerraNova-2*, for example, can be administered repeatedly throughout a student's academic career to determine year-to-year growth.

As explained in Chapter 1, tests may be categorized as either norm referenced or criterion referenced. **Norm-referenced tests**, like the *TerraNova-2*, *Woodcock-Johnson:*

Tests of Achievement—Third Edition (*WJ-III ACH*), or the *Wechsler Individual Achievement Test—Second Edition* (*WIAT-II*), allow a student's score to be compared to those of a group of other students with similar characteristics (i.e., a norm group). This allows the student's performance to be viewed as being above, below, or at the norm (Average). **Criterion-referenced tests**, like the *Brigance* or most teacher-made tests, allow a student's score to be compared to some standard or criterion. This allows the student's performance to be viewed as either meeting or not meeting the criterion for mastery. Some tests, like the *TerraNova-2* or the *Slosson Diagnostic Math Screener* (Erford & Boykin, 1996), can even be adapted to provide both norm- and criterion-referenced information.

Tests can also be categorized as *group administered* and *individually administered*, depending on how many students or clients the examiner is able to administer the test to at a time. Generally speaking, anytime the examiner can administer the test to more than one examinee simultaneously, the test is considered group administered. However, an additional consideration is whether the test was normed through group administration procedures or on individuals. Many tests can be adapted for group administration but were normed via individual administration. Thus, even though the test *can* be administered using a group format, the effects of group administration of the test may be largely unknown and may adversely influence some scores. It is good practice to always follow the standardized procedures listed in the test manual.

Salvia & Ysseldyke (2004) distinguished between single-skill tests and multiple-skills batteries. *Single-skill tests* cover a single academic area, such as reading, mathematics, or written expression. Examples of single-skill tests might include the *KeyMath—Revised/Normative Update* (*KeyMath-R/NU*), which is a diagnostic math test, or the *Woodcock Reading Mastery Test—Revised/Normative Update* (*WRMT-R/NU*), a diagnostic reading assessment. *Multiple-skills tests* measure several academic subject areas in a single administration. These tests vary substantially in breadth and depth of coverage. For example, the *Wide-Range Achievement Test—Third Edition* (*WRAT-3*) measures sight-word vocabulary (i.e., basic reading skill), math calculation, and spelling. The *WRAT-3* covers only two of the eight LD achievement areas listed above, so is quite limited in breadth. Also, the number of items on each subtest is less than that found on most kindergarten through adult achievement tests. On the other hand, the *Wechsler Individual Achievement Test—Second Edition* (*WIAT-II*) measures all seven achievement areas listed within the criteria for a specific learning disability, and the number of items on each subtest is substantial, allowing a good spread of scores for individuals across the kindergarten-to-adulthood range. Both the *WRAT-3* and *WIAT-II* are individually administered, but multiple-subject tests frequently come in a group administration format and are administered in large-scale testing programs (e.g., *TerraNova-2, ITBS-6, Stanford Achievement Test—Tenth Edition* [*SAT-10*]).

Of a somewhat finer distinction, achievement tests can also be classified as screening- and diagnostic-level instruments. In general, **diagnostic tests** have more items to assess specific skills and concepts in depth, often pointing out individual strengths and weaknesses in the process and pinpointing difficulties individuals may be experiencing on a given skill, albeit not always "why" the difficulty exists (Cohen & Swerdlik, 1999; Salvia & Ysseldyke, 2004). Individual diagnostic tests are frequently used to make important placement or eligibility decisions and are normally held to higher psychometric standards (e.g., reliability and validity). For example, norm samples of diagnostic tests frequently have 200 or more participants at each age or grade level, and score reliability is generally expected to be $r = 0.90$ or higher because of the importance of the decisions made using diagnostic tests. In comparison, **screening tests** have fewer items measuring specific skills and are more useful as a general measure of student functioning in a given academic area. Screening tests often have standardization samples of at least 100 participants per age or grade level and desirable reliability coefficients of $r = 0.80$ or higher. Screening tests are helpful for hypothesis testing and validation, but not for making important decisions about a person's life; screening tests are just not as comprehensive, substantively designed, and useful as diagnostic tests.

Regardless of how a test is classified, each has a contribution to make in understanding student achievement. The various categories described above vary in comprehensiveness, administration time, breadth, and depth. The remainder of this chapter reviews commonly used achievement tests professional counselors may encounter in their work with students and clients.

Group-Administered Multi-Skill Achievement Test Batteries

Nitko (2001) outlined several features that standardized survey batteries share in common. The test manuals and other documentation provide information on the content covered, how norms or criterion-referencing procedures were developed, score reliability, and bias analyses. Survey batteries usually are administered in 2 to 3 hours over several time periods or days; provide practice examples to increase student testing sophistication; and include "bubble forms" for older students to enter responses on and response booklets for younger students to enter responses on. Importantly, these batteries provide items that assess a continuum of skills across grade levels, so a student taking the "3rd-grade-level" test will have some items that assess content skills from 1st- and 2nd-grade levels, as well as the 4th-grade and higher levels. Survey tests often feature special norm configurations so that a student's scores can be compared to a total national norm and norms with certain subgroups (e.g., state norm, school system norm, private school norm) or population demographics (e.g., suburban residents). While the design of computerized test scoring features varies, nearly all individual student profile forms provide graphical displays of student performance, an item performance summary, percentile ranks, standard scores (usually representing the extended range rather than an $M = 100$ and $SD = 15$), normal-curve equivalents, stanines, and grade equivalents. Test publishers strive to individualize the student reports and provide information that will be helpful to teachers and parents in addressing individual student needs. Aggregated computerized reports are also usually available in a variety of formats, including single-class, total-grade, and district-wide summaries. Table 12.3 provides a summary of a number of large-scale assessments and the grade levels and content areas covered by each.

Table 12.3   Comparison of large-scale tests of achievement

Test	Levels	Grades	Measures
TerraNova-2	10 (Kindergarten)– 22 (grades 11,12)	K–12	Student achievement in reading and language arts, mathematics, science, social studies
Stanford Achievement Test (*SAT-10*)	*Stanford Early Achievement Test 1 & 2:* Primary 1–3, Intermediate 1–3, Advanced 1 & 2; *Stanford Test of Academic Skills 1 & 2*	K–13	Student achievement in reading, language, spelling, study skills, listening, mathematics, science, social science
Iowa Test of Basic Skills (*ITBS-6*)	5–14	K–8	Student achievement in reading, language arts, mathematics, social studies, science, sources information
Metropolitan Achievement Test (*MAT*)	Preprimer, Primer, Primary 1 & 2, Elementary 1 & 2, Intermediate 1–4, Secondary 1–3	K–12	Student achievement in reading, mathematics, language arts, science, and social studies at appropriate levels
National Achievement Test— Second Edition (*NAT-2*)	A–L	K–12	Student achievement in reading, language, mathematics, and word attack as commonly found in school curricula; higher levels measure science, social studies, reference skills
Science Research Associates Survey of Basic Skills	20–37	K–12	Reading, mathematics, language arts, reference materials, social studies, science, survey of applied skills as based on the learner objectives most commonly taught in the United States

Nitko (2001) also pointed to several important differences between and among survey battery publishers. One important difference is the content emphasized within each subject area. Recall from the discussion of content validity that tests are composed of samples of items representing the domain of knowledge of a given subject or discipline. Great effort is expended to be sure that selected items faithfully represent both the breadth and importance of various subject content. Some disciplines (e.g., math, science) enjoy widespread agreement on essential content among experts and curriculum, others (e.g., literature, social studies) to a lesser degree. A second difference involves the seamlessness of *articulation* (i.e., development over time) within a given content area across grade levels. One purpose of repeated large-scale assessments is to track individual student skill development over time, thus demonstrating that a student's learning trajectory is "on target." Statistical techniques, such as *item response theory,* and test development procedures, such as *equating* or the use of some of the same items administered to students in adjacent grade levels, are two methods that publishers use to facilitate this tracking of learning performance. A final difference involves the types of services that publishers offer to school systems to customize the large-scale assessments to particular needs. Some publishers provide extensive technical support or expert consultation, others do not. Some provide extensive computerized report services, such as comprehensive individualized profile-interpretive reports or classroom/school/district summary reports, while others provide only basic summary information about individual or group performance.

The remainder of this section reviews a number of the major large-scale assessments used in schools today, including the *TerraNova-2*, the *Iowa Test of Basic Skills* (*ITBS*), the *Metropolitan Achievement Test*, the *Science Research Associates* (*SRA*) *Achievement Test*, the *Stanford Achievement Test*, and the *Metropolitan Readiness Tests*.

TerraNova—Second Edition (TerraNova-2)

The *TerraNova-2* (CTB/McGraw Hill, 2001) is a group-administered, multiple-skills battery that provides norm-referenced and objective-mastery scores for students in kindergarten through 12th grade. It takes the place of the *Comprehensive Test of Basic Skills* (*CTBS*-5) and the *California Achievement Test* (*CAT-6*). The survey test battery provides both norm- and criterion-referenced interpretations and is composed of four subtests: Reading/Language Arts, Mathematics, Science, and Social Studies. If more information is desired by the administrator, the supplemental subtests of Word Analysis, Vocabulary, Language Mechanics, Spelling, and Mathematic Computations could be added. School systems can choose both selected response (multiple-choice) and constructed response (short-answer, essay) items. A Spanish version, knows as *Supera,* is also available. Like many other large-scale survey batteries, the *TerraNova-2* used item response theory to calibrate and select items appropriate to a specific grade level. Items were also subjected to differential item functioning, a technique that analyzes between-group item performance. Using this sophisticated technique, items can be analyzed for racial group or sex differences. Total administration time varies based on the grade level of examinees and the number of additional supplemental subtests. Administration times ranged from $1\frac{1}{2}$ hours for kindergarteners to 6 hours and 40 minutes for students in grades 4–12 to complete all of the standard and supplemental subtests. The sample is stratified based on the 2000 U.S. Census (Salvia & Ysseldyke, 2004). Public and parochial and private school samples were stratified according to important population demographics (e.g., socioeconomic status, region of the United States, community size). The sample included more than 200,000 participants. Figure 12.1 provides a sample computer-generated *TerraNova-2* student report profile.

Internal consistency coefficients for the *TerraNova-2* ranged from $r = 0.67$ to $r = 0.91$ for subtests of the survey battery, from $r = 0.64$ to $r = 0.94$ for subtests comprising the complete battery, and from $r = 0.67$ to $r = 0.91$ for the multiple assessments (Salvia & Ysseldyke, 2004). Reliabilities on some subtests were too low for use in making decisions about individuals without other supplemental sources. No data were available on test-retest reliability for the *TerraNova-2*. Content validity was demonstrated by selecting items that were anchored to school curriculums (Salvia & Ysseldyke, 2004), but additional criterion-related correlations were not available.

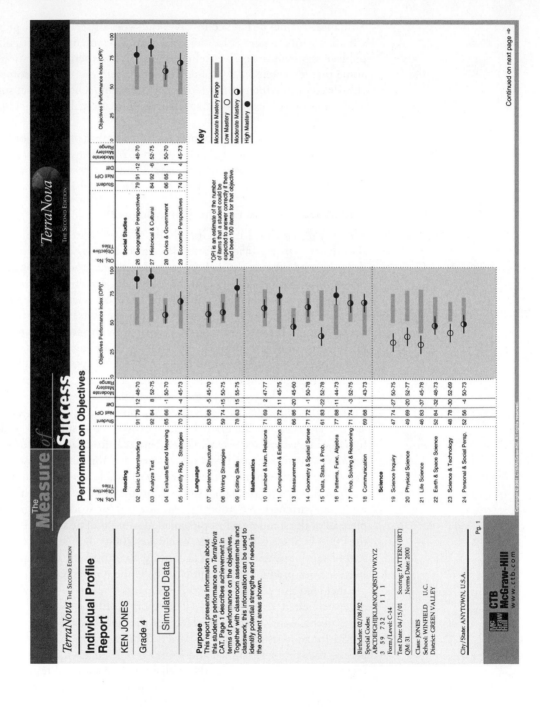

CAT COMPLETE BATTERY

Individual Profile Report

Simulated Data

Purpose
Page 2 of this report presents norm-referenced information as well as descriptions of the skills and abilities the student demonstrated, and the skills and abilities the student can work toward to show academic growth.

Birthdate: 02/08/92
Special Codes:
ABCDEFGHIJKLMNOPQRSTUVWXYZ
3 5 9 7 3 2   1 1 1
Test Date: 04/15/01   Scoring: PATTERN (IRT)
QM: 31   Norms Date: 2000

Class: JONES
School: WINFIELD
District: GREEN VALLEY

City/State: ANYTOWN, U.S.A.

Norm-Referenced Scores

	Scale Score	Grade Equiv.	National Stanine	National Percentile	NP Range
Reading	677	5.8	6	65	55-75
Language	657	4.3	5	53	43-60
Mathematics	699	6.8	7	82	74-89
Total Score**	681	5.8	6	72	60-81
Science	671	4.4	5	55	45-66
Social Studies	669	4.7	5	58	48-68

**Total Score consists of Reading, Language, and Mathematics.

National Percentile Scale
1   10   25   50   75   90   99

National Stanine Scale
1 2 3 4 5 6 7 8 9

Skills and abilities the student demonstrates:

Reading...
Students use context clues and structural analysis to determine word meaning. They recognize homonyms and antonyms in grade-level text. They identify important details; sequence, cause and effect, and lessons embedded in the text. They interpret characters' feelings and apply information to new situations. In written responses, they can express an opinion and support it. Integrate the use of analogies to generalize an idea; identify paraphrases of concepts or ideas in text; indicate specific thought processes that lead to an answer; demonstrate understanding of an implied theme; assess intent of passage information; and provide justification for answers.

The student demonstrated some understanding of the knowledge, skills, and abilities assessed in this content area.

In Language Arts...
Students identify irrelevant sentences in paragraphs and select the best place to insert new information. They recognize faulty sentence construction. They can combine simple sentences with conjunctions and use simple subordination of phrases/clauses. They identify reference sources. They recognize correct conventions for dates, closings, and place names in informal correspondence. Understand logical development in paragraph structure; identify essential information from notes; recognize the effect of prepositional phrases on subject-verb agreement; find and correct errors when editing simple narratives; correct run-on and incomplete sentences; eliminate all errors their own work.

The student demonstrated some understanding of the knowledge, skills, and abilities assessed in this content area.

In Mathematics...
Students identify even and odd numbers; subtract whole numbers with regrouping; multiply and divide by one-digit numbers; identify simple fractions; measure with ruler to nearest inch; tell time to nearest fifteen minutes; recognize symmetry; subdivide shapes; complete bar graphs; extend numerical and geometric patterns; apply simple logical reasoning. Locate decimals on a number line; apply basic number theory; compute with decimals and fractions; measure to the nearest quarter-inch; read scale drawings; identify results of geometric transformations; construct and label bar graphs; find simple probabilities; find averages; use patterns in data to solve problems; use multiple strategies and concepts to solve unfamiliar problems; express mathematical ideas and explain the problem-solving process.

The student demonstrated some of the knowledge, skills, and abilities assessed in this content area.

In Science...
Students are familiar with the life cycles of plants and animals. They can identify an example of a cold-blooded animal. They infer what once existed from fossil evidence. They recognize the term habitat. They understand the water cycle. They know science and society issues such as recycling and sources of pollution. They can sequence technological advances. They extrapolate data, devise a simple classification scheme, and determine the purpose of a simple experiment. Differentiate between instinctive and learned behavior; develop a working understanding of the structure of the Earth; create a better understanding of terms such as decomposers, fossil fuel, eclipse, and buoyancy; interpret more detailed graphs and tables; understand experimentation.

The student demonstrated some of the knowledge, skills, and abilities assessed in this content area.

In Social Studies...
Students demonstrate skills in organizing information. They use time lines, product and global maps, and cardinal directions. They understand simple cause and effect relationships and historical documents. They sequence events, associate holidays with events, and classify natural resources. They compare life in different times and understand some economic concepts related to products, jobs, and the environment. They give some detail in written responses. They synthesize information from sources such as maps and charts; create a better understanding of the democratic process, the basic principles our government was founded on, as well as roles and responsibilities of government and citizens; recognize patterns and similarities in different historical times; understand global and environmental issues; locate continents and major countries; summarize information from multiple sources in early American history; describe how geography affected the development of the colonial economy; thoroughly understand both sides of an issue.

The student demonstrated most of the knowledge, skills, and abilities assessed in this content area.

For more information, refer to the Guide to the Individual Profile Report, or visit CTB's website, www.ctb.com.

Pg. 2

CTB McGraw-Hill
www.ctb.com

Figure 12.1 TerraNova-2 sample profile report

Source: From *TerraNova-2 Individual Profile Report* by CTB/McGraw-Hill, 2001, Monterey, CA: CTB/McGraw-Hill, LLC. Copyright © 2001 by CTB/McGraw-Hill. Reproduced with permission of CTB/McGraw-Hill, LLC.

Table 12.4 *ITBS* subtests and levels within which each is administered

Level/subtest	Levels administered
Vocabulary	5–14
Word Analysis	5–9
Listening	5–9
Reading/Reading Comprehension	6–14
Language	
Spelling	5–14
Capitalization	7–14
Punctuation	9–14
Usage & Expression	9–14
Mathematics	
Concepts & Estimation	5–14
Problem Solving (MPS) & Data Interpretation (DI)	7–14
Computation	7–14
Social Studies	7–14
Science	7–14
Sources of Information	
Maps & Diagrams	7–14
Reference Materials	9–14
Reading	7–14
Vocabulary	7–14
Comprehension	9–14
Pictures	7–8
Sentences	7–8
Stories	7–8
Language	7–14
Spelling	7–8
Capitalization	7–8
Punctuation	7–8
Usage & Expression	7–8
Mathematics	
Concepts & Estimation	7–14
Problem Solving (MPS) & Data Interpretation	7–14
Computation	7–14

Adapted from Hoover et al. (2005).

Iowa Test of Basic Skills (ITBS), *Form A*

The *Iowa Test of Basic Skills* (*ITBS*), Form A (Hoover, Hieronymus, Dunbar, & Frisbie, 2001) provides information about individual student competence in basic school subject areas. The authors divided the sample of students in kindergarten through 8th grade into 14 different levels. The *ITBS* contains 19 different subtests (e.g., Vocabulary, Reading, Math Concepts, Social Studies, Reference Materials), which were administered to each group dependent on grade level (Level 5 = kindergarten through grade 1.5; Level 15 = grade 8) (see Table 12.4.) Administration time

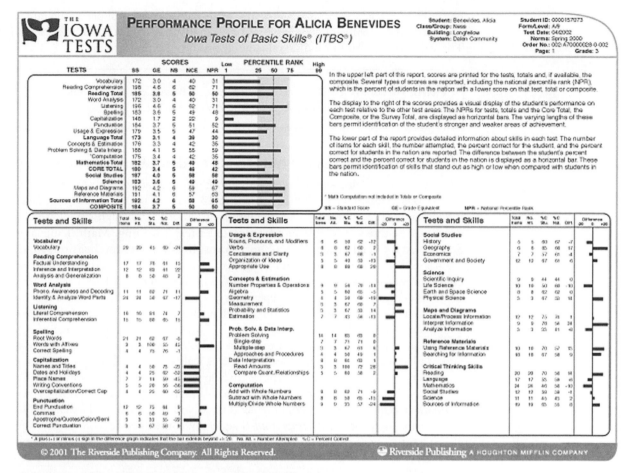

Figure 12.2 *ITBS* Sample performance profile report

Source: From *Iowa Test of Basic Skills (ITBS) Performance Profile,* by H. O. Hoover, A. N. Hieronymus,
S. B. Dunbar, and D. A. Frisbie, 2001, Itasca, IL: Riverside Publishing Company. Copyright © 2001 by
The Riverside Publishing Company. Figure titled "Performance Profile" from the Iowa Tests of Basic Skills®
(ITBS®) reproduced with permission of the publisher. All rights reserved.

ranges from 1½ to 6 hours depending on the battery given (Salvia & Ysseldyke,
2004).

Figure 12.2 provides a sample *ITBS* performance profile report. The *ITBS* involves critical thinking skills rather than factual memorization. Educators often debate whether achievement tests should measure content (e.g., basic facts) or process
(e.g., application of basic facts). The *ITBS* strives to address the latter. Educators
often use the *ITBS* to obtain information in support of instructional decisions or as
a report of individual progress for students and parents. Raw scores are converted to

percentage-correct scores, standard scores, grade equivalents, local percentile ranks, and national percentile ranks as a means of comparison (Salvia & Ysseldyke, 2004). The stratified standardization sample undergoes continuous norming.

Think About It 12.2   Do you think most achievement tests should measure content (fact) or process (application of fact)? Explain.

Metropolitan Achievement Test–Eighth Edition (Metropolitan-8)

The *Metropolitan Achievement Test—Eighth Edition* (*Metropolitan-8*) (Harcourt Educational Measurement, 2001) consists of 13 levels of tests designed for grades kindergarten (Preprimer) through the junior or senior year in high school (Secondary 3). The test is available in a Complete Battery (Reading, Math, Language, Science, and Social Studies) or a Short Form (Reading Comprehension, Math Concepts & Problem Solving, and Language). A separate test of Writing is also included, as well as open-ended response versions for Reading and Math. Each subtest contains between 20 to 50 items, depending on the level of the test, and administration time limits are adjusted accordingly. Total administration time may take from $1\frac{1}{2}$ to over 5 hours, depending on the grade level and test given. Most items are multiple-choice, with the exception of the open-ended items for Reading (e.g., rubrics) and Math. Open-response items are scored on a scale of 0 to 3, although no scoring criteria are given ahead of administration to help prepare students to craft acceptable responses (Lukin, 2005). Scores are used to place students into the performance standard categories of Advanced, Proficient, Basic, and Below Basic (Harwell, 2005).

Norms used for the *Metropolitan-8* generally conformed to U.S. population characteristics, with the critical exception of an overrepresentation of rural schools (51.3%, compared to 29.6% nationally) and an underrepresentation of urban classrooms (10.1%, versus 31.9% nationally). This error in sample representativeness urges caution in interpreting scores for students in urban settings. Internal consistency (KR-20) reliabilities were generally quite high (most exceeding $r = 0.90$), with the exception of the Science and Social Studies subtests in the earlier grades (Harwell, 2005). The majority of test-retest reliabilities were in the $r = 0.70$–0.90 range, with the lower values again associated with the Science and Social Studies subtests. Regarding validity, the test author's primary consideration was a matching of the *Metropolitan-8* to the local school curriculum. This information does not provide compelling evidence that the test scores are valid for their intended use (Lukin, 2005).

Stanford Achievement Test–Tenth Edition (Stanford-10)

The *Stanford Achievement Test—Tenth Edition* (*Stanford-10*) (Harcourt Brace Educational Measurement, 2003) was designed to measure student progress toward high academic standards. It is used in school districts all over the country as a way to inform educators of what their students know and what they are able to achieve. The *Stanford-10* tests the areas of Reading, Mathematics, Language, Spelling, Listening, Science, and Social Studies, from kindergarten through senior year of high school. The *Stanford-10* is an untimed test, but testing guidelines are given to administrators to allow for proper planning (The Psychological Corporation, 2005b). The *Stanford-10* has two equivalent forms (Forms A and B). Figure 12.3 provides a sample computerized profile report for the *Stanford-10*.

All items on the *Stanford-10* are multiple-choice. Raw scores are converted to scaled scores, national and local percentile ranks, stanines, grade equivalents, and normal-curve equivalents. The normative sample generally conformed to 2002 U.S. population demographics (The Psychological Corporation, 2005b). KR-20 reliability coefficients for 8th-grade students ranged from $r = 0.71$ to $r = 0.92$ (median = 0.86) for Form A, and from $r = 0.70$ to $r = 0.91$ (median = 0.86) for Form B. Alternate-form reliability coefficients for subtests ranged from $r = 0.69$ to $r = 0.85$ when comparing Form A to Form B (Harcourt Assessment Inc., 2004a, 2004b).

Metropolitan Readiness Tests—Sixth Edition (MRT-6)

The *Metropolitan Readiness Tests—Sixth Edition* (*MRT-6*) (Nurss & McGauvran, 1995) was designed to assess basic and advanced skills necessary to begin reading and mathematics. It is composed of two levels: Level 1 is individually administered and was developed to assess the evolving literacy and mathematic strategies in pre-kindergarten and beginning kindergarten students; Level 2 is group administered and assesses beginning reading and mathematics strategies and processes (Novak, 2001). Level 1 is composed of six subtests: Auditory Memory, Rhyming, Letter Recognition, Visual Matching, School Language & Listening, and Quantitative Language. Level 2 contains eight subtests: Beginning Consonants, Sound-Letter Correspondence, Visual Matching, Finding Patterns, School Language, Listening, Quantitative Concepts, and Quantitative Operations (Cohen & Swerdlik, 1999). Administration of each level of the *MRT-6* is broken down into four sittings and requires approximately 85 minutes total. Raw scores are converted to percentile ranks, normal-curve equivalents, scaled scores, and standard scores. The standardization sample generally conformed to U.S. population demographics (Novak, 2001).

The *MRT-6* provides information that may be useful in determining early readiness skills in reading and math. However, it should not be used for analysis of individual strengths and weaknesses. Internal consistency estimates determined that Quantitative Concepts and Reasoning subtests may be used for screening purposes. The estimates of the remaining subtests were below $r = 0.80$ and therefore insufficient for decision making regarding individual students. The Story Comprehension subtest was the weakest overall, with coefficients ranging from $r = 0.53$ to $r = 0.77$ (Novak, 2001). There is limited evidence of validity, and what does exist does not support the *MRT-6*'s routine use for the screening of academic achievement (Kamphaus, 2001).

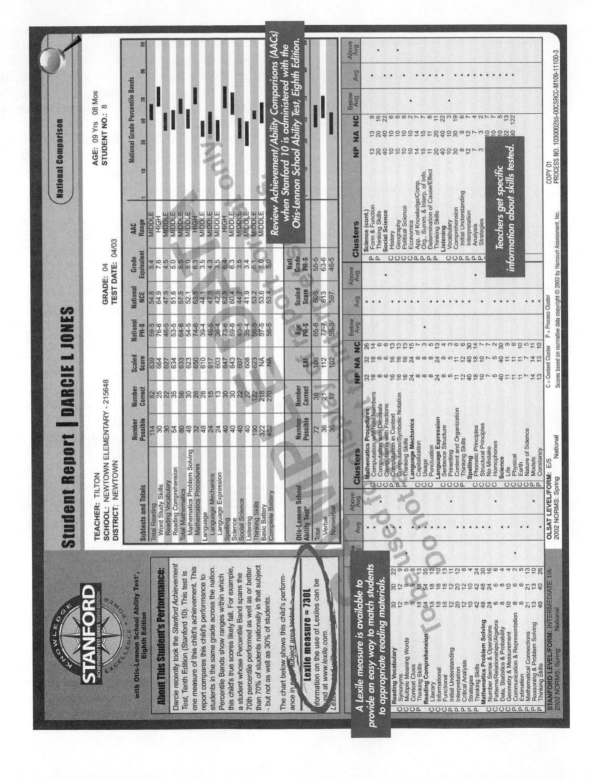

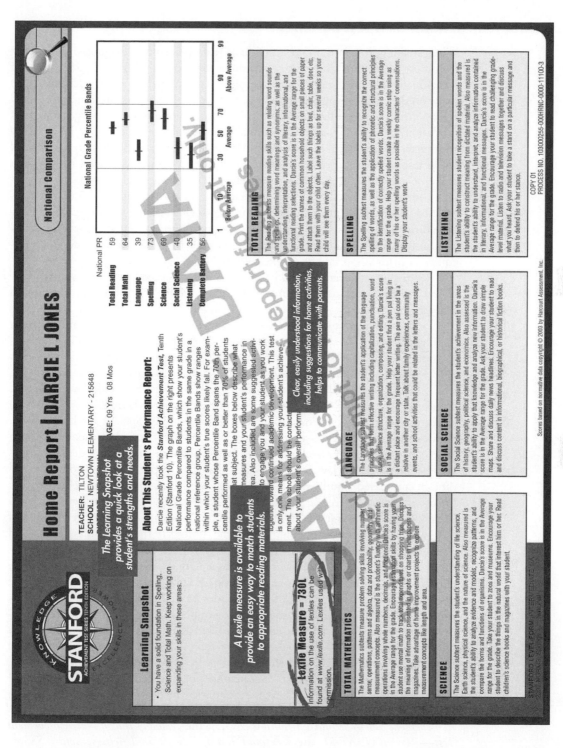

Figure 12.3   *Stanford-10* sample computerized profile report

Source: Figure titled *SAT-10 Student Report* from the *Stanford Achievement Test-Tenth Edition* (*SAT-10*) by Harcourt Brace Educational Measurement, 2003, San Antonio, TX: Author. Copyright © 2003 by Harcourt Assessment, Inc. Reproduced with permission.

Individual Achievement Multi-Skill Test Batteries

When making decisions about individuals (e.g., placement, diagnosis), individual tests must be used. In fact, major educational laws such as IDEIA require the use of individually administered tests and forbid eligibility or placement decisions to be made on the basis of group-administered test scores. In fairness, group-administered achievement tests can often provide helpful information for hypothesis generation or validation, but when making educational decisions about a client's life, individually administered tests are necessary, primarily because the examiner has greater control of the testing environment and is in a much better position to observe the client in a one-on-one situation. Often a client referred for educational reasons will not present with a well-defined academic problem (e.g., reading comprehension, math calculation). Indeed, clients who do present with such a specific learning concern may have difficulties in other academic areas. As a result, many examiners will choose to administer a **multi-skill achievement test battery** to rule in or out academic difficulties in many important academic content areas.

Multi-skill achievement test batteries commonly used today vary substantially in the academic areas assessed and the breadth and depth of coverage. But they all share in common the assessment of more than one important academic area. At this point, it is important to recall the seven academic areas specified within IDEIA for the identification of a specific learning disability: oral expression, listening comprehension, basic reading skill, reading comprehension, written expression, mathematics calculation, and mathematics reasoning. These seven areas, in various combinations, form the core of most individually administered multi-skill achievement batteries. For example, the *Wide-Range Achievement Test—Third Edition* (*WRAT-3*) (Wilkinson, 1993) is composed of three subtests: Reading, Spelling, and Arithmetic. While on the surface, these subtests may appear to cover the major academic content areas, closer inspection reveals that the *WRAT-3* measures only two of the seven areas specified in the public law: basic reading skill and mathematics calculation. Thus, although considered a multi-skill battery, the *WRAT-3* is far from comprehensive. On the other hand, the *Wechsler Individual Achievement Test—Second Edition* (*WIAT-II*) (Psychological Corporation, 2002) was specifically designed to measure all seven of these academic areas (plus spelling). The nine subtests of the *WIAT-II* are even titled to closely align with the IDEIA terminology. The *WIAT-II* is a comprehensive multi-skill battery. Likewise, the *Woodcock-Johnson Tests of Achievement—Third Edition* (*WJ-III-ACH*) (Woodcock, Mather, & McGrew, 2001) more or less covers all of the academic areas specified in IDEIA but includes 22 subtests to provide additional diagnostic support to the major academic areas. Thus the *WJ-III-ACH* is a very comprehensive individually administered multi-skill achievement battery with impressive diagnostic features—no doubt a major reason why it is the most frequently used individually administered achievement battery in schools today.

With these issues as context, the remainder of this section reviews a number of commonly used multi-skill achievement batteries, including the *Woodcock-Johnson Tests of Achievement—Third Edition* (*WJ-III-ACH*), the *Wechsler Individual Achievement Test—Second Edition* (*WIAT-II*), the *Peabody Individual Achievement Test—Revised* (*PIAT-R*), the *Kaufman Test of Educational Achievement—Second*

Table 12.5   Subtests of the *WJ-III-ACH*

Subtest	Summary/examples
1. Letter-Word Identification (76 items)	Measures sight-word vocabulary. Examinees identify letters and pronounce words correctly. Examples: *D, the, new, shut.*
2. Reading Fluency (98 items)	Measures speed in basic reading and comprehension. Examinees quickly read simple sentences, decide if the statement is true or not, and circle Y (Yes) or N (No) for as many items as possible within a 3-minute time limit. Examples: Cats have fur (Y/N). Cars can go fast (Y/N).
3. Story Recall (10 stories, 41 points)	Measures listening comprehension and recall of auditorily presented and processed information. Examinees listen to each story from an audio recording, then tell the story back to the examiner. Example: Julie likes to catch butterflies. Then she lets them go.
4. Understanding Directions (6 pictures, 57 points)	Measures listening comprehension, auditory processing, and short-term auditory memory. Examinees listen to a series of directions from an audio recording related to a picture in front of them and do as the directions ask. Examples: Point to the house. Go. Point to the cat and then the sun. Go.
5. Calculation (45 items)	Measures mathematical computation skills of widely varying difficulty (i.e., single-digit addition to calculus). Examinees perform a series of arithmetic problems. Examples: Make the number *one* in this box. $5 \times 3 = \underline{\quad}$.
6. Math Fluency (160 items)	Measures speed and accuracy of basic mathematical computation skills. Examinees have a 3-minute time limit to complete as many math problems as possible. Examples: $1 - 1 = \underline{\quad}$. $2 \times 9 = \underline{\quad}$.
7. Spelling (59 items)	Measures basic spelling skills. Examinees respond to examiner's directions to either copy what the examiner writes or write what the examiner says to write. Examples: Print the letter *O* (*oh*). Spell the word *green. The grass is green.*
8. Writing Fluency (40 items)	Measures speed and accuracy of basic sentence writing. Examinees have 7 minutes to write as many short sentences as they can about pictures using the words provided in the test booklet. Example: The words *good, cake,* and *is* are listed. The examinee must write a sentence using all of these words (e.g., The cake is good).
9. Passage Comprehension (47 items)	Measures reading comprehension using the "cloze" method. Examinees look at a set of pictures or read a written passage with one word left blank. Examinees infer from context the one word that should go into the blank space.
10. Applied Problems (63 items)	Measures math problem solving with integration of math concepts. Examinees listen as the examiner reads a math story problem and points to visual prompts or passages, then responds with an answer. Examinees are permitted to use paper and pencil to work out the problems.

continued

Table 12.5   continued

Subtest	Summary/examples
11. Writing Samples (30 items, 24 points)	Measures the ability to express ideas in writing. Examinees complete or write sentences based on pictures in the test booklet and directions given by the examiner. Example: Write a good sentence that tells what is happening in the picture.
12. Story Recall—Delayed (10 items, 77 points)	Measures long-term memory of story details the examinee was exposed to earlier in the session. Examinees listen to parts of the stories told earlier in test 3, Story Recall, and are asked to tell what they remember about the rest of the story. Example: Julie likes to catch butterflies. Tell me what you remember.
13. Word Attack (32 items)	Measures ability to follow standard phonetic rules for reading decoding. Examinees are asked to read and correctly pronounce a list of nonsense words. Example: Read each of these words to me. Don't go too fast: *tiff; zoop; nan.*
14. Picture Vocabulary (44 items)	Measures expressive one-word vocabulary knowledge. Examinees pronounce the words represented in pictures presented to them. Example: What is this? (pictured is a watermelon).
15. Oral Comprehension (34 items)	Measures contextual understanding of spoken language using the "cloze" method. Examinees listen to an audio recording and must finish what the person on the recording says. Examples : Candy tastes _____ (*sweet; good*). Dogs are pets, and dolls are ___ (*toys*).
16. Editing (34 items)	Measures examinees' knowledge of correct grammar and punctuation. Examinees are presented with incorrect sentences and asked to tell how to correct them. Example: Robert lost his money. He cannot find it.
17A. Reading Vocabulary—Synonyms (26 items)	Measures verbal analogical reasoning using words with similar meanings. Examinees give synonyms for listed words. Examples: puppy (*dog, doggy, pup*); residence (*home, house, abode*).
17B. Reading Vocabulary—Antonyms (26 items)	Measures verbal analogical reading using words with opposite meanings. Examinees give antonyms for listed words. Examples: "on" (*off, under*); "hinder" (*help, facilitate, promote, allow, encourage, support*).
17C. Reading Vocabulary—Analogies (21 items)	Measures verbal analogical reasoning using word pairs with varying relationships. Examinees look at an incomplete analogy and are asked to complete it. Examples: climb . . . up / fall . . . ___ (*down*) generous . . . stingy / verbose . . . ___ (*quiet, taciturn*).
18A. Quantitative Concepts—Concepts (34 items)	Measures understanding and application of math concepts. Examinees are asked questions about symbols or drawings involving interpretation and analysis of the presented images. Example: The abbreviation *oz.* is presented. The examinee is asked what the abbreviation means.
18B. Quantitative Concepts—Number Series (23 items)	Measures understanding and application of number relationships and reasoning. Examinees are presented with a series of numbers and must use patterns to determine the missing number. Example: 8, 6, 4, ?
19A. Academic Knowledge—Science (28 items)	Measures examinees' knowledge of science. Examinees answer questions about science-related topics. Examples: Point to your knee. Why is fluoride used in water?

Table 12.5   continued

Subtest	Summary/examples
19B. Academic Knowledge—Social Studies (28 items)	Measures examinees' knowledge of social studies. Examinees are asked to pick certain items from a group of pictures or to answer questions related to social studies topics. Examples: Look at the pictures. Put your finger on the comb. What do people call the day they were born?"
19C. Academic Knowledge—Humanities (22 items)	Measures examinees' knowledge of the humanities fields. Examinees are asked to answer questions related to humanities topics. Examples: Look at the colors [five dots of color are presented in the book]. Put your finger on green. How does dialogue differ from narrative?
20. Spelling of Sounds (28 items, 41 points)	Measures phonological awareness and applications for spelling. Examinees are asked to write letters or nonsense words read to them either by the examiner or by means of an audio recording. Examples: Write the letter that makes the /p/ sound, as in *pizza*. Spell the word *gat*.
21A. Sound Awareness—Rhyming (17 items)	Measures phonological awareness and application. Examinees are shown groups of three pictures and are asked to choose the two that rhyme, or to provide a rhyming word for a given word. Examples: Pictured are a tree, a ball, and a bee (examinee should point to the tree and the bee). What rhymes with *meet*?
21B. Sound Awareness—Deletion (10 items)	Measures phonological awareness and application. Examinees are asked to say words without parts of them. Example: Say airplane without air (*plane*).
21C. Sound Awareness—Substitution (9 items)	Measures phonological awareness and application. Examinees will change one sound in a word for another. Example: Change /sm/ in *small to* /st/ (*stall*).
21D. Sound Awareness—Reversal (9 items)	Measures phonological awareness and application. Examinees are given words and must reverse the word order or say the words backwards. Examples: drop . . . rain" (*raindrop*) stop (*pots*).
22. Punctuation and Capitalization (36 items)	Measures knowledge and application of punctuation and capitalization usage. Examinees follow directions regarding punctuation and capitalization. Examples: Make a question mark. Place a colon after this greeting: *Dear Mr. Smith*

Edition (*KTEA-II*), *WRAT-3*, and the *Essential Skills Screener*. Note that each varies according to the age and grade of the intended population as well as the breadth, depth, and general comprehensiveness of content coverage.

Woodcock-Johnson Tests of Achievement—Third Edition (WJ-III-ACH)

The *Woodcock-Johnson Tests of Achievement—Third Edition* (*WJ-III-ACH*) (Mather & Woodcock, 2001; McGrew & Woodcock, 2001; Woodcock, McGrew, & Mather, 2001) is one of the premier batteries for measuring the academic achievement of school-aged school children and adults. It can be used to determine and describe an individual's strengths and weaknesses in academic areas. The *WJ-III-ACH* is available in two alternate forms (Forms A and B) to reduce subject familiarity if readministered on another date. Each of these forms contains 22 tests (see Table 12.5), which are subdivided into two batteries. The Standard Battery consists of subtests 1 through 12 and offers a broad set of scores. The Extended Battery contains subtests 13 through 22 and allows for a more in-depth diagnostic assessment of specific academic strengths and weaknesses. However, it is seldom necessary to administer all 22 tests. The administration time required for the Standard Battery ranges from 60 to 90 minutes, and 5 to 10 minutes should be added for each additional supplemental subtest administered. The *WJ-III-ACH* is mostly scored correct/incorrect (dichotomous scoring), with the exception of a few subtests (i.e., subtests 3, 11, 12, and 20) that require detailed scoring procedures. Items for each subtest are presented in approximate order of increasing difficulty, with basal and ceiling levels specified (e.g., 6 items) for many subtests. Raw scores are converted via a computerized scoring program into age and grade equivalents, percentile ranks, standard scores ($M = 100$; $SD = 15$), and discrepancy scores. The standardization sample generally conforms to U.S. population demographics. Administration of the *WJ-III-ACH* requires some specific training in procedures, and results should be interpreted only by professionals with graduate-level training in relevant areas (Mather & Woodcock, 2001). The *WJ-III-ACH* is considered to be a Level B test.

Test-retest coefficients reported in the technical manual (McGrew & Woodcock, 2001) varied substantially across four age categories (4–7 years, 8–10 years, 11–13 years, and 14–17 years). One-year test-retest correlations ranged from $r = 0.59$ to $r = 0.92$ for the Standard Battery Reading subtests (median = 0.81); from $r = 0.76$ to $r = 0.92$ for the Mathematics subtests (median = 0.88); and from $r = 0.65$ to $r = 0.91$ (median = 0.76) for the Written Language subtests. The internal consistency coefficients generally had ranges in the 0.80s and 0.90s for individual tests and in the 0.90s for clusters (Cizek, 2003). Overall, because of lower subtest reliability, caution is warranted when interpreting subtest scores, particularly when making diagnostic or placement decisions. Confidence is warranted when interpreting domain or cluster scores because these represent combinations of several individual subtests and have much higher reliabilities. For example, the same study resulted in 1-year test-retest correlations of $r = 0.89$–0.93 (median = 0.91) for Broad Math; $r = 0.91$–0.94 (median = 0.92) for the Broad Reading domain; and $r = 0.87$–0.92 (median = 0.90) for Broad Written Language. These broad-domain coefficients allow substantial confidence in score reliability when making diagnostic or placement decisions, confidence that is not warranted when making these same decisions using a single subtest. Evidence of construct validity is shown through factor analysis; however, substantial information on item development, content, and criterion-related score validity was lacking (Cizek, 2003). The examiners and technical manuals are among the most comprehensive on the market. The Compuscore and Profiles Program has replaced the complicated and time-consuming scoring process; however, because conversions are now computerized, it is impossible for examiners to verify the accuracy of converted scores (Sandoval, 2003). Accommodations for students with disabilities are explained in the examiner's manual, and the conorming of the *WJ-III-ACH* with the *Woodcock-Johnson Tests of Cognitive Abilities—Third Edition* (*WJ-III-COG*) allows the cognitive and achievement scores to be compared with greater accuracy (McGrew & Woodcock, 2001).

Additional resources have been developed for interpretation, report writing, and treatment recommendations, including the *Essentials of the WJ-III Tests of Achievement Assessment* (Mather, Wendling, & Woodcock, 2001) and *Woodcock-Johnson III: Reports, Recommendations, and Strategies* (Mather & Jaffe, 2002).

Improvements to this edition of the battery require a greater level of training and a greater degree of sophistication on the part of examiners (Sandoval, 2003). In addition, substantial caution is warranted when using the *WJ-III-ACH* with pre-school children because of a lack of validity studies. Caution is also warranted when interpreting college-aged and adult protocols, because the normative sample was less representative of the population at large, and the recruiting technique was questionable (i.e., posting notices on campus bulletin boards). Finally, although the Writing Samples subtest is a valiant attempt at measuring written expression, low reliability coefficients translate into very broad ranges for standard error of measurement, and lengthy constructed-response items commonly encountered by adolescents and adults were not included.

Wechsler Individual Achievement Test—Second Edition (WIAT-II)

The *Wechsler Individual Achievement Test—Second Edition* (*WIAT-II*) (The Psychological Corporation, 2001) is an individually administered achievement test linked to the *Wechsler* intelligence test series. It was designed to measure the seven areas of learning disabilities defined in the Individuals With Disabilities Education Act (IDEA) (Salvia & Ysseldyke, 2004). The *WIAT-II* is composed of four main academic areas (each with two or three subtests): Reading (Word Reading, Reading Comprehension, Pseudoword Decoding); Mathematics (Numerical Operations, Math Reasoning); Written Language (Spelling, Written Expression); and Oral Language (Listening Comprehension, Oral Expression) (see Table 12.6). Since the number of items administered is dependent on the individual's age, the time required to give the test varies from approximately 45 minutes for very young children (pre-K to Kindergarten) to $1\frac{1}{2}$ to 2 hours for grades 7 to college age. Raw scores can be converted to standard scores, percentile ranks, age and grade equivalents, normal-curve equivalents, stanines, quartiles, and deciles (The Psychological Corporation, 2001).

The stratified norms used for the *WIAT-II* generally conformed to U.S. demographics from the 2000 U.S. Census. These samples yielded excellent content-, construct-, and criterion-related validity. Test-retest reliabilities were above 0.80 for all subtests, but the split-half reliability fell below 0.80 for certain age groups in the Numerical Operations, Written Expression, Listening Comprehension, and Oral Expression subtests (Salvia & Ysseldyke, 2004). Again, these lower reliabilities mean one should use caution when using the *WIAT-II* as the only measure of written or oral language. Overall, the comprehensive nature of the *WIAT-II* allows for a thorough examination of student strengths and weaknesses across several academic domains. Its materials are well organized and accessible. However, some scoring rules are complex and can be confusing (Doll, 2003).

Table 12.6 Subtests of the *WIAT-II*

Subtest	# of Items	Examples	How scored
Word Reading	131	Which letter group makes the /bl/ sounds like in *blue*? OR: Read the following words aloud: *the, when, shout* (words shown on a picture card).	Dichotomous
Reading Comprehension	140	Read this sentence aloud and do what it says: Put your hand on your leg. OR: The student is asked to answer several questions after reading an informative passage.	0, 1, or 2 points based on scoring criteria.
Pseudoword Decoding	55	Say this word: *mub, heb* (words shown on a picture card).	Dichotomous
Numerical Operations	54	$8 + 5 = \underline{\quad}$. $\frac{2}{3} - \frac{1}{2} = \underline{\quad}$.	Dichotomous
Math Reasoning	67	When you are counting, which number comes after 15? OR: Cindy has scores of 75, 95, and 85 on her spelling tests. What is her average test score?	Dichotomous
Spelling	53	Spell the word *new*. The student was *new* to the school. *New*.	Dichotomous
Written Expression	17	Here is a picture of two boys. Write one well-written sentence that describes what is happening in the picture. Do not use the word *the* in your sentence. Write only one sentence and be sure to use correct punctuation.	Alphabet writing is scored dichotomously. Constructed-response items are scored based on separate criteria.
Listening Comprehension	41	Which picture [of the four color pictures] matches the sentence? 'Bill hurries to the parking lot because he thinks it might start raining.'	Dichotomous
Oral Expression	15	Show the examinee a four-paneled cartoon strip with no words and say, Look carefully at each of the pictures, then tell your story from beginning to ending. Remember to include details to make your story interesting.	0, 1, or 2 points for each of multiple scoring criteria

Peabody Individual Achievement Test-Revised (PIAT-R)

The *Peabody Individual Achievement Test-Revised* (*PIAT-R*) (Markwardt, 1998) is a survey of scholastic attainment for students ages 5 to 18 years and takes about 60 minutes to administer. The test is composed of six subtests, each with 100 possible raw score points or items: General Information, Reading Recognition, Reading Comprehension, Spelling, Mathematics, and Written Expression. Some *PIAT-R* items follow a multiple-choice format, others a free-response format. Items on each subtest are arranged in order of increasing difficulty. The basal score is established for each subtest through five consecutive correct responses, and the ceiling is composed of seven consecutive responses that contain five errors (because of the multiple-choice format). Raw scores are converted into age- and grade-based standard scores, age and grade equivalents, percentile ranks, and stanines. The standardization sample generally conforms to the U.S. population estimates (Markwardt, 1998).

According to the manual (Markwardt, 1998), test-retest reliability for subtests and the total battery for selected grades ranged from $r = 0.67$ to $r = 0.98$ (median = 0.91). Internal consistency coefficients ranged from $r = 0.87$ to $r = 0.98$ (median = 0.95). The large number of items in each subtest led to very stable score reliability. However, this may be because all items below the basal level are counted as correct, and all items above the ceiling level are considered incorrect (Cross, 2001). Importantly, the Written Expression subtest displayed an extremely small range of scores and poor psychometrics; thus norm-referenced scores were not derived for this subtest. Construct validity is demonstrated through correlations with the original *PIAT* and the *Peabody Picture Vocabulary Test—Revised* (PIAT-R) (Dunn & Dunn, 1997). The *PIAT-R* is a well-written test constructed to give a greater understanding of an individual's achievement, as well as to pinpoint the examinee's strengths and weaknesses in basic academic areas (Cross, 2001).

Kaufman Test of Educational Achievement—Second Edition (KTEA-II)

The *Kaufman Test of Educational Achievement—Second Edition* (*KTEA-II*) (Kaufman & Kaufman, 2005) is used in the screening and diagnosis of academic achievement for children in grades 1–12, or ages 6–22 years. It is available in two formats: brief and comprehensive. The Brief Form contains three subtests: Reading (word recognition and reading comprehension); Mathematics (computation and application problems); and Written Expression (written language and spelling). The Comprehensive Form contains six components, each with two or more subtests: Reading Composite (Letter & Word Recognition and Reading Comprehension); Reading-Related Subjects (Phonological Awareness, Nonsense Word Decoding, Word Recognition Fluency, Decoding Fluency, Associational Fluency, and Naming Facility); Math Composite (Math Concepts & Applications and Math Computation); Written Language Composite (Written Expression and Spelling); Oral Language Composite (Listening Comprehension and Oral Expression); and the Comprehensive Achievement Composite. The grade level of the individual determines the starting point for each subtest, and testing stops (i.e., ceiling) if the student fails every item in one unit of the subtest. Depending on a client's grade and ability level, the Brief Form may take 20 to 30 minutes to administer, while the Comprehensive Form may take between 30 and 80 minutes. Scoring is dichotomous. Interpretive scores include standard scores ($M = 100$; $SD = 15$), age and grade equivalents, percentile ranks, stanines, and normal-curve equivalents (Salvia & Ysseldyke, 2004).

The authors of the *KTEA-II* did an excellent job of describing and documenting the characteristics of the normative sample. It was shown in detail to generally conform to the U.S. population (Salvia & Ysseldyke, 2004). While Venn (1994) reported that the original *K-TEA* was well designed and provided a complete system for measuring academic achievement, a measure of written expression was noticeably absent. This was corrected in the second edition. Internal consistency and test-retest reliability for scores on subtests were acceptable for screening-level purposes. Both forms showed evidence of content validity (Kaufman & Kaufman, 2005). Miller (1999) reported that detailed procedures for error analyses in the previous

K-TEA allowed examiners to compare a student's errors to that of grade mates. However, he cautioned that "neither the brief or comprehensive forms appear to have a sufficient number of items at the level of emerging academic abilities to discriminate between deficient and low-normal achievements" (p. 153). New research on the *KTEA-II* will determine whether scale improvement will address this concern.

Wide-Range Achievement Test–Third Edition (WRAT-3)

The *Wide-Range Achievement Test—Third Edition WRAT-3* (Wilkinson, 1993) is a brief (15- to 30-minute) screening test of achievement with three subtests: Basic Arithmetic (55 items); Spelling (55 items); and Reading (sight-word vocabulary, 57 items). The Reading subtest must be administered individually, but the Arithmetic and Spelling subtests can be administered to individuals or groups. Alternate forms (Blue Form and Tan Form) are available, and the test can be used with clients ages 5–75 years. The Spelling and Reading subtests are untimed, but the Arithmetic subtest has a 15-minute time limit. Items are scored correct (1 point) or incorrect (0 points). The "5/10 rule" is used to determine basal (5 consecutive correct items) and ceiling levels (10 consecutive incorrect items). The stratified standardization sample (n = 4,443) generally conformed to U.S. population demographics based on the 1990 U.S. Census.

The *WRAT-3* is an inexpensive, easy-to-administer screening test but lacks the comprehensiveness to identify specific learning deficiencies. Raw scores are converted to standard scores (M = 100; SD = 15), percentile ranks, and age and grade equivalents. Internal consistency estimates ranged from r = 0.69 to r = 0.92 for the Arithmetic subtest; from r = 0.83 to r = 0.95 for the Spelling subtest; and from r = 0.88 to r = 0.95 for the Reading subtest across all age categories (Wilkinson, 1993)—very acceptable for a screening-level test. Venn (1994) indicated that scores on the *WRAT-3* had "mediocre" concurrent validity. Knoop (2004) pointed to the *WRAT-3*'s versatility in distinguishing difficulties in the initial stages of basic academic skills, and in vocational or rehabilitation counseling when questions are raised over a client's ability to function adequately in the workplace. Salvia and Ysseldyke (2004) reported the *WRAT-3* correctly classified more than 80% of gifted students and students with mental retardation and learning disabilities. Miller and Barona (1997) reported the *WRAT-3* correctly classified 80% of students as learning disabled or nondisabled. It appears to also be a robust instrument across cultures (Kaplan, 1996).

Essential Skills Screener (ESS)

The *Essential Skills Screener* (*ESS*) (Erford, Vitali, Haas, & Boykin,1995) was designed to identify 3- to 11-year-old children who may be at risk of educational problems or failures. It is composed of reading, math, and writing screening tests for each of three age levels: preschool, early elementary, and upper elementary (see Table 12.7). Each test typically takes less than 10 minutes to administer and score. Dichotomous scoring is used, and raw scores are converted into standard scores, percentile ranks, and age and grade equivalents. The standardization sample is generally representative of the U.S. population (Erford et al., 1995).

Table 12.7   *Essential Skill Screener* test format

Screener	Age/grade of students	# of items	Facets assessed
Preschool			
Reading ESS—Preschool Version (*RESS-P*)	Ages 3–5	51 items	(1) Picture Vocabulary (2) Visual Discrimination (3) Visual Figure-Ground (4) Letter Identification (5) Experience with Books
Math ESS—Preschool Version (*MESS-P*)	Ages 3–5	24 items	(1) Recognition of Shapes (2) Oral Counting (3) Identifying Quantities (4) Identifying Numerals (5) Equalities/Inequalities (6) Word Problems
Writing ESS—Preschool Version (*WESS-P*)	Ages 4–5	23 items	(1) Form Copying (2) Copying Speed (3) Letter/Number Copying (4) Name Writing
Early Elementary			
Reading ESS—Elementary Version (*RESS-E*)	Ages 6–7, Grades 1–3	67 items	(1) Letter Identification (2) Consonant Letter-Sound Association (3) Digraphs and Blends (4) Sight-Word Vocabulary (5) Oral Reading/Passage Comprehension
Math ESS—Elementary Version (*MESS-E*)	Ages 6–8, Grades 1–3	27 items	(1) Writing Numerals (2) Addition Calculations (3) Subtraction Calculations (4) Time (5) Money (6) Fractions (7) Word Problems
Writing ESS—Elementary Version (*WESS-E*)	Ages 6–8, Grades 1–2	13 items	(1) Name Writing (2) Writing Speed (3) Spelling (4) Sentence Writing
Upper Elementary			
Reading ESS—Upper Elementary Version (*RESS-U*)	Ages 8–11, Grades 4–6	35 items	(1) Sight-Word Vocabulary (2) Digraphs and Blends (3) Oral Reading/Passage Comprehension
Math ESS—Upper Elementary Version (*MESS-U*)	Ages 9–11, Grades 4–6	31 items	(1) Place Value (2) Computation (3) Time (4) Money (5) Fractions (6) Word Problems
Writing ESS—Upper Elementary Version (*WESS-U*)	Ages 9–11, Grades 3–6	14 items	(1) Writing Speed (2) Spelling (3) Story Composition

Internal consistency for all nine screeners ranged from 0.87 to 0.95 (median = 0.93), and test-retest coefficients ranged from 0.83 to 0.93 (median = 0.90), indicating acceptable levels of reliability for a screening-level purpose. Sufficient evidence of score validity has been amassed (Erford, 1997b, 1999, 2004; Erford, Ivey, & Dorman, 1999; Erford, Ivey, Dorman, & Wingeart, 2001; Erford & Stephens, 2005; Erford et al., 1995; Erford et al., 1998).

Individual and Group-Administered Single-Skill Achievement Tests for Reading

In contrast to multi-skill batteries, **single-skill achievement tests** focus on a single academic area. This section reviews commonly used reading achievement tests. Reading is a critical academic skill, and students who struggle with reading will frequently struggle with most academic areas as they encounter increasing expectations for independent work during late elementary school years and, of course, through middle and high school. Tremendous emphasis is placed on reading in the early elementary grades, and most individuals with reading problems or a learning disability in reading are identified and receive remedial services while still in elementary school. While most of the tests reviewed in this section assess reading skills, attention also should be paid to reading readiness skills that develop during the preschool and early elementary grades.

Reading readiness is dependent on a variety of factors, including motivation, intellectual ability, visual perception, auditory perception, visual-motor coordination, and general knowledge (Mehrens & Lehmann, 1991). Usually, children between ages 6 and 8 have sufficient capabilities in each of these areas and begin to read using normal instructional strategies, which may include a phonetic or whole-word approach. A substantial deficit in one or more readiness areas can inhibit normal reading progress. While some of these readiness skills (i.e., intelligence, motivation) have been discussed elsewhere in this book, several warrant further explanation.

The term **visual perception** refers to several specific facets of one's ability to receive, perceive, and make sense of visual stimulation. The term does not include visual acuity, which is the ability to see things clearly, and which is frequently measured by a school nurse or optometrist using a Snellen eye chart or some mechanical variation. Commonly identified facets of visual perception include visual discrimination, visual figure-ground, and visual closure. *Visual discrimination* involves the ability to distinguish characteristics of a visual stimulus, such as the difference between the letters *b* and *d,* or a square and a rectangle. *Visual figure-ground* involves the ability to extract the relevant visual detail(s) from a background of visual stimulation. For example, when looking at a page of printed text, most older children have no difficulty focusing on a single letter, word, or even a phrase, while younger children often cannot. Age-appropriate text for children in kindergarten and 1st grade is therefore of a larger print and spaced in wider lines to help young children focus on letters and words without the confusion of competing visual stimulation. *Visual closure,* frequently referred to as "inferring from context," involves the ability to discern from part of a drawing, word, or sentence what the rest would look like. Adults seldom "read" an entire word or sentence by focusing on every letter or phrase; they see part of the word or sentence, make sense of it within the given context, and move quickly on. For example, few continue to "see" the main character's name page after page in a novel, but quickly move past it because it is "obvious" (i.e., makes sense in context).

In sum (and simply put), reading is a process that involves visually picking words, phrases, and even whole sentences up off the page, quickly discriminating relevant details and closing on others to extract meaning from the symbols, then dropping this visual stimulation back onto the page as the process repeats itself on the next set of visual information. The process becomes so automatic that most people rarely think about it (textbook authors and reading specialists excepted, of course). A number of tests have been developed to assess visual perceptual skills, including the *Slosson-Visual Perceptual Skill Screener* (Erford, 2006) and the *Test of Visual Perceptual Skills—Revised* (Gardner, 1996a).

Visual-motor integration (VMI) involves the ability to visually discriminate forms and reproduce them with some motor response, usually by drawing a copy of the visual stimulus. Thus a child might be shown a picture of a circle and asked to copy it with a pencil onto paper. Such a task gives insight into at least three potential areas of difficulty: (1) visual discrimination, (2) fine-motor coordination, and (3) the integration of these (i.e., visual-motor integration). Importantly, a weakness in VMI should be followed up on with additional assessment in each of these three areas, because individuals are more likely to have poor visual discrimination or fine-motor incoordination rather than a deficiency in the integration of the two (i.e., VMI). Commonly used tests to measure visual-motor integration include the *Developmental Test of Visual-Motor Integration—Fourth Edition, Revised(VMI-4)* (Beery, 1997), the *Bender Visual-Motor Gestalt Test* using the Koppitz developmental scoring system (Koppitz, 1975), and the *Slosson Visual-Motor Performance Test (S-VMPT)* (Nicholson, 1999).

The term **auditory perception** refers to several specific facets of one's ability to receive, perceive, and make sense of auditory stimulation. The term does not include auditory acuity, which is the ability to hear things clearly, and which is frequently measured by a school nurse or audiologist using a puretone audiometer or some variation that measures sensitivity to different sound frequencies. Commonly identified facets of auditory perception include auditory discrimination and auditory figure-ground. *Auditory discrimination* involves the ability to distinguish characteristics of an auditory stimulus, such as the difference between two similar sounds (e.g., *ch* and *t*) or words (e.g., *mice* and *nice*). *Auditory figure-ground* involves the ability to extract the relevant auditory detail(s) from a background of auditory stimulation. For example, conversations between friends often occur in the context of background noises, or students frequently need to attend to what a teacher is saying even though other noises or activities may be occurring in the immediate environment. A number of tests have been developed to assess auditory perceptual skills, including the *Slosson Auditory Perceptual Skill Screener (S-APSS)* (Erford, 2007) and the *Test of Auditory Perceptual Skills—Revised (TAPS-R* (Gardner, 1996b).

An example of a group-administered readiness test battery, the *Metropolitan Readiness Tests* (*MRT*), has been discussed earlier in the chapter. An example of an individually administered readiness test is the *Gesell School Readiness Test* (Ilg, 1978).

As a student's reading readiness skills are developing, more traditional types of reading tests can be used to determine how well a student is learning to read and is applying these skills to new situations. IDEIA indicates that basic reading skills and reading comprehension are two essential academic areas in which a child may possess a learning disability. In the parlance of the *DSM-IV-TR*, a learning disability in reading is referred to as a Reading Disorder. Terminology such as dyslexia is outdated and should be avoided.

Basic reading skills determine a student's proficiency at recognizing or decoding a given word. For example, most novice readers sound out and blend the phonemes *d-o-g* to read the word *dog*. Eventually, when a child has encountered this word a number of times, the child recognizes it as the word *dog* and no longer needs to decode, sound, and blend. How quickly a child is able to recognize a word is a function of the reading readiness skills reviewed above, as well as the child's memory (one facet of intelligence). Usually, a child needs to encounter a word about 20 times before automatically recalling it, although great variation is observed among children and words. Some very proficient readers may need only one to several exposures to master a given word, whereas some children with learning disabilities may require hundreds of exposures.

Reading comprehension is the understanding of what is read. Reading comprehension can be assessed by a number of techniques, but nearly all involve reading a passage and performing some task to demonstrate understanding. For example, the *Woodcock Reading Mastery Tests—Revised/Normative Update* (*WRMT-R/NU*) (Woodcock, 1998) measure reading comprehension using the "cloze" method, in which the student reads a passage with a word missing and replaced by a blank space. The student must infer from context what the missing word is. Of course, if the student's basic reading skills are poor and the student cannot recognize many of the words in a given passage, inferring from context will be even more difficult because rather than encountering one blank space, additional word clues will be unknown to the student. Perhaps a more common reading comprehension technique is to have the student read a passage and answer questions stemming from the passage content. The format for answering the question may involve a multiple-choice question or a constructed-response format (e.g., "What color was the horse?" "What emotion did Marcus display?"). Still others (Erford et al., 1995) use a story detail recall procedure in which the student reads a passage aloud and then recalls as many details from the passage as possible. Luftig (1989) identified five levels of reading comprehension: (1) understanding facts (recall); (2) reorganizing (classify, categorize, summarize); (3) inferring (interpret, predict); (4) evaluating (judging); and (5) critiquing (opinion, question, determining feelings). Each is important in its own right, and various tests of reading comprehension measure one or more of these levels.

A third important reading area often discussed is **reading fluency**, a function of oral or silent reading proficiency. Having students read from a list of words can be helpful in understanding their reading skills, but in real life people read passages or stories, not single words out of context. Fluency can be assessed by having students read many simple sentences and answer whether each sentence is true or false within a certain limit of time, such as is done on the *WJ-III-ACH* Reading Fluency subtest. The more sentences answered correctly in the 3-minute time limit, the more fluent the student's reading proficiency. Silent reading speed is another way to measure fluency. For example, the *Nelson-Denny Reading Test* provides norms for speed in reading an initial passage, reported in words per minute. Reading fluency is often related to the more global construct of *processing speed,* which is measured by several individual intelligence tests. Thus, if a student has good oral reading skills and comprehension, but poor reading fluency (slow reading speed), the student may require additional time to complete reading-laden tasks. Many such individuals receive time accommodations on standardized tests, such as the *Scholastic Assessment Test* (*SAT-I*).

Finally, when listening to oral reading, examiners often analyze patterns in errors to diagnose potential reading difficulties. Reading errors generally take the form of *mispronunciations* (e.g., "kitten" rather than "cotton"); *omissions* (e.g., "generally take form of" rather than "generally take the form of"); *insertions* (e.g., "generally take a the form of" rather than "generally take the form of"); and *repetitions* (e.g., "generally take, take the form of" rather than "generally take the form of") (Venn, 1994).

Following are reviews of commonly used standardized reading tests professional counselors should be familiar with. Each measures one to several of the above-mentioned reading facets and in a somewhat different manner. Some can be group administered, others must be administered individually.

Think About It 12.3   Why would it be important to take all of the above-mentioned reading facets into account when selecting the appropriate reading test to administer?

Gray Oral Reading Test–Fourth Edition (GORT-4)

The *Gray Oral Reading Test—Fourth Edition* (*GORT-4*) (Weiderholf & Bryant, 2001) was designed to measure growth in oral reading as well as aid in the diagnosis of oral reading difficulties. It measures the rate, accuracy, fluency, and comprehension of student oral reading ability for ages 6-0 to 18-11. The *GORT-4* is composed of two parallel forms, each containing 14 separate stories with five multiple-choice comprehension questions for each story. It takes 20 to 30 minutes to administer and score. The norms used are considered representative of the current U.S. population (Crompton, 2003).

According to Crompton (2001), the revision of the *GORT-4* has led to an edition that meets technical challenges. It provides the test user with accurate information reflecting the current theoretical rationale in measuring reading ability. However, the examiner should have considerable practice prior to administering the *GORT-4* to be able to sufficiently prompt the reader, time the reader's rate, and mark deviations from the print while testing. Reliability was sufficient, with test-retest scores ranging from $r = 0.85$ to $r = 0.95$. Coefficient alphas from 13 age groups averaged from $r = 0.91$ to $r = 0.97$. Equivalence of parallel forms was documented (Crompton, 2001).

Nelson-Denny Reading Test, *Forms G and H*

The *Nelson-Denny Reading Test* (Brown, Fishco, & Hanna, 1993) was designed to provide an assessment of ability in vocabulary, reading comprehension, and reading rate for students in grades 9 through college age. It is composed of two subtests: Vocabulary (80 items) and Comprehension (38 items), and two equivalent forms exist (Forms G and H). Students are given 15 minutes to complete the vocabulary subtest and 20 minutes for the comprehension subtest, with the first minute being used to determine the reading rate of the student. The total administration time, including answer sheet preparation, is approximately 45 minutes. Raw scores are converted to standard scores, grade equivalents, percentile ranks, stanines, and normal-curve equivalents (Brown, Fishco, & Hanna, 1993).

The standardized sample was somewhat dated and therefore unrepresentative of the U.S. population today (Smith, 1998). Because of this, a basis for normative comparisons is highly questionable (Murray-Ward, 1998). Alternate-form reliability studies (conducted using Forms E and F) yielded coefficients of $r = 0.90$. Content validity was questionable since limited information was provided on the sources of words and passages and on the criteria for their selection. Test-retest data and concurrent validity studies are lacking (Smith, 1998). In general, the *Nelson-Denny* is an easy-to-use test that can be administered in one class period. However, other tests should be used along with the *Nelson-Denny* to properly assess the student's vocabulary and reading comprehension ability.

Woodcock Reading Mastery Tests—Revised/Normative Update (WRMT-R/NU)

The six subtests of the *Woodcock Reading Mastery Tests—Revised/Normative Update* (*WRMT-R/NU*) (Woodcock, 1998) (Letter Identification, Word Identification, Word Attack, Word Comprehension, Passage Comprehension, and Visual-Auditory Learning) combine to measure several important aspects of reading ability. The *WRMT-R/NU* was designed to test individuals ages 5–75 years and requires about 45 minutes to administer. A short scale, consisting of the Word Identification and Passage Comprehension subtests, may also be given in about 15 minutes. The scoring is dichotomous, and raw scores can be converted to percentile ranks, standard scores, age and grade equivalents, and instructional ranges (Crocker, 2001).

The *WRMT-R/NU* contains the same items as the 1987 edition but has been updated to 1998 norms. It shows good technical quality and diagnostic value (Overton, 1996). However, economizing by using the same normative study participants for multiple batteries has introduced context effect and scale-equating issues that test users should take note of (Crocker, 2001). Internal consistency coefficients ranged from $r = 0.68$ to $r = 0.98$ (median = 0.91). Split-half reliability estimates ranged from $r = 0.86$ to $r = 0.99$ (median = 0.97). Content and concurrent validity were shown, as well as intercorrelations with other tests (*Woodcock-Johnson Tests of Achievement—Revised [WJ-R], Iowa Test of Basic Skills [ITBS], Peabody Individual*

Achievement Test [PIAT], and Wide-Range Achievement Test—Third Edition [WRAT-3]) (American Guidance Services, Inc., 2005b). It should be mentioned that the reliability and validity were not derived from the current normative update sample (Crocker, 2001).

Stanford Diagnostic Reading Test–Fourth Edition (SDRT-4)

The *Stanford Diagnostic Reading Test—Fourth Edition* (*SDRT-4*) (Karlsen & Gardner, 1996) helps to determine a student's strengths and weaknesses in the major skills of reading. It can also be used to find patterns of reading skills in schools or districts (Engelhard, 1998). The main categories tested are Decoding or Phonetic Analysis, Vocabulary, Comprehension, and the Rate of Reading or Scanning. There are six levels of the test, and the upper three levels have two alternate forms. These levels can be used for students from 1st grade through the first semester of college (Swerdlik & Bucy, 1998). Norm-referenced and criterion-referenced information is provided in the manual, in addition to a detailed and comprehensive explanation of the standardization sample (Engelhard). Raw scores can be converted into progress indicators, which help to identify students who have or have not demonstrated basic proficiency in certain skills important to the developmental sequence of reading, as well as percentile ranks, stanines, grade equivalents, and scaled scores using the tables provided in the manual. The instructions for the examiner are clear and detailed, and the teacher's manual gives some helpful information and tips for teaching reading. The alternate-form reliability ranged from $r = 0.62$ to $r = 0.82$, and content validity, criterion-related validity, and construct validity are all presented. Overall, the psychometric results are sufficient, but low enough on some subtests to rule out using the *SDRT-4* for individual diagnosis (Engelhard).

Slosson Oral Reading Test–Revised (SORT-R)

The *Slosson Oral Reading Test—Revised* (*SORT-R*) (Slosson & Nicholson, 1990) was designed to give a quick estimate of word recognition levels for children and adults. It consists of 200 words arranged in ascending order of difficulty by groupings of 20 words from a primer list for grades 1–8 and a high school list. The basal is established when an individual is able to correctly pronounce each of the 20 items of a group. The ceiling is reached when the individual cannot pronounce any of the items in a grouping. The *SORT-R* is a dichotomously scored test and can be administered in approximately 3 to 10 minutes (Slosson & Nicholson, 1990).

The normative population referenced for the *SORT-R* generally conform to the U.S. population. However, the percentage of White individuals (82%) was high in comparison to the U.S. population (74%), and the percentage of individuals falling into the "other" category (4%) was low in comparison to the U.S. population (12%). Split-half reliability coefficients for the total scale by grade ranged from $r = 0.92$ to $r = 0.99$ (median = 0.98). Concurrent validity was established through comparisons with the *Woodcock-Johnson's* Letter-Word Identification ($r = 0.90$) and Passage Comprehension ($r = 0.68$) subtests (Slosson & Nicholson, 1990). The *SORT*-R is a quick test of word recognition and is easy to administer and score. However, it is not a diagnostic test and should be used only for initial screening or research purposes (Shaw, 1995).

Individual and Group-Administered Single-Skill Achievement Tests for Mathematics

In general, a comprehensive assessment of mathematical skills involves assessment of **mathematical computation** (e.g., addition, subtraction, multiplication, division); **problem solving** (i.e., story problems involving application of computations, measurement, time, money, estimation, geometry, etc.); and **mathematical fluency**. Sometimes basic mathematical concepts (e.g., numeration, geometry) are assessed as a separate category, but these skills are usually (and best) assessed in the context of some application or story problem format. The academic content areas of calculation and problem solving are the same as found in IDEA and align with most group- and individually administered tests of math achievement. In the parlance of the *DSM-IV-TR,* a learning disability in math is referred to as a Mathematics Disorder.

From a diagnostic perspective, math items have the advantage of being relatively easy to cast in the language of an educational objective (e.g., 2×2 measures "single-by single-digit multiplication"). Even screening-level mathematics tests may therefore have some value in indicating student strengths and limitations, and in planning treatment. Of course, whether a professional counselor can use a mathematics inventory for establishing treatment strategies depends on the professional counselor's level of expertise in mathematics instruction. Math fluency is also an important consideration in the assessment of math achievement. Generally, math fluency is assessed by having students respond to as many simple calculation problems (e.g., $1 + 5$, 2×3, $10 - 6$) as possible during a specified time period (e.g., 3 minutes). In this way, math fluency provides a measure of speed of basic calculation skills. As with reading fluency, slow processing speed can also influence a student's math fluency. The remainder of this section reviews the group- and individually administered standardized tests of mathematics with which professional counselors should be familiar.

KeyMath Revised: A Diagnostic Inventory of Essential Mathematics (KeyMath-R/NU)

The *KeyMath Revised: A Diagnostic Inventory of Essential Mathematics* (*KeyMath-R/NU*) (Connolly, 1998) was designed to assess an individual's (ages 5–22 years) understanding and application of mathematic concepts and skills in 3 primary areas, which are subdivided into 14 subareas: Basic Concepts (Numeration, Rational Numbers, and Geometry); Operations (Addition, Subtraction, Multiplication, Division, and Mental Computation); and Applications (Measurement, Time, Money, Estimation, Interpreting Data, and Problem Solving) (Wollack, 2001). The test has a free-response format and takes 35 to 50 minutes to administer. Scoring is dichotomous, and raw scores are converted to age and grade equivalents, standard scores, and percentile ranks. The basal scores are determined by an individual's score on the first subarea (Numeration), and the ceilings are established after three consecutive incorrect answers are made in a subarea (Kingsbury, 2001).

Evidence of reliability of scores for the individual subareas of the *KeyMath-R/NU* included split-half coefficients ranging from $r = 0.26$ to $r = 0.94$ (median =

0.81) and alternate-form coefficients ranging from $r = 0.53$ to $r = 0.80$ (Kingsbury, 2001). Thus decisions based on subarea performance should be made with extreme caution. Reliability coefficients for the three primary areas were more substantial (e.g., split-half of $r = 0.65–0.97$). Correlations were reported between the original *KeyMath* and mathematics scales of the *California Tests of Basic Skills* ($r = 0.66$) and *Iowa Test of Basic Skills* ($r = 0.76$). Overall, the *KeyMath-R/NU* is considered to be one of the best test batteries for assessing student knowledge and understanding of basic mathematic skills, as well as for providing useful diagnostic information to the teacher (Wollack, 2001).

Stanford Diagnostic Mathematics Test—Fourth Edition (SDMT-4)

The *Stanford Diagnostic Mathematics Test—Fourth Edition* (*SDMT-4*) (Beatty, Madden, Gardner & Karlsen, 1996) was designed to measure a student's mastery of basic math skills and concepts. The *Directions for Administering* state that "the primary purpose of *SDMT* is to determine specific areas in which each pupil is having difficulty," so clients can be given the help they need on an individualized basis (Beatty, Gardner, Madden, & Karlsen, 1984, p. 5). The test can be given to individuals or to a small group. Nagy (1998) indicated that the test tries to be diagnostic and normative at the same time but does not have great success doing either; although it is probably better used diagnostically. The test consists of six levels: (1) Red (grades 1.5–2.5); (2) Orange (grades 2.5–3.5); (3) Green (grades 3.5–4.5); (4) Purple (grades 4.5–6.5); (5) Brown (grades 6.5–8.9); and (6) Blue (grades 9–13). Each of the three lower levels has one form, and the three upper levels have two alternate forms (Lehmann, 1998). On each level, the questions test the student's understanding of concepts and applications (32 multiple-choice and 30 free-response questions) and computation (20 multiple-choice and 20 free-response questions). Problem solving and strategies are emphasized (Lehmann), but the content focused on at each level differs. This test has more low-difficulty questions than most mathematics achievement tests, which makes it especially helpful for assessing the performance of below-average students, because they will have some success. Because this test is designed specifically to find weaknesses, it is less helpful for higher-achieving students. Each level is accompanied by a manual that is well laid out and has clear instructions. The *SDMT-4* can be hand-scored or sent to The Psychological Corporation for computer scoring. Three of four reports are given as part of the Basic Scoring Service, and the fourth, the Group Roster Summary, is optional. Raw scores can be converted into progress indicators that help to identify students who have or have not demonstrated basic proficiency in certain skills important to the developmental sequence of reading, percentile ranks, stanines, grade equivalents, and scaled scores using tables provided in the manual. Numeric, graphic, and verbal information can be obtained for the class as well as information on where the class falls according to national norms. The standardization sample was generally representative of U.S. demographics, and the test items have been well researched and developed. In addition, the content validity is adequate, as is the reliability, although it may indicate that the test is adequate only for screening purposes because of the small numbers of items (Lehmann).

Slosson-Diagnostic Math Screener (S-DMS)

The *Slosson Diagnostic Math Screener* (*S-DMS*) (Erford & Boykin, 1996) is a basic assessment of a child's mathematics skills, including calculation skill, math concepts, and math problem solving. The *S-DMS* is a five-level test matched to a child's age or grade. The test can be group- or individually administered to children ages 6–13 years (grades 1–8). Levels 1 to 3 are designed to have the administrator read the items aloud, while Levels 4 and 5 are designed for each student to read the items to themselves. Items are open ended and are scored right or wrong. Open-ended questioning yields a more accurate score than multiple-choice questioning. Very specific administration and scoring procedures are provided in the test manual. Raw scores can be converted into standard scores, percentile ranks, grade equivalents, and interpretive ranges.

According to the manual, the standardization sample was representative of U.S. population demographics, although it was slightly overrepresentative of students from areas of greater than 2,500 residents and slightly underrepresentative of students from lower socioeconomic groups. Test-retest reliability coefficients ranged from 0.85 to 0.96, and internal consistency coefficients ranged from 0.85 to 0.97. The *S-DMS* had moderate correlation coefficients at all levels with the *Woodcock-Johnson—Revised (WJ-R)*, KeyMath-R Operations Area, and the *WRAT-R1*. Overall, reliability and validity studies seemed to yield more than adequate results, especially considering the complexity of the studies with five separate test levels to interpret. The *S-DMS* can be adapted for criterion-referenced assessment and provides well-defined instructional objectives for diagnostic use. See Table 12.8 for sample behavioral objectives from the *S-DMS*.

Individual and Group-Administered Single-Skill Achievement Tests for Written Expression

The ability to express ideas in written form is one of the most critical communication skills that students are required to master. Failure to master basic written communication skills puts one at a severe disadvantage in the work force, and this disadvantage will become more profound as computer and technological skill demands become integrated even more into job and educational functions.

A comprehensive assessment of **written expression** involves assessment of wide-ranging skills, including quality of expression (e.g., writing maturity, style, contextual mechanics); writing mechanics (e.g., capitalization, punctuation, grammar, spelling); and writing fluency. The academic content area of written expression is found in IDEA under the specific learning disability category, and most group- and individually administered tests of written expression strive to align with this content area. In the parlance of the *DSM-IV-TR,* a learning disability in written expression is referred to as a Disorder of Written Expression.

The diagnosis of written expression can be complex because, of all the basic academic content areas, the quality of written expression is the one that most often requires examiner judgment. Indicators of quality requiring judgment typically have

Table 12.8   Sample behavioral objectives from the *Slosson Diagnostic Math Screener*—Level 3

Math Concepts
1. The student can identify and write three-digit numerals with zero as a place holder.
2. The student can identify and write four-digit numerals with zero as a place holder.
3. The student can identify a sequence of three-digit numbers with zero as a placeholder.

Problem Solving
1. The student can solve word problems using addition of two-digit numbers with regrouping.
2. The student can solve word problems using subtraction of two-digit numbers with regrouping.
3. The student can solve word problems using multiplication of one-digit numbers.
4. The student can solve two-step word problems using addition of two-digit numbers with regrouping and multiplication.

Computation
1. The student can add two two-digit numbers without regrouping.
2. The student can add three-digit numbers requiring three regroupings for a four-digit stem.
3. The student can add money (decimals) with regrouping.
4. The student can add fractions with unlike denominators.
5. The student can subtract two-digit numbers with regrouping.

Source: From *Manual for the Slosson Diagnostic Math Screening Test (S-DMST)*, by B. T. Erford and R. R. Boykin, 1996, East Aurora, NY: Slosson Educational Publications. Copyright 1995 by Slosson Educational Publications. Reprinted with permission.

lower levels of score reliability and, subsequently, lower levels of score validity. Thus test developers go to great lengths to create objective scoring systems and minimize subjectivity. For example, in developing the *Slosson Written Expression Test (SWET)*, Hofler, Erford, and Amoriell (2001) measured writing maturity of three alternate forms of student compositions using two mathematically defined objective measures: *average sentence length* and *type-token ratio*. It was reasoned that less mature writers use simple sentence structure, while more mature writers use compound, complex, or compound-complex sentence structure. Therefore, after correcting for run-on sentences, the average length of a person's sentence (in words per sentence) could be easily determined (i.e., by dividing the number of words in a composition by the number of corrected sentences) and compared to a normative sample. Likewise, type-token ratio, a measure of vocabulary density, can be derived by determining the number of different words used within the sample of the first 50 words of a composition. It was reasoned that less mature writers use the same words repeatedly, while more mature writers have a richer, more diverse writing vocabulary. The type-token ratio can be determined mathematically and objectively from a writing sample and subsequently compared to the norm group performance. On the *SWET,* type-token ratio and average sentence length are combined to form an objectively derived measure of writing maturity. Alternatively, educators often will create basic to intricate rubrics to enhance scorer agreement of written-expression quality.

Writing fluency is also an important consideration in the assessment of writing achievement and is often overlooked as a concern with behaviorally disordered or unmotivated students. After about the 3rd grade, writing becomes a primary focus of the curriculum, and students with difficulties in writing speed often lose motivation to perform in the classroom. Generally, writing fluency is assessed through two methods. The first involves measuring speed in copying sentences. This can be done either in manuscript (i.e., printing) or cursive writing. Many school curricula begin cursive by grade 2, and it is not widely known that many students can print in manuscript substantially faster than in cursive. Thus students with writing speed deficiencies may experience less frustration when allowed to print in manuscript or to use the computer to type notes and assignments. Indeed, the computer has the potential for revolutionizing intervention for clients with writing disorders, both through the speed keyboarding allows, as well as through the invention of voice-activated writing programs (e.g., Dragon NaturallySpeaking) that allow individuals to dictate compositions into a computerized word processing file, such as Microsoft Word.

The second commonly used method for measuring writing fluency is to require students to quickly construct simple sentences from several provided words (e.g., *dog, barking, is* becomes, "The dog is barking"). Generally, students must construct as many sentences as possible within a given time limit (e.g., 5 minutes) by writing each sentence in a designated space on the paper using pen or pencil.

Again, whether a professional counselor can use a written-expression test for establishing treatment strategies depends on the professional counselor's level of expertise in written-expression instruction. The remainder of this section reviews the group- and individually administered standardized tests of written expression professional counselors should be familiar with.

Think About It 12.4   What are some methods for objectively scoring written-expression tests? Why are these techniques important for enhancing the reliability of the test scores?

Test of Written Language–Third Edition (TOWL-3)

The *Test of Written Language—Third Edition* (*TOWL-3*) (Hammill & Larsen, 1996) is a diagnostic test of written language, designed to help 7- to17-year-old students who may need specialized help with writing. The most recent version of the test consists of eight subtests: Vocabulary, Spelling, Style, Logical Sentences, Sentence Combining, Contextual Conventions, Contextual Language, and Story Construction (see Table 12.9). The test has no set time limits, except for the story writing section (Contextual Conventions), which is limited to 15 minutes. Administration normally takes more than 1 hour, and scoring about 15 minutes, assuming the examiner is qualified and well trained for this test. Subtest raw scores are transformed into scaled scores for individual subtests ($M = 10$; $SD = 3$). Three com-

Table 12.9 Subtest format of the *TOWL-3*

Subtest	What is being measured?	How is it measured?
Vocabulary	Use of vocabulary in sentence construction	Student writes a sentence with a presented stimulus word.
Spelling	Spelling ability	Student writes a sentence that is dictated.
Style	Mastery of punctuation and capitalization rules	Student writes a sentence that is dictated.
Logical Sentences	Ability to compose paragraphs and sentences that make sense	Student edits an illogical sentence so that it makes better sense.
Sentence Combining	Syntactic knowledge	Student integrates the meaning of several short sentences into a longer, grammatically correct sentence.
Contextual Conventions	Spelling, punctuation, and capitalization in context	Student writes a story in response to a stimulus picture.
Contextual Language	Vocabulary, grammar, syntax in context.	Student's story is evaluated relative to the quality of vocabulary, sentence construction, and grammar.
Story Construction	Maturity of prose, presence of a plot, use of a theme, development of characters, other conceptual aspects of a composition	Student's story is evaluated relative to the quality of plot, prose, character development, interest to the reader, and compositional aspects.

posite scores are generated: Overall Writing, Contrived Writing, and Spontaneous Writing, each presented as a standard score (M = 100; SD = 15). "These composite scores enable the examiner to estimate a student's general writing proficiency and determine any strength or weakness relative to contrived or spontaneous testing formats" (Hammill & Larsen, 1996, p. 6). The manual is complete and clearly written and is easy to use, although scoring and interpretation can be complicated and time consuming (Hansen, 1998). The reliability statistics are comprehensive, and most meet desired standards for a diagnostic test, except for the Contextual Conventions subtest, which was r = 0.70 (Hammill & Larsen). The validity information is also very comprehensive in the manual and achieves sufficient standards. The norming sample is acceptable, although a larger sample would have been more appropriate (Hansen).

Slosson Written Expression Test (SWET)

The *Slosson Written Expression Test* (*SWET*) (Hofler, Erford, & Amoriell, 2000) is a screening tool used to assess skills of written expression in children ages 8–17 years. The *SWET* can be administered both individually as well as in a group setting and can be helpful for screening children at risk for writing problems, children new to a school, and for curriculum evaluation. Three alternate-form writing prompts are available. Students are presented with a black-and-white picture prompt and are asked to write a story about that picture (see Figure 12.4). Specific administration and scoring guidelines are written in the manual. Children are given

SWET
The Slosson Written Expression Test

Student Response Form B

Name: _____   **Age:** _____

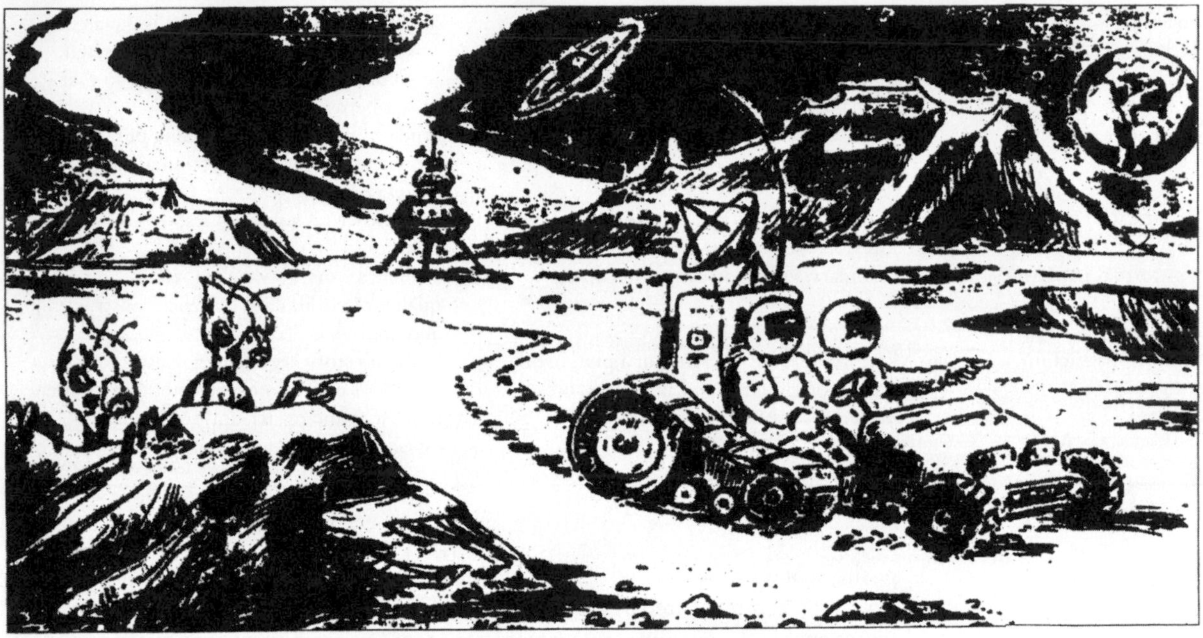

Figure 12.4   *Slosson Written Expression Test (SWET)* sample picture prompt

Source: From the *Slosson Written Expression Test (SWET)*, by D. B. Hofler, B. T. Erford, & W. J. Amoriell, 2001, East Aurora, NY: Slosson Educational Publications, Inc. Copyright © 2000 by Donald B. Hofler, William J. Amoriell, & Bradley T. Erford. All rights reserved. Reproduced with permission.

exactly 15 minutes to write a good story about the picture. The authors assert that the *SWET* provides a more authentic assessment of written expression than most tests because of the composition format, which reduces the likelihood of guessing and false elevation of scores. Specific scoring criteria are presented in the manual's scoring protocol. Raw scores can be converted into scaled scores, percentile ranks, and interpretive ranges. Two subscores (Writing Maturity Index and Writing Mechanics Index) as well as a composite score (Written Expression total standard score) can be determined. The Writing Maturity Index score is composed of two objectively determined measures of writing maturity: average sentence length and type-token ratio (i.e., a measure of vocabulary density). The Writing Mechanics Index is composed of spelling, capitalization, and punctuation as determined by proportions of these skills in the context of the composition.

According to the test manual, normative data generally conformed to U.S. population demographics. Test-retest coefficients ranged from 0.80 to 0.95 for a large sample of children in grades 3–10 after a 2-week period. Alternate-form reliability correlation coefficients were also strong, ranging from 0.73 to 0.95. The *SWET* had moderate criterion-validity correlation coefficients with the *Woodcock-Johnson—Revised* (*WJ-R*) Broad Written Expression domain as well as the *WJ-R* Dictation subtest and the *WJ-R* Writing Samples subtest.

Tests of English Language Proficiency

In the United States, many students enter the K–12 public school system and university system each year. To better serve students entering K–12 schools, several **English proficiency tests** have been developed to ensure that these students are identified early and receive necessary language and academic support services. At the university level, tens of thousands of students enter the United States to study each year, and universities frequently use oral and written English fluency examinations to ensure that these students have the English language skills to be successful at the university level. Following are reviews of some of the more commonly used tests of English proficiency.

Secondary Level English Proficiency Test (SLEP)

The *Secondary Level English Proficiency Test* (*SLEP*) (ETS, 2004) is a norm-referenced test to determine nonnative speakers' understanding of the English language. It is an individual or group-administered test for students in grades 7–12 and is generally used to make decisions regarding placement into or out of English as a Second Language (ESL) classes (ETS, 2005a). The test is divided into two sections, one that measures understanding of spoken language (Listening Comprehension) and one that measures understanding of written language (Reading Comprehension). Each section is divided into four subsections made up of eight types of multiple-choice questions and totaling 150 questions (see Table 12.10 for sample questions). The test can be administered in one or two sessions but usually takes about 85 minutes total, and can only be hand-scored using the manual. The first three alternate forms (Forms 1–3) of the test are no longer used, and three new forms (Forms 4–6) are now used (ETS, 2005a).

Raw scores are converted into scaled scores (range: 10–32 for Listening Comprehension, 10–35 for Reading Comprehension), which are combined to form the total scaled score. Percentile ranks are given in table format in the manual (Loyd, 1985). The pilot study was administered to 1,650 nonnative English-speaking students, but the *Technical Supplement* provides few details about the sample's demographic makeup. Reliability of scores for each section and the overall test for all three forms is very good, ranging from $r = 0.88$ to $r = 0.96$. The manual provides sample questions for each of the eight subsections of the test (ETS, 2004). To determine validity, native English speakers were given one of the new forms, and teachers rated participating students on their listening and reading skills to see how well the two were correlated. The *SLEP Technical Supplement,* the *SLEP Test Manual,* and a *Research Report* are available for download from the Educational Testing Service's website (ETS, 2005a).

Table 12.10   Sample questions from the *SLEP*

Part B—Match the printed sentence with one of four drawings.
The bigger circle is in the lower left corner.

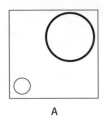 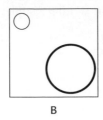 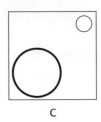 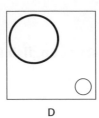

A   B   C   D

A B C D

Part C—Conversations between students or announcements made by teachers in a school are
read aloud. The questions are given before the conversation reading begins, allowing students to
direct their attention to listening for the correct answer. The questions and answers are printed
in the test book. For each question, students must choose one of four answers.

On tape:
(Narrator) *Listen for the answer to the following question. What did the girl think the homework
    assignment was for math class? Here is the conversation.*
(Boy) *Did you figure out the answer to problem number ten in the math homework?*
(Girl) *Number ten? I thought we were only supposed to do the first eight problems.*
(Boy) *That's what the teacher said at the beginning of class, but right before the bell rang she changed
    the assignment to the first twelve problems.*
(Narrator) *What did the girl think the homework assignment was for math class?*

In the test book:
What did the girl think the homework assignment was for math class?

   (A) Only problem number 10
   (B) Problem numbers 1 though 8
   (C) Problem numbers 1 through 10
   (D) Problem numbers 1 through 12

Source: ETS materials were selected from the *SLEP Test Manual* for use with forms 4, 5, and 6 only.
Copyright 2004, Educational Testing Service. Reprinted by permission of Educational Testing Service, the
copyright owner. Permission to reprint ETS materials does not constitute review or endorsement by
Educational Testing Service of this publication as a whole or of any other testing information it may contain.

Test of English as a Foreign Language (TOEFL)

The *Test of English as a Foreign Language* (*TOEFL*) (ETS, 2005b) is an individual or
group-administered test designed to determine proficiency of nonnative English language speakers. It is used primarily with students who are applying for college, and
whose scores on other standardized achievement or aptitude tests are not as high as
they might be if the student had grown up with English as a primary language.

Table 12.11   Sample problems from the Grammar and Vocabulary sections of the *MELAB*

Grammar Problem Example:
"Your clothes are all wet!"
"Yes, I didn't come _____ the rain soon enough."
  a. away to
  b. over to
  c. down with
  d. in from

Vocabulary Problem Example:
Bill Collins *launched* his restaurant last June.
  a. moved
  b. started
  c. sold
  d. bought

Source: University of Michigan, Ann Arbor, English Language Institute, July 2003, *MELAB* sample test items. Retrieved January 17, 2005, from the Michigan English Language Assessment Battery website: http://www.lsa.umich.edu.

The TOEFL integrates all four basic communication skills—Reading, Listening, Speaking, and Writing—and requires the test taker to demonstrate how language is really used (ETS, 2005b). Each of the four sections is scored with a possible range of 0–30 points for a combined total of 120 possible points. Administration requires approximately 4 hours. The TOEFL is delivered via the Internet at test centers. Also, students are able to download practice versions of the test from the website. Since the new version of the test was just released, reliability and validity information is not available.

Michigan English Language Assessment Battery (MELAB)

The *Michigan English Language Assessment Battery* (*MELAB*) (English Language Institute, 1998) is a test for nonnative speakers of the English language and measures how well they might do in an American college or university. It is often used as an alternative to the *TOEFL*. The *MELAB* is composed of three sections: Composition, Listening, and Grammar/Cloze/Vocabulary/Reading, and requires from 2 ½ to 3 ½ hours to complete. There is also an optional Speaking section. The Listening section has 50 questions, and the Reading section has 100 questions. The Composition section consists of a writing sample on one of two given topics (see Table 12.11 for sample problems). Each section is scored slightly differently. The Composition section is scored on 10 levels. The range of scores for the Composition section is from 53 to 97, with an average score of about 73. The Listening section and the Reading section use the number correct, which is converted to a scaled score based on the difficulty of the questions answered. The range of scores for the Listening section is from 30 to 100, with an average score of around 77. The range for the Reading section is from 15 to 100, with an average score of around 75. The examinee's final score is an average of the first three parts (not including the optional Speaking section), with an average final score of around 76. Final scores usually range from the 50s (elementary-level English proficiency) to the 90s (native adult English speakers). Universities set standards for admission into their schools, but the scores are used additionally to measure a student's preparedness for individual academic programs (English Language Institute, 2004). Protocols must be sent to the English Language Institute at the University of Michigan to be scored, a process usually requiring about 5–8 weeks. Internal consistency coefficients ranged from $r = 0.87$ to $r = 0.95$ across the scales, and interrater reliability for the composition section was approximately $r = 0.90$. Content and construct validity studies provided strong evidence that the test measures English language proficiency (Garfinkel, 2001). Garfinkel stated that the test's psychometrics are strong enough to deserve the confidence given it by the academic and professional groups using it across the United States.

SUMMARY/CONCLUSION

Achievement tests are the most commonly used type of tests used in schools, and professional counselors must be familiar with their use. Professional counselors must be familiar with IDEIA and Section 504 to advocate effectively for clients with special needs, and with tests of English proficiency to aid students for whom English may be a second language. Achievement tests are frequently categorized as group- or individually administered, norm- or criterion-referenced, screening or diagnostic, single- or multiple-level, and single- or multi-skill tests. Large-scale testing programs in schools provide assessments of students' developmental progress but also may take the form of high-stakes testing that has consequences for students and schools. Program and placement decisions about students with special needs must be made using individually administered achievement tests. These tests generally measure one or more of the primary academic content areas: oral language, listening comprehension, written expression, mathematics computation, mathematics problem solving, basic reading skills, and reading comprehension. The professional counselor knowledgeable about assessment in these areas can be of great help to clients of all ages as they transition through educational and career pathways.

KEY TERMS

ability	grade-equivalent discrepancies
achievement	handicapped persons
achievement test	high stakes
advocate	IDEIA
auditory perception	individual diagnostic achievement tests
content validity	mathematical computation
criterion-referenced test	mathematical fluency
diagnostic test	minimum-level skills test
English proficiency test	multilevel battery

multi-skill achievement test battery
norm-referenced test
problem solving
reading comprehension
reading fluency
reading readiness
screening test
Section 504
single-level test

single-skill achievement test
specific learning disability
standard score point discrepancy
statistical regression
survey batteries
visual-motor integration
visual perception
written expression

CHAPTER **13**

Assessment in Career Counseling

by Deborah Newsome, Bradley T. Erford,
and Kathleen McNinch

C areer counseling is a complex process that continues to evolve in our rapidly changing society. To meet the needs of clients seeking help with career-related issues, professional counselors need to be skilled in several areas, including assessment. The National Career Development Association (NCDA) has developed and revised a set of career counseling competency statements to guide the practice of professional career counselors. The competencies, which can be accessed at www.ncda.org/pdf/counselingcompetencies.pdf, focus on a broad range of general counseling and specific career-related skills. One of those skills is the ability to conduct career-related assessment. This chapter describes the purposes of career assessment, reviews some of the frequently used formal and informal methods of career assessment, and discusses ways professional counselors can use these assessment tools to help clients with career-related issues.

PURPOSES OF CAREER ASSESSMENT

It is not uncommon for clients seeking career counseling to believe incorrectly that professional counselors will administer and interpret tests that will magically reveal the client's perfect career match (Gladding & Newsome, 2004). Perhaps this misconception stems from the early days of **trait-and-factor theory**, when Frank Parson's model of career guidance was the standard. Parsons (1909) outlined a three-step process of occupational decision making that emphasized the following guidelines:

- Develop a clear understanding of your aptitudes, interests, resources, limitations, and other qualities.
- Acquire knowledge about the world of work, including the requirements and conditions of success, compensation, and opportunities in a given field.
- Use "true reasoning" to relate self-knowledge to knowledge about the world of work, resulting in occupational choice.

The trait-and-factor approach to career counseling "dominated the 20th century in helping individuals with career choice" (Niles & Harris-Bowlsbey, 2005, p. 147). The volume of standardized assessment tools designed to enhance self-understanding increased significantly, with individuals such as Edward Strong, Frederick Kuder, Donald Super, John Holland, and others making important contributions to the field of test development.

However, the complex process of career counseling and assessment interpretation goes well beyond the "test and tell" method that often is associated with early trait-and-factor approaches, and professional counselors recognize the limitations associated with standardized testing. Consequently, it is essential for professional counselors working with clients on career-related issues to clarify the role of the professional counselor from the outset so that clients understand the purposes and limits of career assessment and the counseling process.

With this caveat in mind, professional counselors recognize that assessment does serve a key role in the career counseling process. The primary purpose of assessment in career counseling is to facilitate self-exploration and self-understanding (Duckworth, 1990; Swanson & Fouad, 1999). Niles and Harris-Bowlsbey (2005) remind us that assessment in the 21st century should be valued as a tool used to help clients gather data about themselves at a *given point in time* to assist in career planning. Assessment results are just one piece of data; hence, many other sources of data, including the client's self-knowledge, past educational and vocational experiences, and knowledge about the work demands of the future, need to be a part of the career counseling process.

To aid clients with career planning, professional counselors use formal and informal assessments to help clients learn about their interests, abilities, values, and personality. Assessment tools also are used to help evaluate where clients are in the career development or decision-making process. In this chapter, we describe several of the instruments, both formal and informal, that have been developed to assess each of these areas. Unless stated otherwise, the psychometric properties associated with the formal assessment instruments have been well researched and deemed acceptable. For more in-depth information about these and other career assessment tools, readers are encouraged to consult *A Counselor's Guide to Career Assessment Instruments* (Kapes & Whitfield, 2002); the *Mental Measurements Yearbook* (Plake, Impara, & Spies, 2003); and the website of the Buros Institute (www.unl.edu/buros).

Think About It 13.1   Before beginning the next section on assessing interests, make a short list of the activities, tasks, and even jobs or careers that you find interesting. Is this list diverse or narrow? Given that you may be currently in a graduate program that prepares professional counselors, do your interests align with this career path?

ASSESSING INTERESTS

Interest inventories are often used in career counseling to help determine clients' likes and dislikes, particularly as they relate to occupations. Interests are important determinants of career choice and are assessed to help clients with academic or career planning. Interest inventories can help clients explore new academic or career possibilities, differentiate among various alternatives, and/or confirm a choice that has already been made (Hood & Johnson, 2002).

Interests often are categorized as expressed, manifest, and inventoried (Crites, 1999; Drummond, 2004; Herr, Cramer, & Niles, 2004; Whiston, 2005). **Expressed interests** refer to those activities individuals state that they prefer—for example, they may state that they enjoy playing soccer or painting. **Manifest interests** are inferred by examining how individuals spend their time—for example, playing the piano or volunteering in a hospital. **Inventoried interests** are identified when clients complete assessment instruments, such as the ones described in this section. One of the limits of interest inventories is that only a limited number of interests are represented on any given instrument. Consequently, professional counselors will want to use other methods, including interviewing and qualitative approaches, to assess a client's patterns of interest (Nitko, 2001).

Many of the interest inventories used in career counseling base their measurements on John Holland's (1966, 1985, 1997) theory that career interests are largely an expression of an individual's personality type. His theory states that people and work environments can be described in terms of their resemblance to six types (known as the RIASEC model): Realistic (R), Investigative (I), Artistic (A), Social (S), Enterprising (E), or Conventional (C) (see Table 13.1). Individuals typically are not "pure" types; rather, they are more likely to be a combination of several types, with one type being more dominant (Swanson & Fouad, 1999). People search for environments that will allow them to use their skills, express their values, and implement their problem-solving styles effectively (Holland, 1997). Personality and environment interact to produce work-related behavior, such as vocational choice, job tenure, satisfaction, and achievement.

In addition to these theoretical assumptions, Holland (1997) proposed that the six personality types can be depicted in a hexagonal structure (see Figure 13.1). Adjacent types have more in common than do types farther away on the hexagon. For example, Realistic and Investigative types share similarities, whereas Realistic and Social types tend to be dissimilar. Many interest inventories provide people with a

Table 13.1   Holland's personality codes and work environment models

Type	Personality	Work Environment
Realistic	Prefers concrete versus abstract work tasks. Enjoys working outdoors doing manual activities. May enjoy building and repairing things. Sees self as practical, physically strong, rugged, stable, and mechanically and physically skilled.	Characterized by manipulation of objects, tools, machines, and animals. Mechanical and technical abilities are used to produce things. Examples of occupations include construction, forestry, mechanics, farming, technology, and certain engineering specialties and military jobs.
Investigating	Enjoys research activities that involve ideas in math and science fields. Enjoys working on abstract problems that require analytical thinking. Sees self as intellectual, curious, original, critical, and talented in mathematics and science.	Characterized by research and exploration of physical, biological, or cultural knowledge. Workers are rewarded for demonstrating scientific values and the ability to view the world in complex and abstract ways. Examples of occupations include scientist, research laboratory worker, medical technologist, design engineer, and computer programmer.
Artistic	Appreciates opportunities for self-expression and artistic creation in writing, music, art, dance, and theater. Often tries to avoid highly structured situations. Sees self as expressive, intuitive, imaginative, creative, talented, and aesthetically oriented.	Characterized by artistic creations in writing, music, art, dance, and theater. Workers are rewarded for demonstrating originality, independence, artistic values, and unconventionality. Examples of occupations include dancer, author, actor, composer, musician, and interior designer.
Social	Enjoys working cooperatively with others. Likes to train or inform others and/or help others solve personal problems. Likes situations that involve establishing relationships, being with groups, and resolving problems by talking them out.	Characterized by interaction with other people to inform, train, develop, cure, or enlighten. Workers are rewarded for displaying social values, cooperating, and demonstrating flexibility and sociability. Examples of occupations include teacher, counselor, religious worker, and recreation specialist.
Enterprising	Views self as cooperative, friendly, humanistic, tactful, and understanding. Enjoys activities that involve leading, controlling, or persuading others. May be concerned about power and status. Views self as energetic, ambitious, enthusiastic, self-confident, adventurous, and skilled in leadership and speaking.	Characterized by the manipulation of others to attain personal and organizational goals. Workers are rewarded for demonstrating the enterprising values of money, power, and status and are encouraged to view the world in terms of power, status, and responsibility. Examples of occupations include lawyer, business executive, politician, salesperson, buyer, realtor, television producer, and insurance agent.
Conventional	Prefers structured jobs and activities. Wants to know expectations and values order. May be uncomfortable in leadership positions. Views self as careful, obedient, dependable, orderly, systematic, persistent, efficient, and skilled in clerical and numerical tasks.	Characterized by detailed, orderly, systematic manipulation of data. Workers are rewarded for conformity, dependability, and working carefully and precisely. Examples of occupations include accountant, bank teller, bookkeeper, administrative assistant, file clerk, tax expert, and computer operator.

three-letter profile, which can be examined to determine the consistency of their interests. To illustrate, the interests of individuals with an SAI profile would be considered consistent; however, the interests of individuals with an SRC profile would be considered inconsistent. Finding work environments that match inconsistent pro-

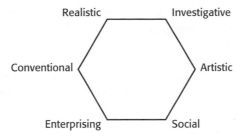

Figure 13.1   Holland's six personality types: The hexagon model

files is more challenging than finding environments that match consistent typologies. It is important for professional counselors who use interest inventories based on Holland's typology to be skilled in understanding the many implications associated with his person-environment fit theory.

Before examining some of the more frequently used interest inventories, it is helpful to consider some suggestions regarding their use in counseling. Hood and Johnson (2002) and Mehrens and Lehmann (1991) summarized research and provided the following guidelines:

- Interest inventories measure likes and dislikes, not abilities. They may suggest what a client will find satisfying in a career or work setting, but they do not indicate how successful the client will be in that setting. Moreover, although interest inventories may be good predictors of future academic and career choices, they do not guarantee that upon selecting a particular choice, individuals will find it satisfying (Whiston, 2005).

- Interests tend to become progressively more stable with age, but they are never permanently fixed. In particular, interest patterns of young adolescents may change with development. Interests are most likely to change when people under age 20 years experience significant changes in their work or school experiences.

- Interest inventories are subject to response set and faking. Clients may respond to inventories in regard to what they think others would like them to say, or they may respond hastily or insincerely. Furthermore, depending on the nature of the inventory, items listed may not be familiar to the client, making the resulting scores invalid.

- General interest inventories have limited value for clients who are trying to make fine distinctions within a broad career category, such as medicine. Questionnaires designed specifically for these situations, such as the *Medical Specialty Preference Inventory* for medical students (Savickas, Brizzi, Brisbin, & Pethtel, 1988) may prove helpful.

- Interest inventories may not be appropriate for clients with certain emotional problems, including depression, as the clients may be more likely to respond negatively to items. Hood and Johnson (2002) and others emphasize the need to address emotional difficulties before proceeding with career planning.

- Interest inventories may be susceptible to bias, particularly sex bias. To address this issue, some inventories, such as the *Strong Interest Inventory*, provide different norms for men and women.
- Interest inventories provide just one piece of information about a client's interests. It is important to consider other approaches, such as interest card sorts or interviews, to explore the client's underlying reasons for particular choices.

Although the focus of this section is on assessment of interests, many instruments designed to measure interests also include measures of perceived ability. For example, the *Strong Interest Inventory* (Harmon , Hansen, Borgen, & Hammer, 1994) often is paired with the *Skills Confidence Inventory* (Betz, Borgen, & Harmon, 1996), and the *Campbell Interest and Skill Survey* (Campbell, 1992) measures interests and self-reported skills. Whereas tools designed to measure interests assess what activities and subjects a client finds appealing, tools designed to measure perceptions of ability assess clients' self-efficacy in regard to those activities and subjects. **Self-efficacy** refers to the beliefs a person has about his or her ability to successfully complete certain tasks (Bandura, 1986). Self-perceptions of ability differ from objective measurements of ability and are more likely to be used in counseling than are objective measures of ability, which are typically used for selection and placement purposes (Hood & Johnson, 2002).

Tests Measuring Interests

Strong Interest Inventory (SII)

The *Strong Interest Inventory* (Harmon et al., 1994), also known as the *Strong* or the *SII,* is one of the most widely used interest inventories. It is a vocational interest questionnaire designed for use by high school students, college students, and adults. The *SII,* which was originally introduced in 1927, has evolved considerably over the past 75 years. The 1994 revision (Form T317) is composed of 317 items: 282 from the 1985 version and 35 additional items. Individuals are asked to indicate whether they *like, dislike,* or are *indifferent to* a wide range of occupations, school subjects, leisure activities, and types of people. They also are asked to state a preference between two activities among several listed pairs.

The *SII* is composed of four sets of scales: General Occupational Themes, Basic Interest Scales, Occupational Scales, and Personal Style Scales. The General Occupation Themes (GOT) are based on the six vocational interest types proposed by John Holland (Realistic, Investigative, Artistic, Social, Enterprising, and Conventional). Results of the inventory provide a three-letter theme code, such as SAI (Social, Artistic, Investigative) or CER (Conventional, Enterprising, Realistic). The Basic Interest Scales (BIS) report consistency of interests or aversions in 25 specific areas, such as religious activities, computer activities, or public speaking. The Occupational Scales indicate similarities between a respondent's interests and the interests of individuals working in specific occupations. The four Personal Style Scales are used to explore preferences concerning working style, learning environment, leadership style, and propensity toward risk taking and adventure.

In addition to the scales, the *SII* provides a summary of item responses, which helps counselors to examine patterns of responses and to determine whether the inventory results are valid. The total number of responses, the index of infrequent responses, and the pattern of response percentages are used to guide decisions about validity. Negative scores on the index of infrequent responses may signal invalidity. Also, as a rule of thumb, at least 300 items need to be answered for scores to be considered valid (Harmon et al., 1994; Whiston, 2005).

Consulting Psychologists Press (CPP) (www.cpp.com) publishes several versions of the *SII,* including a standard, college, and high school edition. It also offers the option of taking the *Skills Confidence Inventory* in conjunction with the *SII.* Paper-and-pencil forms and online administrations are available. Paper-and-pencil forms are sent to the publisher for scoring, and profiles are returned to the professional counselor for interpretation. Online administrations are managed by CPP's online system, SkillsOne (www.skillsone.com), which provides professional counselors with a way to purchase, administer, score, and share interpretive reports with clients.

All scales of the *SII* yield T scores ($M = 50$; $SD = 10$) (Harmon et al., 1994). Scores are based on the combined male and female General Reference Sample (the 18,951 norming sample), with the exception of the Occupational Scales, which provide two sets of standard scales derived from gender-based samples. Professional counselors are encouraged to use the *Application and Technical Guide* to facilitate the interpretation of clients' scores.

The *Strong Interest Inventory* has been described as a model for other interest inventories because of its strong psychometric properties (Whiston, 2005). It provides a valuable measure of vocational interests and presents information to clients in a clear and understandable form. Some concerns have been expressed about the high level of education reflected in the norming sample (e.g.,Vacc & Newsome, 2002; Worthen & Sailor, 1995), and professional counselors need to make responsible decisions about the instrument's suitability for individual clients. In general, however, the *SII* is "a robust career-assessment instrument that provides a valuable measure of vocational interests for the test taker" (Vacc & Newsome, 2002, p. 296).

The main reasons for using the *SII* are to identify the client's interests, provide a framework for organizing interests into categories within the world of work, and help the client identify potential occupations that may not have been considered previously. The *SII* can be used to help people select majors or training programs, choose occupations, determine midcareer changes, plan for retirement, or understand reasons for job dissatisfaction (Harmon et al., 1994).

Scores on the *SII* profile are presented so that interpretation moves from general to more specific information (see Figure 13.2). Steps for interpretation are outlined in the *Application and Technical Guide,* which also provides assistance in interpreting unusual profiles and in using the *SII* with different age groups, cultures, genders, and special populations. Scores are reported on a six-page profile sheet. Interpretation focuses on each of the four scales, beginning with the General Occupational Themes. Prince and Heiser (2000) suggested that professional counselors present the client with an overview of Holland's theory before interpreting the six-page profile sheet.

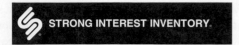 **STRONG INTEREST INVENTORY**

Profile report for:	**JANE SAMPLE**
ID:	**6316950**
Age:	**25**
Gender:	**Female**

Page 1 of 6

Date tested: **6/18/05**
Date scored: **6/18/05**

SNAPSHOT: A SUMMARY OF RESULTS FOR JANE SAMPLE

VH = very high interest	VS = very similar
H = high interest	S = similar
A = average interest	M-R = mid-range
L = little interest	D = dissimilar
VL = very little interest	VD = very dissimilar

GENERAL OCCUPATIONAL THEMES

The General Occupational Themes describe interests in six very broad areas, including interest in work and leisure activities, kinds of people, and work settings. Your interests in each area are shown at the right in rank order. Note that each Theme has a code, represented by the first letter of the Theme name.

You can use your Theme code, printed below your results, to identify school subjects, part-time jobs, college majors, leisure activities, or careers that you might find interesting.

THEME CODE	THEME	VL	L	A	H	VH	TYPICAL INTERESTS
I	INVESTIGATIVE	☐	☐	☐	☐	☑	**Researching, analyzing**
A	ARTISTIC	☐	☐	☑	☐	☐	**Creating or enjoying art**
C	CONVENTIONAL	☐	☐	☑	☐	☐	**Accounting, processing data**
S	SOCIAL	☐	☐	☑	☐	☐	**Helping, instructing**
R	REALISTIC	☐	☐	☑	☐	☐	**Building, repairing**
E	ENTERPRISING	☑	☐	☐	☐	☐	**Selling, managing**

Your Theme code is IAC—(see explanation at left).

You might explore occupations with codes that contain any combination of these letters.

BASIC INTEREST SCALES

The Basic Interest Scales measure your interests in 25 specific areas or activities. Only those 5 areas in which you show the *most* interest are listed at the right in rank order. Your results on all 25 Basic Interest Scales are found on page 2.

To the left of each scale is a letter that shows which of the six General Occupational Themes this activity is most closely related to. These codes can help you to identify other activities that you might enjoy.

THEME CODE	BASIC INTERESTS	VL	L	A	H	VH	TYPICAL ACTIVITIES
I	SCIENCE	☐	☐	☐	☐	☑	**Conducting scientific research**
I	MATHEMATICS	☐	☐	☐	☐	☑	**Working with numbers or statistics**
R	NATURE	☐	☐	☐	☐	☑	**Appreciating nature**
S	RELIGIOUS ACTIVITIES	☐	☐	☐	☑	☐	**Participating in spiritual activities**
A	MUSIC/DRAMATICS	☐	☐	☑	☐	☐	**Performing or enjoying music/drama**

OCCUPATIONAL SCALES

The Occupational Scales measure how similar your interests are to the interests of people who are satisfied working in those occupations. Only the 10 scales on which your interests are *most* similar to those of these people are listed at the right in rank order. Your results on all 211 of the Occupational Scales are found on pages 3, 4, and 5.

The letters to the left of each scale identify the Theme or Themes that most closely describe the interests of people working in that occupation. You can use these letters to find additional, related occupations that you might find interesting.

THEME CODE	OCCUPATION	VD	D	M-R	S	VS
IRA	BIOLOGIST	☐	☐	☐	☐	☑
IRC	MATHEMATICIAN	☐	☐	☐	☐	☑
IR	CHEMIST	☐	☐	☐	☐	☑
IR	COMPUTER PROGR./ SYSTEMS ANALYST	☐	☐	☐	☐	☑
IAR	COLLEGE PROFESSOR	☐	☐	☐	☐	☑
A	LIBRARIAN	☐	☐	☐	☐	☑
IS	AUDIOLOGIST	☐	☐	☐	☐	☑
IRA	PHYSICIST	☐	☐	☐	☐	☑
CI	ACTUARY	☐	☐	☐	☐	☑
IRA	GEOLOGIST	☐	☐	☐	☐	☑

PERSONAL STYLE SCALES *measure your levels of comfort regarding Work Style, Learning Environment, Leadership Style, and Risk Taking/Adventure. This information may help you make decisions about particular work environments, educational settings, and types of activities you would find satisfying. Your results on these four scales are on page 6.*

Figure 13.2   Sample *Strong Interest Inventory* profile sheets

Modified and reproduced by special permission of the Publisher, CPP, Inc., Mountain View, CA 94043 from the Strong Interest Inventory® Instrument. © 1933, 1945, 1946, 1966, 1968, 1974, 1981, 1985, 1994, by CPP, Inc. Further reproduction is prohibited without the Publisher's written consent. Strong Interest Inventory is a registered trademark of CPP, Inc.

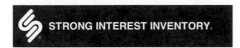 **STRONG INTEREST INVENTORY.**

GENERAL OCCUPATIONAL THEMES

BASIC INTEREST SCALES

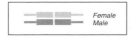

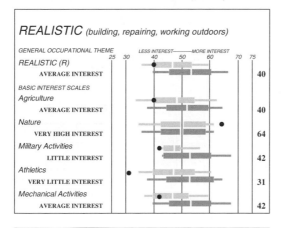

REALISTIC (building, repairing, working outdoors)

REALISTIC (R) AVERAGE INTEREST	40
Agriculture AVERAGE INTEREST	40
Nature VERY HIGH INTEREST	64
Military Activities LITTLE INTEREST	42
Athletics VERY LITTLE INTEREST	31
Mechanical Activities AVERAGE INTEREST	42

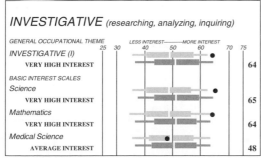

INVESTIGATIVE (researching, analyzing, inquiring)

INVESTIGATIVE (I) VERY HIGH INTEREST	64
Science VERY HIGH INTEREST	65
Mathematics VERY HIGH INTEREST	64
Medical Science AVERAGE INTEREST	48

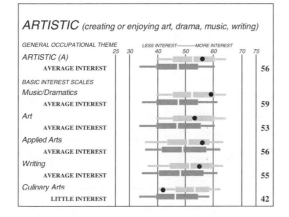

ARTISTIC (creating or enjoying art, drama, music, writing)

ARTISTIC (A) AVERAGE INTEREST	56
Music/Dramatics AVERAGE INTEREST	59
Art AVERAGE INTEREST	53
Applied Arts AVERAGE INTEREST	56
Writing AVERAGE INTEREST	55
Culinary Arts LITTLE INTEREST	42

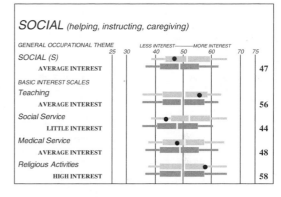

SOCIAL (helping, instructing, caregiving)

SOCIAL (S) AVERAGE INTEREST	47
Teaching AVERAGE INTEREST	56
Social Service LITTLE INTEREST	44
Medical Service AVERAGE INTEREST	48
Religious Activities HIGH INTEREST	58

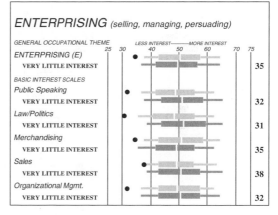

ENTERPRISING (selling, managing, persuading)

ENTERPRISING (E) VERY LITTLE INTEREST	35
Public Speaking VERY LITTLE INTEREST	32
Law/Politics VERY LITTLE INTEREST	31
Merchandising VERY LITTLE INTEREST	35
Sales VERY LITTLE INTEREST	38
Organizational Mgmt. VERY LITTLE INTEREST	32

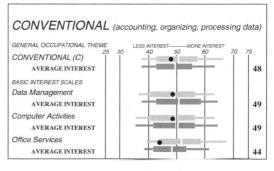

CONVENTIONAL (accounting, organizing, processing data)

CONVENTIONAL (C) AVERAGE INTEREST	48
Data Management AVERAGE INTEREST	49
Computer Activities AVERAGE INTEREST	49
Office Services AVERAGE INTEREST	44

Figure 13.2   continued

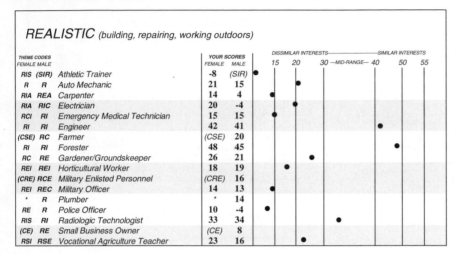

OCCUPATIONAL SCALES

NOTES

REALISTIC (building, repairing, working outdoors)

THEME CODES FEMALE MALE			YOUR SCORES FEMALE MALE	
RIS	(SIR)	Athletic Trainer	-8	(SIR)
R	R	Auto Mechanic	21	15
RIA	REA	Carpenter	14	4
RIA	RIC	Electrician	20	-4
RCI	RI	Emergency Medical Technician	15	15
RI	RI	Engineer	42	41
(CSE)	RC	Farmer	(CSE)	20
RI	RI	Forester	48	45
RC	RE	Gardener/Groundskeeper	26	21
REI	REI	Horticultural Worker	18	19
(CRE)	RCE	Military Enlisted Personnel	(CRE)	16
REI	REC	Military Officer	14	13
*	R	Plumber	*	14
RE	R	Police Officer	10	-4
RIS	RI	Radiologic Technologist	33	34
(CE)	RE	Small Business Owner	(CE)	8
RSI	RSE	Vocational Agriculture Teacher	23	16

DISSIMILAR INTERESTS———————SIMILAR INTERESTS
15   20   30 —MID-RANGE— 40   50   55

INVESTIGATIVE (researching, analyzing, inquiring)

THEME CODES FEMALE MALE			YOUR SCORES FEMALE MALE	
IS	IA	Audiologist	53	46
IRA	IA	Biologist	66	65
IR	IR	Chemist	61	60
IR	IRA	Chiropractor	30	20
IAR	IAS	College Professor	56	60
IR	IAR	Computer Progr./Systems Analyst	57	54
IRA	IR	Dentist	34	31
IES	(SEC)	Dietitian	23	(SEC)
IRA	IA	Geographer	45	57
IRA	IRA	Geologist	51	58
IRC	ICA	Mathematician	62	60
IRC	IRE	Medical Technician	26	27
IRC	IRC	Medical Technologist	44	35
IR	IR	Optometrist	42	30
ICR	ICE	Pharmacist	48	33
IAR	IAR	Physician	49	51
IRA	IRA	Physicist	53	53
IA	IA	Psychologist	42	53
IR	IRC	Research & Development Manager	49	29
IRA	IRS	Respiratory Therapist	30	33
IRS	IRS	Science Teacher	41	33
IAR	(AI)	Sociologist	36	(AI)
IRA	IR	Veterinarian	46	37

DISSIMILAR INTERESTS———————SIMILAR INTERESTS
15   20   30 —MID-RANGE— 40   50   55

Figure 13.2   continued

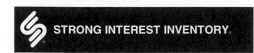

OCCUPATIONAL SCALES *(continued)*

NOTES

ARTISTIC *(creating or enjoying art, drama, music, writing)*

THEME CODES FEMALE MALE		Occupation	YOUR SCORES FEMALE	MALE
AE	AE	Advertising Executive	12	24
ARI	ARI	Architect	26	35
ARI	A	Artist, Commercial	21	27
AR	A	Artist, Fine	38	40
ASE	AS	Art Teacher	10	31
AE	AE	Broadcaster	19	19
AES	AES	Corporate Trainer	18	20
ASE	ASE	English Teacher	30	39
(EA)	AE	Interior Decorator	(EA)	28
A	A	Lawyer	17	23
A	A	Librarian	54	67
AIR	AIR	Medical Illustrator	23	22
A	A	Musician	47	50
ARE	ARE	Photographer	32	14
AER	ASE	Public Administrator	10	14
AE	AE	Public Relations Director	-2	19
A	A	Reporter	24	30
(IAR)	AI	Sociologist	(IAR)	41
AIR	AI	Technical Writer	49	60
A	AI	Translator	46	64

DISSIMILAR INTERESTS —————— SIMILAR INTERESTS
15 20 30 —MID-RANGE— 40 50 55

SOCIAL *(helping, instructing, caregiving)*

THEME CODES FEMALE MALE		Occupation	YOUR SCORES FEMALE	MALE
(RIS)	SIR	Athletic Trainer	(RIS)	-4
S	*	Child Care Provider	17	*
SE	SE	Community Serv. Organization Dir.	8	9
(IES)	SEC	Dietitian	(IES)	17
S	S	Elementary School Teacher	24	43
SAE	SA	Foreign Language Teacher	33	41
SE	SE	High School Counselor	18	30
SE	*	Home Economics Teacher	12	*
SAR	SA	Minister	20	30
SCE	SCE	Nurse, LPN	13	20
SI	SAI	Nurse, RN	33	38
SAR	SA	Occupational Therapist	33	36
SE	SE	Parks and Recreation Coordinator	13	13
SRC	SR	Physical Education Teacher	0	1
SIR	SIR	Physical Therapist	21	16
SEA	SEC	School Administrator	15	17
SEA	SEA	Social Science Teacher	24	18
SA	SA	Social Worker	31	36
SE	SEA	Special Education Teacher	31	41
SA	SA	Speech Pathologist	41	43

DISSIMILAR INTERESTS —————— SIMILAR INTERESTS
15 20 30 —MID-RANGE— 40 50 55

Figure 13.2   continued

STRONG INTEREST INVENTORY.

OCCUPATIONAL SCALES (continued)

ENTERPRISING (selling, managing, persuading)

THEME CODES FEMALE MALE			YOUR SCORES FEMALE	MALE	DISSIMILAR INTERESTS 15	20	30	—MID-RANGE— 40	50	55 SIMILAR INTERESTS
*	ECR	Agribusiness Manager	*	2						
EC	EC	Buyer	-17	-4	●					
ERA	ER	Chef	-3	11	●					
EIS	*	Dental Hygienist	11	*	●					
EAS	ESA	Elected Public Official	9	6	●					
EAS	EAS	Flight Attendant	6	23	●					
EAC	EAC	Florist	-10	8	●					
EC	EA	Hair Stylist	0	19	●					
ECS	ECS	Housekeeping & Maintenance Supr.	8	8	●					
EAS	ES	Human Resources Director	9	16	●					
EA	(AE)	Interior Decorator	3	(AE)	●					
EIR	ECI	Investments Manager	29	18			●			
E	E	Life Insurance Agent	-1	-3	●					
EA	EA	Marketing Executive	19	29		●				
ECR	ER	Optician	10	8	●					
ECR	ECR	Purchasing Agent	5	5	●					
E	E	Realtor	-9	4	●					
ECR	ECR	Restaurant Manager	-4	0	●					
ECA	ECS	Store Manager	2	2	●					
ECA	ECA	Travel Agent	4	11	●					

CONVENTIONAL (accounting, organizing, processing data)

THEME CODES FEMALE MALE			YOUR SCORES FEMALE	MALE	DISSIMILAR INTERESTS 15	20	30	—MID-RANGE— 40	50	55 SIMILAR INTERESTS
CE	CE	Accountant	24	12			●			
CI	CI	Actuary	51	48					●	
CE	CE	Banker	23	13			●			
C	C	Bookkeeper	21	8		●				
CES	CES	Business Education Teacher	17	23	●					
CE	CE	Credit Manager	13	10	●					
CSE	*	Dental Assistant	12	*	●					
CSE	(RC)	Farmer	20	(RC)		●				
CES	CES	Food Service Manager	21	14		●				
CIR	CIS	Mathematics Teacher	39	36				●		
C	C	Medical Records Technician	38	40				●		
CRE	(RCE)	Military Enlisted Personnel	17	(RCE)	●					
CES	CES	Nursing Home Administrator	13	25	●					
CE	CA	Paralegal	15	20	●					
CES	*	Secretary	5	*	●					
CE	(RE)	Small Business Owner	18	(RE)	●					

NOTES

Figure 13.2   continued

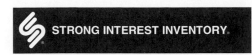

PERSONAL STYLE SCALES

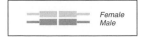

Female
Male

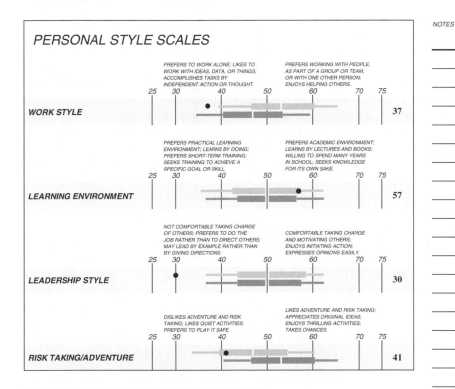

PERSONAL STYLE SCALES

WORK STYLE

PREFERS TO WORK ALONE; LIKES TO WORK WITH IDEAS, DATA, OR THINGS; ACCOMPLISHES TASKS BY INDEPENDENT ACTION OR THOUGHT.

PREFERS WORKING WITH PEOPLE, AS PART OF A GROUP OR TEAM, OR WITH ONE OTHER PERSON; ENJOYS HELPING OTHERS.

25   30   40   50   60   70   75   **37**

LEARNING ENVIRONMENT

PREFERS PRACTICAL LEARNING ENVIRONMENT; LEARNS BY DOING; PREFERS SHORT-TERM TRAINING; SEEKS TRAINING TO ACHIEVE A SPECIFIC GOAL OR SKILL.

PREFERS ACADEMIC ENVIRONMENT; LEARNS BY LECTURES AND BOOKS; WILLING TO SPEND MANY YEARS IN SCHOOL; SEEKS KNOWLEDGE FOR ITS OWN SAKE.

25   30   40   50   60   70   75   **57**

LEADERSHIP STYLE

NOT COMFORTABLE TAKING CHARGE OF OTHERS; PREFERS TO DO THE JOB RATHER THAN TO DIRECT OTHERS; MAY LEAD BY EXAMPLE RATHER THAN BY GIVING DIRECTIONS.

COMFORTABLE TAKING CHARGE AND MOTIVATING OTHERS; ENJOYS INITIATING ACTION; EXPRESSES OPINIONS EASILY.

25   30   40   50   60   70   75   **30**

RISK TAKING/ADVENTURE

DISLIKES ADVENTURE AND RISK TAKING; LIKES QUIET ACTIVITIES; PREFERS TO PLAY IT SAFE.

LIKES ADVENTURE AND RISK TAKING; APPRECIATES ORIGINAL IDEAS; ENJOYS THRILLING ACTIVITIES; TAKES CHANCES.

25   30   40   50   60   70   75   **41**

NOTES

Total responses out of 317:   **317**
Infrequent responses: **5**

SUMMARY OF ITEM RESPONSES

ADMINISTRATIVE INDEXES (response percentages)

OCCUPATIONS	20	%L	16	%I	64	%D
SCHOOL SUBJECTS	49	L	18	I	33	D
ACTIVITIES	24	L	19	I	57	D
LEISURE ACTIVITIES	34	L	14	I	52	D
TYPES OF PEOPLE	45	L	25	I	30	D
CHARACTERISTICS	42	Y	16	?	42	N
SUBTOTAL	29	%	17	%	54	%
PREFERENCES: ACTIVITIES	43	L	10	=	47	R
PREFERENCES: WORK	50	L	17	=	33	R

Figure 13.2   continued

The first page of the profile provides a "snapshot" summary of the client's General Occupational Themes, highest-ranked Basic Interests, and top Occupational Scale similarities. On the second page of the profile, the client's scores on the Basic Interest Scales, which are grouped according to General Occupational Themes, are presented in detail. Terms ranging from Very Little Interest to Very High Interest are used to describe the client's scores on each scale, and shaded interpretive bars graphically illustrate norms for men and women, allowing clients to compare their scores with those norms. Professional counselors can use the information provided by the BIS to expand the client's understanding of the world of work as well as to initiate discussion of nonvocational interests (Hansen, 2000).

The next three pages of the profile depict scores on the Occupational Scales. There are 211 scales, representing 109 different occupations (107 for women and 104 for men). The occupations are grouped by Holland's themes and include professional and nonprofessional occupations. High scores on a particular scale, such as biologist, indicate a similarity in interest patterns between the client and individuals who have been working in, and are satisfied with, that occupation. Harmon et al. (1994) recommended examining areas of high and low interest to identify interest patterns. After examining these three scales, professional counselors can encourage clients to examine additional sources, such as the *Dictionary of Holland Occupational Codes* (Gottfredson & Holland, 1996) or the *Occupations Finder* (Holland, 1994), to explore other occupations that have codes similar to the client's (Zunker & Osborn, 2002).

The final page of the *SII* profile includes the Personal Style Scales and the Summary of Item Responses. As stated earlier, the Summary of Item Responses provides a way to evaluate the validity of the client's score and depicts frequencies of *like, dislike,* and *indifferent* responses. Scores on the four Personal Style Scales indicate whether the client prefers (a) working with people or working with data, things, or ideas; (b) an academic learning environment or a practical learning environment; (c) taking charge and motivating others or leading by example; and (d) taking risks and seeking adventurous activities or "playing it safe." Scores fall on a continuum, and, as with interests, preferences do not imply abilities.

Skills Confidence Inventory (SCI)

A relatively new addition to the *Strong Interest Inventory* is the *Skills Confidence Inventory* (*SCI*) (Betz et al., 1996). The 60-item *SCI* measures a respondent's self-perceived ability to successfully complete a variety of tasks, activities, and coursework. Items correspond to the *SII*'s General Occupational Themes, with 10 items constituting each theme scale. Scores on each scale range from 1 to 5, with scores of 3.5 or higher representing areas of high skill confidence.

The *SCI* is designed for use with college students and adults who have some amount of work experience. Results are reported on a single-page profile that compares the respondent's perceived capabilities with expressed interests in each of the six General Occupational Themes. Scores are reported on two levels: Levels of Skills Confidence by Theme, which reports the client's level of skills confidence with respect to the General Occupational Themes, and the Skills Confidence-Interest Comparison, which compares levels of confidence with levels of interest.

Career professionals using the *Skills Confidence Inventory* can help clients examine their interests and perceived abilities simultaneously to interpret vocational interest patterns. The combined use of the *SII* and *SCI* provides information that neither inventory provides alone. The integrated profile categorizes each theme area by priority for exploration. High confidence and interest in a theme signal a need for further exploration. When confidence is higher than interest or vice versa, the professional counselor can help the client explore reasons for the discrepancy. It is important to note that confidence in a particular area does not necessarily reflect actual ability or the potential to develop ability (Betz et al., 1996).

Research on career self-efficacy has supported its role as an important predictor of academic performance and career decision-making intentions (Betz et al., 1996). The *SCI* provides a way to coordinate a measure of career self-efficacy with measures of vocational interest, thereby paving the way for further exploration of career options.

Self-Directed Search (SDS)

Another widely used measure of interests and perceived abilities is the *Self-Directed Search* (*SDS*) (Holland, Fritzche, & Powell, 1994). The *SDS* was developed by John Holland and is based on his theory of vocational choice. Like the *SII,* the *SDS* provides test takers with a three-letter Holland code, which then is matched with occupations and/or college majors with codes identical to or similar to that code. The *SDS* is a 228-item, self-administered, self-scored, and self-interpreted instrument that is available in paper-and-pencil, computerized, and online forms (Osborn, 2002). Several versions of the *SDS* are available, including Form R (for high school students, college students, and adults); Form E (for individuals with limited education or reading skills); Form CP (for professionals or adults in transition); and the Career Explorer (for middle school–aged students). Each of these versions is designed to help individuals identify their personality types and discover careers or fields of study that are compatible with those types.

The most commonly used form of the *SDS,* Form R, was revised in 1994 and consists of an assessment booklet and several supplemental materials, including *The Educational Opportunities Finder, You and Your Career, The Occupations Finder,* and *The Leisure Activities Finder.* Clients complete the assessment booklet first. The booklet consists of several sections, including a section for describing occupational daydreams and sections composed of four different scales: Activities, Competencies, Occupations, and Self-estimates. Responses to these four scales yield a three-letter RIASEC Summary Code. This code is used with *The Occupations Finder* to identify matching occupations from a list of over 1,300 occupations classified according to Holland's system (Ciechalski, 2002).

As stated earlier, the *SDS* is self-administered and self-scored. After responding to the four scales (Activities, Competencies, Occupations, and Self-estimates), test takers total their scores for each of the six "personality types" that are represented in

Table 13.2   Sample *Self-Directed Search* raw scores report

	R	I	A	S	E	C
Activities	8	2	5	4	6	3
Competencies	7	2	2	5	8	2
Occupations	5	2	0	3	5	2
Self-Estimates	6	3	3	4	8	1
Total Scores	26	9	10	16	27	8
Summary Code:	ERS (Enterprising, Realistic, Social)					

Note: In Holland's RIASEC model; R = Realistic; I = Investigative; A = Artistic; S = Social; E = Enterprising; and C = Conventional.

the four scales. Unlike most assessment tools, raw scores are used to determine results. *SDS* summary code scores range from 2 to 50, and the top three scores are used to determine the individual's three-letter type (see Table 13.2). Results can be calculated immediately, and although the instrument can be self-interpreted, it is helpful for counselors to be involved in the process (Brown, 2001; Whiston, 2005).

As when interpreting the *SII,* counselors will want to help clients understand Holland's framework before discussing assessment results. The Holland typology provides a framework for clients to conceptualize their vocational personality and observe how it may coincide with the world of work (Swanson & Fouad, 1999).

After explaining Holland's theory, professional counselors can use a series of questions to guide clients in interpreting and discussing the *SDS.* Rayman (1998) suggested using the following set of questions, first posed by Johnston and Rakes (1992), to shape the interpretation of a client's *SDS* profile:

- *What are the client's expressed career choices, based on the client's list of occupational daydreams?* These choices can be coded to help determine an individual's predominant personality characteristics.
- *Is there anything about the client's current situation or background that might help with understanding or interpreting the SDS scores?* Environmental and experiential influences are likely to have shaped the client's current values, attitudes, and aspirations.
- *How do the client's vocational aspirations compare with the SDS summary code?* Do the careers the client is considering contain the high-point codes that are part of the client's summary profile?
- *What does the application of the "Rule of Eight" suggest about the predictability of the SDS summary code?* When scores between any two RIASEC scales differ by less than 8 points, that difference may be due to measurement error. Therefore, it is important to look at all the permutations of the client's predominant codes when comparing them to occupational codes (e.g., for SEA, consider ESA, AES, EAS, SAE, and ASE).

- *What does the "Rule of Asymmetrical Distribution of Types" tell about the client's summary code?* Counselors can refer to the tables in Appendix A of the *SDS Professional User's Guide* (Holland et al., 1994) to examine the distribution of *SDS* codes among and within the six Holland categories. This information can help determine whether a particular code is common or unusual. In some cases, unusual codes may make it more difficult for the client to find a congruent work environment.

- *What traits, values, aptitudes and competencies, and identifications are implied by the client's SDS code?* What salient personality characteristics are identified by the client's predominant Holland type, and how well do those characteristics match the client's self-perception? (Refer to Table 1 in the *SDS* manual for a listing of personality characteristics associated with each personality type.)

- *How consistent is the client's SDS summary code?* Consistency refers to the degree of distance between two types as they are represented on the Holland hexagonal model. Adjacent types, such as R and I, are considered the most consistent; alternate types, such as R and A, are less consistent; and opposites, such as R and S, are least consistent.

- *What does the degree of differentiation of the SDS code imply about the client's behavior?* **Differentiation** refers to how much the highest and lowest code scores differ from one another. Scores that differ by less than 8 points may indicate that the differences are meaningless. People may be highly differentiated, closely resembling one type, or they may be undifferentiated, resembling many types. Many high, undifferentiated scores may indicate multipotentiality, multiple interests, or, in some cases, indecisiveness. In contrast, many low, undifferentiated scores may indicate undeveloped or minimal interests that could reflect a lack of work-related experience or the presence of negative self-talk (Zunker & Osborn, 2002).

- *What other diagnostic information is available?* What other assessments has the client completed, and what do the results of those assessments indicate? What additional information would help the client in exploring career options?

The Self-Directed Search and Related Holland Career Materials: A Practitioner's Guide (Reardon & Lenz, 1998) is a resource that counselors can use to help guide the interpretation of *SDS* results. Reardon and Lenz review the *SDS* and the theory behind it and also provide an overview of all of Holland's assessment materials. The book helps professional counselors make the most efficient use of a client's *SDS* results and provides suggestions for working holistically with clients as they make career decisions (Consolvo, 2001).

In summary, the *SDS* is considered a sound vocational interest inventory that has a long history of use, strong psychometric properties, and a variety of career development applications (Brown, 2001). The manuals are comprehensive and well written, and the materials are attractive, comprehensive, and easy to use. One concern is that using the instrument superficially may oversimplify the process of career choice. Thus it is essential for professional counselors to have a solid background in career counseling to avoid underestimating the complexity of either the instrument or the overall process of career development.

Kuder Interest Inventories

The *Kuder Interest Inventories* have a rich tradition that began with the publication of the *Kuder Preference Survey* by Frederic Kuder in 1939. Since that time, the Kuder instruments have evolved through three generations of interest inventories and have been a source of extensive empirical study (Zytowski, 1992). The instruments that currently are used to assess career-related interests include the *Kuder Occupational Interest Survey,* Form DD (*KOIS*) (Kuder & Zytowski, 1991); the *Kuder General Interest Survey,* Form E (*KGIS*) (Kuder, 1988): and the *Kuder Career Search With Person Match* (*KCS*) (Kuder & Zytowski, 1999; Zytowski, 2004). In addition, the *Kuder Career Planning System* (*KCPS*) is an online, interactive program that includes the *KCS,* a skills assessment, and a work values inventory. All of the Kuder instruments are published by National Career Assessment Services, which can be accessed through its website, www.kuder.com.

The *Kuder Occupational Interest Survey* (*KOIS-DD*) (Kuder & Zytowski, 1991) can be used with adolescents in grades 10 through 12, college students, and adults who are making career changes or reentering school or the work force. Similar to other interest inventories, its purpose is to assess interests to help people select college majors and/or potential careers. Unlike the interest inventories described previously, the *KOIS* does not directly match interests with Holland codes; instead, interests are aligned with 10 vocational interest categories: Outdoor, Mechanical, Computational, Scientific, Persuasive, Artistic, Literary, Musical, Social Service, and Clerical.

The instrument consists of 100 triad items representing 300 different activities (Kelly, 2002a). For example, a sample *KOIS* triad set includes these activities: "*Write a book, Sell a book, Print a book.*" Individuals are asked to select their most and least preferred item from each set of three. Responses are computer-scored, and narrative reports are compiled. In addition to providing information about the 10 vocational interest scales (reported as vocational interest estimates), the report includes information about 109 occupational scales and 40 college major scales.

Vocational interest estimates are categorized as High (above the 75th percentile), Average (25th–75th percentile), and Low (below 25th percentile). Interest estimates are listed by gender (i.e., "compared with men" and "compared with women"). Occupational scales also are listed by gender and compare the test taker's interest patterns with the interest patterns of individuals in 109 different occupations. Of these, 33 are normed with both female and male occupational groups, 32 are normed for males only, and 11 are normed for females only (Kuder & Zytowski, 1991). The scales are rank ordered and placed in one of three categories: Most Similar, Next Most Similar, and The Rest Listed in Order of Similarity.

The 40 college major scales also are presented in rank order according to level of similarity. As with the other scales, comparisons are made to both male and female criterion groups. In addition to the college major scales, occupational scales, and vocational interest estimates, the *KOIS* report includes a dependability statement, which indicates whether the results are reliable. The report also includes the descriptions of 8 experimental scales, for which there currently is little interpretive information (Kelly, 2002a).

One of the concerns related to the *KOIS* is that the occupational scales and college major scales are based on normative groups that are dated and that are not representative of the racial and ethnic composition of the United States (Kelly, 2002a). Kelly described the *KOIS* as a "beautifully constructed measurement device that needs to be updated" (p. 273). Consequently, career counselors may be better served by using the *Kuder Career Search With Person Match* (*KCS*), described below.

The *Kuder General Interest Scale* (*KGIS-E*) (Kuder, 1988) is designed for students in grades 6 to 12. Like the *KOIS,* the instrument assesses interests in 10 vocational areas: Outdoor, Mechanical, Computational, Scientific, Persuasive, Artistic, Literary, Musical, Social Service, and Clerical. The purpose of the *KGIS* is to stimulate career exploration and open up career options, rather than suggest specific occupational options (Kuder, 1988; Pope, 2002). Students respond to 168 triad items, indicating which activities they prefer most and least. Scores are matched with the 10 vocational interest areas, and responses also can be converted to Holland codes. A verification score (V score) is reported, which can be used to determine the dependability of results. Profiles with V scores at or above 15 may be problematic (Hood & Johnson, 2002).

Answer sheets for the *KGIS* may be hand-scored or computer-scored. However, errors have been reported as fairly common on self-scored answer sheets (Pope, 2002). Although the instrument may be a helpful way to help youth explore career interests, Pope cautions that the *KGIS-E* normative data are dated and that culture-specific data are lacking. Indeed, the *Kuder Career Search* (*KCS*) (Zytowski, 2004), which is based on more current normative information, may be a better choice for assessing the interests of adolescents. D. G. Zytowski (personal communication, October 12, 2004) indicated that there are plans to discontinue production of the *KGIS* once current stock is exhausted.

The *Kuder Career Search with Person Match* (*KCS*) is the most current version of the Kuder interest surveys (Kuder & Zytowski, 1999; Zytowski, 2004). The primary purpose of the *KCS* is to help individuals generate a list of reasonable occupational possibilities (Ihle-Helledy, Zytowski, & Fouad, 2004). The *KCS* helps individuals discover career interests, explore occupations beyond job titles, and apply personal interests to career plans. The instrument is innovative in that individuals are not compared to a representative group of members of particular occupations but instead are compared to 25 possible individuals within an occupation (Zytowski, 2004). Most often, the *KCS* is taken online; however, it also can be taken in paper-and-pencil format.

The *KCS* consists of 60 forced-choice triads, 48 of which were taken from the *KOIS.* For each triad, individuals rank their first, second, and last preference. The Internet-based version takes approximately 20 minutes to complete and provides immediate online scoring, a self-interpretive report of career interests, and occupational biographies for the 14 highest person matches. The instrument is designed to help people recognize their multipotentiality; that is, patterns of interests may be satisfied in several possible occupations or careers (Zytowski, 2004).

The *KCS* differs from the *KOIS* in four significant ways (Kelly, 2002b). First, the *KOIS* vocational interest estimates have been updated and renamed the Activity

Preference scales: Nature, Mechanical, Science/Technical, Art, Music, Communications, Human Services, Sales/Management, Computations, and Office Detail. Second, the online version provides an interactive report that links the user with the online version of the *Occupational Outlook Handbook,* occupational news groups, and a college search engine (Zytowski, 2004). A third innovation is the inclusion of results for six career clusters that match the six Holland (1997) interest types: Outdoor/Mechanical (Realistic), Science/Technical (Investigative), Arts/Communication (Artistic), Social/Personal Services (Social), Sales/Management (Enterprising), and Business Detail (Conventional). Clusters are reported in rank order of percentile scores based on a norming group of 8,489 males and females, from middle school aged to adult (Zytowski, 2002). The fourth innovation is the Person Match scoring system, which compares the test taker's activity preferences to a database of approximately 2000 individuals working in specific occupations. First-person occupational descriptions are presented for the 14 closest matches within the individual's top two clusters.

The *KCS* is a relatively new instrument, particularly the online version. Consequently, information about its psychometric properties is still being gathered. The online user's manual provides evidence of various types of validity, including content, substantive, structural, and consequential (Zytowski, 2004). Initial reports of temporal (test-retest) reliability for activity preference scales range from 0.79 (Nature) to 0.92 (Art, Human Services) (Ihle-Helledy, Zytowski, & Fouad, 2004). The user's manual states that "the development of the *KCS* emphasizes utility over elegant psychometrics" (Zytowski, 2004, p. 11). Kelly (2002a) cautioned professional counselors to view findings as tentative and subject to error. However, as researchers continue to gather supporting evidence of the *KCS*'s psychometric properties, this caution may not be necessary.

Other Interest and Skill Inventories

Many other assessment instruments that measure interests and skills are available to professional counselors. A brief description of some of the more commonly used instruments follows. Professional counselors can refer to Kapes and Whitfield's (2002) *A Counselor's Guide to Career Assessment Instruments* (4th ed.) and to the website of the Buros Institute (www.unl.edu/buros) to gather additional information about these and other measures of interest and perceived ability.

Abilities Explorer (AE)

The *Abilities Explorer* (*AE*) (Harrington & Harrington, 1996) assesses 14 work-related abilities that are measured on a 6-point Likert scale. The instrument, which consists of 280 items, includes statements about work-related activities, past performance on various activities, and academic coursework. The assessment is available in two forms: Level 1 for middle school–aged students and Level 2 for high school students and adults. It may be hand-scored (yielding raw scores) or machine-scored (yielding percentile ranks).

Campbell Interest and Skill Survey (CISS)

The *Campbell Interest and Skill Survey* (*CISS*) (Campbell, 1992) is designed to measure self-reported interests and skills and focuses mainly on careers that require post-secondary education. It is most useful for college-bound students, adults with college educations, and adults making career transitions. The assessment includes interest and skill scores for 7 orientation scales, 25 basic scales, and 60 occupational scales. The orientation scales correspond to RIASEC themes and represent the major subsets of the world of work: Influencing, Organizing, Helping, Creating, Analyzing, Producing, and Adventuring. The *CISS* is published by Pearson Assessments (formerly NCS Assessments), which can be accessed at www.pearsonassessments.com.

Career Assessment Inventory: Vocational Version (CAI-VV) and Enhanced Version (CAI-EV)

The two versions of the *CAI* (Johannson, 1984, 1986) are designed to measure occupational interests for use in career exploration and decision making. The *CAI-VV* provides options for individuals who aspire to technical or nonprofessional careers. The *CAI-EV* is somewhat longer and covers 111 occupations requiring various levels of education, thereby meeting the needs of both non-college-bound and college-bound individuals. Profile reports yield scores on six general theme scales that correspond with Holland's RIASEC areas, basic interest area scales, occupational scales, administrative indices, and special scales. Both versions of the CAI are published by Pearson Assessments (www.pearsonassessments.com).

Career Occupational Preference System (COPSystem)

The *Career Occupational Preference System* (*COPSystem*) (Knapp, Knapp, & Knapp-Lee, 1990) is an integrated career assessment system that includes interrelated assessments of interests, abilities, and work values. The three assessments are keyed to 14 *COPSystem* Career Clusters: Professional, Science Skilled, Technology Professional, Technology Skilled, Consumer Economics, Outdoor, Business Professional, Business Skilled, Clerical, Communication, Arts Professional, Arts Skilled, Service Professional, and Service Skilled. *COPSystem* is geared toward middle school students, high school students, college students, and adults. Unlike the other instruments described in this section, the abilities assessment (Career Abilities Placement Survey) measures observed abilities, rather than perceived abilities, in eight areas. However, the measures are not comprehensive and should be interpreted cautiously. Although concerns have been expressed about the lack of validity evidence (Whiston, 2005), Wickwire (2002) encouraged professional counselors to become actively involved in the use of the *COPSystem,* which is published by EdITS (Educational and Industrial Testing Service, www.edits.net).

Jackson Vocational Interest Survey (JVIS)

The *Jackson Vocational Interest Survey* (*JVIS*) (Jackson, 1999) was designed to assist with educational and career planning and may be used with adolescents and adults. The instrument measures vocational interest areas using 34 scales, each with

17 items. It consists of 289 pairs of statements representing work-related activities and focuses primarily on professional occupations or jobs that require some training (Shute, 2002). The *JVIS* is unique in that it measures interests in different types of work environments as well as different types of work activities. It takes approximately 45 minutes to complete and is published by Sigma Assessment Systems (www.sigmaassessmentsystems.com).

Kuder Skills Assessment (KSA)

The *Kuder Skills Assessment* (*KSA*) (Zytowski & Luzzo, 2002) is a relatively new assessment of self-reported abilities. The instrument measures perceptions of skills in six areas that correspond to the six clusters comprising the Kuder Career Search (Zytowski, 1992, 2004). It can be taken online in about 15 minutes and is designed for middle school and high school students, college students, and adults. Its psychometric properties are still in the process of being established. Internal consistency reliabilities are high, ranging from 0.90 to 0.94 (Zytowski & Luzzo, 2002). The *KSA* is part of the online, interactive Kuder Career Planning system, which includes the *KCS,* the *KSA,* and a work values inventory. The instrument can be accessed via the Kuder website at www.kuder.com.

ASSESSING VALUES AND LIFE ROLE SALIENCE

Whereas interests refer to what a person *likes to do,* **values** define what an individual *thinks is important.* In multiple areas of life, including work, our choices reflect our values. Values direct behavior toward particular life goals and serve as the basis by which people evaluate their actions and the actions of others (Brown, 2002). Values have been found to correlate more highly with work satisfaction than interest (Brown; Rounds, 1990). It therefore is helpful for professional counselors to be familiar with ways to assess work and life values, which have implications for career choice and satisfaction.

Values can be assessed in multiple ways, including formal and informal methods. Examples of standardized measures of values include the *Values Scale* (*VS*) (Nevill & Super, 1989); the *Minnesota Importance Questionnaire* (*MIQ*) (Rounds, Henly, Dawis, Lofquist, & Weiss, 1981); the *Work Values Inventory* (*WVI*) (Zytowski, 2002); and the *O*NET Work Importance Profiler* (United States Employment Service, 2003). Informal methods of assessing values include card sorts, values clarification exercises, checklists, and forced-choice activities.

When assessing values, it is important to keep in mind that no single instrument adequately represents all work and life values. Moreover, individuals define values differently, so it is essential for professional counselors to encourage clients to clarify the meanings they assign to particular values. Also, professional counselors will want to use the results of values inventories in tandem with other data that measure interests, abilities, previous experiences, and career development (Hood & Johnson, 2002).

Table 13.3 The *Values Scale:* Measures of intrinsic and extrinsic values

Values	Sample statements
1. Ability Utilization	Use all my skills and knowledge.
2. Achievement	Have results that show that I have done well.
3. Advancement	Get ahead.
4. Aesthetics	Make life more beautiful.
5. Altruism	Help people with problems.
6. Authority	Tell others what to do.
7. Autonomy	Act on my own.
8. Creativity	Discover, develop, or design new things.
9. Economic Rewards	Have a high standard of living.
10. Life Style	Live according to my own ideas.
11. Personal Development	Develop as a person.
12. Physical Activity	Get a lot of exercise.
13. Prestige	Be admired for my knowledge or skills.
14. Risk	Do risky things.
15. Social Interaction	Do things with other people.
16. Social Relations	Be with friends.
17. Variety	Have every day be different in some way.
18. Working Conditions	Have good space and light in which to work.
19. Cultural Identity	Live where my religion and race are accepted.
20. Physical Prowess	Work hard physically.
21. Economic Security	Be where employment is regular and secure.

Source: Modified and reproduced by special permission of the publisher, CPP, Inc., Mountain View, CA 94043, from the *Values Scale: Theory, Application, and Research,* by Dorothy D. Nevill, Ph.D., and Donald E. Super, Ph.D. Copyright 1986. All rights reserved. Further reproduction is prohibited without the publisher's written consent.

> **Think About It 13.2**   Why are career values and beliefs important facets to assess when counseling a client? What are your most important career and leisure values?

Commonly Used Tests Assessing Values and Life Role Salience

The Values Scale—Second Edition

The *Values Scale—Second Edition* (Nevill & Super, 1989) assesses 21 different values, of which 15 are work related and 6 are more general in nature (see Table 13.3). The *VS* consists of 106 items with four response choices, ranging from 1 (Of Little or No Importance) to 4 (Very Important). The instrument can be completed in 30 to 45 minutes and may be hand-scored or machine-scored. Although scores can be calculated for normative interpretation, the authors recommend using an ipsative interpretation, which means that an individual's scores are compared with each other in reference to that individual, not to a normative group.

The *Values Scale* categorizes values as intrinsic and extrinsic. For **intrinsic values**, the objective is attained while engaging in the behavior, whereas for **extrinsic values**, the objective is a consequence of the behavior. Altruism and creativity are examples of intrinsic values, and economic reward and prestige are examples of extrinsic values (Schoenrade, 2002). In addition to these two categories, the 21 values can also be classified into five factors or orientations: Utilitarian, Self-Actualization, Individualist, Social Orientation, and Adventurous.

When using the *Values Scale* with clients, it is helpful for the professional counselor to show clients a list of the 21 values (unranked) and ask them to predict their top 5 and lowest 5 values. It also helps to ask clients to explain what the values mean to them personally. For example, *autonomy* carries different connotations for different people. Next, professional counselors can share the ranked scores with clients and then discuss how the scores match the clients' predictions. Professional counselors can then help clients think about the connections between their values and potential careers.

Schoenrade (2002) describes the *Values Scale* as an easy-to-administer instrument with simply worded, straightforward items that can help clients who are uncertain of appropriate career directions. The instrument can help individuals identify values and priorities and take an in-depth look at what they seek from careers.

Other Measures of Career Values and Life Role Salience

Minnesota Importance Questionnaire (MIQ)

The *Minnesota Importance Questionnaire* (*MIQ*) (Rounds, Henly, Dawis, Lofquist, & Weiss, 1981) measures clients' values and needs in the workplace and how each correlates with specific occupations (Vocational Psychology Research, 2004). Six categories of values are assessed: Achievement, Comfort, Status, Altruism, Safety, and Autonomy (the latter used only in the Ranked Form of the questionnaire). Twenty psychological needs are assessed as well, including Security, Social Status, Compensation, Achievement, Authority, Creativity, and Moral scales (Drummond, 2000). The test is administered only in pencil-and-paper format to anyone who can read at the 5th-grade level or above, although it is most often used for college students (Thompson & Blain, 1992). It is also gender-neutral, and because it is based primarily in theory, sex bias is relatively nonexistent. There are two forms, the Paired Form, which is usually used for individual administrations, and the Ranked Form, which is often used for individuals or group administrations of the inventory. The Paired Form asks the client to choose one of two vocational needs statements that is more important. This form takes about 30 to 40 minutes to complete. The Ranked Form provides groups of five statements that the client must rank according to importance. This form takes about 15 to 25 minutes to complete. The *MIQ* manual provides more information about the administration, interpretations, and strategies for using the test in counseling situations.

The technical manual provides more information on the development of the instrument and reliability and validity information. The reliability coefficients, taken for the original 1967 test, ranged from 0.30 to 0.95, with the median coefficients between 0.77 and 0.81. The median scale test-retest reliability correlations ranged from 0.89 for immediate retesting to 0.53 for retesting after 10 months. It would be useful to update this information for current users (Lachar, 1992). The validity information originally was not helpful at all, but in the 1971 manual, discriminant and convergent validity were demonstrated and appear to be sufficient for a vocational test (Layton, 1992). The inventory cannot be reasonably scored by hand, but the test taker is given a computer-generated, interpretive profile with each vocational value, a graphic profile, and an overall consistency-of-response score. The Standard Report uses 90 occupations, and the Extended Report uses 185 occupations to find appropriate matches for the individual.

O*NET Work Importance Profiler (WIP)

The *O*NET Work Importance Profiler* (*WIP*) (U.S. Department of Labor, 2005) is similar to the *MIQ* in that it helps individuals determine what is most important for them in potential occupations. It is generally administered via computer (although a pencil-and-paper version is available), and test takers decide which work needs are most important. The work values are broken down into six categories: Achievement, Independence, Recognition, Relationships, Support, and Working Conditions. The first step has individuals rank 21 work need statements by importance. For the second part, individuals rate whether the work needs are important, dependent, or independent of the other needs. The two parts take about 30 minutes to complete. The resulting computer-based profile provides information about client work values, helps increase career awareness, and links clients to the O*NET (www.onetcenter.org/WIP.html) online website, which gives 900 or more occupations. This instrument has been used for over 30 years, and extensive research supports its relevance and usefulness. It can be self-administered and self-interpreted, and the user's guide provides supplemental information.

Life Values Inventory (LVI)

The *Life Values Inventory* (*LVI*) (Crace & Brown, 1994) measures 14 positive life values and helps the client to determine the priority and influence those values have on decision making (www.life-values.com). The inventory was developed to be sensitive to cultural differences, has well-established reliability and validity, and helps connect personal values to life roles. The inventory can be self-scored and takes about 20 minutes to administer. A *Facilitator's Guide* discusses the definition of values; how the inventory was developed; how to administer, score and interpret the results; and ways to use the inventory in different counseling situations. It can meet many counseling needs, including career development, life role planning, adjustment and transition, retirement and leisure counseling, team building, organizational development, and more. A four-page supplement, *Understanding Your Values,* provides information and descriptions of values and how they are involved in decisions clients make.

Salience Inventory

Similar to the *Life Values Inventory*, the *Salience Inventory* (Hagin, 1992) requires clients to mark how important their life roles are in relation to one another. The inventory consists of three scales (Value Expectations, Participation, and Commitment) and five life roles (student, worker, citizen, homemaker, and leisurite). There are a total of 170 statements for which the individual must determine relative importance or **salience**. For example, the first question on the Participation scale reads: "I have spent or do spend time in . . . 1. studying, 2. working, 3. community service, 4. home and family, 5. leisure activities." The individual will answer each categorical question (numbers 1–5) on a scale of 1–4 (1 being least amount of time, 4 being most amount of time). The inventory helps to determine the individual's participation in and commitment to life roles (www.psychometrics.com/). Upper elementary students up through adults can benefit from this scale, and it can be administered individually or in a group. Also, the *Salience Inventory* was developed to be culturally sensitive and is useful in cross-cultural research. It can be administered and scored (by hand or machine) easily within the 30- to 45-minute time requirement. The test manual gives detailed and clear instructions, and a section on interpretation is included as well. The major weakness of this inventory is a lack of representative sampling used in the original norming of the test. Two thousand subjects were used, more for convenience of sampling than for representativeness of the U.S. population. Internal consistency of test scores is satisfactory, but the validity of scores required for the test to be useful in counseling is slightly less than desirable. Test-retest reliabilities were less than 0.70 for 10 of the 15 scales, but internal consistency is acceptable (Hagin). The *Salience Inventory* is considered to be a useful and efficient device for determining an individual's major life roles (Osberg, 1992).

Informal career assessment measures

A **forced-choice activity** asks individuals to choose one of two quite different options or to rank three or more activities. Forced-choice activities can be used to determine values, interests, or compatible job characteristics or work settings (Niles & Harris-Bowlsbey, 2002).

In a **card sort**, an individual is given a stack of cards, all related to career choice (i.e., work value, work task, skill). The person can either rank the cards (depending on the number and time available) or sort them into three categories. These categories are usually things that are very important, somewhat important, and not important. It is essential to make sure that the entire range of choices individuals are likely to select is included. This technique can require a great deal of research and thought (Niles & Harris-Bowlsbey, 2002).

A **structured interview** consists of a professional counselor's asking the client questions aligned with a theory. For instance, a professional counselor might ask for the client's work history, extracurricular activities, volunteer experiences, and so forth and then organize those answers according to the particular theory being used. This type of information does not compare the individual to anyone else, but it does give the professional counselor some idea of where the individual's interests, abilities, or values lie (Niles & Harris-Bowlsbey, 2002).

ASSESSING CAREER DEVELOPMENT AND CAREER MATURITY

A number of inventories have been developed to assess the maturity of a client's thoughts and career development progression. In general, the group of instruments reviewed in this section strives to help clients clarify and analyze beliefs and values so that career goals can be developed, agreed to, and pursued. Professional counselors can refer to Kapes and Whitfield's (2002) *A Counselor's Guide to Career Assessment Instruments* (4th ed.) and to the website of the Buros Institute (www.unl.edu/buros) to gather additional information about these and other measures of interest and perceived ability.

Tests Used to Assess Career Development and Career Maturity

Career Maturity Inventory (CMI)

The *Career Maturity Inventory* (*CMI*) is similar to the *Salience Inventory* but is much more psychometrically sound (Kaplan & Saccuzzo, 2001). The *Career Maturity Inventory* is designed to measure vocational maturity and is best used for students of high school age and older. Measured categories include Vocational Maturity, Attitude, Self-Knowledge or Vocational Competence, Choosing a Job, Problem Solving, Occupational Information, and Looking Ahead (Kaplan & Saccuzzo, p. 389).

Career Decision Scale (CDS)

The *Career Decision Scale* (*CDS*) (Osipow, Carney, Winer, Yanico, & Hoschier, 1980) allows an examination of the thought processes involved with career decision making. The interest inventories use drawings and pictures for those who do not read well (Cohen & Swerdlik, 1999). The subtests are Job Satisfaction, Work Involvement, Skill Development, Career Worries, Interpersonal Abuse, Family Commitment, Risk-Taking Style, and Geographic Barriers. This scale is best used with high school and college-aged students (Sax, 1997). The test can be given to individuals or groups and takes approximately 10 to 15 minutes to administer. The test is very well researched and developed, as evidenced by the reliability and validity results. For instance, the test-retest reliabilities for a 2-week period are 0.90 and 0.82, and for a 6-week period they are reported as 0.70 (Harmon, 1985). The *CDS* manual is complete and clearly written and provides a great deal of information. It is recommended for use in assessing groups of clients thinking about career interventions (Harmon).

Career Beliefs Inventory (CBI)

The *Career Beliefs Inventory* (*CBI*) (Krumboltz, 1997) helps a client to clarify and solidify beliefs about work so career goals can be developed. It is recommended for students in their junior year of high school and above (Bolton, 1995). There are 96 items, divided among 25 scales, and they are measured using a 5-point Likert scale ranging from Strongly Disagree to Strongly Agree (Krumboltz, 1997). The manual is easy to use, but the instructions are incomplete, and scoring can be done only through a scoring service. Several reviewers believed the inventory to be more of a jumping-off point for a discussion or interview than a measurement tool (Bolton, 1995; Guion, 1995). Since this is the case, sending the test away to be scored might prove cumbersome and waste too much time to be of substantial use in counseling. The psychometric properties are not up to standards acceptable for a screening test (only 3 of 78 reliability coefficients were 0.70 or above, and 9 were less than 0.40), and the norm group is not representative of the U.S. population. The test can be a useful tool to provide insights into assumptions and beliefs inhibiting good career decisions (Guion, 1995).

Career Thoughts Inventory (CTI)

The *Career Thoughts Inventory* (*CTI*) (Sampson, Peterson, Lenz, Reardon, & Saunders, 1996) is a cognitive test used to help individuals understand their thoughts on careers and decision making by identifying dysfunctional thought patterns. There are three scales: Decision Making Confusion, Commitment Anxiety, and External Conflict (Fontaine, 2001). These scales are divided into 48 questions that the test taker will rank with one of four choices ranging from strongly agree to strongly disagree. The questions are negatively worded to help determine dysfunctional thoughts (Pickering, 1998). The inventory is most appropriate for students of high school age and above and can be administered to individuals or groups. It is relatively short, taking only about 7 to 15 minutes. A comprehensive workbook is included that provides exercises to help the practitioner or the person self-administering to find "dysfunctional career thinking" (Fontaine), although the instructions could be more clear. The test has appropriate psychometric measures, and a representative normative sample was used in the development of the instrument. The overall reliability measures had a median range of 0.90–0.94, and high face validity, content validity, and concurrent criterion-related validity were all found (Fontaine).

Adult Career Concerns Inventory (ACCI)

The *Adult Career Concerns Inventory* (*ACCI*) (Super, Thompson, & Lindeman, 1988) is used for individuals ages 24 years and older to determine where the person is along the career development path. Sixty-one questions are arranged into 12 subscales, which are then split among four career stages: Exploration, Establishment, Maintenance, and Disengagement. The items are answered on a 5-point scale ranging from No Concern to Great Concern (Johnson, 1995). Taking this inventory will help students determine which career stage they are currently in and can help adults explore career choices and development (Manuele-Adkins, 1995). The test takes about 15 to 30 minutes to administer and is taken and scored by the individual, although it can be machine-scored as well (Manuele-Adkins). The estimates of score reliability and validity received mixed reviews; some studies found the *ACCI* to be appropriate, while other reviews were less favorable. The *alpha* coefficients ranged from 0.92 to 0.96, but no test-retest reliabilities were reported (Johnson). More information is needed to make a better determination of the technical adequacy of scores on this inventory. According to Johnson (1995, p. 47), the "ACCI is limited in scope. It principally assesses the adult's needs for career planning and adaptation. It does not measure career planning competencies such as decision-making skills, job-hunting skills, and work-effectiveness skills," so examiners may need to administer supplemental tests or information on interests, values, or abilities.

Think About It 13.3   Think about an acquaintance or client who is experiencing a career transition. Which of the inventories in this chapter would you select to assess this individual's current career development? Consider how you might use these instruments in career counseling with this individual.

SUMMARY/CONCLUSION

The use of assessment in career counseling is changing rapidly. The influence of the Internet and the multitude of available inventories has ensured that assessment will continue to be a critical skill for professional counselors in this specialty area for decades to come. This chapter has reviewed numerous formal and informal career interest, values, and salience inventories, with a focus on their usefulness in facilitating a client's career development. The integration of these inventories into the career counseling process leads to an efficient approach with measurable outcomes.

KEY TERMS

card sort
differentiation
expressed interests
extrinsic values
forced-choice activity
interest inventory
intrinsic values

inventoried interests
manifest interests
salience
self-efficacy
structured interview
trait-and-factor theory
values

14

Assessing Couples and Families

by Debbie W. Newsome, Jon-Michael Brasfield,
and Catherine Flemming

This chapter describes some of the factors that differentiate family assessment
from individual assessment and discusses areas that frequently are assessed in
family counseling. It focuses on two broad categories of assessment: formalized assessment instruments for couples and families and qualitative assessment techniques. Professional counselors frequently use a combination of these two approaches in their assessment and treatment of couples and families.

PURPOSES OF COUPLES AND FAMILY COUNSELING

People come to couples and family counseling for a variety of reasons. Some may
seek premarital counseling to help prepare for an upcoming marriage. Others may
want to find ways to deal more effectively with a child who is acting out. Still others
may seek couples counseling to understand why they feel distanced from each other
after years of marriage. In each of these cases, assessment techniques can be used effectively by professional counselors to gather information, develop hypotheses, evaluate treatment progress and outcomes, and facilitate change.

During the past several decades, the practice of couples and family counseling
has evolved substantially. Likewise, the practice of assessing families has made notable advances, as evidenced by an increase in formal and informal measures of interpersonal relationships. Indeed, few methods of assessing couples and families existed prior to the 1960s (Deacon & Piercy, 2001). Prior to that time, assessment

methods were typically designed for one person, not an entire family. Behavior checklists, rating scales, individual interviews, personality inventories, and projective tests were the primary evaluation methods used by counselors working with couples or families.

Assessing couples and families differs in a number of ways from assessing individuals, due largely to the influence of family systems theory. According to systems theory, families are interacting systems composed of interdependent members. Systems theorists view problems as relationship issues associated with the system itself rather than with specific individuals. Consequently, the family, not the individual, is the unit of change. Rather than assessing individual constructs, family counselors focus on assessing the family system. Family relationships, patterns, structure, and level of functioning are the primary areas of focus (Edwards, 2003). Determining what to assess in a family depends on the nature of the family, the presenting issue, and the professional counselor's theoretical orientation.

Because family counselors assess dynamic systems, the process can be more challenging than individual assessment. Several issues make family assessment challenging:

- It is likely that family members will view issues differently and will bring differing perspectives to the table. Consequently, it may be difficult to make sense of the divergent information gathered (Whiston, 2005).
- Some family practitioners view empirically based, structured methods of assessment as static measures that do not capture the dynamic process of family interactions. Many of the variables assessed, such as communication styles, family roles, and levels of cohesion, are fluid and likely to fluctuate (Whiston, 2005). For example, a couple's response to an assessment of emotional closeness may differ depending on whether the couple spent the weekend relaxing at a beach cottage or disagreeing over the family budget.
- There is no unified theory of family functioning, no consensus about the definition of healthy or dysfunctional family relationships, and no agreement about the key processes that need to be assessed (Bray, 1995). Furthermore, at this time, the *DSM-IV-TR* (APA, 2000) provides diagnostic categories for individuals, not families, with the exception of V-codes (normal or developmental problems), which are not reimbursable by most insurance companies.
- Many of the formal assessment measures were developed for research rather than for clinical practice (Bray, 1995). Moreover, many of the measures are based on inadequate norming samples that may not be clinically relevant and that are often predominantly Caucasian (Whiston, 2005).

Rationale for Family Assessment

Despite the inherent challenges, there are many reasons clinicians will want to become skilled in using formal and informal methods of family assessment. Deacon and Piercy (2001) compare family counseling without assessment to a car trip without a map. Family counselors need to know where the family has been, where the family is now, and where the family hopes to go. Family assessment offers a systematic method for making those determinations. Assessment can provide a rich source of information that can be used to develop initial hypotheses about the nature of the problem, the causes of the problem, family members' varying perceptions of the problem, and potential areas of strength (Bray, 1995; McPhatter, 1991).

Assessment also provides clinicians with baseline data by which progress in counseling can be measured. Without a baseline, it is difficult to document intervention-related changes. L'Abate (1994) suggested that clinicians use a variety of measures to obtain baseline data; a single approach cannot sufficiently assess the complexity of a particular family. Throughout counseling, assessment can be used to evaluate the family's progress. It also can be used at the end of counseling to evaluate outcomes (Sporakowski, 1995).

In addition to providing information, measuring progress, and evaluating outcomes, the assessment process can facilitate change. Counselors can use assessment to help join with families, provide feedback and support, validate concerns, and engender hope (Floyd, Weinand, & Cimmarusti, 1989). The process can help families to view the presenting issue from a systems perspective rather than as an individual family member's problem (Bray, 1995). Many informal assessment techniques, described below, involve active family participation and have therapeutic potential.

Yet another reason for including formal and informal assessment methods in family counseling is to help clinicians to avoid bias. Assessment supplements subjective clinical impressions with objective data (L'Abate, 1994) and provides a way to collect information that otherwise might be overlooked (Bray, 1995). Data collected through assessment can be used to help corroborate, strengthen, or weaken hypotheses or conclusions that clinicians make based on their subjective impressions.

What Is Assessed?

Family assessment is conducted to understand a family, not to pathologize or stereotype (L'Abate, 1994). The method of assessment selected is based on several factors, including the professional counselor's theoretical orientation and the family's presenting issue. Professional counselors are responsible for determining what data are needed to understand the family and to plan effective treatment. They also need to make decisions about when and how data will be collected (Deacon & Piercy, 2001). Nichols and Schwartz (2001) noted that just as there are many ways to conduct counseling, there are many ways to conduct assessment. A combination of methods, intentionally selected for the family seeking counseling, helps professional counselors to avoid bias, focus on interactions, and effectively plan and evaluate treatment.

Marriage and family counselors typically follow a holistic systems approach. Consequently, data are collected about relationships, interactions, and family dynamics. From a systems perspective, there is no single best method to evaluate, because it is often necessary to evaluate multiple aspects of the family system. What is assessed depends on the context, purpose, and specific aspects of family functioning that are being evaluated (Bray, 1995).

In considering family evaluation, it is important to keep in mind that many theoretical orientations are subsumed under the broad category of **systems**

approach. The family dimensions, processes, and structures that are selected for assessment are influenced by the clinician's theoretical orientation. Theoretical orientation and beliefs about human nature, specific to the given family situation, will "inform choices in the types and thoroughness of the assessment function" (Sporakowski, 1995, p. 61). For example, professional counselors following a Bowenian approach will assess family history, transgenerational patterns, and levels of self-differentiation. A structural family therapist will assess family structure, subsystem boundaries, and hierarchy. An experiential family counselor is more likely to use informal, rather than formal, methods of assessment, such as family sculpting. For each theoretical perspective, specific areas that contribute to family functionality are assessed.

While we recognize that there are differences in approaches to family assessment, there is also much overlap among the constructs believed to contribute to functional and dysfunctional families. Some of the general areas of marital and family assessment include factors related to the presenting issue, family composition, family process, family affect, family organization, strengths and resources, and goals for change (Bray, 1995; Deacon & Piercy, 2001; L'Abate, 1994).

The presenting issue

Gathering information about the presenting issue begins during the initial interview. L'Abate (1994, pp. 65–66) recommends using the following questions as guidelines to assess the presenting issue:

- What is the problem as the family views it?
- Who has defined the problem?
- Who is more involved in the problem than others?
- Who is uninvolved and why?
- How do various definitions (perceptions, views) of the problem agree or disagree?
- What experiences and discussions have led the family to define the problem in the way they do?
- What unresolved questions remain?
- What expectations for the future does the family have that are relevant to the present problem?
- Is there any unresolved mourning or grief left over from the past?
- What solutions have been tried in the past?
- What made the family decide to seek help now?
- What kind of help does the family expect?

Family composition

Family composition, which may be the most straightforward factor to assess, refers to membership (e.g., couple only, couple with children, single-parent family) and to general structure (e.g., nuclear family, nuclear family with extended family members living in the home, grandparent and child family, blended family). In some cases, family composition may include "non-kin" members who are significantly involved with the family.

Family process

Family processes are those behaviors and interactions that characterize family functioning. Examples of process factors include ways families manage conflict and solve problems. Other examples of process-related constructs include differentiation, individuation, communication, and control.

Family affect

Family affect refers to the manner in which emotion is expressed and received in the family. Is emotional expression open or restricted? To what degree do family members view themselves as emotionally close or distant from each other? A family's emotional climate has a major impact on how members experience communications. Family affect is indicated by the mood or emotional tone of the family, ranging from positive to negative, and may vary in intensity (Bray, 1995).

Family organization

Family organization encompasses several different constructs related to family functioning. Examples of family organization factors include roles, rules, expectations for behavior, boundaries surrounding the family and its subsystems, and levels of hierarchy (Bray, 1995).

Think About It 14.1   Think about your family. How are family processes, affect, and organization demonstrated? How does each influence family member interaction?

Strengths and resources

All families have unique strengths, some readily evidenced and others not yet recognized. Clinicians can help families articulate, acknowledge, and build on those strengths. One particular type of strength is **family resilience**, which refers to a family's ability to self-repair and which develops as a family masters or overcomes challenging situations (Worden, 2003). **Resources** refer to those tangible or intangible supports within the family, community, and extended environment. Assessing a family's strengths and resources can engender hope and also provide pathways for therapeutic change.

Goals for change

Family members frequently enter counseling with differing perspectives about the nature of the presenting issues and with unclear goals for change. Solution-focused therapists emphasize the importance of involving the family in collaboratively defining goals for treatment as early as the first session (O'Hanlon & O'Hanlon, 2002). It is important that the goals are not superimposed by the clinician but stem directly from the family. Equally important is the need for goals to be specific and attainable. Throughout the course of therapy, goals should be revisited, accomplishments noted, and changes made as needed.

Other areas of assessment

In addition to the areas already described, professional counselors may choose to gather information about family members' personality characteristics, coping and adaptation strategies, values, stressors, life cycle stages, and daily routines (Deacon & Piercy, 2001). A fundamental purpose of family assessment is to inform treatment planning; consequently, professional counselors will make decisions about what data are needed based on the specific family seeking treatment. After determining what information is needed, clinicians then must decide what methods to use for gathering that information.

Methods of Assessment

Just as there are multiple areas of family assessment, there also are multiple methods that can be used to evaluate families (Bray, 1995). Methods include individual self-reports of family interactions, reports of family members about their views of others in the family, and observational methods, which can include clinical ratings. Sporakowski (1995) categorized assessment methods as

- Observational methods (live or taped simulated situational examinations of family interactions)
- Graphic representations of relationships (genograms, kinetic drawings)
- Measures of temperament, character, or personality (personality inventories and checklists, such as the *Myers-Briggs Type Indicator*)
- Techniques to assess levels of marital satisfaction, quality, or happiness
- Family adaptation measures
- Stress and coping appraisals (life events, expectations, disruptions)
- Parenting and family skills
- Other areas (e.g., sexual functioning)

Rather than address each of these categories separately, the remainder of this chapter focuses on two broad classifications of family assessment: (1) formal, standardized methods used to assess interpersonal relationships; and (2) less formal, qualitative methods of assessment, including tasks and observations. Instruments designed for individual assessment, which sometimes are used in family or couples counseling (e.g., *MBTI, 16-PF*), are not addressed in depth in this chapter because they are described in greater detail in Chapter 8.

FORMALIZED ASSESSMENT INSTRUMENTS

A plethora of instruments has been developed to evaluate couples and families (L'Abate, 1994). Touliatos, Perlmutter, and Straus (2001) compiled a description of approximately 1,300 instruments. Other family researchers also have published descriptions of various quantitative instruments (e.g., Fredman & Sherman, 1987; Grotevant & Carlson, 1989; L'Abate & Bagarrozzi, 1993). However, there are indications that most of these instruments are used in family research rather than clinical practice. A survey of marriage and family therapists revealed that less than 40%

of them used standardized instruments on a regular basis, and no single assessment instrument was used by more that 8% of the sample (Boughner, Hayes, Bubenzer, & West, 1994). In addition, many of the therapists who reported using standardized instruments used measures developed for individuals, such as the *California Personality Inventory* (*CPI*) and the *Myers-Briggs Type Indicator* (*MBTI*).

Gold (1997) cited three factors that might contribute to the infrequent use of standardized assessment in marriage and family counseling: (1) individual attitudes of clinicians toward testing; (2) the assessment practices of employment sites; and (3) professional counselor assessment education. Floyd et al., (1989) suggested that many quantitative instruments reduce holistic data into linear constructs that do not adequately capture the dynamic nature of the family. Others (e.g., Greene & Vosler, 1992) have suggested that quantitative assessment information can be misleading. However, when selected and employed by skilled clinicians, standardized assessment can enhance the work of marriage and family counselors.

The instruments described in the next section can be categorized as couples-marital and family-parenting assessment tools. They represent just a few of the many measures that have been developed for clinical practice with couples and families.

Assessment of Couples

PREPARE/ENRICH *inventories*

The *PREPARE/ENRICH* inventories (Olson, 2004) are designed to assess couples in various stages of relationships. Five different instruments are part of the *PREPARE/ENRICH* Program: (1) *PREPARE* (PREmarital Personal and Relationship Evaluation) for premarital couples; (2) *PREPARE-MC* for premarital couples with children; (3) *PREPARE-CC* for cohabiting couples with or without children; (4) *ENRICH* (Enriching Relationship Issues, Communication, and Happiness) for married couples; and (5) *MATE* (Mature Age Transitional Evaluation) for couples over the age of 50. The *PREPARE/ENRICH* Program is used by over 50,000 professional counselors, and over 1,000,000 (nearly all heterosexual) couples have taken the inventories (Olson & Gorall, 2003). *PREPARE* also has been adapted for use in other cultures—for example, with premarital couples in Japan (Asai & Olson, 2004).

The original *PREPARE* inventory was created in 1978. Revisions of the inventory in 1982, 1986, and 1996 increased the original number of 125 items to 165. The inventory highlights areas of strength and conflict for couples and also provides them with practical ways to apply communication and problem-solving skills through activities and exercises.

Each version of the inventory consists of 12 content area scales, 4 family-of-origin scales, and 4 personality scales. The content areas relate to significant relationship issues, such as financial concerns, communication, spiritual beliefs, leisure activities, conflict resolution, and several others. The family-of-origin analysis gauges flexibility and closeness, and the personality section of the inventory assesses assertiveness, avoidance, self-confidence, and partner dominance. An idealistic distortion scale exists to uncover instances in which partners might have responded in socially acceptable, rather than truthful, ways. Some versions of *PREPARE/ENRICH* have scales

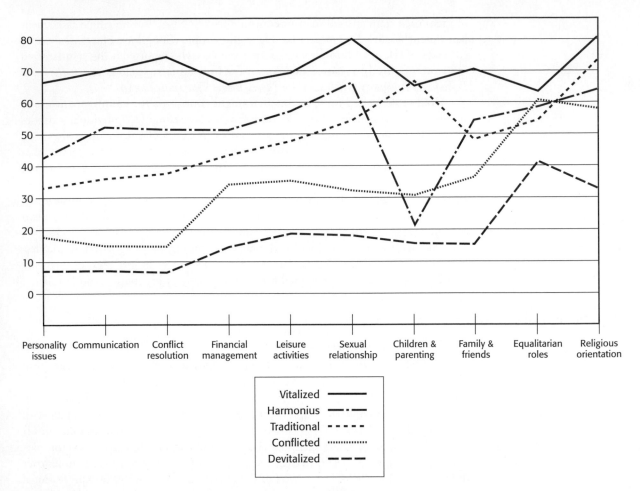

Figure 14.1   Five types of married couples based on *ENRICH*

Source: Olson, D. H., & A. Olson-Sigg (2000), *Empowering Couples,* Minneapolis, MN: Life Innovations, Inc. Reprinted with permisison.

unique to their particular population. For example, both the *PREPARE* and the *PREPARE-MC* include sections related to partner expectations; *ENRICH* addresses marital satisfaction; and *MATE* deals with issues related to life transition.

In addition to charting individuals on the 20 scales, *PREPARE, ENRICH,* and *MATE* categorize couples according to the convergence of individual responses. According to *PREPARE,* there are four types of premarital couples: Vitalized, Harmonious, Traditional, and Conflicted. *ENRICH* and *MATE* include an additional couple type, Devitalized (see Figure 14.1). The designation of a type occurs in accordance with the couple's Positive Couple Agreement (PCA) score, which is created by comparing the two individuals' responses on each question to assess whether they agree with each other on positive items and disagree on negative items.

The inventories are typically taken in paper-and-pencil format, though online administration has recently become available. Professional counselors can register clients and manage administration at the Life Innovations website (www.lifeinnovations.com). Ideally, partners complete the forms in separate locations to avoid influencing each other's responses. Paper-and-pencil forms typically take 2 weeks to process after submission to the publisher, while online scoring occurs immediately. Client reports are sent to the professional counselor for use in counseling. Each report includes a guide to facilitating feedback, which typically takes from four to six sessions.

The client report is particularly in-depth and includes a personality assessment for both partners, a detailed description of areas of agreement and disagreement for all scales, a grid that maps ways partners experience their families of origin and their current relationship, and a linear graph of the couple's typology in relation to the predetermined categories. The professional counselor does not give the written copy of the client report to the couple either during or after counseling. Instead, the professional counselor interprets results for the couple during feedback sessions.

In addition to addressing the couple's strength and growth areas, the feedback sessions include a skills-based component. Couples receive a workbook, which they keep, with six activities designed to improve listening and communication skills, financial management, and other areas of potential difficulty, including ones that the couple indicate as particularly pressing.

The *PREPARE/ENRICH* inventories report coefficients of internal consistency for all subscales as ranging from 0.73 to 0.90. Test-retest reliability was reported as 0.80 for *PREPARE* and 0.86 for *ENRICH*; however, the temporal interval was not specified. Some concerns have been expressed about the lack of evidence supporting the validation of the current *PREPARE/ENRICH* inventories, although validity evidence has been provided for earlier versions of the inventories (Fitzpatrick, 2001).

The main reason for using the *PREPARE, ENRICH,* and *MATE* inventories is to illuminate areas in which a couple's relationship functions well and areas in which a change would increase relational satisfaction. The client report highlights areas in which partners do not agree on perceptions of their relationship, expectations of their or their partner's role, or satisfaction with interpersonal dynamics.

- *Use of the subscales.* The relationship subscales (e.g., Financial Concerns, Communication, Spiritual Beliefs, Conflict Resolution) are composed of items such as, "Sometimes I wish my partner were more careful about spending money," and "I go out of my way to avoid conflict with my partner." Partners' responses to these questions highlight specific areas of agreement or disagreement, with the goal of either resolving the current conflict or preventing future conflict. The inventory is especially useful because it assesses areas the couple may fail to address through deliberate or unconscious omission.
- *Use of the personality assessment.* The personality assessment indicates to the professional counselor possible relational dynamics in play. For example, should one client score low on assertiveness and high on avoidance, the professional counselor has an indication that communication skills might be an area in which the

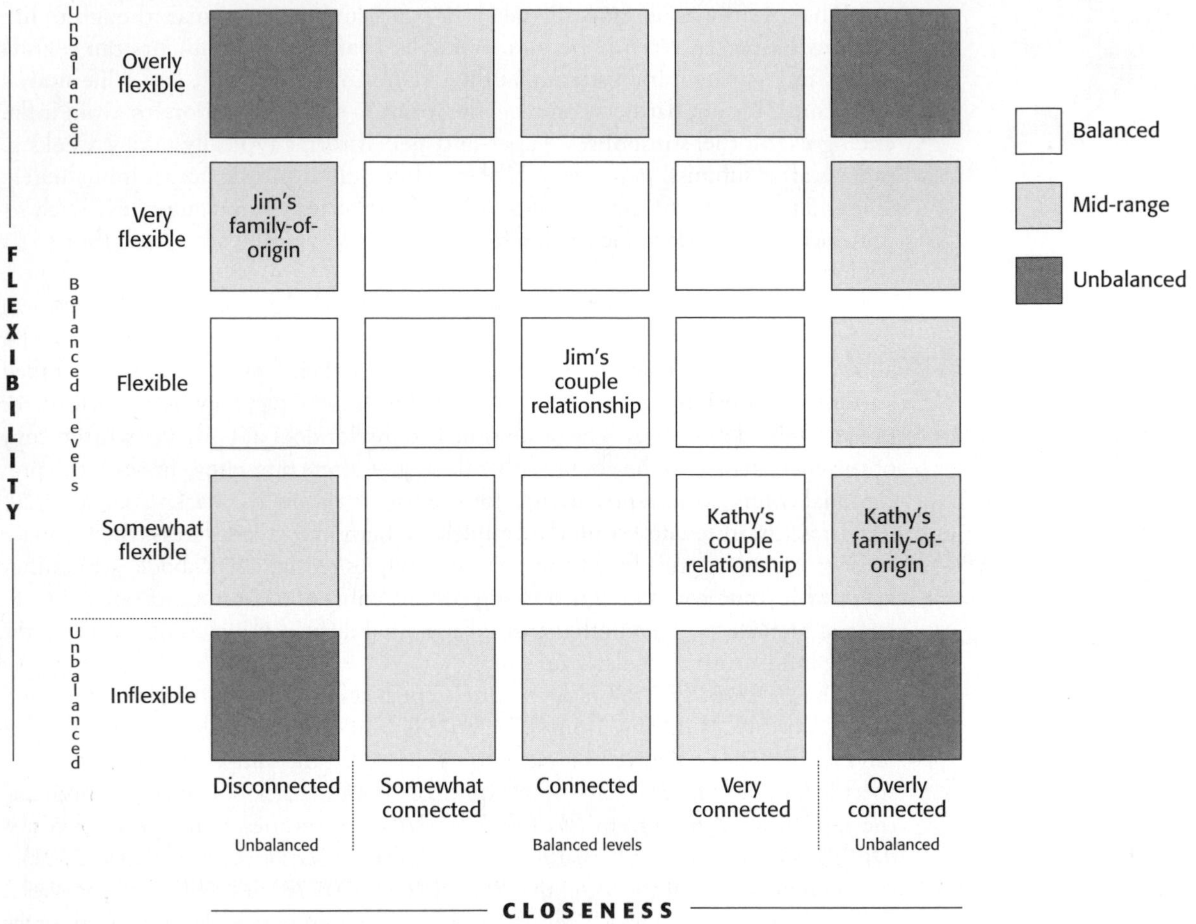

The couple and family map

Figure 14.2 The couple and family map

Source: From *PREPARE/ENRICH Counselor's Manual,* by D. H. Olson, 2004, Minneapolis, MN: Life Innovations. Copyright 2004 by Life Innovations. Reprinted with permission. Further reproduction prohibited without written permission from the publisher.

couple needs attention. The information can be disseminated to the client in a way that allows the less assertive partner to feel safe sharing feelings, and the professional counselor can be sensitive to attempts to avoid difficult issues.

■ *Use of the couple and family map.* The couple and family map indicates, through the plot of the family of origin and of the current relationship, possible expectations partners bring into their current relationship (see Figure 14.2). The professional counselor might find it useful to discuss with each partner how they perceive differences and similarities between their family of origin and their current relationship. Also, large differences between the two partners' plots of the current relationship can indicate a disparity in perceptions or expectations, which can be addressed in counseling.

PREPARE is endorsed by the American Association of Marriage and Family Therapists (Larson, 2002). The *PREPARE/ENRICH* inventories provide professional counselors with rich sources of information about various dimensions of a couple's relationship and offer practical ways for professional counselors to help couples to improve their interactions.

Marital Satisfaction Inventory–Revised (MSI-R)

The *Marital Satisfaction Inventory—Revised Edition* (*MSI-R*) (Snyder, 1997) is a self-report inventory with 150 true-false items designed to provide insight into respondents' areas of distress within their interpersonal relationships. Both hand-scored and computer-based forms exist, and scores are reported on 13 factors of interpersonal relationships: Conventionalization, Global Distress, Affective Communication, Problem-Solving Communication, Aggression, Time Together, Disagreements About Finances, Sexual Dissatisfaction, Role Orientation, Family History of Distress, Dissatisfaction With Children, Conflict Over Child Rearing, and Inconsistency. Between 9 and 19 items are scored for each subscale.

The original *MSI* was published in 1981 by Western Psychological Services (WPS) and was designed for couples who had been together for a minimum of 6 months. The *MSI-R,* the first complete revision, was published in 1997 with a larger norming sample (1,020 couples), 150 items instead of 280 (129 items for couples without children), the "aggression" factor added, and "inconsistency" added as a false-report indicator.

Moderate to high-moderate test-retest reliability of scores was found for the *MSI-R* after an interval of 6 weeks, with temporal stability coefficients ranging from $r = 0.74$ (Disagreement About Finances) to $r = 0.88$ (Role Orientation). Internal consistency scores also were acceptable, with all subscales providing a mean *alpha* of 0.79 (a range of $r = 0.70$ to $r = 0.93$).

Validity of scores on the *MSI-R* are likewise high, with correlations between subscales of the original and revised forms ranging from $r = 0.94$ to $r = 0.98$. In addition, the original *MSI* subscales were found to be significantly correlated with both the *Locke-Wallace Marital Adjustment Test* and the *Global Distress Scale.* Discriminant and convergent validity has been demonstrated by studies using the *MSI-R* to differentiate between clinical and nonclinical couples, as well as between pre- and post-treatment couples, married and divorced couples, and battered women and women from the general community, among others. Results of a recent study that used the *MSI-R* to measure satisfaction scores among cohabiting homosexual couples showed that these couples and cohabiting heterosexual couples were more alike than different in their responses, and that their scores were more like those of nonclinical married couples than of those presenting for treatment (Means-Christensen, Snyder, & Negy, 2003).

The original *MSI* was regarded as one of the best instruments of its kind (Bernt, 2001), and the revision includes changes that should keep it at the front of the field for professional counselors, including a shorter form for more time-efficient administration. The *MSI-R* offers three different scoring options. Forms are available for computer scoring and interpretation, mail-in scoring and interpretation, and paper-and-pencil on-site scoring without automatic interpretation. The first two options allow professional counselors who desire the benefits of administering the *MSI-R* but who may not be very familiar with the interpretation to receive interpretation assistance from Western Psychological Services.

Both members of the couple take the instrument separately, and results are provided in the form of T scores ($M = 50$; $SD = 10$) normed separately for men and women. The couple's scores are plotted together on the *MSI-R* Profile Form, allowing the professional counselor and couple to compare scores and trends. In most cases, higher scores indicate problem areas or areas of dissatisfaction with the relationship. Scores provide both a quantitative general assessment of the quality of the relationship and a starting point for therapeutic discussions on areas seen as particularly troublesome by either member of the couple. See Box 14.1 for an example of how the MSI-R can be used in couples counseling.

The large number of subscales and relative brevity of the instrument make it an appealing option for marriage and family professionals. The *MSI-R* is regarded as a thorough, well-normed instrument that can go a long way in assessing the strengths and weaknesses of a couple's relationship.

Box 14.1   Using the *MSI-R* in counseling: A case study

Confidential Evaluation
Names: Mr. and Mrs. Borders
Instrument: *Marital Satisfaction Inventory–Revised*

Description of the Couple:

Mr. and Mrs. Borders, both aged 37 years, have been married 14 years at the time of evaluation. This is the first marriage for each. The couple has two children: Chris (age 11 years) and Ashley (age 6 years). Mr. Borders graduated from a local junior college. Recently, he earned his B.A. degree after attending evening classes for several years. Mrs. Borders has completed her B.S. degree in communications. She has also completed some graduate work in business administration. For the past 12 years, Mr. Borders has owned and operated an upholstery shop, a business that has proved quite successful. Prior to having children, Mrs. Borders worked as an assistant manager in retail, as the owner of a house cleaning agency, and as an assistant to her husband. For the past 11 years, she has been a homemaker.

Presenting Problems:

Mrs. Borders requested the evaluation because of some marital difficulties she was experiencing. Recently, she and Mr. Borders have disagreed over their financial situation. Although the couple has managed money well in the past, they are currently in debt. This is due in part to the fact that both children are now attending private school. In addition, the couple recently purchased a new van and had two rooms in their house renovated.

Because both of her children are now in school, Mrs. Borders is considering embarking on a new career. Due to the fact that she has been home for the past 11 years, she is not certain where to start. One option is to complete a master's degree in business administration. Mrs. Borders believes that the payoff for completing her degree will ultimately benefit the family financially. She also believes that it will provide her with a sense of fulfillment.

Mr. Borders says that he supports Mrs. Borders in whatever decision she makes. However, he holds a traditional view of men and women's roles, and Mrs. Borders is uncertain about his response should she choose to pursue a career. Also, because of financial issues, neither spouse feels that Mrs. Borders can return to school without financial assistance. Moreover, the couple expressed concern about who would care for the children if Mrs. Borders was not home when they returned from school.

Changes Sought by the Couple:

Both spouses want to resolve their financial difficulties. The issue is complicated by the problems they have discussing the subject. Mrs. Borders expressed an interest in improving communication skills that relate to problem-solving. She also wants to work through role-orientation issues. Mr. Borders thinks that their problem-solving skills could be improved, but is not certain that counseling is necessary.

Other Significant Issues:

Mr. and Mrs. Borders's families of origin differed significantly in regard to level of functioning and degree of nurturing. Mr. Borders was adopted as an infant. His adoptive mother died of cancer when he was 11 years old. His father emotionally distanced himself from the two children during this time by immersing himself in his career. Two years later, he remarried a woman who never attached herself to the children. Mr. Borders reports a conflicted relationship with his stepmother.

Mrs. Borders, on the other hand, came from a warm, relatively affluent family. Although she was frequently in conflict with her father, she had a close relationship with her mother. Both Mr. and Mrs. Borders speak positively of Mrs. Borders's parents, whom they see on a regular basis.

Clinical Assessment:

MSI-R scores for this couple are provided in Table 14.1. Mr. and Mrs. Borders completed the *Marital Satisfaction Inventory* separately. Mrs. Borders approached the test in an open, nondefensive manner. Mr. Borders distorted his score somewhat in a socially desirable direction. Mr. Borders reported

continued

Box 4.1 continued

very positive feelings about his marriage. Mrs. Borders indicated strong commitment to the marriage, but she also indicated a moderate degree of dissatisfaction. Her most elevated scores were in the area of time spent together and affective communication. She states that she and Mr. Borders do not share many common interests and that they are often going in different directions. She also feels that although he has improved, her husband is somewhat reluctant to express his feelings. Mr. Borders reported some concerns in these two areas as well. He would like to develop better affective communication skills. To enhance their leisure time together, he would like for Mrs. Borders to participate in more recreational activities.

Both spouses indicated some dissatisfaction related to finances. Mr. Borders's responses indicated that this is a problem area in the marriage. He feels that the family outlives its financial means, but that working out a family budget is more trouble than it is worth. Mrs. Borders is less concerned

Table 14.1   Robert and Leah Borderss scores on the *Marital Satisfaction Inventory—Revised*

Subscale	ROBERT'S SCORES		LEAH'S SCORES	
	Raw scores	T scores	Raw scores	T scores
Inconsistency (INC)	3	47	3	48
Conventionalization (CNV)	7	55	2	42
Global Distress (GDS)	1	46	*5*	54
Affective Communication (AFC)	*3*	51	*6*	56
Problem-Solving Communication (PSC)	3	45	*6*	51
Aggression (AGG)	1	48	1	48
Time Together (TTO)	*4*	52	*6*	58
Disagreement About Finances (FIN)	8	67	*3*	52
Sexual Dissatisfaction (SEX)	0	34	1	41
Role Orientation (ROR)	2	38	8	51
Family History of Distress (FAM)	6	58	1	42
Dissatisfaction with Children (DSC)	*3*	54	1	44
Conflict Over Child Rearing (CCR)	0	41	1	47

Interpretive key—only raw scores have been colored:

Good [ ]   Possible Problem *X*   Problem [ ]

about the family's financial situation, although she believes that her husband buys too much on credit. She would like to see a budget established.

The couple also evidenced a difference in gender role orientation, with Mr. Borders espousing a more conventional view of marital roles than his wife. It is possible that Mrs. Borders is aware of these differences and that she resents her husband's attitudes to some extent. Because she desires marital stability, she may find it difficult to pursue a career until the unspoken family rules regarding gender roles become overt and are subjected to change.

A strong sense of satisfaction with the sexual relationship was expressed, as well as with the manner in which they are raising their children. Overall, both husband and wife are satisfied with their relationships with their children, although Mrs. Borders expressed a slightly greater level of satisfaction than did her spouse. Finally, Mr. Borders indicated that issues related to his family of origin are problematic.

Hypotheses:

- Mr. Borders does not want his wife to return to work because of the traditional views he holds about gender roles and because he views himself as the breadwinner.
- Mr. Borders's view of himself as breadwinner and the pressure of owning his own business contribute to his spending more time at work than with his family.
- Financial issues are complicated in part by difficulties Mr. Borders has in expressing his feelings to his wife.
- Mrs. Borders has spent the past 11 years as a homemaker meeting the needs of her husband and children. She would like to expand her opportunities but feels guilty about neglecting the homemaker role that has been hers for so long.
- Mr. Borders experienced distancing in his family of origin and has a tendency to deal with conflict by denial or withdrawal.
- The couple is committed to the marriage. Mr. Borders is more satisfied with the marriage than is Mrs. Borders, but he recognizes that he has difficulty expressing his feelings and is willing to work in that area.

Recommendations:

Marital therapy for this couple is recommended. It will be important to address the presenting problems (e.g., financial concerns, issue of Mrs. Borders's career) from a systems perspective. Some gender role restructuring may be indicated, as well as communication training, particularly in the area of affective communication. Attention should also be given to ways the family spends time together, both as a couple and as a family. The couple's strong commitment to the marriage and their children provides a good foundation for continued growth toward marital satisfaction.

Dyadic Adjustment Scale (DAS)

The *Dyadic Adjustment Scale* (*DAS*) (Spanier, 1989) was designed to measure the quality of adjustment in relationships of two committed individuals. Described as "the first of the current generation of marital adjustment and satisfaction measures" (Fowers, 1990, p. 371), the *DAS* has been used in over 1,000 studies and is considered one of the most frequently used and best-researched measures of marital satisfaction (Budd & Heilman, 1992).

The *DAS* is a relatively brief instrument, consisting of 32 items. Some items ask respondents about their perceived level of agreement with their partner on subjects such as religion, physical affection, and choice of friends. Other items request responses regarding how often respondents engage in specific activities with their partners. These final items were identified as items that discriminated between married and divorced couples in Spanier's original 1976 study.

The 32 items are scored on four subscales (Dyadic Consensus, Dyadic Satisfaction, Affectional Expression, and Dyadic Cohesion) and as a total. Responses are recorded along a series of 5- and 6-point Likert scales, with the exception of two yes-no questions and one forced-choice question. Raw scores are converted to T scores ($M = 50$; $SD = 10$) before being reported to clients.

The *DAS* is available from Multi-Health Systems, Inc., both in paper-and-pencil format with score sheets and in disk format with computer-based administration and scoring. Both formats require an estimated 5 to 10 minutes for administration and a similar amount of time for scoring. Included with the *DAS* is a 55-page manual, which has been noted for its clear, easy-to-follow instructions for administering, scoring, and interpreting the instrument (Budd & Heilman, 1992). Although the scoring procedure was most recently updated in 1989, the instrument itself remains unchanged from its original 1976 form.

Reliability and validity scores for the *DAS* are high, although substantial concerns about the initial norming sample have been raised. The *DAS* has an 11-week test-retest reliability coefficient of $r_{tt} = 0.96$, and coefficient *alpha*s for the subscales range from $r_{ic} = 0.73$ to $r_{ic} = 0.96$, with Affectional Expression being the only subscale below $r_{ic} = 0.90$. In addition, several studies provide evidence supporting the validity of the *DAS* (O'Rourke & Cappeliez, 2001). Convergent validity has been demonstrated by an $r = 0.86$ correlation with the *Locke-Wallace Marital Adjustment Test* (Spanier, 1989). In addition, data provide evidence of the *DAS*'s concurrent and predictive validity in regard to domestic violence, couples' communication, depression, and family dysfunction (Stuart, 1992).

As mentioned earlier, concerns have been raised over the norming sample, thereby calling into question the T scores provided to test takers (Budd & Heilman, 1992; Stuart, 1992). The norming sample consisted of 109 married, White, middle class, heterosexual couples in one Pennsylvania county. Despite these concerns, the *DAS* has been used in studies and clinical settings for many years, and has been described as "the most frequently used measure in the study of marital satisfaction" (Rosen-Grandon, Myers, & Hattie, 2004, p. 60).

Because of its brevity and clarity, the *DAS* is an effective instrument both for research and for clinical purposes. Although the author provided no cutoff score for distinguishing well-adjusted couples from distressed couples, many clinicians have adopted the admittedly arbitrary total raw score of 100 as a rough guideline (Fowers, 1990; Stuart, 1992). Because this score is arbitrary, the author and others have suggested that the *DAS* may be better suited as a global assessment of marital satisfaction than as a true multidimensional scale and model (Fowers, 1990). In contrast, Prouty, Markowski, and Barnes (2000) advocated for using scores on each of the four scales to structure the content of therapy.

In a counseling setting, the *DAS* may have an effective use beyond that of a quantitative assessment of satisfaction. The instrument items call for respondents to indicate their perceived level of agreement with their partner on various aspects of the relationship. When both partners have completed the form, many avenues for discussion may open. Items with a large score discrepancy between partners may signal areas the partners have not discussed in the past and could benefit from discussing in a counseling setting. In addition, items with similar scores between partners that indicate strong disagreement in a particular area may qualitatively highlight "problem areas" for discussion in counseling. As with any quantitative assessment, it is important to view the results in the context of what a counselor already knows about a couple and as simply one more tool in the overall assessment process.

Other Instruments Used in Assessing Couples

Myers-Briggs Type Indicator (MBTI)

The *Myers-Briggs Type Indicator* (*MBTI*) (Myers, McCaulley, Quenk, & Hammer, 1998) is one of the most frequently used assessment tools in marriage and family counseling (Boughner et al., 1994). The *MBTI* measures individual preferences for each of four dichotomous pairs of personality characteristics: Extraversion-Introversion, Sensing-Intuition, Thinking-Feeling, and Judging-Perceiving. Professional counselors can use the *MBTI* with couples to facilitate discussion about how differences in perceiving and processing information can affect their communication (Whiston, 2005). For a more complete description of the *MBTI,* readers are referred to Chapter 8.

Facilitating Open Couple Communication, Understanding and Study—Third Edition (FOCCUS)

Facilitating Open Couple Communication, Understanding and Study—Third Edition (*FOCCUS*) (Markey, Micheletto, & Becker, 2000) is a 156-item instrument that is widely used by Protestant and Catholic churches as well as by nondenominational counseling services (Larson, Newell, Topham, & Nichols, 2002). It consists of 19 scales that measure four major content areas: Matches of Personality, Lifestyles, and Friends; Communication and Problem-Solving skills; Bonders and Integrators (e.g., Religion, Values, and Finances); and Summary Categories (e.g., Key Problem Indicators, Family-of-origin, and Dual Career Issues).

Premarriage Awareness Inventory (PAI)

The *Premarriage Awareness Inventory* (*PAI*) (Velander, 1993) comes in three forms (F, C, and R) to assist clergy and professional counselors with premarital counseling. Form F is for couples who have never been married and are not living together. Form C is for couples who are living together and plan to get married. Form R is for couples planning to marry in which one or both partners have been previously married. The purpose of the *PAI* is to help couples identify the unique strengths and challenges in their relationship. The inventory consists of 119 items designed to assess 10 relationship categories: Sound Beginnings, Expectations, Communication, Sharing Feelings, Personality/Relating Style, Conflict Resolution/Problem Solving, Family and Friends, Finances and Legal Issues, Sexuality, and Religion. The manual is user-friendly and provides specific, session-by-session directions for interpretation and counseling.

RELATionship Evaluation (RELATE)

The *RELATionship Evaluation* (*RELATE*) (Loyer-Carlson, Busby, Holman, Klein, & Larson, 2002) (formerly known at the *PREP-M*) is a 270-item instrument designed to measure relationship satisfaction and stability. Four general domains are assessed: Individual (personality, values, interaction styles), Family (past and present), Cultural (race, religion, social class, geographical location), and Couple (patterns of interaction). *RELATE* can be accessed online at www.relate.byu.edu.

Taylor-Johnson Temperament Analysis (T-JTA)

The *Taylor-Johnson Temperament Analysis* (*T-JTA*) (Taylor & Morrison, 1996) was designed for general use in personality testing and premarital and marital counseling. It has a long history, with its original predecessor dating back to 1941. The *T-JTA* measures nine bipolar traits: Nervous vs. Composed; Depressive vs. Lighthearted; Active-Social vs. Quiet; Expressive-Responsive vs. Inhibited; Sympathetic vs. Indifferent; Subjective vs. Objective; Dominant vs. Submissive; Hostile vs. Tolerant; and Self-Disciplined vs. Impulsive. When the test is used with couples, individuals rate their views of themselves and of their partners, resulting in a "criss-cross" production of profiles that can enhance premarital or marital counseling.

Assessment of Families

Many standardized instruments have been developed to assess various dimensions of family functioning. Some of the instruments were developed primarily for research purposes; others have clinical application as well. The instruments described next are examples of standardized tools that can be used effectively in a clinical setting.

Family Environmental Scale (FES)

The *Family Environment Scale* (*FES*) (Moos & Moos, 1994) is a self-administered 90-item true-false family assessment instrument that provides test takers with scores related to their perceived, ideal, and/or expected familial environments. The *FES*

Table 14.2   The *Family Environmental Scale* (*FES*): Subscales and dimension descriptions

Subscale	Relationship dimensions
1. Cohesion	The degree of commitment, help, and support family members provide for one another.
2. Expressiveness	The degree to which family members are encouraged to act openly and express their feelings directly.
3. Conflict	The amount of openly expressed anger, aggression, and conflict among family members.
	Personal growth dimensions
4. Independence	The extent to which family members are assertive, self-sufficient, and make their own decisions.
5. Achievement Orientation	The extent to which activities (such as school or work) are cast into an achievement-oriented or competitive framework.
6. Intellectual-Cultural Orientation	The degree of interest in political, social, intellectual, and cultural activities.
7. Active-Recreational Orientation	The extent of participation in social and recreational activities.
8. Moral-Religious Emphasis	The degree of emphasis on ethical and religious issues and values.
	System maintenance dimensions
9. Organization	The degree of importance of clear organization and structure in planning family activities and responsibilities.
10. Control	The extent to which set rules and procedures are used to run family life.

scores items on 10 subscales, with nine items attributed to each. For each item, clients respond to statements such as "being on time is important in my family." The measured subscales are Cohesion, Expressiveness, Conflict, Independence, Achievement Orientation, Intellectual-Cultural Orientation, Active-Recreational Orientation, Moral-Religious Emphasis, Organization, and Control (see Table 14.2 and Figure 14.3). Scores also are provided on two 27-item indices: the Family Relationships Index and the Family Social Integration Index. Although the manual is currently in its third edition, the scale itself remains unchanged from its original publication in 1974.

Unlike many marriage and family assessments, the *FES* focuses on relationships between members of an entire family, rather than simply a particular couple or dyad. In addition, the *FES* is designed for use by a single respondent, rather than multiple family members. Of course, multiple family members may take this assessment within any counseling session, but results would be reported for each test-taking member individually.

The *FES* is offered in four forms: Form R (Real) measures the respondent's perceived current family condition; Form I (Ideal) measures the respondent's preferred family situation; Form E (Expectations) measures the respondent's familial expectations; and Form C (Children's) is a pictorial version designed for children ages 5–11.

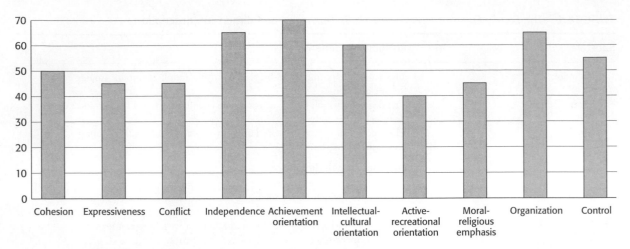

Figure 14.3   Profile from the *Family Environment Scale (FES)*

Test-retest reliability of scores at a 2-month interval ranged from 0.68 (Independence) to 0.86 (Cohesion). Internal consistency of scores ranged across subscales from 0.61 to 0.78. Validity for the *FES* has been evidenced by moderate correlations between its subscales and those of instruments such as the *Locke-Wallace Marital Adjustment Scale,* the *Family Routines Inventory,* and other measures (Buboltz, Johnson, & Woller, 2003).

The *FES* has seen widespread use for 25 years and is regularly touted as one of the most commonly used family assessment instruments, indicating trust among members of the clinical community. It is primarily recommended for times when a clinician desires a global assessment of a family member's view of his or her family (Mancini, 2001). The multiple forms allow for insight into possible discrepancies between the client's perception of the family's current state and expected or ideal states, which would be useful in goal setting and in assessing changes in perception over time. The manual for the *FES* features many illustrations of how to use the instrument in various family settings and situations.

In addition to its use in serving as a starting point for discussions related to individuals' perceptions of their family environment, subscales on the *FES* also have recently been used to predict psychological reactance (resistance when one's freedoms are restricted) in adolescents, predicting adolescents' satisfaction in meeting leisure needs, and predicting test and trait anxiety in children (Buboltz et al., 2003; Garton, Harvey, & Price, 2004; Peleg-Popko & Klingman, 2002).

Family Assessment Measure–Version III (FAM-III)

The *Family Assessment Measure* (*FAM-III*) (Skinner, Steinhauer, & Santa-Barbara, 1995) is a self-report assessment tool that evaluates family strengths, weaknesses, and processes. It is based on the process model of family functioning (Satir, 1982) and

Table 14.3   The *Family Assessment Measure—Version III (FAM-III)*: Scales and contrived sample items

Respondents answer each item with Strongly Agree, Agree, Disagree, or Strongly Disagree

General scale	Dyadic scale	Self-report
Family duties are shared.	I can tell when this person is upset.	My family expects too much of me.
You don't get a chance to be an individual in our family.	This person gets too involved in my affairs.	I do my share of duties in the family.
We feel loved in our family.	I can count on this person to help me in a crisis.	I stay out of other family members' business.

consists of three interrelated instruments: the General Scale (50 items), the Dyadic Relationship Scale (42 items), and the Self-Rating Scale (42 items). Table 14.3 provides examples of items that comprise these scales.Each of the scales provides scores for the following family process areas: (1) Task Accomplishment, (2) Role Performance, (3) Communication, (4) Affective Expression, (5) Involvement, (6) Control, and (7) Values and Norms. In addition to these scores, the General Scale also provides scores on social desirability and defensiveness, which serve as validity checks.

Each family member is asked to complete the *FAM-III* battery. For the Dyadic Relationship Scale, individuals complete separate forms describing their relationships with each member of the family, which can be somewhat cumbersome in a large family. The test authors suggest administering the questionnaires as part of an intake assessment rather than part of the first family counseling session (Skinner et al., 1995). Questions are listed on three color-coded, hand-scorable carbon sheets and typically take between 30 and 40 minutes to complete. One reviewer stated that the scoring is time consuming, and that evaluators should count on 2 hours for scoring and interpretation for a four-member nuclear family (Manges, 2001). In addition to the format just described, the *FAM-III* can be administered and scored on the computer. Brief *FAM* versions also are available, which can reduce the time involved in administration and scoring.

The *FAM-III* manual (Skinner et al., 1995) reports evidence of construct, content, and predictive validity. Reported coefficient *alpha*s range from 0.86 to 0.95, and test-retest reliability for the subscales ranges from 0.57 to 0.66 over a 12-day period. The instrument was normed on groups of 247 adults and 65 adolescents.

Family counselors can use the *FAM-III* as part of an intake assessment, for outcome evaluation, for general family research, or simply as a tool within the counseling process. It is important to remember, especially if the *FAM-III* is used as part of a forensic evaluation, that the items are all self-report and can be manipulated by the test taker (Manges, 2001). As is true for all assessment tools, the *FAM-III* can supplement, but not substitute for, clinical observations (Spillane, 2001).

Family Adaptability and Cohesion Evaluation Scale–Fourth Edition (FACES IV)

The Family Adaptability and Cohesion Evaluation Scale—Fourth Edition (*FACES IV*) (Olson, Gorall, & Tiesel, 2002) represents the fourth revision of the *Family Adaptability and Cohesion Scales* (*FACES I, II,* and *III*), which are all based on the circumplex model of family functioning (Olson & Gorall, 2003; Olson, Russell, & Sprenkle, 1989). Its predecessor, *FACES III,* has been described as "one of the state-of-the-art family assessment instruments in the field" (Franklin, Streeter, & Springer, 2001, p. 576). The current version, *FACES IV,* is more comprehensive than previous versions. The purpose of *FACES IV* is to assess dimensions of family cohesion, flexibility, communication, and satisfaction. The instrument consists of 62 items and can be answered by all family members over the age of 12. Representative items from *FACES IV* are depicted in Box 14.2.

FACES IV is composed of eight scales, six of which specifically measure family cohesion and family flexibility. Of these six scales, two are *balanced scales* (linear scales, so the higher the score, the more positive the attribute), and four are *unbalanced scales* (designed to assess the high and low extremes of cohesion and flexibility). Scores on the six scales identify families as one of six types: Balanced, Rigidly Cohesive, Midrange, Flexibly Unbalanced, Chaotically Unbalanced, and Unbalanced.

Family communication is measured by a 10-item scale that addresses various aspects of communication in a family system. Family satisfaction is measured by another 10-item scale that assesses family members' satisfaction in regard to their perceived cohesion, flexibility, and communication. After the instrument is scored, scores are graphically plotted as part of the Family Profile Summary.

Scores on the *FACES IV* scales "have been found to be reliable and valid for research use and clinical use" (Olson & Gorall, 2003, p. 532), with internal consistency *alpha* coefficients ranging from 0.80 to 0.93 on all scales. *FACES IV* is part of the new *Family Inventories Package* (*FIP*) (Olson et al., 2002). Two other instruments included in the *FIP* are the *Family Strengths Scale* (Olson, Larsen, & McCubbin, 1989) and the *Family Stress Scale,* which taps the levels of stress experienced by individuals within their family system and which was adapted from the *Coping and Stress Profile* (*CSP*) (Olson, 1997).

Parent-Child Relationship Inventory (PCRI)

The *Parent-Child Relationship Inventory* (*PCRI*) (Gerard, 1994) is a 78-item, self-report questionnaire that assesses parents' attitudes toward parenting and toward their children. It is designed for use with mothers or fathers of 3- to 15-year-old children and provides a quantified description of the parent-child relationship. The *PCRI* is composed of seven content scales and two validity indicators (see Table 14.4). Content scales assess specific aspects of the parent-child relationship, with higher scores indicating good parenting skills on six of the seven scales. The Role Orientation scale indicates attitudes toward egalitarian values and traditional role values and does not denote parenting skills. The two indicators of validity, Social

---

Box 14.2   *FACES IV* Package: Sample Items

Directions to Family Members:

1. All family members over the age 12 can complete a *FACES IV.*
2. Family members should complete the instrument independently, not consulting or discussing their responses until they have been completed.

FACES IV: Sample Items

1	2	3	4	5
DOES NOT describe our family at all	SLIGHTLY describes our family	SOMEWHAT describes our family	GENERALLY describes our family	VERY WELL describes our family

1. Family members are involved in each other's lives.
5. There are strict consequences for breaking the rules in our family.
10. Family members feel pressured to spend most free time together.
15. Family members feel closer to people outside the family than to other family members.
20. In solving problems, the children's suggestions are followed.
25. Family members like to spend some of their free time with each other.
30. There is no leadership in this family.
35. It is important to follow the rules in our family.
40. Family members feel guilty if they want to spend time away from the family.

Family Communication: Sample Items

44. Family members are very good listeners.
45. Family members are able to ask each other for what they want.
50. Family members try to understand each other's feelings.

Family Satisfaction: Sample Items

1	2	3	4	5
Very Dissatisfied	Somewhat Dissatisfied	Generally Dissatisfied	Very Satisfied	Extremely Satisfied

54. Your family's ability to cope with stress
58. Your family's ability to resolve conflict.
62. Family members concern for each other.

*The above items are only a
sample of the 62 items in the FACES IV package.*

Source: Retrieved August 3, 2005, from www.facesiv.com/pdf/sample_items.pdf. Used with permission from Life Innovations.

Table 14.4   The *Parent-Child Relationship Inventory (PCRI):* Content scales

Scale	Explanation
Parental Support	Measures the practical help and emotional support the client receives as a parent.
Satisfaction with Parenting	Measures the enjoyment a parent receives from parenting.
Involvement	Measures a parent's propensity to seek out his or her children, demonstrate interest in their activities, and spend time with them.
Communication	Measures a parent's awareness of how well he or she communicates with the children in a variety of situations.
Autonomy	Measures the parent's willingness to promote the child's independence.
Role Orientation	Unlike the other scales, this scale does not have positive or negative dimensions. Instead, the two poles represent the parent's attitude toward current egalitarian values and traditional role values.

Desirability and Inconsistency, measure the degree toward which responses may be biased or inconsistent.

The *PCRI* uses a carbon-backed, hand-scorable questionnaire that can be completed in approximately 15 minutes. Parents respond, using a 4-point Likert scale, to items such as "I spend a great deal of time with my child" or "I sometimes feel overburdened by my responsibilities as a parent." Alternatively, the *PCRI* can be administered and scored on a microcomputer disk, or answer sheets can be mailed or faxed for computerized scoring and interpretation. Scores are converted to T scores and percentiles. T scores above 40 are congruent with good parenting, whereas scores below 40 may indicate areas of concern.

The *PCRI* was normed on a sample of over 1,100 mothers and fathers representing 13 school and day-care centers in the United States. Overall, the sample was better educated and less culturally diverse than the U.S. population at large (Gerard, 1994). Internal consistency for the seven *PCRI* scales ranged from 0.70 (Parental Support) to 0.88 (Limit Setting). Test-retest reliability estimates ranged from 0.68 (Communication) to 0.93 (Limit Setting) after a 1-week interval. Estimates after 5 months ranged from 0.44 (Autonomy) to 0.71 (Parental Support, Role Orientation). Although evidence of content, construct and predictive validity has been demonstrated (Gerard, 1994), the author and others (e.g., Marchant & Paulson, 1998) have noted that the construct of parenting is complex and difficult to define. Also, what constitutes "good" parenting in a middle-class Caucasian family may not necessary match what is considered "good parenting" in families from different ethnic and social class groups (Marchant & Paulson).

The *PCRI,* having been developed only a decade ago, has quickly gained respect as a reliable and useful assessment of parent-child relationships, both clinically and in research. It can be used as a catalyst to identify areas of concern, as well as areas of strength, in parents' relationships with their children.

Other Measures of Family Assessment

Family Assessment Device (FAD)

The *Family Assessment Device* (*FAD*) (Epstein, Baldwin, & Bishop, 1983) is a 60-item measure of family functioning based on the McMaster model of family functioning. It is used to assess emotional relationships and functioning along seven dimensions: Problem Solving, Communication, Roles, Affective Responsiveness (sharing of affection), Affective Involvement (emotional sensitivity), Behavior Control, and General Functioning (boundaries).

Global Assessment of Relational Functioning (GARF)

While not a standardized measurement of family functioning, the *Global Assessment of Relational Functioning* (*GARF*) (American Psychiatric Association, 2000) was designed to measure relational health and dysfunction in couple and family systems (Ross & Doherty, 2001) and can be found in Appendix B of the *Diagnostic and Statistical Manual of Mental Disorders* (*DSM-IV-TR*) (APA, 2000). The *GARF* is patterned after the Global Assessment of Functioning (GAF) scale, which is used for individual evaluation. The *GARF* assesses three dimensions of relational functioning: (1) Problem Solving (skills in negotiating goals, rules, and routines; adaptability to stress; communication skills; the ability to resolve conflict); (2) Organization (maintenance of interpersonal roles and subsystem boundaries; hierarchical functioning; coalitions and distribution of power, control and responsibility); and (3) Emotional Climate (tone and range of feelings; quality of caring, empathy, involvement, and attachment/commitment; sharing of values, mutual affective responsiveness, respect, and regard; quality of sexual functioning (APA, 2000).

Like the *GAF*, the *GARF* uses a 100-point scale to assess interpersonal functioning. Anchor points are given at five levels of functioning, ranging from Very Poor (low scores) to Satisfactory (high scores), with a 20-point range within each. The *GARF* assesses healthy functioning as well as unhealthy functioning, requires no formal training, and is designed to be used by a wide range of professionals. Its inclusion in the *DSM-IV-TR* "marks progress for the field of family therapy, as it is a first step toward recognition and inclusion of relational disorders in the *DSM*" (Ross & Doherty, 2001, p. 242).

Parenting Stress Index—Third Edition (PSI-3)

The *Parenting Stress Index—Third Edition* (*PSI-3*) (Abidin, 1995) is published by Psychological Assessment Resources and was developed to identify problem areas in parent-child relationships. The instrument assesses three general sources of stress: sources associated with the child's characteristics, sources associated with parent characteristics, and life event stressors. In addition to the 120-item self-report form, there is a short form (*PSI-SF*) consisting of 36 items that measure maternal esteem, parent-child interaction, and child self-regulation.

As stated earlier, there are hundreds of other instruments available for assessing family relationships. Limited psychometric information is available for many of those instruments, so it is essential for professional counselors to evaluate them carefully before selecting and administering them to clients (Whiston, 2005).

Whereas standardized instruments provide one way of assessing family functioning, qualitative approaches offer another useful form of family assessment. One is not a substitute for the other; both types of assessment, when used intentionally and skillfully, can be integrated into the counseling process to gather information about families and facilitate change.

QUALITATIVE ASSESSMENT OF FAMILY RELATIONSHIPS

Characteristics of Qualitative Assessment

Qualitative assessment procedures involve nonstandardized, nonquantitative approaches to evaluating families (Goldman, 1990, 1992). Examples of qualitative approaches include structured exercises, creative activities, genograms, timelines, card sorts, and a host of other open-ended activities. Some qualitative approaches have a projective quality; that is, family members reveal personal values, beliefs, and needs as they respond to an unstructured stimulus situation (Goldman, 1992). However, qualitative assessment is not a covert process, nor is it used to diagnose or categorize families. Instead, these methods help professional counselors learn from families and help families increase their understanding of themselves (Deacon & Piercy, 2001).

In general, qualitative methods are holistic and integrated, which complements the systemic approach that is used by many family counselors. Goldman (1990, 1992) outlined some of the characteristics of qualitative assessment methods that tend to make them useful in counseling:

- Qualitative approaches tend to be more informal than standardized assessment, allowing for greater professional counselor and client flexibility.
- Qualitative approaches actively involve the clients and lead readily into counseling interactions.
- Qualitative approaches usually are not restricted to preset scales and scoring categories. Instead, they emphasize holistic study of families. Interpretations tend to be open ended and divergent.
- Because qualitative methods do not attempt precise measurement or normative comparison, they may be modified, both in content and in interpretation, to meet the needs of the family being assessed.
- Because qualitative methods can be modified, they can be more easily adapted for clients of different cultural backgrounds than can standardized methods of assessment.
- Qualitative approaches emphasize the concepts of learning about oneself within a developmental framework, such as understanding where a family is in the family life cycle.
- Qualitative approaches can serve as interventions, thereby reducing the distinction between assessment and counseling.

Deacon and Piercy (2001) offer additional reasons for using qualitative assessment in evaluating families:

- Qualitative assessment empowers clients as they become active partners in the assessment process.
- Because family members are involved in generating and making sense of their own assessment data, their commitment to the therapy process is likely to increase.
- When family members share their qualitative assessment data, they learn about the different perspectives that are part of their dynamic family system. In so doing, communication and understanding are enhanced.
- Qualitative assessment helps professional counselors gain a contextually rich sense of the family in ways that measuring discrete variables may not.
- Qualitative assessment helps professional counselors understand the personal constructs, stories, and meanings that families attach to their experiences.

In general, the areas that qualitative methods evaluate parallel those that standardized measures assess, including the presenting issue; the family structure and organization; family functioning, strengths and stressors; and goals for change. Qualitative approaches can be used to help clarify the nature of the family's problems, understand family members' subjective perceptions, develop hypotheses, and clarify goals. The process helps create a picture of the structure, functioning, and influences of family dynamics.

Qualitative Assessment Methods

Interviews represent the most common form of qualitative assessment in family counseling (L'Abate & Bagorozzi, 1993). However, a host of other qualitative methods have been used by therapists, many of which are described in depth elsewhere (e.g., Deacon & Piercy, 2001; Edwards, 2003; Kinston, Loader, & Sullivan, 1985; L'Abate, 1994). In this section, examples are provided of a few of the many informal methods of assessment that clinicians can use to evaluate families.

Drawing and art assessments

Art activities can be used with family members of all ages. By engaging them in activities that involve drawing, painting, coloring, or modeling with clay, professional counselors can learn about their clients in a manner that is typically considered nonthreatening (Deacon & Piercy, 2001). The focus shifts from the "identified patient" or problem to the art process and product. Drawings by family members can reveal feelings, thoughts, and attitudes that are difficult to put into words. There are multiple ways to integrate art into the assessment process, some of which are described below.

Family Circle

The purpose of the *Family Circle* activity, originally described by Thrower (1982) and later adapted by Edwards (2003), is to give family members and the professional counselor a graphic representation of ways family members view each other in regard to closeness, power, and centrality. The professional counselor gives each family member a piece of paper on which a large circle is drawn. The family is then instructed as follows:

> Place your family on the paper. You can put them inside or outside the circle, you can put them close together or far apart, and you can draw them large or small. Please indicate each person with a circle; that is, don't draw the person's face or body. (Edwards, 2003, p. 125)

Family members should draw their pictures independently. After they finish, the professional counselor asks each person to show the drawing so that everyone can see it. The professional counselor then makes comments about each drawing, asks questions, and encourages discussion. No interpretations are made about the drawings; instead, observations are noted (e.g., "I notice that you put yourself closest to your mother and your brother closest to your father"). Depending on the family and the nature of the presenting problem, the professional counselor may want to ask family members to turn the page over and draw the family the way they would like it to be. At the end of the session, the professional counselor may want to ask to keep the drawings for later reference.

Kinetic Family Drawing

The *Kinetic Family Drawing* (*KFD*) (Burns, 1982; Burns & Kaufman, 1970, 1972) is a widely used method of assessing family dynamics. The activity can be completed by individual family members (typically children) or by family members working together. A third variation involves asking everyone in the family to complete a drawing independently, then guiding a joint family discussion of the various perceptions represented in the different pictures (Thompson & Nurse, 1999).

Basic instructions for completing the *KFD* are as follows: "Draw a picture of everyone in your family, including you, doing something. Try to draw whole people, not cartoons or stick people. Remember, make everyone doing something—some kind of action" (Burns & Kaufman, 1970, pp. 19–20). It may be necessary for the clinician to encourage family members to include themselves in the picture.

The *KFD* has been used extensively with children, adolescents, and adults (Thompson & Nurse, 1999). Burns and Kaufman (1972) introduced a formal scoring system for the *KFD* that focused on actions, styles, and symbols. Burns (1982) later adapted the scoring system to focus on actions; distances, barriers, and positions; physical characteristics of the figures; and styles. However, according to Thompson & Nurse, scoring individual signs in this manner "has not proved particularly productive" (p. 125). Instead, an integrative, holistic approach that focuses on family dynamics is encouraged. Although the *KFD* lacks extensive empirical and experimental data supporting its validity, when used as a qualitative assessment instrument, it consistently taps into family interrelationships, providing a helpful way to evaluate family functioning.

Joint family drawings

There are many ways to use **joint family drawings** in family assessment. Asking families to collaborate in a drawing task provides opportunities for the professional counselor to observe interactions, form hypotheses, and plan interventions (Gladding, 2005; Riley, 1987). One drawing activity that is especially nonthreatening is the Joint Family Scribble (Kwiatkowska, 1978), in which family members are asked to make scribbles and then integrate their scribbles into a unified family picture. Alternatively, family members may be asked to draw a mural together of whatever they choose (e.g., their home, an activity). In this enactment, the clinician "observes how family members cooperate and communicate with each other, how they make decisions, what roles individual members play, and what problems arise" (Deacon & Piercy, p. 361). After the mural is complete, the professional counselor asks questions about the mural, the process, and the observed interactions.

A variation to the mural activity is the Joint Family Holiday Drawing, described by Jordan (2001). The family is asked to work together on a joint drawing of one of their family holidays. The family is instructed to decide together which holiday they want to draw and how they will do so, involving all the family members. After the instructions are given and the family selects a holiday, the drawing is created nonverbally. Afterwards, the professional counselor discusses the experience with the family, asking questions such as, "What did you experience as you worked together?" "How were decisions made?" "What role did everyone take in this exercise?" "What was the most challenging (fun, difficult, surprising) part of the activity?"

Jordan (2001) proposes that the *Joint Family Holiday Drawing* can be used with a variety of families, regardless of ethnicity, socioeconomic status, or language ability. However, she cautions that it may not be suitable for highly conflicted families.

Mapping Activities

Genogram

The **genogram** (pronounced *JEN-uh-gram*), represents one of the best-known and most frequently used methods of qualitative family assessment. It is a powerful tool that enables professional counselors to record family information and processes for the purposes of hypothesizing and planning interventions (Coupland, Serovich, & Glenn, 1995). Family members and the clinician coconstruct the genogram in sessions, following a standardized format. The format "records information about family members and their relationships over at least three generations" (McGoldrick, Gerson, & Shellenberger, 1999, p. 1). Like many qualitative methods, the genogram serves both as an assessment tool and as a therapeutic intervention. It is most closely associated with Bowen family systems theory (Bowen, 1978), although it is used by marriage and family counselors from a wide range of theoretical orientations (Whiston, 2005).

Genograms provide tangible, graphic representations of intergenerational family patterns (McGoldrick et al., 1999). Genograms provide a way to organize a large amount of family data by illustrating family history, patterns, and events that may have ongoing significance. McGoldrick et al. (1999, p. 2) stated that "gathering genogram information should be seen as an integral part of a comprehensive, clinical assessment." From a Bowenian stance, relationship styles are transmitted from one generation to the next, and unresolved issues from one generation may surface in later generations (Bowen, 1978). When clients recognize these patterns of behavior, they can learn ways to interrupt patterns that are counterproductive and create new patterns of relating that promote health (Magnuson & Shaw, 2003; Searight, 1997).

Dunn and Levitt (2000) recommended using a mutually collaborative and process-oriented approach to genogram construction. Genogram information can be gathered by interviewing one family member or several. In either case, it is important to respect the family's expertise and to use the genogram in a way that not only provides the professional counselor with information but also gives voice to the family's concerns and facilitates the therapeutic process.

McGoldrick et al. (1999) suggested constructing genograms by: (1) mapping the family structure, (2) recording important family information, (3) delineating family relationships, and (4) examining family patterns. Symbols that are commonly used to map the family structure are depicted in Figure 14.4. Specific dates that are recorded on the genogram include births, deaths, marriages or partnerships, and divorces. Other data often include ages, names, occupations, educational background, medical conditions, religious practices, and significant events (McGoldrick et al., 1999). Patterns of functioning are noted, such as alcoholism, violence, success, failure, and resilience.

In addition to factual information, descriptions of dyadic relationships are illustrated on the genogram. Different lines are used to symbolize various types of relationships. For example, a zigzag line between two squares could illustrate a hostile relationship between brothers. McGoldrick et al. (1999) note that this task is inferential and subjective and that relationships in a family often change over time.

Once the initial genogram is constructed, professional counselors can use it to help families understand their experiences within the context of family patterns. Patterns of family functioning—healthy and unhealthy—may repeat themselves across several generations. Examples of negative patterns include addiction, violence, incest, and conflictual relationships (McGoldrick et al., 1999). Positive patterns include resilience, resourcefulness, healthy nurturing, and close (not enmeshed) relationships. It is helpful to keep the genogram available throughout the course of counseling so that it can be used therapeutically and so that information can be modified as needed (Dunn & Levitt, 2000).

Magnuson and Shaw (2003) cited multiple studies that described the effective use of genograms with couples and families. They report that genograms can be used for premarital counseling and to address a wide range of issues, including intimacy, gender dynamics, sexual orientation, addictions, grief and loss, and career concerns. As with any assessment tool, professional counselors need to experience and practice genogram construction to become proficient in its use (Dunn & Levitt, 2000).

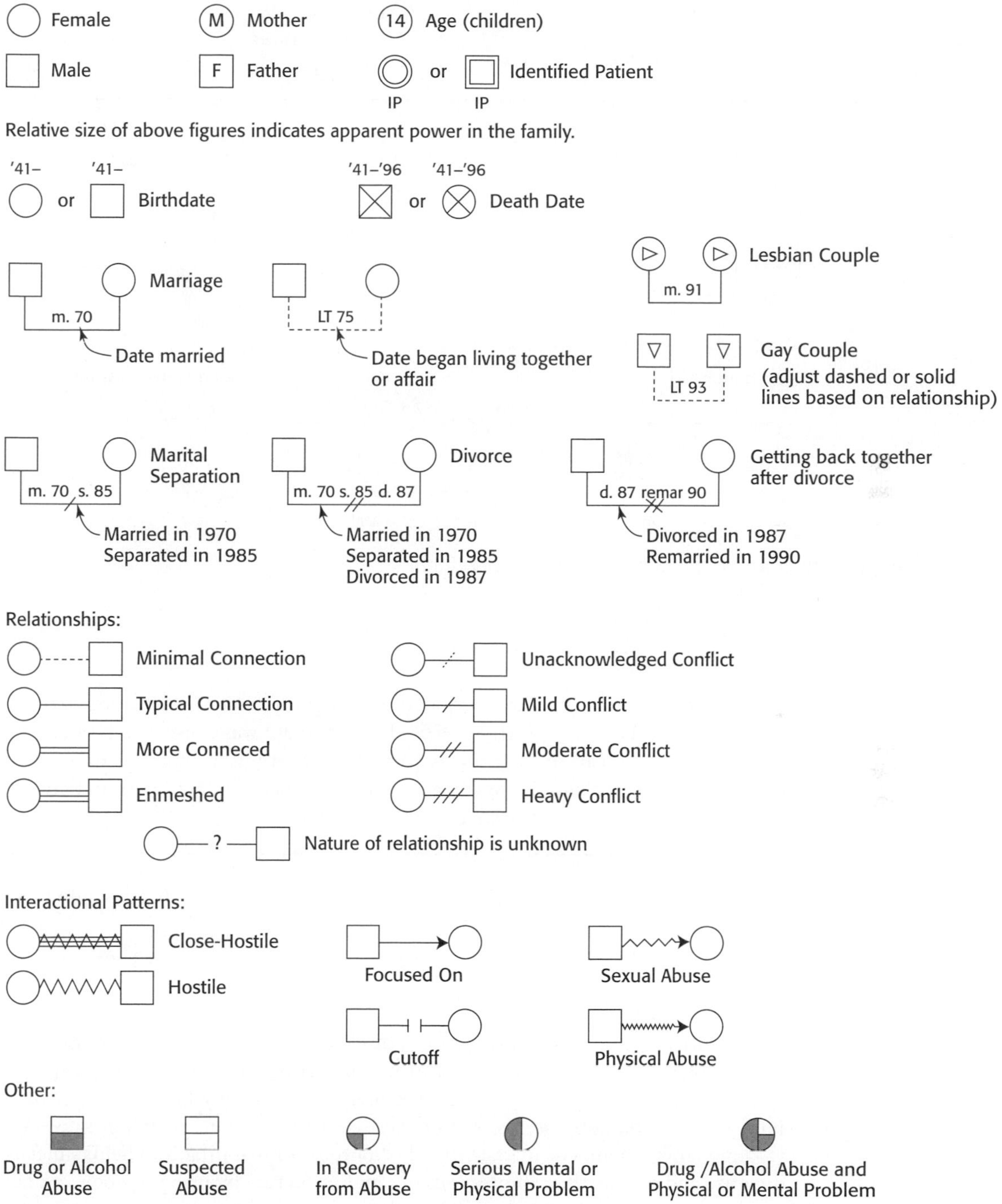

Female   (M) Mother   (14) Age (children)

Male   F Father   Identified Patient
IP   IP

Relative size of above figures indicates apparent power in the family.

'41–   '41–
or   Birthdate

'41–'96   '41–'96
or   Death Date

Marriage   Lesbian Couple
m. 70   m. 91
Date married

LT 75   Date began living together
or affair

Gay Couple
(adjust dashed or solid
LT 93   lines based on relationship)

Marital
Separation   Divorce   Getting back together
after divorce
m. 70 s. 85   m. 70 s. 85 d. 87   d. 87 remar 90
Married in 1970   Married in 1970   Divorced in 1987
Separated in 1985   Separated in 1985   Remarried in 1990
Divorced in 1987

Relationships:

○------□ Minimal Connection   ○—/—□ Unacknowledged Conflict

○——□ Typical Connection   ○—/—□ Mild Conflict

○══□ More Conneced   ○—//—□ Moderate Conflict

○══□ Enmeshed   ○—///—□ Heavy Conflict

○—?—□ Nature of relationship is unknown

Interactional Patterns:

○ΛΛΛΛ□ Close-Hostile   □——►○ Focused On   □〜〜〜►○ Sexual Abuse

○〜〜〜□ Hostile   □—⊦—○ Cutoff   □〜〜〜►○ Physical Abuse

Other:

Drug or Alcohol   Suspected   In Recovery   Serious Mental or   Drug /Alcohol Abuse and
Abuse   Abuse   from Abuse   Physical Problem   Physical or Mental Problem

Figure 14.4   Common symbols used for genograms

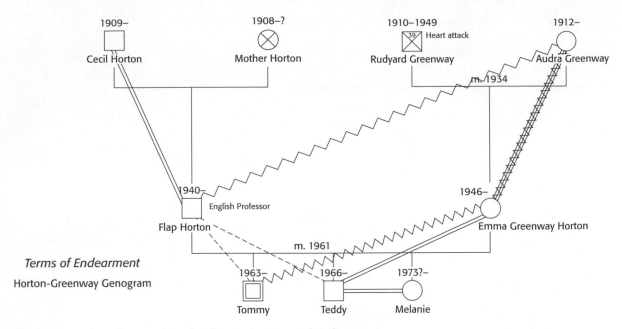

Figure 14.5   Sample genogram for the movie *Terms of Endearment*

Note: Data were selected based on the novel.

Figure 14.5 illustrates an example of a genogram based on the novel *Terms of Endearment,* by Larry McMurtry (1975). The genogram was completed by a student in a counselor education program as part of her training in marriage and family counseling. Drawing and discussing genograms representing families from fiction is one way to become better versed in effective genogram use.

> **Think About It 14.2**   How could you use genograms when you counsel couples, families, and individual clients?

Family mapping

The **family mapping** technique is a form of structural mapping, which is associated with Salvador Minuchin (1974) and his model of structural family therapy. Structural family therapy is based on the premise that family functioning involves family structure, subsystems, boundaries, and hierarchies, which are revealed through family members' interactions. The purpose of mapping is to help clinicians organize and display their impressions of family structure by using symbols to draw relationship patterns (Edwards, 2003). The family map differs from the genogram in that it is subjective rather than factual, is constructed by the professional counselor

What's an "Ideal" Family Supposed to Look Like?

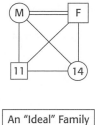

An "Ideal" Family

Mapping an "ideal" family reveals our assumptions about how family relationships function best. The map to the left shows the following:

1. The mother-father bond is strongest in the family.
2. Mother and father are of equal size.
3. Children are below the parent-child boundary.
4. Children are smaller than parents.
5. The older child is slightly larger than the younger (a little more power).
6. The map has no conflict lines.

Figure 14.6   Map of an "ideal" family

Source: From *Working With Families: Guidelines and Techniques* (6th ed.), by J. T. Edwards, 2003, Durham, NC: Foundation Place Publishing. Copyright © 2003 by J. T. Edwards. Reprinted with permission.

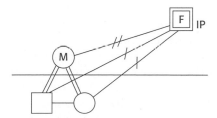

Figure 14.7   Map of a family with a chemically dependent father

Source: From *Working With Families: Guidelines and Techniques* (6th ed.), by J. T. Edwards, 2003, Durham, NC: Foundation Place Publishing. Copyright © 2003 by J. T. Edwards. Reprinted with permission.

without directly involving the family, and provides little social or multigenerational history. However, maps include more information than genograms about current relationships between family members.

Edwards (2003) used some of the symbols depicted in Figure 14.4 to illustrate family relationships. The family map helps clarify what the professional counselor currently believes about the family organization and about what may be contributing to the issue. Figures 14.6 and 14.7 provide examples of a model depicting an "ideal" family and a family with a chemically dependent father, respectively. Other examples of what might be considered "ideal" depend on the family's structure and cultural background. Family maps help organize and display information about the family, help the professional counselor maintain a systems focus, and help indicate goals for the counseling process.

Ecomap

The **ecomap** represents a way to illustrate families within an ecological system. One variation of the ecomap, described by L'Abate (1994), involves a collaborative effort by everyone in the family. The family begins by drawing their home in the center of a large piece of paper. Then they are asked to draw schools, grocery stores, churches, recreational sites, significant people, and other resources in the community that are important to them. Distances between the home and the various sites and resources are recorded as well. During the process, the professional counselor may make observations and ask questions to help with clarification and elaboration. The process of creating the ecomap provides insight about ways family members interact and spend their time. It also provides information about sources of support within the larger community.

Another variation of the ecomap is illustrated in Figure 14.8. This type of ecomap is completed in collaboration with the professional counselor, but rather than involving the entire family, it typically involves a single family member or subsystems of the family (e.g., siblings). Figure 14.8 also provides a legend of symbols commonly used in an ecomap.

In this example, an adolescent ("Janet") drew a circle representing herself in the center of the paper. Surrounding the circle, she drew symbols of activities, interests, and specific areas of concern. The lines connecting her with the surrounding images illustrate the nature of her relationship with those items. For example, her relationship with school is depicted as "tenuous." She has a history of making poor grades, but during the current year she has made improvements. Her relationship with her 88-year-old grandparents is positive, as indicated by the "energy in, energy out" connector. The degree of stress caused by the issues with which she is dealing is depicted by the number of vertical lines drawn on the connector lines. For Janet, the abuse she experienced as a child and her compulsive hand washing are considered quite stressful. In contrast, painting and participating in church represent sources of strength.

One of the drawbacks of having an individual, rather than the family, draw the ecomap is that the focus is taken away from the family system. However, for family therapists who spend part of their time working with different segments of the family, using an individualized ecomap such as this one can provide a wealth of contextual information that can be effectively incorporated into family work. As with any assessment activity, the therapist will need to make clinical judgments about what methods are most likely to benefit a particular family (Deacon & Piercy, 2001).

Sculpting Activities

Sculpting is a technique associated with experiential family therapy models that can be used not only as an intervention but also as a way to gather information about family relationships (Deacon & Piercy, 2001). A standard method of using sculpting is to ask one family member to physically arrange others to represent the sculptor's picture of relationships in the family at a given point in time (Duhl, Kantor, & Duhl, 1973). One way of doing this is to say:

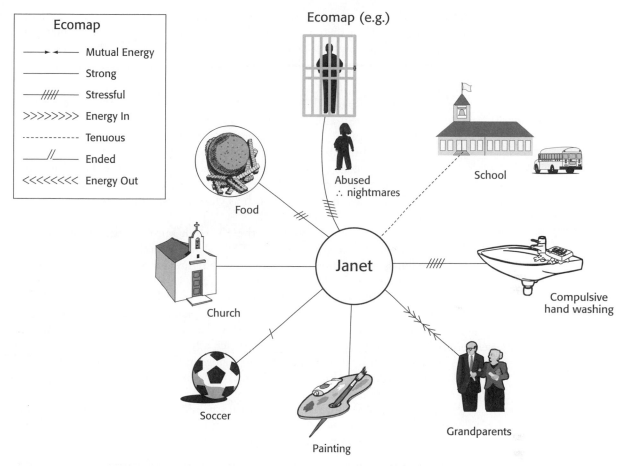

Figure 14.8 Ecomap completed by an adolescent with common ecomap symbols illustrating relationships and connections

Source: Ecomap courtesy of Arpana Gupta (M.A.Ed., NCC). Reprinted with permission.

Imagine that you are a sculptor and that your family is made of clay. Make a sculpture of your family. You can place them anywhere, in any position (illustrate by touching and moving the sculpture as you explain). Go ahead and be the sculptor. I want to see how your family looks to you. (Edwards, 2003, p. 145)

Sculptors can use distance, posture, facial expressions, and even props to illustrate their perceptions of relationships. After the sculpture is complete, the clinician asks questions and makes objective comments about the scene (Edwards, 2003). For example, the clinician may ask each person, "What is it like for you in this sculpture?" or "What about the sculpture surprises you?" In some cases, it may be helpful to ask the family to sculpt the scene again, this time depicting how they would like it to be. Throughout the process, the clinician gains insight into family members' perceptions of relationships, family issues, and potential goals for change.

Multiple variations of sculpting include the following:

- To assess family history, sculpt the family at some time in the past. Deacon and Piercy (2001) suggested that the family choose a time when things were peaceful or, alternatively, a time of crisis.

- Use linear sculpture to depict feelings, relationships, and other constructs that fall along a continuum (Constantine, 1978; Edwards, 2003). For example, ask members to arrange themselves along an imaginary line on the floor that represents a continuum of power (Deacon & Piercy, 2001). Other constructs that might be assessed include traits such as cheerfulness, talkativeness, and protectiveness.

- A unique form of sculpting is the Kvebaek family sculpting technique (Cromwell, Fournier, & Kvebaek, 1980). A board similar to a chessboard but containing 100 squares and several wooden figures representing different family members are needed for this sculpting exercise. Initially, the professional counselor meets individually with family members and asks them to place the figures representing the family on the board. Each person is asked to arrange the figures according to how close he or she feels to the other members and according to how close he or she thinks they feel to each other. Next, the same person is asked to show what he or she would like to change in the family and to move the figures accordingly. After each individual has completed the activity, the professional counselor invites the whole family to create their version of what the family actually looks like and of what they would like it to resemble. For some families, using a game board and small figures may feel less threatening than creating sculptures with actual family members.

> **Think About It 14.3**   How would you "sculpt" your family? What might your sculpting indicate about family relationships and interactions?

Other Qualitative Methods

Multiple methods of qualitative assessment besides those already mentioned can be used by skilled clinicians to gather family information. Examples include *timelines of family history* (e.g., Arrington, 1991; Goldman, 1990, 1992); *psychodrama* (Minuchin & Fishman, 1981; Moreno, 1945/1999); *photographic collages* (Deacon & Piercy, 2001); and the *Family Task Interview* (Kinston et al., 1985). Clinical judgment is essential for determining which, if any, qualitative assessment methods to use with a given family.

In making decisions about selecting qualitative assessment methods, it is helpful to ask the following questions:

- Does the activity relate to the family's unique personality and current concerns?
- Does each family member have an opportunity to tell his or her story?
- Does the assessment help the family draw on its strengths and resources?

It also is important to remember that some professional counselors will want to take into account family members' sensitivity, openness, groundedness in reality, physical limitations, and need for crisis intervention (Deacon & Piercy, 2001). In selecting and carrying out any assessment activity, it is the clinician's responsibility to protect the family members and act in their best interest. Moreover, clinicians are reminded that interpretations based on qualitative assessment are merely hypotheses, and that additional confirming evidence should be gathered to support or refute those hypotheses.

SUMMARY/CONCLUSION

Although challenging, assessing couples and families is a key component of effective marriage and family counseling. Professional counselors can use formal and informal methods of assessment to gather information, develop hypotheses, evaluate progress and outcomes, and facilitate change. Comprehensive assessment methods provide ways to combine objective data with subjective impressions, thus facilitating treatment planning and intervention.

Professional counselors who work with couples and families are typically guided by a holistic, systemic approach. Consequently, when they assess families, they are assessing systems rather than individuals. Constructs assessed often include the presenting problem, family composition, family process, family affect, family organization, strengths and resources, and goals for change.

There are a variety of ways to assess families. This chapter has focused on two broad categories: formalized assessment instruments and qualitative assessment techniques. Using multiple methods of assessment, which may involve combining formal and informal methods, is more effective than relying on a single approach. Professional counselors will want to acquire the knowledge and skills necessary to determine what assessment approaches to use when and with whom, so that they can work effectively with couples and families.

KEY TERMS

ecomap
family affect
family circle
family composition
family mapping
family organization
family processes

family resilience
genogram
joint family drawing
qualitative assessment
resources
sculpting
systems approach

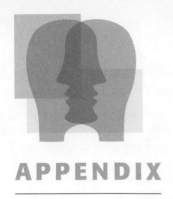

Responsibilities of Users of Standardized Tests (RUST) (3rd Edition)

Association for Assessment in Counseling (AAC)

Many recent events have influenced the use of tests and assessment in the counseling community. Such events include the use of tests in the educational accountability and reform movement, the publication of the *Standards for Educational and Psychological Testing* (American Educational Research Association [AERA], American Psychological Association [APA], National Council on Measurement in Education [NCME], 1999), the revision of the *Code of Fair Testing Practices in Education* (Joint Committee on Testing Practices [JCTP], 2002), the proliferation of technology-delivered assessment, and the historic passage of the *No Child Left Behind Act* (HR1, 2002) calling for expanded testing in reading/language arts, mathematics, and science that are aligned to state standards.

The purpose of this document is to promote the accurate, fair, and responsible use of standardized tests by the counseling and education communities. RUST is intended to address the needs of the members of the American Counseling Association (ACA) and its Divisions, Branches, and Regions, including counselors, teachers, administrators, and other human service workers. The general public, test developers, and policy makers will find this statement useful as they work with tests and testing issues. The principles in RUST apply to the use of testing instruments regardless of delivery methods (e.g., paper/pencil or computer administered) or setting (e.g., group or individual).

The intent of RUST is to help counselors and other educators implement responsible testing practices. The RUST does not intend to reach beyond or reinterpret the principles outlined in the *Standards for Educational and Psychological Testing* (AERA et al., 1999), nor was it developed to formulate a basis for legal action. The intent is to provide a concise statement useful in the ethical practice of testing. In addition, RUST is intended to enhance the guidelines found in ACA's *Code of Ethics and Standards of Practice* (ACA, 1997) and the *Code of Fair Testing Practices in Education* (JCTP, 2002).

Organization of Document: This document includes test user responsibilities in the following areas:

- Qualifications of Test Users
- Technical Knowledge
- Test Selection
- Test Administration
- Test Scoring
- Interpreting Test Results
- Communicating Test Results

QUALIFICATIONS OF TEST USERS

Qualified test users demonstrate appropriate education, training, and experience in using tests for the purposes under consideration. They adhere to the highest degree of ethical codes, laws, and standards governing professional practice. Lack of essential qualifications or ethical and legal compliance can lead to errors and subsequent harm to clients. Each professional is responsible for making judgments in each testing situation and cannot leave that responsibility either to clients or others in authority. The individual test user must obtain appropriate education and training, or arrange for professional supervision and assistance when engaged in testing in order to provide valuable, ethical, and effective assessment services to the public. Qualifications of test users depend on at least four factors:

- **Purposes of Testing:** A clear purpose for testing should be established. Because the purposes of testing direct how the results are used, qualifications beyond general testing competencies may be needed to interpret and apply data.
- **Characteristics of Tests:** Understanding of the strengths and limitations of each instrument used is a requirement.
- **Settings and Conditions of Test Use:** Assessment of the quality and relevance of test user knowledge and skill to the situation is needed before deciding to test or participate in a testing program.
- **Roles of Test Selectors, Administrators, Scorers, and Interpreters:** The education, training, and experience of test users determine which tests they are qualified to administer and interpret.

Each test user must evaluate his or her qualifications and competence for selecting, administering, scoring, interpreting, reporting, or communicating test results. Test users must develop the skills and knowledge for each test he or she intends to use.

TECHNICAL KNOWLEDGE

Responsible use of tests requires technical knowledge obtained through training, education, and continuing professional development. Test users should be conversant and competent in aspects of testing including:

- **Validity of Test Results:** Validity is the accumulation of evidence to support a specific interpretation of the test results. Since validity is a characteristic of test results, a test may have validities of varying degree, for different purposes. The concept of instructional validity relates to how well the test is aligned to state standards and classroom instructional objectives.
- **Reliability:** Reliability refers to the consistency of test scores. Various methods are used to calculate and estimate reliability depending on the purpose for which the test is used.
- **Errors of Measurement:** Various ways may be used to calculate the error associated with a test score. Knowing this and knowing the estimate of the size of the error allows the test user to provide a more accurate interpretation of the scores and to support better-informed decisions.
- **Scores and Norms:** Basic differences between the purposes of norm-referenced and criterion-referenced scores impact score interpretations.

TEST SELECTION

Responsible use of tests requires that the specific purpose for testing be identified. In addition, the test that is selected should align with that purpose, while considering the characteristics of the test and the test taker. Tests should not be administered without a specific purpose or need for information. Typical purposes for testing include:

- **Description:** Obtaining objective information on the status of certain characteristics such as achievement, ability, personality types, etc. is often an important use of testing.
- **Accountability:** When judging the progress of an individual or the effectiveness of an educational institution, strong alignment between what is taught and what is tested needs to be present.
- **Prediction:** Technical information should be reviewed to determine how accurately the test will predict areas such as appropriate course placement; selection for special programs, interventions, and institutions; and other outcomes of interest.
- **Program Evaluation:** The role that testing plays in program evaluation and how the test information may be used to supplement other information gathered about the program is an important consideration in test use.

Proper test use involves determining if the characteristics of the test are appropriate for the intended audience and are of sufficient technical quality for the purpose at hand. Some areas to consider include:

- **The Test Taker:** Technical information should be reviewed to determine if the test characteristics are appropriate for the test taker (e.g., age, grade level, language, cultural background).
- **Accuracy of Scoring Procedures:** Only tests that use accurate scoring procedures should be used.
- **Norming and Standardization Procedures:** Norming and standardization procedures should be reviewed to determine if the norm group is appropriate for the intended test takers. Specified test administration procedures must be followed.
- **Modifications:** For individuals with disabilities, alternative measures may need to be found and used and/or accommodations in test taking procedures may need to be employed. Interpretations need to be made in light of the modifications in the test or testing procedures.
- **Fairness:** Care should be taken to select tests that are fair to all test takers. When test results are influenced by characteristics or situations unrelated to what is being measured. (e.g., gender, age, ethnic background, existence of cheating, unequal availability of test preparation programs) the use of the resulting information is invalid and potentially harmful. In achievement testing, fairness also relates to whether or not the student has had an opportunity to learn what is tested.

TEST ADMINISTRATION

Test administration includes carefully following standard procedures so that the test is used in the manner specified by the test developers. The test administrator should ensure that test takers work within conditions that maximize opportunity for optimum performance. As appropriate, test takers, parents, and organizations should be involved in the various aspects of the testing process including.

Before administration it is important that relevant persons

- are informed about the standard testing procedures, including information about the purposes of the test, the kinds of tasks involved, the method of administration, and the scoring and reporting;
- have sufficient practice experiences prior to the test to include practice, as needed, on how to operate equipment for computer-administered tests and practice in responding to tasks;
- have been sufficiently trained in their responsibilities and the administration procedures for the test;
- have a chance to review test materials and administration sites and procedures prior to the time for testing to ensure standardized conditions and appropriate responses to any irregularities that occur;
- arrange for appropriate modifications of testing materials and procedures in order to accommodate test takers with special needs; and
- have a clear understanding of their rights and responsibilities.

During administration it is important that

- the testing environment (e.g., seating, work surfaces, lighting, room temperature, freedom from distractions) and psychological climate are conducive to the best possible performance of the examinees;
- sufficiently trained personnel establish and maintain uniform conditions and observe the conduct of test takers when large groups of individuals are tested;
- test administrators follow the instructions in the test manual; demonstrate verbal clarity; use verbatim directions; adhere to verbatim directions; follow exact sequence and timing; and use materials that are identical to those specified by the test publisher;
- a systematic and objective procedure is in place for observing and recording environmental, health, emotional factors, or other elements that may invalidate test performance and results; deviations from prescribed test administration procedures, including information on test accommodations for individuals with special needs, are recorded; and
- the security of test materials and computer-administered testing software is protected, ensuring that only individuals with a legitimate need for access to the materials/software are able to obtain such access and that steps to eliminate the possibility of breaches in test security and copyright protection are respected.

After administration it is important to

- collect and inventory all secure test materials and immediately report any breaches in test security; and
- include notes on any problems, irregularities, and accommodations in the test records.

These precepts represent the basic process for all standardized tests and assessments. Some situations may add steps or modify some of these to provide the best testing milieu possible.

TEST SCORING

Accurate measurement necessitates adequate procedures for scoring the responses of test takers. Scoring procedures should be audited as necessary to ensure consistency and accuracy of application.

- Carefully implement and/or monitor standard scoring procedures.
- When test scoring involves human judgment, use rubrics that clearly specify the criteria for scoring. Scoring consistency should be constantly monitored.
- Provide a method for checking the accuracy of scores when accuracy is challenged by test takers.

INTERPRETING TEST RESULTS

Responsible test interpretation requires knowledge about and experience with the test, the scores, and the decisions to be made. Interpretation of scores on any test should not take place without a thorough knowledge of the technical aspects of the test, the test results, and its limitations. Many factors can impact the valid and useful interpretations of test scores. These can be grouped into several categories including psychometric, test taker, and contextual, as well as others.

- **Psychometric Factors:** Factors such as the reliability, norms, standard error of measurement, and validity of the instrument are important when interpreting test results. Responsible test use considers these basic concepts and how each impacts the scores and hence the interpretation of the test results.
- **Test Taker Factors:** Factors such as the test taker's group membership and how that membership may impact the results of the test is a critical factor in the interpretation of test results. Specifically, the test user should evaluate how the test taker's gender, age, ethnicity, race, socioeconomic status, marital status, and so forth, impact on the individual's results.
- **Contextual Factors:** The relationship of the test to the instructional program, opportunity to learn, quality of the educational program, work and home environment, and other factors that would assist in understanding the test results are useful in interpreting test results. For example, if the test does not align to curriculum standards and how those standards are taught in the classroom, the test results may not provide useful information.

COMMUNICATING TEST RESULTS

Before communication of test results takes place, a solid foundation and preparation is necessary. That foundation includes knowledge of test interpretation and an understanding of the particular test being used, as provided by the test manual.

Conveying test results with language that the test taker, parents, teachers, clients, or general public can understand is one of the key elements in helping others understand the meaning of the test results. When reporting group results, the information needs to be supplemented with background information that can help explain the results with cautions about misinterpretations. The test user should indicate how the test results can be and should not be interpreted.

CLOSING

Proper test use resides with the test user—the counselor and educator. Qualified test users understand the measurement characteristics necessary to select good standardized tests, administer the tests according to specified procedures, assure accurate scoring, accurately interpret test scores for individuals and groups, and ensure productive applications of the results. This document provides guidelines for using tests responsibly with students and clients.

REFERENCES AND RESOURCE DOCUMENTS

American Counseling Association. (1997). *Code of ethics and standards of practice.* Alexandria, VA: Author.

American Counseling Association. (2003). *Standards for qualifications of test users*. Alexandria, VA: Author.

American Educational Research Association, American Psychological Association, National Council on Measurement in Education. (1999). *Standards for educational and psychological testing*. Washington, DC: American Educational Research Association.

American School Counselor Association & Association for Assessment in Counseling (1998). *Competencies in assessment and evaluation for school counselors*. Alexandria, VA: Author.

Joint Committee on Testing Practices. (2000) *Rights and responsibilities of test takers: Guidelines and expectations*, Washington, DC: Author.

Joint Committee on Testing Practices. (2002). *Code of fair testing practices in education*. Washington, DC: Author.

RUST Committee

Janet Wall, Chair	Brad Erford
James Augustin	David Lundberg
Charles Eberly	Timothy Vansickle

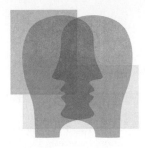

References

Abidin, R. (1995). *Parenting Stress Index* (3rd ed.). Odessa, FL: Psychological Assessment Resources.

Achenbach, T. M., & Rescorla, L. A. (2001). *Manual for the Achenbach System of Empirically Based Assessment* (*ASEBA*). Burlington, VT: ASEBA.

Achenbach System of Empirically Based Assessment (ASEBA). (2004). *ASEBA Products*. Retrieved June 15, 2004, from www.aseba.org/products/forms.html.

Alban, T. R., Lissitz, R. W., & Croninger, R. G. (2003, April). *Holding schools and teachers accountable: A comparison of analytic approaches and their implications for policy.* Paper presented at the annual meeting of the American Educational Research Association, San Diego, CA.

Albanese, M. A. (2001). Review of the *Hay Aptitude Test Battery.* In B. S. Plake & J. C. Impara (Eds.), *The fourteenth mental measurements yearbook* (pp. 529–532). Lincoln, NE: Buros Institute of Mental Measurements.

Alberto, P. A., & Troutman, A. C. (2003). *Applied behavior analysis for teachers* (6th ed.). Upper Saddle River, NJ: Pearson Education.

Alexopoulos, D. S., & Foudoulaki, E. (2002). Construct validity of the *Piers-Harris Children's Self-Concept Scale. Psychological Reports, 91,* 827–838.

Algozzine, B., Eaves, R. C., Mann, L., & Vance, H. R. (1993). *Slosson Full-Range Intelligence Test: Examiner's manual.* East Aurora, NY: Slosson Educational Publications.

Allen, M. J., & Yen, W. M. (1979). *Introduction to measurement theory*. Monterey, CA: Brooks/Cole.

Allport, G. W. (1937). *Personality: A psychological interpretation.* New York: Holt, Rinehart & Winston.

Allport, G. W., & Odbert, H. S. (1936). Trait-names, a psycholexical study. *Psychological Monographs, 47* (Whole No. 211).

Ambrosini, P., & Dixon, J. F. (1996). *Schedule for Affective Disorders and Schizophrenia for School-Age Children* (*K-SADS-IVR*). Philadelphia: Allegheny University of Health Success.

American College Testing, Inc. (2004). *The American College Testing (ACT) Assessment* Student Report. Iowa City, IA: Author.

American College Testing, Inc. (2005). *The American College Testing Assessment*. Retrieved January 24, 2005, from www.act.org.

American Counseling Association. (2005a). *Code of ethics and standards of practice*. Alexandria, VA: Author.

American Counseling Association. (2005b). *Position Statement On High Stakes Testing*. Alexandria, VA: Author.

American Educational Research Association. (2000). *AERA position statement concerning high-stakes testing in preK-12*. Washington, DC: Author.

American Educational Research Association, American Psychological Association, & National Council on Measurement in Education. (1974). *Standards for educational and psychological tests and manuals.* Washington, DC: American Psychological Association.

American Educational Research Association, American Psychological Association, & National Council on Measurement in Education. (1985). *Standards for educational and psychological testing* (2nd ed.). Washington, DC: American Psychological Association.

American Educational Research Association, American Psychological Association, & National Council on Measurement in Education. (1999). *Standards for educational and psychological testing* (3rd ed.). Washington, DC: American Psychological Association.

American Guidance Services. (1969). *Minnesota Rate of Manipulation Test: Examiner's manual.* Circle Pines, MN: Author.

American Guidance Services. (2005a). *Catalog.* Circle Pines, MN: Author.

American Guidance Services. (2005b). *WRMT-R/NU technical information.* Retrieved on January 7, 2005, from www.agsnet.com/assessments/technical/ wrmt.asp#a.

American Heritage College Dictionary. (1992). Boston: Houghton Mifflin.

American Psychiatric Association. (1987). *Diagnostic and statistical manual of mental disorders* (3rd ed., rev.). Washington, DC: Author.

American Psychiatric Association. (1994). *Diagnostic and statistical manual of mental disorders* (4th ed.). Washington, DC: Author.

American Psychiatric Association. (2000). *Diagnostic and statistical manual of mental disorders* (4th ed., text rev.). Washington, DC: Author.

American Psychological Association. (1954). *Technical recommendations for psychological tests and diagnostic techniques.* Washington, DC: Author.

American School Counselor Association. (1999). *Position statement: Multicultural counseling.* Alexandria, VA: Author.

American School Counselor Association. (2003). *The national model for school counseling programs.* Alexandria, VA: Author.

Anastasi, A. (1976). *Psychological testing* (4th ed.). New York: Macmillan.

Anastasi, A. (1985). Interpreting results from multiscore batteries. *Journal of Counseling and Development, 64,* 84–86.

Anastasi, A., & Urbina, S. (1997). *Psychological testing* (7th ed.). Upper Saddle River NJ: Prentice Hall.

Anderson, W. (1995). Ethnic and cross-cultural differences on the MMPI-2. In J. C. Duckworth & W. P. Anderson, *MMPI and MMPI-2 interpretation manual for counselors and clinicians* (pp. 382–395). Bristol, PA: Accelerated Press.

Andrew, D. M., Paterson, D. G., & Longstaff, H. P. (1979). *Minnesota Clerical Test.* San Antonio, TX: Psychological Corporation.

Angold, A., Cox, A., Prendergast, M., Rutter, M., Simonoff, E. (1996). *The Child and Adolescent Psychiatric Assessment (CAPA).* Duke University School of Medicine, Durham, NC.

Archer, R. P., & Handel, R. W. (2001). The effectiveness of *MMPI-A* items in discriminating between normative and clinical samples. *Journal of Personality Assessment, 77,* 420–435.

Archer, R. P., & Krishnamurthy, R. (2002). *Essentials of MMPI-A assessment.* New York: Wiley.

Ardovino, J., Hollingsworth, J., & Ybarra, S. (2000). *Multiple measures: Accurate ways to assess student achievement.* Thousand Oaks, CA: Corwin Press.

Arenth, P. M., Bogner, J. A., Corrigan, J. D., & Schmidt, L. (2001). The utility of the *Substance Abuse Subtle Screening Inventory-3* for use with individuals with brain injury. *Brain Injury, 15,* 499–510.

Arredondo, D. E., & Butler, F. S. (1994). Affective comorbidity in psychiatrically hospitalized adolescents with conduct disorder or oppositional defiant disorder: Should conduct disorder be treated with mood stabilizer? *Journal of Child and Adolescent Psychopharmacology, 4,* 151–158.

Arrington, D. (1991). Thinking systems—seeing systems: An integrative model for systemically oriented art therapy. *Arts in Psychotherapy, 18,* 201–211.

Arter, J. (2004). Assessment for learning: Classroom assessment to improve student achievement and well-being. In J. E. Wall & G. R. Walz (Eds.), *Measuring up: Assessment issues for teachers, counselors, and administrators* (pp. 463–484). Greensboro, NC: CAPS Publications.

Arvy, R. D., & Campion, J. E. (1982). The employment interview: A summary and review of recent research. *Personnel Psychology, 35,* 281–322.

Asai, S., & Olson, D. (2004). Culturally sensitive adaptation of *PREPARE w*ith Japanese premarital couples. *Journal of Marital and Family Therapy, 30,* 411–426.

Association for Assessment in Counseling and Education (AACE). (2003a) *Responsibilities of Users of Standardized Tests—Third Edition* (*RUST-3*). Alexandria, VA: Author.

Association for Assessment in Counseling and Education (AACE). (2003b). *Standards for multicultural assessment.* Alexandria, VA: Author.

Atkinson, M. J. (2003). Review of the *California Psychological Inventory.* In B. S. Plake, J. C. Impara, & R. A. Spies (Eds.), *The fifteenth mental measurements yearbook* (pp. 160–161). Lincoln, NE: Buros Institute of Mental Measurements.

Atlas, J. A. (2001). Review of the *Test of Nonverbal Intelligence—Third Edition.* In B. S. Plake & J. C. Impara (Eds.), *The fourteenth mental measurements yearbook* (pp. 1259–1260). Lincoln, NE: Buros Institute of Mental Measurements.

Baldwin, A. L., Kalhorn, J., & Breese, F. H. (1945). Patterns of parent behavior. *Psychological Monographs, 58* (Whole No. 268).

Bandura, A. (1986). *Social foundations of thought and action.* Upper Saddle River, NJ: Prentice Hall.

Barak, A. (2003). Ethical and professional issues in career assessment on the Internet. *Journal of Career Assessment, 11,* 3–21.

Baughman, E. E., & Dahlstrom, W. B. (1968). *Negro and white children: A psychological study in the rural south.* New York: Academic Press.

Bayley, N. (1993). *Bayley Scales of Infant Development—Second Edition* (*Bayley-II*). San Antonio, TX: PsychCorp.

Beatty L. S., Gardner, E. F., Madden, R., & Karlsen, B. (1984). *Stanford Diagnostic Mathematics Test, 3rd Edition*: *Directions for administering.* San Antonio, TX: Psychological Corporation.

Beatty, L. S., Madden, R., Gardner, E. F., & Karlsen, T. (1996). *Stanford Diagnostic— Mathematics Test—Fourth Edition.* San Antonio, TX: Psychological Corporation.

Beck, A. T. (1991). *Manual for the Beck Scale for Suicide Ideation.* San Antonio, TX: Psychological Corporation.

Beck, A. T. (1993). *Beck Anxiety Inventory.* San Antonio, TX: Psychological Corporation.

Beck, A. T., Epstein, N., Brown, G., & Steer, R. A. (1988). An inventory for measuring clinical anxiety: Psychometric properties. *Journal of Consulting and Clinical Psychology, 56,* 893–897.

Beck, A. T., Kovacs, M., & Weissman, A. (1979). Assessment of suicide intention: The *Scale for Suicide Ideation. Journal of Consulting and Clinical Psychology, 47,* 343–352.

Beck, A. T., & Steer, R. (1993). *Manual for the Beck Hopelessness Scale.* San Antonio, TX: Psychological Corporation.

Beck, A. T., Steer, R. A., & Brown, G. K. (1996). *Manual for the Beck Depression Inventory— Second Edition.* San Antonio, TX: Psychological Corporation.

Beery, K. E. (1997). *Manual for the Beery-Buktenica Developmental Test of Visual-Motor Integration* (*VMI*). Parsippany, NJ: Modern Curriculum Press.

Bell, N. L., Lassiter, K. S., Matthews, T. D., & Hutchinson, M. B. (2001). Comparison of the *Peabody Picture Vocabulary Test—Third Edition* and *Wechsler Adult Intelligence Scale—Third Edition* with university students. *Journal of Clinical Psychology, 57,* 417–422.

Bellak, L. (1992). *The TAT, CAT and SAT in clinical use* (Rev. ed.). New York: Grune & Stratton.

Bellak, L., & Bellak, S. S. (1992). *Manual for the Children's Apperception Test—Revised*. Larchmont, NY: Children's Apperception Test.

Beller, M., & Gafni, N. (1996). The 1991 international assessment of educational progress in mathematics and sciences: The gender differences and perspectives. *Journal of Educational Psychology, 88,* 365–377.

Benes, K. M. (1995). Review of the *Social Skills Rating System*. In J. C. Conoley & J. C. Impara (Eds.), *The twelfth mental measurements yearbook*. Lincoln, NE: Buros Institute of Mental Measurements.

Benet, W. E. (2005). Review of the *Forer Structured Sentence Completion Test*. Benet Clinical Assessment webpage. Retrieved January 25, 2005 from http://cps.nova.edu/~cpphelp/FSSCT .html.

Bennett, G. K. (1980). *Bennett Mechanical Comprehension Test* (2nd ed.). San Antonio, TX: Psychological Corporation.

Bennett, G. K. (1985). *Bennett Hand-Tool Dexterity Test*. San Antonio, TX: Psychological Corporation.

Bennett, G. K., Seashore, H. G., & Wesman, A. G. (1990). *Manual for the Differential Aptitude Test*. San Antonio, TX: Psychological Corporation.

Bernt, F. (2001). Review of the *Marital Satisfaction Inventory—Revised*. In B. S. Plake & J. C. Impara (Eds.), *The fourteenth mental measurements yearbook* (pp. 711–712). Lincoln, NE: Buros Institute of Mental Measurements.

Bessai, F. (2001). Review of the *Peabody Picture Vocabulary Test*. In B. S. Plake & J. C. Impara (Eds.), *The fourteenth mental measurements yearbook* (pp. 908–909). Lincoln, NE: Buros Institute of Mental Measurements.

Betz, N. E., Borgen, F. H., & Harmon, L. W. (1996). *Skills Confidence Inventory: Applications and technical guide*. Palo Alto, CA: Consulting Psychologists Press.

Bijou, S. W., Peterson, R. F., & Ault, M. H. (1968). A method to integrate descriptive and experimental field studies at the level of data and empirical concepts. *Journal of Applied Behavioral Analysis, 1,* 175–191.

Binet, A., & Henri, V. (1895a). La memoire des mots. *L'Année Psychologique, 1,* 1–23.

Binet, A., & Henri, V. (1895b). La memoire des phrases. *L'Année Psychologique, 1,* 24–59.

Binet, A., & Henri, V. (1895c). La psychologie individuelle. *L'Année Psychologique, 2,* 411–465.

Binet, A., & Simon, T. (1905). Methodes nouvelles pour le diagnostic du niveau intellectual des anormaux. *L'Année Psychologique, 11,* 191–244.

Binet, A., & Simon, T. (1908). La development de l'intelligence chez les enfants [The development of intelligence in children] (E. S. Kite, Trans.). In J. J. Jenkins & D. G. Paterson (reprint Eds.), *Studies in individual differences: The search for intelligence* (pp. 90–96). New York: Appleton-Century-Crofts (reprinted in 1961).

Birmaher, B., Ryan, N. D., Williamson, D. E., Brent, D. A., & Kaufman, J. (1996). Childhood and adolescent depression: A review of the past 10 years: Part II. *Journal of the American Academy of Child and Adolescent Psychiatry, 35,* 1575–1583.

Birren, J. E. (1968). Increments and decrements in the intellectual status of the aged. *Psychiatric Research Reports, 23,* 207–214.

Birren, J. E., & Schaie, K. W. (1985). *Handbook of psychology of aging* (2nd ed.). New York: Van Nostrand Reinhold.

Blair, J. (2005). Review of the *Reynolds Adolescent Depression Scale, Second Edition*. In B. S. Plake, J. C. Impara, & R. A. Spies (Eds.), *The sixteenth mental measurements yearbook*. Lincoln, NE: Buros Institute of Mental Measurements.

Bloom, B. S. (1956). *Taxonomy of educational objectives: The classification of educational goals. Handbook 1. Cognitive domain*. New York: David McKay.

Bohrnstedt, G. W. (1983). Measurement. In P. H. Rossi, J. D. Wright, & A. B. Anderson (Eds.), *Handbook of survey research* (pp. 69–121). New York: Academic Press.

Bolton, D. L. (1995). Review of the *Career Beliefs Inventory*. In. J. C. Conoley & J. C. Impara (Eds.), *The twelfth mental measurements yearbook* (pp. 159–160). Lincoln, NE: Buros Institute of Mental Measurements.

Born, M., Bleichrodt, N., & van der Flier, H. (1987). Cross-cultural comparison of sex-related differences on intelligence tests: A meta-analysis. *Journal of Cross-Cultural Psychology, 18,* 283–314.

Botwin, M. D. (1995). Review of the *Revised NEO Personality Inventory.* In J. C. Impara & B. S. Plake (Eds.), *The twelfth mental measurements yearbook* (pp. 862–863). Lincoln, NE: Buros Institute of Mental Measurements.

Boughner, S. R., Hayes, S. F., Bubenzer, D. L., & West, J. D. (1994). Use of standardized assessment instruments by marital and family therapists: A survey. *Journal of Marital and Family Therapy, 20,* 69–75.

Bourne, S. K., Bryant, R. A., Griffiths, R. A., Touyz, S. W., & Beumont, P. J. V. (1998). Bulimia Nervosa, restrained, and unrestrained eaters: A comparison of non-binge eating behavior. *International Journal of Eating Disorders, 24,* 185–192.

Bowen, M. (1978). *Family therapy in clinical practice.* New York: Jason Aronson.

Bowman, M. L. (1989). Testing individual differences in ancient China. *American Psychologist, 44,* 576–578.

Boyle, G. J. (1995). Review of the *Personality Assessment Inventory*. In J. C. Conoley & J. C. Impara (Eds.), *The twelfth mental measurements yearbook* (pp. 746–766). Lincoln, NE: Buros Institute of Mental Measurements.

Brace, C. (1995). Race and political correctness. *American Psychologist, 50,* 725–726.

Bracey, G. W. (1994). Finding gifted kids. *Phi Delta Kappan, 76,* 252.

Bradley, R. H. (1985). Review of *Gesell School Readiness Test*. In J. V. Mitchell (Ed.), *The ninth mental measurements yearbook* (pp. 609–610). Lincoln, NE: Buros Institute of Mental Measurements.

Bradway, K. P., Thompson, C. W., & Cravens, R. B. (1958). Preschool IQs after twenty-five years. *Journal of Educational Psychology, 49,* 278–281.

Branden, J. B. (1995). Review of the *Wechsler Intelligence Scale for Children—Third Edition.* In J. C. Conoley & J. C. Impara (Eds.), *The twelfth mental measurements yearbook* (pp. 1098–1102). Lincoln, NE: Buros Institute of Mental Measurements.

Bray, J. H. (1995). Family assessment. *Family Relations, 44,* 469–477.

Brennan, R. L. (2000). Performance assessment from the perspective of generalizability theory. *Applied Psychological Measurement, 24,* 339–353.

Brennan, R. L. (2001a). *Generalizability theory.* New York: Springer-Verlag.

Brennan, R. L. (2001b). *Manual for mGENOVA.* Iowa City: Iowa Testing Programs, University of Iowa.

Brennan, R. L. (2001c). *Manual for urGENOVA.* Iowa City: Iowa Testing Programs, University of Iowa.

Brennan, R. L., & Kane, M. T. (1977). An index of dependability for mastery tests. *Journal of Educational Measurement, 14,* 277–289.

Brennan, R. L., & Lee, W. C. (1999). Conditional scale-score standard errors of measurement under binomial and compound binomial assumptions. *Educational and Psychological Measurement, 59,* 5–24.

Brooks, S. J., & Kutcher, S. (2001). Diagnosis and measurement of adolescent depression: A review of commonly utilized instruments. *Journal of Child and Adolescent Psychopharmacology, 11,* 341–376.

Brown, A. (1996, Winter). Mood disorders in children and adolescents. *NARSAD Research Newsletter.*

Brown, D. (2002). The role of work values and cultural values in occupational choice, satisfaction, and success: A theoretical statement. In D. Brown & Associates (Eds.), *Career choice and development* (4th ed., pp. 465–509). San Francisco: Jossey-Bass.

Brown, J. I., Fishco, V. V., & Hanna, A. (1993). *Nelson-Denny Reading Test, Forms G & H.* Itasca, IL: Riverside Publishing.

Brown, L., Sherbenou, R. J., & Johnsen, S. K. (1997). *Manual for the Tests of Nonverbal Intelligence—Third Edition (TONI-III).* Austin, TX: PRO-ED.

Brown, M. B. (2001). Review of the *Self-Directed Search: Fourth Edition.* In B. S. Plake & J. C. Impara (Eds.), *The fourteenth mental measurements yearbook* (pp. 1105-1107). Lincoln, NE: Buros Institute of Mental Measurements.

Brown, R. (1998). Review of the *Tennessee Self-Concept Scale—Second Edition.* In J. C. Impara & B. S. Plake (Eds.), *The thirteenth mental measurements yearbook* (pp. 1010–1011). Lincoln, NE: Buros Institute of Mental Measurements.

Brown, V., Hammill, D., & Weiderholt, J. L. (1995). *Manual for the Test of Reading Comprehension—Third Edition (TORC-3).* Austin, TX: PRO-ED.

Bubenzer, D. L., Zimpfer, D. G., & Mahrle, C. L. (1990). Standardized individual appraisal in agency and private practice: A survey. *Journal of Mental Health Counseling, 12,* 51–66.

Buboltz, W. C., Jr., Johnson, P., & Woller, K. M. P. (2003). Psychological reactance in college students: Family-of-origin predictors. *Journal of Counseling and Development, 81,* 311–317.

Buck, J. (1964). *Manual for the House-Tree-Person.* Los Angeles: Western Psychological Services.

Budd, K. S., & Heilman, N. (1992). Review of the *Dyadic Adjustment Scale.* In J. J. Kramer & J. C. Conoley (Eds.), *The eleventh mental measurements yearbook* (pp. 296–297). Lincoln, NE: Buros Institute of Mental Measurements.

Burgemeister, B. B., Blum, L. H., & Lorge, I. (1972). *The Columbia Mental Maturity Scale.* San Antonio, TX: Psychological Corporation.

Burns, R. (1982). *Self-growth in families: Kinetic Family Drawings (K-F-D) research and application.* New York: Brunner/Mazel.

Burns, R., & Kaufman, H. (1970). *Kinetic family drawings K-F-D: An introduction to understanding children through kinetic drawings.* New York: Brunner/Mazel.

Burns, R., & Kaufman, H. (1972). *Actions, styles, and symbols in Kinetic Family Drawings (K-F-D).* New York: Brunner/Mazel.

Buros, O. K. (Ed.) (1938). *The 1938 mental measurements yearbook.* New Brunswick, NJ: Rutgers University Press.

Bussing, R., Schuhmann, E., & Belin, T. (1998). Diagnostic utility of two commonly used ADHD screening measures among special educational students. *Journal of the American Academy of Child and Adolescent Psychiatry, 37,* 74–82.

Bussing, R., Zima, B. T., Perwien, A. R., Belin, T. R., & Widawski, M. (1998). Children in special education: Attention Deficit Hyperactivity Disorder, use of services, and unmet need. *American Journal of Public Health, 88,* 1–7.

Butcher, J. N., Graham, J. R., Ben-Porath, Y. S., Tellegen, A., Dahlstrom, W. G., & Kaemmer, B. (1989). *The Minnesota Multiphasic Personality Inventory—Second Edition (MMPI-2).* Minneapolis: University of Minnesota Press.

Butcher, J. N., Graham, J. R., Ben-Porath, Y. S., Tellegen, A., Dahlstrom, W. G., & Kaemmer, B. (2001). *Manual for administration, scoring, and interpretation of the Minnesota Multiphasic Personality Inventory—Second Edition.* Minneapolis: University of Minnesota Press.

Butcher, J. N., & Han, K. (1995). Development of an *MMPI-2* scale to assess the presentation of self in a superlative manner: The *S* Scale. In J. N. Butcher & C. D. Spielberger (Eds.), *Advances in personality assessment* (Vol. 10, pp. 25–50). Hillside, NJ: Erlbaum.

Butcher, J. N., Williams, C. L., Graham, J. R., Archer, R. P., Tellegen, A., & Ben-Porath, Y. S. (1992). *The Minnesota Multiphasic Personality Inventory—Adolescent* (*MMPI-A*): *Manual for administration, scoring, and interpretation.* Minneapolis: University of Minnesota Press.

Campbell, D. P. (1992). *Campbell Interest and Skills Survey manual.* Minneapolis, MN: National Computer Systems.

Campbell, G. A., & Ashmore, R. J. (1995). Test review: The *Slosson Intelligence Test—Revised* (*SIT-R*). *Measure and Evaluation in Counseling and Development, 28*, 116–119.

Campbell, M., Cueva, J. E., & Hallin, A. (1996). Autism and pervasive developmental disorders. In J. M. Wiener (Ed.), *Diagnosis and psychopharmacology of childhood and adolescent disorders* (2nd ed., pp. 151–192). New York: Wiley.

Campbell, V. L. (2000). A framework for using tests in counseling. In C. E. Watkins & V. L. Campbell (Eds.), *Testing and assessment in counseling practice* (2nd ed., pp. 3–11). Mahwah, NJ: Erlbaum.

Campos, L. P. (1989). Adverse impact, unfairness, and bias in the psychological screening of Hispanic peace officers. *Hispanic Journal of Behavioral Sciences, 11*, 122–135.

Canivez, G. L., & Watkins, M. N. (1998). Long-term stability of the *Wechsler Intelligence Scale for Children—Third Edition. Psychological Assessment, 10,* 285–291.

Cantwell, P. D. (1996). Attention Deficit Disorder: A review of the past 10 years. *Journal of the American Academy of Child and Adolescent Psychiatry, 35,* 978–987.

Capraro, R. M., & Capraro, M. M. (2002). *Myers-Briggs Type Indicator* score reliability across studies: A meta-analytic reliability generalization study. *Educational and Psychological Measurement, 62,* 590–602.

Carey, M. P., Gresham, F. M., Ruggiero, L., Faulstich, M. E., & Engart, P. (1987). *Children's Depression Inventory*: Construct and discriminate validity across clinical and non-referred (control) populations. *Journal of Consulting and Clinical Psychology, 55,* 755–761.

Cattell, J. M. (1890). Mental tests and measurements. *Mind, 15,* 373–381.

Cattell, P. (1946). *Cattell Infant Intelligence Scale.* San Antonio, TX: PsychCorp.

Cattell, R. B. (1943). The measurement of adult intelligence. *Psychological Bulletin, 40,* 153–193.

Cattell, R. B. (1963). Theory of fluid and crystallized intelligence: A critical experiment. *Journal of Educational Psychology, 54,* 1–22.

Cattell, R. B. (1971). *Abilities: Their structure, growth, and action.* Boston: Houghton Mifflin.

Cattell, R. B. (1979). Are culture fair intelligence tests possible and necessary? *Journal of Research and Development in Education, 12,* 3–13.

Cattell, R. B., & Cattell, A. K. S. (1950). *The Culture Fair Intelligence Test* (*CFIT*). Champaign, IL: Institute for Personality and Ability Testing.

Cattell, R. B., Cattell, A. K. S., & Catell, H. E. P. (1993). *16PF* (5th ed.). Champaign, IL: Institute for Personality and Ability Testing.

Chase, C. (1996). Estimating the reliability of criterion-referenced tests before administration. *Mid-Western Educational Researcher, 9,* 2–4.

Chernyshenko, O., Stark, S., & Chan, K. (2001). Investigating the hierarchical factor structure of the fifth edition of the *16PF*: An application of the Schmid-Leiman orthogonalization procedure. *Educational and Psychological Measurement, 61,* 290–302.

Chipuser, H. M., Rovine, M., & Plomin, R. (1990). LISREL modeling: Genetic and environmental influences on IQ revisited. *Intelligence, 14,* 11–29.

Chiu, L. (1988). Testing the test: Measures of self-esteem for school-aged children. *Journal of Counseling and Development, 66,* 298–301.

Choca, J. P. (2001). Review of the *Millon Clinical Multiaxial Inventory—Third Edition.* In B. S. Plake & J. C. Impara (Eds.), *The fourteenth mental measurements yearbook* (pp. 765–766). Lincoln, NE: Buros Institute of Mental Measurements.

Ciechalski, J. C. (2002). *Self-Directed Search*. In J. T. Kapes & E. A. Whitfield (Eds.), *A counselor's guide to career assessment instruments* (4th ed., pp. 276–287). Tulsa, OK: National Career Development Association.

Cizek, G. J. (2003). Review of the *Woodcock-Johnson III*. In B. S. Plake, J. C. Impara, & R. A. Spies (Eds.), *The fifteenth mental measurements yearbook* (pp. 1020–1024). Lincoln, NE: Buros Institute of Mental Measurements.

Claiborn, C. D. (1995). Review of the *Minnesota Multiphasic Personality Inventory—Adolescent*. In J. C. Conoley & J. C. Impara (Eds.), *The twelfth mental measurements yearbook* (pp. 627–328). Lincoln, NE: Buros Institute of Mental Measurements.

Clark, B. (1979). *Growing up gifted* (3rd ed.). Columbus, OH: Merrill.

Clark, D. C., & Fawcett, J. (1992). Review of empirical risk factors for evaluation of the suicidal patient. In B. Bongar (Ed.), *Suicide: Guidelines for assessment, management, and treatment* (pp. 16–48). New York: Oxford University Press.

Clark, L. A., Watson, D., & Reynolds, S. (1995). Diagnosis and classification in psychopathology: Challenges to the current system and future directions. *Annual Review of Psychology, 46,* 121–153.

Clark, P., McCallum, R. S., Edwards, R. P., & Hildman, L. K. (1987). Use of the *Slosson Intelligence Test* in screening of gifted children. *Journal of School Psychology, 25,* 189–192.

Cliff, N. (1987). *Analyzing multivariate data*. San Diego, CA: Harcourt Brace Jovanovich.

Cohen, J. (1988). *Statistical power analysis for the behavioral sciences* (2nd ed.). Hillsdale, NJ: Erlbaum.

Cohen, R. J., & Swerdlik, M. E. (1999). *Psychological testing and assessment: An introduction to tests and measurements* (4th ed.). Mountain View, CA: Mayfield.

College Board (2005a). *The Graduate Record Exam*. Princeton, NJ: Educational Testing Service. Retrieved January 24, 2005, from www.collegeboard.com.

College Board. (2005b). The *Preliminary Scholastic Assessment Test / National Merit Scholarship Qualifying Test (PSAT/NMSQT)*. Princeton, NJ: Author.

College Board. (2005c). *The Scholastic Assessment Test (SAT)*. Princeton, NJ: Educational Testing Service. Retrieved January 24, 2005, from www.collegeboard.com.

College Entrance Examination Board. (2002). *Guidelines and uses of College Board test scores and related data*. Princeton, NJ: Author.

Compton, C. (1984). *A guide to 75 tests for special education*. Belmont, CA: Fearon Education.

Conn, M. R., & Rieke, S. L. (1994). *Technical manual for 16PF*. Champaign, IL: Institute for Personality and Ability Testing.

Conners, C. K. (1997). *Manual for the Conners' Rating Scales—Revised*. North Tonawanda, NY: Multi-Health Systems.

Conners, C. K., Erhardt, D., & Sparrow, E. P. (1999). *Manual for the Conners' Adult ADHD Rating Scales (CAARS)*. North Tonawanda, NY: Multi-Health Systems.

Conners, C. K., & Wells, S. (1997). *Conners-Wells Adolescent Self-Report Scale (CASS)*. North Tonawanda, NY: Multi-Health Systems.

Connolly, A. J. (1998). *Manual for the KeyMath—Revised: A diagnostic inventory of essential mathematics—1998 Normative Update* (KeyMath-R/NU). Circle Pines, MN: American Guidance Services.

Consolvo, C. (2001). Book review of the *Self-Directed Search* and related Holland career materials: A practitioner's guide. *Counselor Education and Supervision, 40,* 230–233.

Constantine, L. (1978). Family sculpture and relationship mapping techniques. *Journal of Marriage and Family Counseling, 4,* 13–23.

Constantine, M. (2001). Theoretical orientation, empathy, and multicultural counseling competence in school counselor trainees. *Professional School Counseling, 4,* 342–348.

Cooley, E. J., & Ayres, R. R. (1988). Cluster scores for the *Piers-Harris Children's Self-Concept Scale*: Reliability and independence. *Educational & Psychological Measurement, 48,* 1019–1024.

Cooper, C. (2001). Review of the *Devereux Scales of Mental Disorders*. In B. S. Plake & J. C. Impara (Eds.), *The fourteenth mental measurements yearbook* (pp. 408–410). Lincoln, NE: Buros Institute of Mental Measurements.

Coopersmith, S. (1981). *The antecedents of self-esteem*. Palo Alto, CA: Consulting Psychologists Press.

Coopersmith, S. (1989). *Self-Esteem Inventories manual*. Palo Alto, CA: Consulting Psychologists Press.

Cosden, M. (2001). Review of the *Roberts Apperception Test for Children*. In B. S. Plake & J. C. Impara (Eds.), *The fourteenth mental measurements yearbook* (pp. 1030–1032). Lincoln, NE: Buros Institute of Mental Measurements.

Costa, P. T., Jr., & McCrae, R. R. (1990). Personality disorders and the five-factor model. *Journal of Personality Disorders, 4,* 362–371.

Costa, P. T., Jr., & McCrae, R. R. (1992). *Revised NEO Personality Inventory (NEO-PI-R) and NEO Five-Factor Inventory (NEO-FFI) professional manual*. Odessa, FL: Psychological Assessment Resources.

Costello, J. & Dickie, J. (1970). *Leiter* and *Stanford-Binet* IQ's of preschool disadvantaged children. *Developmental Psychology, 2,* 314.

Council for Accreditation of Counseling and Related Educational Programs. (2001). *Council for Accreditation of Counseling and Related Educational Programs—2001 accreditation manual*. Alexandria, VA: Author.

Coupland, S. K., Serovich, J., & Glenn, J. E. (1995). Reliability in constructing genograms: A study among marriage and family therapy doctoral students. *Journal of Marital and Family Therapy, 18,* 323–333.

Crace, R. K., & Brown, D. (1994). *Life Values Inventory* [Electronic version]. Williamsburg, VA: Applied Psychological Resources. Retrieved January 6, 2005, from www.life-values.com.

Craighead, W. E., Curry, J. F., & Ilardi, S. S. (1995). Relationship of *Children's Depression Inventory* factors to major depression among adolescents. *Psychological Assessment, 7,* 171–176.

Crawford, J. E., & Crawford, D. M. (1985). *Crawford Small Parts Dexterity Test*. San Antonio, TX: Psychological Corporation.

Crick, J. E., & Brennan, R. L. (1983). *Manual for GENOVA: A generalized analysis of variance system*. Iowa City, IA: ACT.

Crites, J. O. (1999). Operational definitions of vocational interests. In M. L. Savickas & A. R. Spokane (Eds.), *Vocational interests: Meaning, measurement, and counseling use*. Palo Alto, CA: Davies-Black.

Crocker, L. (2001). Review of the *Woodcock Reading Mastery Tests—Revised/Normative Update (WRMT-R/NU)*. In B. S. Plake & J. C. Impara (Eds.), *The fourteenth mental measurements yearbook* (pp. 1370–1371). Lincoln, NE: Buros Institute of Mental Measurements.

Crocker, L., & Algina, J. (1986). *Introduction to classical and modern test theory*. Fort Worth, TX: Harcourt Brace Jovanovich College Publishers.

Crompton, N. L. (2003). Review of the *Gray Oral Reading Test—Fourth Edition (GORT-4)*. In B. S. Plake, J. C. Impara, & R. A. Spies (Eds.), *The fifteenth mental measurements yearbook* (pp. 417–419). Lincoln, NE: Buros Institute of Mental Measurements.

Cromwell, R., Fournier, D., & Kvebaek, D. (1980). *The Kvebaek Family Sculpture Technique: A diagnostic and research tool in family therapy*. Jonesboro, TN: Pilgrimage Press.

Cronbach, L. J. (1951). Coefficient alpha and the internal structure of a test. *Psychometrika, 16,* 297–334.

Cronbach, L. J. (1984). *Essentials of psychological testing* (4th ed.). New York: Harper & Row.

Cronbach, L. J., & Furby, L. (1970). How should we measure change—or should we? *Psychological Bulletin, 74,* 68–80.

Cross, L. H. (2001). *Review of the Peabody Individual Achievement Test—Revised.* In B. S. Plake & J. C. Impara (Eds.), *The fourteenth mental measurements yearbook* (pp. 904–906). Lincoln, NE: Buros Institute of Mental Measurements.

CTB/McGraw-Hill (2001). *TerraNova—Second Edition* (*TerraNova 2*). Monterey, CA: Author.

CTB/McGraw-Hill (2005). *TerraNova 2.* Monterey, CA.: Author.

Cull, J. G., & Gill, W. S. (1992). *Suicide Probability Scale.* Los Angeles: Western Psychological Services.

Cundick, B. P. (1976). Measures of intelligence on Southwest Indian students. *Journal of Social Psychology, 81,* 151–156.

Cundick, B. P. (1989). Review of the *Kinetic Drawing System for Family and School.* In J. C. Conoley & J. J. Kramer & (Eds.), *The tenth mental measurements yearbook* (pp. 422–423). Lincoln, NE: Buros Institute of Mental Measurements.

Curtis, J. W. (n.d.) *Curtis Verbal-Clerical Skills Tests.* Murfreesboro, TN: Psychometric Affiliates.

Dana, R. H. (1993). *Multicultural assessment perspectives for professional psychology.* Boston: Allyn & Bacon.

Darley, J. M., & Fazio, R. H. (1980). Expectancy confirmation processes arising in the social interaction sequence. *American Psychologist, 35,* 867–881.

Davis, N. L. F. (1990). The *Reynolds Adolescent Depression Scale. Measurement and Evaluation in Counseling and Development, 23,* 88–91.

Davis, R. N. (1999). Web-based administration of a personality questionnaire: Comparison with traditional methods. *Behavior Research Methods, Instruments, & Computers, 31,* 572–577.

Dawes, R. (1971). A case study of graduate admission: Application of three principles of human decision-making. *American Psychologist, 26,* 180–188.

Dawes, R., & Corrigan, B. (1974). Linear models in decision making. *Psychological Bulletin, 81,* 95–106.

De Ayala, R. J. (2001). Review of the *Computer-Based Test of English as a Foreign Language* and the *Test of Written English.* In B. S. Plake & J. C. Impara (Eds.), *The fourteenth mental measurements yearbook* (pp. 319–323). Lincoln, NE: Buros Institute of Mental Measurements.

Deacon, S. A., & Piercy, F. P. (2001). Qualitative methods in family evaluation: Creative assessment techniques. *The American Journal of Family Therapy, 29,* 355–373.

Deffenbacher, J. L., Lynch, R. S., Oetting, E. R., & Swaim, R. C. (2002). The *Driving Anger Expression Inventory:* A measure of how people express their anger on the road. *Behavior Research and Therapy, 40,* 717–737.

DeFur, S. (2003). Review of the *Test of Early Reading Ability, Third Edition.* In B. S. Plake, J. C. Impara, & R. A. Spies (Eds.), *The fifteenth mental measurements yearbook* (pp. 940–943). Lincoln, NE: Buros Institute of Mental Measurements.

Demaray, M. K., & Elting, J. (2003). Assessment of Attention-Deficit/Hyperactivity Disorder (ADHD): A comparative evaluation of five commonly used, published rating scales. *Psychology in the Schools, 40,* 341–361.

DeMauro, G. E. (2001). Review of the *Test of Nonverbal Intelligence, Third Edition.* In B. S. Plake & J. C. Impara (Eds.), *The fourteenth mental measurements yearbook* (pp. 1260–1262). Lincoln, NE: Buros Institute of Mental Measurements.

DeMauro, G. E. (2003). Review of the *Test of Written Spelling-4.* In B. S. Plake, J. C. Impara, & R. A. Spies (Eds.), *The fifteenth mental measurements yearbook* (pp. 965–968). Lincoln, NE: Buros Institute of Mental Measurements.

Derogatis, L. R. (1990). *SCL-90-R* (*Symptom Checklist-90-Revised*). Minneapolis, MN: NCS Pearson Assessments.

Derogatis, L. R. (1992). *Manual for the Symptom Checklist-90-Revised*. Minneapolis: NCS Pearson.

DeStephano, L. (2001). Review of the *Otis-Lennon School Abilities Test, 7th Edition*. In B. S. Plake & J. C. Impara (Eds.), *The fourteenth mental measurements yearbook* (pp. 875–878). Lincoln, NE: Buros Institute of Mental Measurements.

Digman, J. M. (1990). Personality structure: Emergence of the five-factor model. *Annual Review of Psychology, 41,* 417–440.

Digman, J.M., & Inouye, J. (1986). Further specification of the five robust factors of personality. *Journal of Personality and Social Psychology, 50,* 116–123.

Dimitrov, D. M. (2002). Reliability: Arguments for multiple perspectives and potential problems with generalization across studies. *Educational and Psychological Measurement, 62,* 783–801.

Dipboye, R. (1982). Self-fulfilling prophecies in the selection-recruitment interview. *Academy of Management Review, 7,* 579–586.

Doll, B. J. (2003). Review of the *Wechsler Individual Achievement Test* (*WIAT-II*). In B. S. Plake, J. C. Impara, & R. A. Spies (Eds.), *The fifteenth mental measurements yearbook* (pp. 996–999). Lincoln, NE: Buros Institute of Mental Measurements.

Downs, C. W., Smeyak, G. P., & Martin, E. (1980). *Professional interviewing*. New York: Harper & Row.

Dresser, N. (1996). *Multicultural manners*. New York: Wiley.

Drummond, R. J. (2000). *Appraisal procedures for counselors and helping professionals* (4th ed.). Upper Saddle River, NJ: Prentice Hall.

Drummond, R. J. (2004). *Appraisal procedures for counselors and helping professionals* (5th ed.). Upper Saddle River, NJ: Merrill/Prentice Hall.

Dryfoos, J. (1994). *Full-service schools: A revolution in health and social services for children, youth and families*. San Francisco: Jossey-Bass.

DuBois, P. H. (1966). A test-dominated society: China 1115 BC–1905 AD. In A. Anastasi (Ed.), *Testing problems in perspective* (pp. 29–36). Washington, DC: American Council on Education.

DuBois, P. H. (1970). *A history of psychological testing*. Boston: Allyn & Bacon.

Duckworth, J. C. (1990). The counseling approach to the use of testing. *Counseling Psychologist, 18,* 198–204.

Duckworth, J. C., & Anderson, W. P. (1995). *MMPI and MMPI-2: Interpretation manual for counselors and clinicians* (4th ed.). Bristol, PA: Accelerated Development.

Duhl, F., Kantor, D., & Duhl, B. (1973). Learning space and action in family therapy. In D. Block (Ed.), *Techniques of family psychotherapy: A primer* (pp. 69–76). New York: Grune & Stratton.

Dunn, A. B., & Levitt, M. M. (2000). The genogram: From diagnostics to mutual collaboration. *The Family Journal: Counseling and Therapy for Couples and Families, 8,* 236–244.

Dunn, L. M., & Dunn, L. M. (1997). *Manual for the Peabody Picture Vocabulary Test—Third Edition* (*PPVT-III*). Circle Pines, MN: American Guidance Services.

Dunst, C. J. (1998). Review of *Bayley Scales of Infant Development: Second Edition*. In J. C. Impara & B. S. Plake (Eds.), *The thirteenth mental measurements yearbook* (pp. 92–93). Lincoln, NE: Buros Institute of Mental Measurements.

Eaves, S. H., & Sheperis, C. J. (2006). Review of the *Eyberg Child Behavior Inventory* (*ECBI*) and *Sutter-Eyberg Student Behavior Inventory—Revised* (*SESBI-R*). In B. T. Erford (Ed.), *Counselor's guide to clinical, personality, and behavioral assessment* (pp. 143–147). Boston: Lahaska/Houghton Mifflin.

Ebbinghaus, H. (1897). Über eine neue Methode zur Prüfung geistiger Fähigkeiten und ihre Awendung bei Schulkindern. *Zeitschrift fur Angewandte Psychologie, 13,* 401–459.

Ebel, R. L. (1976). The paradox of educational testing. *Measurement in Education, 7*(4), 1–8.

Educational Testing Service. (2004). *SLEP test manual*. Princeton, NJ: Author.

Educational Testing Service. (2005a). SLEP web page. Retrieved January 15, 2005, from www.ets.org/slep/englishprograms/overview.html.

Educational Testing Service. (2005b). TOEFL web page. Retrieved January 15, 2005, from www.ets.org/toefl/nextgen/index.html.

Edwards, J. T. (2003). *Working with families: Guidelines and techniques* (6th ed.). Durham, NC: Foundation Place Publishing.

Elmore, P. B., Ekstrom, R., Diamond, E. E., & Wittaker, S. (1993). School counselors' test use patterns and practices. *School Counselor, 41,* 73–80.

Endler, N. S. (1997). Stress, anxiety and coping: The multidimensional interaction model. *Canadian Psychology, 38,* 136–153.

Engelhard, G., Jr., (1998). Review of the *Stanford Diagnostic Reading Test, Fourth Edition.* In J. C. Impara & B. S. Plake (Eds.), *The thirteenth mental measurements yearbook* (pp. 939–941). Lincoln, NE: Buros Institute of Mental Measurements.

English Language Institute (1998). *Michigan English Language Assessment Battery.* Ann Arbor: University of Michigan.

English Language Institute. (2004). *Michigan English Language Assessment Battery.* Ann Arbor: University of Michigan. Retrieved January 16, 2005, from www.lsa.umich.edu/eli/melab.htm.

Epstein, J. (1985). Review of the *Piers-Harris Self-Concept Scale.* In J. V. Mitchell Jr. (Ed.), *The ninth mental measurements yearbook* (pp. 1168–1169). Lincoln, NE: Buros Institute of Mental Measurements.

Epstein, N. B., Baldwin, L. M., & Bishop, D. S. (1983). The *McMaster Family Assessment Device. Journal of Marital and Family Therapy, 9,* 171–180.

Erford, B. T. (1993). *Manual for the Disruptive Behavior Rating Scale.* East Aurora, NY: Slosson Educational Publications.

Erford, B. T (1996). Reliability and validity of mother responses to the *Disruptive Behavior Rating Scale—Parent Version (DBRS-P). Diagnostique, 21,* 17–33.

Erford, B. T. (1997a). Reliability and validity of scores on the *Disruptive Behavior Rating Scale—Teacher Version (DBRS-T). Educational and Psychological Measurement, 57,* 329–339.

Erford, B. T. (1997b). Reliability and validity of the *Writing Essential Skills Screener—Preschool Version (WESS-P). Diagnostique, 23,* 213–223.

Erford, B. T. (1998). Technical analysis of father responses to the *Disruptive Behavior Rating Scale—Parent Version (DBRS-P). Measurement and Evaluation in Counseling and Development, 30,* 199–210.

Erford, B. T. (1999). Development and psychometric properties of the *Math Essential Skills Screener—Preschool Version (MESS-P). Educational Research Quarterly, 23,* 37–43.

Erford, B. T. (2004). *The Reading Essential Skill Screener—Preschool Version (RESS-P):* Studies of reliability and validity. *Assessment for Effective Intervention, 29*(3), 19–34.

Erford, B. T. (Ed.) (2006). *The counselor's guide to clinical, personality, and behavioral assessment.* Boston: Lahaska/Houghton Mifflin.

Erford, B. T. (2007). *Manual for the Slosson—Visual Perceptual Skills Screener (S-VPSS).* East Aurora, NY: Slosson Educational Publications.

Erford, B. T. (in press a). *Manual for the Slosson—Auditory Perceptual Skills Screener (S-APSS).* East Aurora, NY: Slosson Educational Publications.

Erford, B. T. (in press b). *Research and evaluation in counseling.* Boston: Lahaska/Houghton Mifflin.

Erford, B. T., Bagley, D. L., Hopper, J. A., Lee, R. M., Panagopulos, K. A., & Preller, D. B. (1998). Reliability and validity of the *Math Essential Skills Screener—Elementary Version (MESS-E). Psychology in the Schools, 35*(2), 1–9.

Erford, B. T., & Boykin, R. R. (1996). *Manual for the Slosson Diagnostic Math Screening Test (S-DMST).* East Aurora, NY: Slosson Educational Publications.

Erford, B. T., Ivey, E. A., & Dorman, S. L. (1999). The *Writing Essential Skill Screener—Upper Elementary Version:* A technical analysis. *Psychological Reports, 84,* 917–926.

Erford, B. T., Ivey, E. A., Dorman, S. L., & Wingeart, L. (2001). The *Writing Essential Skill Screener—Elementary Version (WESS-E):* A technical analysis. *Assessment for Effective Intervention, 26,* 133–140.

Erford, B. T., & McKechnie, J. A. (2006). Review of the *Personality Inventory for Children—Second Edition (PIC-2).* In B. T. Erford (Ed.), *The counselor's guide to clinical, personality, and behavioral assessment* (pp. 50–54). Boston: Lahaska/Houghton Mifflin.

Erford, B. T., & Stephens, V. M. (2005). The *Reading Essential Skill Screener Elementary Version (RESS-E):* Studies of reliability and validity. *Measurement and Evaluation in Counseling and Development,* 38, 104-114.

Erford, B. T., Vitali, G., Haas, R., & Boykin, R. R. (1995). *Manual for the Essential Skills Screener.* East Aurora, NY: Slosson Educational Publications.

Erford, B. T., Vitali, G., & Slosson, S. (1999). *Manual for the Slosson Intelligence Test—Primary.* East Aurora, NY: Slosson Educational Publications.

Erickson, D. (1995). Review of the *Minnesota Manual Dexterity Test.* In J. C. Conoley & J. C. Impara (Eds.), *The twelfth mental measurements yearbook* (p. 624). Lincoln, NE: Buros Institute of Mental Measurements.

Erk, R. R. (1995). The evolution of Attention Deficit Disorders terminology. *Elementary School Guidance and Counseling, 29,* 243–248.

Essau, C. A., Condradt, J., & Peterman, F. (2000). Frequency, comorbidity, and psychosocial impairment of depressive disorders in adolescents. *Journal of Adolescent Research, 15,* 470–481.

Exner, J. (2002). *The comprehensive system for administering, scoring, and interpreting the Rorschach.* New York: Wiley.

Eyberg, S. M., & Pincus, D. (1999). *Eyberg Child Behavior Inventory and Sutter-Eyberg Student Behavior Inventory—Revised professional manual.* Lutz, FL: Psychological Assessment Resources.

Farmer, R. F. (2001). Review of the *Beck Depression Inventory—II.* In B. S. Plake & J. C. Impara (Eds.), *The fourteenth mental measurements yearbook* (pp. 123–126). Lincoln, NE: Buros Institute of Mental Measurements.

Farr, R. C., & Tone, B. (1994). *Growing to meet your needs.* New York: Harcourt Brace College.

Feingold, A. (1993). Cognitive gender differences: A developmental perspective. *Sex Roles, 29,* 91–112.

Feldman, S. E., & Sullivan, D. S. (1960). Factors mediating the effects of enhanced rapport on children's performances. *Journal of Consulting and Clinical Psychology, 36,* 302.

Feldt, L. S., & Brennan, R. L. (1989). Reliability. In R. L. Linn (Ed.), *Educational measurement* (3rd ed., pp. 105–146). New York: Macmillan.

First, M. B., Gibbon, M., Spitzer, R. L., Williams, J. B. W., & Benjamin, L. S. (1997). *The Structured Clinical Interview for DSM-IV Axis II Personality Disorders (SCID-II).* Washington, DC: American Psychiatric Press.

First, M. B., Spitzer, R. L., Gibbon, M., & Williams, J. B. W. (1997). *The Structured Clinical Interview for DSM-IV Axis I Disorders—Clinical Version (SCID-CV).* Washington, DC: American Psychiatric Press.

Fischer, L. Y., & Sorenson, G. P. (1997). *School law for counselors, psychologists, and social workers* (3rd ed.). White Plains, NY: Longman.

Fishkin, A. S., & Kampsnider, J. J. (1996). Exploring the *WISC-III* as a measure of giftedness. *Roeper Review, 18,* 226–231.

Fitts, W. H., & Warren, W. L. (1996). *Manual for the Tennessee Self-Concept Scale—Second Edition.* Los Angeles: Western Psychological Services.

Fitzpatrick, C. (2001). Review of the *PREPARE-ENRICH*. In B. S. Plake & J. C. Impara (Eds.), *The fourteenth mental measurements yearbook* (pp. 951–953). Lincoln, NE: Buros Institute of Mental Measurements.

Flanagan, C. (1993). Gender and social class: Intersecting issues in women's achievement. *Educational Psychologist, 28,* 357–378.

Flanagan, D., Ortiz, S. O., Alfonso, V. C., & Mascolo, J. T. (2002). *The achievement test desk reference (ATDR): Comprehensive assessment and learning disabilities.* Boston: Allyn & Bacon.

Fleenor, J. W. (2001). Review of the *Myers-Briggs Type Indicator, Form M.* In B. S. Plake & J. C. Impara (Eds.), *The fourteenth mental measurements yearbook* (pp. 816–818). Lincoln, NE: Buros Institute of Mental Measurements.

Fletcher, J. M., Shaywitz, S. E., Shankweiler, D. P., Katz, L., Liberman, I. Y., Stuebing, K. K., Francis, D. J., Fowler, A. E., & Shaywitz, B. A. (1994). Cognitive profiles of reading disability: Comparisons of discrepancy and low achievement definitions. *Journal of Educational Psychology, 25,* 6–23.

Floden, R.E. (1985). Review of the *Basic Achievement Skills Individual Skills Screener (BASIS).* In J. V. Mitchell Jr. (Ed.), *The ninth mental measurements yearbook* (pp. 134–135). Lincoln, NE: Buros Institute of Mental Measurements.

Floyd, F. J., Weinand, J. W., & Cimmarusti, R. A. (1989). Clinical family assessments: Applying structured measurement procedures in treatment settings. *Journal of Marital and Family Therapy, 9,* 171–180.

Flynn, J. R. (1991). *Asian-American: Achievement beyond IQ.* Hillsdale, NJ: Erlbaum.

Folstein, M. F., Folstein, S. E., McHugh, P. R., & Fanjiang, G. (2001). *Mini-Mental State Examination (MMSE): User's guide.* Lutz, FL: Psychological Assessment Resources.

Fong, M. L. (1995). Assessment and *DSM-IV* diagnosis of personality disorders: A primer for counselors. *Journal of Counseling and Development, 73,* 635–639.

Fontaine, J. H. (2001). Review of the *Career Thoughts Inventory.* In B. S. Plake & J. C. Impara (Eds.), *The fourteenth mental measurements yearbook* (pp. 228–230). Lincoln, NE: Buros Institute of Mental Measurements.

Forer. (1967). *The Forer Structured Sentence Completion Test (FSSCT).* Los Angeles: Western Psychological Services.

Forest, D. W. (1974). *Francis Galton: The life and work of a Victorian genius.* New York: Taplinger.

Forester-Miller, H. & Davis, T. (1996) A practioner's guide to ethical decision making. Retrieved on February 20, 2006 at http://www.counseling.org/content/navigationmenu/RESOURCES/ETHICS/APractionersGuidetoEthicalDecisionMaking/Practioner_s_Guide.htm

Fouad, N., & Chan, P. (1999). Gender and ethnicity: Influence on test interpretation and reception. In J. W. Lichtenberg & R. K. Goodyear (Eds.), *Scientist-practitioner perspectives on test interpretation* (pp. 31–58). Boston: Allyn & Bacon.

Fowers, B. J. (1990). An interactional approach to standardized marital assessment: A literature review. *Family Relations, 39,* 368–377.

Frances, A. J., First, M. B., & Pincus, H. A. (1995). *DSM-IV guidebook.* Washington, DC: American Psychiatric Press.

Frankenburg, W. K., Dodds, J., Archer, P., Bresnik, B., Maschka, P., Edelman, N., & Shapiro, H. (1990). *Denver II.* Denver, CO: Denver Developmental Materials.

Franklin, C., Streeter, C. L., & Springer, D. W. (2001). Validity of the *FACES-IV* family assessment measure. *Research on Social Work Practice, 11,* 576–571.

Frary, R. B. (1995). Review of the *Miller Analogies Test.* In J. C. Conoley & J. C. Impara (Eds.), *The twelfth mental measurements yearbook* (pp. 617–619). Lincoln, NE: Buros Institute of Mental Measurements.

Frauenhoffer, D., Ross, M. J., Gfeller, J., Searight, H. R., & Piotrowski, C. (1998). Psychological test usage among licensed mental health practitioners: A multidisciplinary survey. *Journal of Psychological Practice, 4,* 28–33.

Fredman, N., & Sherman, R. (1987). *Handbook of measurements for marriage and family therapy.* New York: Brunner/Mazel.

Freud, S. (1956). Those wrecked by success. In J. Strachey (Ed. & Trans.), *Standard edition of the complete psychological works of Sigmund Freud* (Vol. 14, pp. 316–331). London: Hogarth Press.

Freud, S. (1961a). The Ego and the Id. In J. Strachey (Ed. & Trans.) *Standard edition of the complete psychological works of Sigmund Freud* (Vol. 19, pp. 3-66). London: Hogarth Press. (Original work published 1923)

Freud, S. (1961b). The disillusion of the Oedipus complex. In J. Strachey (Ed. & Trans.), *Standard edition of the complete psychological works of Sigmund Freud* (Vol. 19, pp. 173–179). London: Hogarth Press. (Original work published 1924)

Fristad, M. A., Emery, B. L., & Beck, S. J. (1997). Use and abuse of the *Children's Depression Inventory. Journal of Consulting and Clinical Psychology, 65,* 699–702.

Fuchs, D., & Fuchs, L. S. (1986). Test procedure bias: A meta-analysis of examiner familiarity effects. *Review of Educational Research, 56,* 243–262.

Furlong, M., & Karno, M. (1995). Review of the *Social Skills Rating System.* In J. C. Conoley & J. C. Impara (Eds.), *The twelfth mental measurements yearbook.* Lincoln, NE: Buros Institute of Mental Measurements.

Gailbreath, R. D., Wagner, S. S., Moffett, R. G., & Hein, M. B. (1997). Homogeneity in behavioral preferences among U.S. Army leaders. *Group Dynamics, 1,* 220–230.

Galton, F. (1869). *Hereditary genius.* London: Macmillan. (Republished in 1892)

Gans, A. M., Kenny, M. C., & Ghany, D. L. (2003). Comparing the self-concept of students with and without learning disabilities. *Journal of Learning Disabilities, 36,* 287–296.

Gardner, H. (1983). *Frames of mind: The theory of multiple intelligences.* Cambridge: Cambridge University Press.

Gardner, H. (1993). *Frames of mind: The theory of multiple intelligences.* New York: Basic Books.

Gardner, M. (1996a). *Manual for the Test of Auditory Perceptual Skills—Revised (TAPS-R).* Hydesville, CA: Psychological and Educational Publications.

Gardner, M. (1996b). *Manual for the Test of Visual Perceptual Skills (nonmotor)—Revised (TVPS-R).* Hydesville, CA: Psychological and Educational Publications.

Gardner, W. L., & Martinko, M. J. (1996). Using the *Myers-Briggs Type Indicator* to study managers: A literature review and research agenda. *Journal of Management, 22,* 45–83.

Garfinkel, A. (2001). Review of the *Michigan English Language Assessment Battery.* In B. S. Plake & J. C. Impara (Eds.), *The fourteenth mental measurements yearbook* (pp. 756–757). Lincoln, NE: Buros Institute of Mental Measurements.

Garner, D. M. (2004). *Eating Disorder Inventory-3.* Lutz, FL: Psychological Assessment Resources.

Garton, A. F., Harvey, R., & Price, C. (2004). Influence of perceived family environment on adolescent leisure participation. *Australian Journal of Psychology, 56,* 18–24.

Gates, A. I., McKillop, A. S., & Horowitz, E. C. (1981). *Reading Diagnostic Tests—Second Edition.* New York: Teachers College Press.

Gerard, A. B. (1994). *Parent-Child Relationship Inventory (PCRI) manual.* Los Angeles: Western Psychological Services.

Gerry, M. H. (1973). Cultural myopia: The need for a corrective lens. *Journal of School Psychology, 11,* 307–315.

Ghiselli, E. E. (1973). The validity of aptitude tests in personnel selection. *Personnel Psychology, 26,* 461–477.

Gianarris, W. J., Golden, G. J., & Greene, L. (2001). The *Conners' Parent Rating Scales:* A critical review of the literature. *Clinical Psychology Review, 21,* 1061–1093.

Gibson, R. L., & Mitchell, M. H. (1999). *Introduction to counseling and guidance* (5th ed.). Upper Saddle River, NJ: Merrill/Prentice Hall.

Ginsburg, H. P., & Baroody, A. J. (1990). *Manual for the Test of Early Mathematics Ability—Second Edition.* Austin, TX: PRO-ED.

Giordano, F. G., & Schweibert, V. L. (1997). School counselors' perceptions of the usefulness of standardized tests, frequency of their use, and assessment training needs. *School Counselor, 44,* 198–206.

Gladding, S. T. (2001). *The counseling dictionary: Concise definitions of frequently used terms.* Upper Saddle River, NJ: Prentice Hall.

Gladding, S. T. (2005). *Counseling as an art: The creative arts in counseling* (3rd ed.). Alexandria, VA: American Counseling Association.

Gladding, S. T., & Newsome, D. W. (2004). *Community and agency counseling* (2nd ed.). Upper Saddle River, NJ: Merrill/Prentice Hall.

Gold, J. M. (1997). Assessing education in marriage and family counseling. *Family Journal: Counseling and Therapy for Couples and Families, 5,* 159–163.

Goldberg, L. R. (1970). Man versus model of man: A rationale plus evidence for a method of improving clinical inference. *Psychological Bulletin, 73,* 422–432.

Goldberg, L. R. (1992). The development of markers for the big five-factor structure. *Psychological Assessment, 4,* 26–42.

Goldman, L. (1990). Qualitative assessment. *Counseling Psychologist, 18,* 205–213.

Goldman, L. (1992). Qualitative assessment: An approach for counselors. *Journal of Counseling and Development, 70,* 616–621.

Goleman, D. (1995). *Emotional intelligence: Why it can matter more than IQ.* New York: Bantam.

Goodenough, D. B., & Harris, F. L. (1963). *The Goodenough Harris Drawing Test.* San Antonio, TX: PsychCorp.

Goodyear, R. K. (1990). Research on the effects of test interpretation: A review. *Counseling Psychologist, 18,* 240–257.

Gordon, E. E. (1995). *Musical Aptitude Profile.* Chicago: GIA Publications.

Gordon, H. W., & Lee, P. (1986). A relationship between gonadotroins and visuospatial function. *Neuropsycholia, 24,* 563–576.

Gottfredson, G. D., & Holland, J. L. (1996). *Dictionary of Holland occupational codes* (3rd ed.). Odessa, FL: Psychological Assessment Resources.

Gottfried, A. W. (Ed.) (1984). *Home environment and early cognitive development: Longitudinal research.* New York: Academic Press.

Gough, H. G., & Bradley, P. (1996). *California Personality Inventory* (*CPI*) *manual* (3rd ed.). Palo Alto, CA: Consulting Psychologists Press.

Graduate Record Examination Board. (1997). *GRE 1997–1998 guide to the use of scores.* Princeton, NJ: Educational Testing Service.

Gratus, J. (1988). *Successful interviewing.* Harmondsworth, England: Penguin Books.

Graves, M. E. (1948). *Graves Design Judgment Test.* New York: Psychological Corporation.

Green, A. (1986). True and false allegations of sexual abuse in child custody disputes. *Journal of the American Academy of Child Psychology, 23,* 449–456.

Green, F. J. (1998). Review of the *Test of Reading Comprehension—Third Edition* (*TORC-3*). In J. C. Impara & B. S. Plake (Eds.), *The thirteenth mental measurements yearbook.* Lincoln, NE: Buros Institute of Mental Measurements.

Greene, R. G., & Vosler, N. R. (1992). Issues in the assessment of family practice: An empirical study. *Journal of Social Service Research, 13,* 1–19.

Gregory, R. J. (1999). *Foundations of intellectual assessment.* Boston: Allyn & Bacon.

Gresham, F. M. (1984). Behavioral interviews in school psychology: Issues in psychometric adequacy and research. *School Psychology Review, 13,* 17–25.

Gresham, F. M. (1989). Review of the *Revised Children's Manifest Anxiety Scale*. In J. C. Conoley & J. J. Kramer (Eds.), *The tenth mental measurements yearbook* (pp. 695–697). Lincoln, NE: Buros Institute of Mental Measurements.

Gresham, F. M., & Elliott, S. N. (1987). The relationship between adaptive behavior and social skills: Issues in definition and assessment. *Journal of Special Education, 21,* 167–181.

Gresham, F. M., & Elliott, S. N. (1990). *Social Skills Rating System Manual.* Circle Pines, MN: American Guidance Services.

Gresham, F. M., Watson, T. S., & Skinner, C. H. (2001). Functional behavioral assessments: Principles, procedures, and future directions. *School Psychology Review, 30,* 156–172.

Grotevant, H. D., & Carlson, C. I. (1989). *Family assessment: A guide to methods and measures.* New York: Guilford.

Guilford, J. P. (1967). *The nature of human intelligence.* New York: McGraw-Hill.

Guilford, J. P. (1988). Some changes in the Structure-of-Intellect Model. *Educational & Psychological Measurement, 48,* 1–4.

Guilford, J. P., & Hoepfner, R. (1971). *The analysis of intelligence.* New York: McGraw-Hill.

Guion, R. M. (1995). Review of the *Career Beliefs Inventory.* In. J. C. Conoley & J. C. Impara (Eds.), *The twelfth mental measurements yearbook* (pp. 160–161). Lincoln, NE: Buros Institute of Mental Measurements.

Gunsalus, A. J. C., & Kelly, K. R. (2001). Korean cultural influences on the *Millon Clinical Multiaxial Inventory III. Journal of Mental Health Counseling, 23,* 151–161.

Hagin, R. A. (1992). Review of the *Salience Inventory.* In J. J. Kramer & J. C. Conoley (Eds.), *The eleventh mental measurements yearbook* (pp. 777–778). Lincoln, NE: Buros Institute of Mental Measurements.

Haladyna, T. (1999). *Developing and validating multiple-choice test questions.* Mahwah, NJ: Lawrence Erlbaum.

Hall, J., & Kimura, D. (1995). Sexual orientation and performance on sexually dimorphic motor tasks. *Archives of Sexual Behavior, 24,* 395–407.

Halpern, D., & Wright, T. (1996). A process oriented model of cognitive sex differences. *Learning and Individual Differences, 8,* 3–24.

Hammill, D. D., & Larsen, S. C. (1996). *Manual for the Test of Written Language* (3rd ed.). Austin, TX: PRO-ED.

Handler, L. (1996). The clinical use of figure drawings. In C. S. Newmark (Ed.), *Major psychological assessment instruments* (2nd ed., pp. 206–293). Boston: Allyn & Bacon.

Hanna, G. S. (2001). Review of the *Slosson Full-Range Intelligence Test.* In B. S. Plake & J. C. Impara (Eds.), *The fourteenth mental measurements yearbook* (pp. 1147–1150). Lincoln, NE: Buros Institute of Mental Measurements.

Hansen, J. B. (1998). Review of the *Test of Written Language—Third Edition.* In J. C. Impara & B. S. Plake (Eds.), *The thirteenth mental measurements yearbook* (pp. 1070–1072). Lincoln, NE: Buros Institute of Mental Measurements.

Hansen, J. C. (1999). Test psychometrics. In J. W. Lichtenberg & R. K. Goodyear (Eds.), *Scientist-practitioner perspectives on test interpretation* (pp. 15–30). Sydney: Allyn & Bacon.

Hansen, J. C. (2000). Interpretation of the *Strong Interest Inventory.* In C. E. Watkins Jr. & V. L. Campbell (Eds.), *Testing and assessment in counseling practice* (2nd ed., pp. 227–262). Mahwah, NJ: Erlbaum.

Hansen, J. C. (2001). Interest assessment. In G. R. Walz & J. C. Blcucr (Eds.) *Assessment: Issues and challenges for the millennium* (pp. 305–308). Greensboro, NC: CAPS Publications.

Hansen, J. C., & Ncuman, J. L. (1997). Comparison of user reaction to two methods of *Strong Interest Inventory* administration and report feedback. *Measurement and Evaluation in Counseling and Development, 30,* 115–137.

Harcourt Assessment. (2004a). Harcourt: Welcome to HarcourtAssessment.com. Retrieved June 15, 2004, from https://marketplace.psychcorp.com/PsychCorp/International.aspx.

Harcourt Assessment. (2004b). *Stanford 10* technical data report. San Antonio, TX: Author.

Harcourt Assessment. (2005). *Miller Analogies Test (MAT)*. San Antonio, TX: Harcourt. Retrieved January 24, 2005, from www.milleranalogies.com.

Harcourt Brace Educational Measurement. (2003). *Stanford Achievement Test—Tenth Edition (Stanford 10)*. San Antonio, TX: Author.

Harcourt Educational Measurement. (2001). *Metropolitan Achievement Test—Eighth Edition (Metropolitan8)*. San Antonio, TX: Author.

Hardy, J. B., Welcher, D. W., Mellitis, E. D., & Kagan, J. (1976). Pitfalls in the measurement of intelligence: Are standardized intelligence tests valid for measuring the intellectual potential of urban children? *Journal of Psychology, 94,* 43–51.

Harmon, L. W. (1985). Review of *Career Decision Scale.* In J. V. Mitchell (Ed.), *The ninth mental measurements yearbook* (p. 270). Lincoln, NE: Buros Institute of Mental Measurements.

Harmon, L. W., Hansen, J. C., Borgen, F. H., & Hammer, A. L. (1994). *Strong Interest Inventory application and technical guide.* Palo Alto, CA: Consulting Psychologists Press.

Harrington, J. C., & Harrington, T. F. (1996). *Ability Explorer: Preliminary technical manual.* Chicago, IL: Riverside Publishing.

Harrington, R. G. (1998). Review of the *AAMR Adaptive Behavior Scale-School, Second Edition.* In J. C. Impara & B. S. Plake (Eds.), *The thirteenth mental measurements yearbook* (pp. 5–9). Lincoln, NE: Buros Institute of Mental Measurements.

Harrington, T. F., & Feller, R. (2004). Facilitating career development assessment and interpretation practices. In J. E. Wall & G. R. Walz (Eds.) *Measuring up: Assessment issues for teachers, counselors, and administrators* (pp. 581–594). Greensboro, NC: CAPS Publications.

Harrington, T. F., & O'Shea, A. J. (1993). *The Harrington-O'Shea Career Decision-Making System—Revised manual.* Circle Pines, MN: American Guidance Services.

Harris, D. J. (2004). Reporting and interpreting test results. In J. E. Wall & G. R. Walz (Eds.) *Measuring up: assessment issues for teachers, counselors, and administrators* (pp. 53–64). Greensboro, NC: CAPS Publications.

Harris, M. B. (1998). *Basic statistics for behavioral science research* (2nd ed.). Needham Heights, MA: Allyn & Bacon.

Harris, S. L. (1995). *The Vineland Adaptive Behavior Scales* for young children with autism. *Special Services in the Schools, 10,* 45–54.

Harrison, P. (1985). *Manual for the Vineland Adaptive Behavior Scales—Teacher Interview.* Circle Pines, MN: American Guidance Services.

Hart, B., & Risley, T. R. (1992). American parenting of language-learning children: Persisting differences in family-child interactions observed in natural home environments. *Developmental Psychology, 28,* 1096–1105.

Harwell, M.R. (2005). Review of the *Metropolitan Achievement Test—Eighth Edition (Metropolitan8).* In B. S. Plake, J. C. Impara, & R. A. Spies (Eds.), *The sixteenth mental measurements yearbook.* Lincoln, NE: Buros Institute of Mental Measurements.

Hassin, D. S., Trautman, K. D., Miele, G. M., Same, S., Smith, M., & Endicott, J. (1996). *Psychiatric Research Interview for Substance Abuse and Mental Disorders (PRISM)*: Reliability for substance abusers. *American Journal of Psychiatry, 153,* 1195–1201.

Hattie, J. (1992). *Self-concept.* Hillsdale, NJ: Erlbaum.

Hattrup, K. (1995). Review of the *Differential Aptitude Tests, Fifth Edition.* In J. C. Conoley & J. C. Impara (Eds.), *The twelfth mental measurements yearbook* (pp. 302–304). Lincoln, NE: Buros Institute of Mental Measurements.

Hattrup, K. (2003). Review of the *California Psychological Inventory.* In B. S. Plake, J. C. Impara,

& R. A. Spies (Eds.), *The fifteenth mental measurements yearbook* (pp. 161–163). Lincoln, NE: Buros Institute of Mental Measurements.

Hay, E. N. (1999). *Hay Aptitude Test Battery—Revised.* Libertyville, IL: Wonderlic.

Hayes, S. C. (1999). Comparison of the *Kaufman Brief Intelligence Test* and the *Matrix Analogies Test—Short Form* in an adolescent forensic population. *Psychological Assessment, 11,* 108–110.

Healy, C. C., & Woodward, G. A. (1998). The *Myers-Briggs Type Indicator* and career obstacles. *Measurement and Evaluation in Counseling and Development, 31,* 74–85.

Hearst, E. (1979). *The first century of experimental psychology.* Hillsdale, NJ: Erlbaum.

Hedges, L. V., & Nowell, A. (1995). Sex differences in mental test scores, variability, and numbers of high-scoring individuals. *Science, 269,* 41–45.

Herlihy, B., & Corey, G. (1996). *ACA ethical standards casebook* (5th ed.). Alexandria, VA: American Counseling Association.

Hernstein, R., & Murray, C. (1994). *The bell curve: Intelligence and class structure in American life.* New York: Free Press.

Herr, E. L. (1998). *Counseling in a dynamic society: Contexts and practices in the 21st century* (2nd ed.). Alexandria, VA: American Counseling Association.

Herr, E. L., Cramer, S. H., & Niles, S. G. (2004). *Career guidance and counseling through the lifespan* (6th ed.). Boston: Allyn & Bacon.

Herring, R. (1997). *Multicultural counseling in schools: A synergetic approach.* Alexandria, VA: American Counseling Association.

Hess, A. K., Zachar, P., & Kramer, J. (2001). Review of the *Rorschach Inkblot Test.* In B. S. Plake & J. C. Impara (Eds.), *The fourteenth mental measurements yearbook* (pp. 1033–1038). Lincoln, NE: Buros Institute of Mental Measurements.

Hines, M. (1990). Gonadal hormones and human cognition development. In J. Balthazart (Ed.), *Hormones, brains, and behaviors in vertebrates: I. Sexual differentiation, neuroanatomical aspects, neurotransmitters, and neuropeptides* (pp. 51–63). Basel, Switzerland: Karger.

Hinkle, J. S. (1994). Practitioners and cross-cultural assessment: A practical guide to information and training. *Measurement and Evaluation in Counseling and Development, 27,* 103–115.

Hoagwood, K., Kelleher, K. J., Feil, M., & Comer, D. M. (2000). Treatment services for children with AD/HD. A national perspective. *American Academy of Child and Adolescent Psychiatry, 39,* 198–206.

Hodges, K. (1990). Depression and anxiety in children: Comparison of self-report questionnaires to clinical interview. *Psychological Assessment, 2,* 376–381.

Hodges, K. (1993). Structured interviews for assessing children. *Journal of Child Psychology and Psychiatry, 34,* 49–68.

Hodges, K. (1997). *Child Adolescent Schedule* (*CAS*). Ypsilanti: Eastern Michigan University.

Hofler, D. B., Erford, B. T., & Amoriell, W. J. (2001). *Manual for the Slosson Written Expression Test.* East Aurora, NY: Slosson Educational Publications.

Hohensil, T. H. (1993). Teaching the *DSM-III-R* in counselor education. *Counselor Education and Supervision, 32,* 267–275.

Hohensil, T. H. (1996). Editorial: Role of assessment and diagnosis in counseling. *Journal of Counseling and Development, 75,* 64–67.

Holland, J. L. (1966). *The psychology of vocational choice.* Waltham, MA: Blaisdell.

Holland, J. L. (1985). *Making vocational choices: A theory of vocational personalities and work environments* (2nd ed.). Upper Saddle River, NJ: Prentice Hall.

Holland, J. L. (1994). *The occupations finder.* Odessa, FL: Psychological Assessment Resources.

Holland, J. L. (1997). *Making vocational choices: A theory of vocational personalities and work environments* (3rd ed.). Odessa, FL: Psychological Assessment Resources.

Holland, J. L. (2000). *Occupations finder* (Rev. ed.). Odessa, FL: Psychological Assessment Resources.

Holland, J. L., Fritzche, B. A., & Powell, A. B. (1994). *Self-Directed Search: Technical manual.* Odessa, FL: Psychological Assessment Resources.

Honzik, M. P. (1967). Environmental correlates of mental growth: Prediction from the family setting at 21 months. *Child Development, 38,* 337–364.

Honzik, M. P., McFarlane, J. W., & Allen, L. (1948). The stability of mental test performance between 2 and 18 years. *Journal of Experimental Education, 17,* 309–324.

Hood, A. B., & Johnson, R. W. (2002). *Assessment in counseling: A guide to the use of psychological assessment procedures* (3rd ed.). Alexandria, VA: American Counseling Association.

Hoover, H. D., Hieronymus, A. N., Dunbar, S. B., & Frisbie, D. A. (2001). *Iowa Test of Basic Skills* (*ITBS*). Itasca, IL: Riverside Publishing.

Hopkins, K. D. (1996). *Educational and psychological measurement and evaluation* (8th ed.). Boston: Allyn & Bacon.

Houts, P. (1977). *The myth of measurability.* New York: Hart Publishing.

Hresko, W. P., Herron, S. R., & Peak, P. K. (1996). *Manual for the Test of Early Written Language—Second Edition.* Austin, TX: PRO-ED.

Hsu, L. M. (1986). Implications of differences in elevations of K-corrected and non-K-corrected *MMPI* T scores. *Journal of Consulting and Clinical Psychology, 54,* 552–557.

Hughes, S. (1995). Review of the *Denver II.* In J. C. Conoley & J. C. Impara (Eds.), *The twelfth mental measurements yearbook* (pp. 264–265). Lincoln, NE: Buros Institute of Mental Measurements.

Humphreys, L. G. (1962). The organization of human abilities. *American Psychologist, 17,* 475–483.

Humphreys, L. G. (1970). A skeptical look at the factor pure test. In C. Lunneborg (Ed.), *Current problems and techniques in multivariate psychology* (pp. 23–32). Seattle: University of Washington Press.

Hunt, J. M. (1961). *Intelligence and experience.* New York: Ronald Press.

Hurford, D. P. (1998). Review of the *Test of Early Written Language.* In J. C. Impara & B. S. Plake (Eds.), *The thirteenth mental measurements yearbook* (pp. 1027–1030). Lincoln, NE: Buros Institute of Mental Measurements.

Hyde, J. S., Fennema, E., & Lamon, S. J. (1990). Gender differences in mathematics performance: A meta-analysis. *Psychological Bulletin, 107,* 139–155.

Ihle-Helledy, K., Zytowski, D. G., & Fouad, N. A. (2004). *Kuder Career Search:* Test-retest reliability and consequential validity. *Journal of Career Assessment, 12,* 285–297.

Ilg, F. (1978). *Manual for the Gesell School Readiness Test.* Lumberville, PA: Programs for Education.

Individuals with Disabilities Education Act Amendments of 1997, 20 U.S.C.,1401 et. seq., 1415 (k) (1) (b) (1997).

Ivens, S. H. (1995). Review of the *Miller Analogy Test.* In J. C. Conoley & J. C. Impara (Eds.), *The twelfth mental measurements yearbook* (pp. 619–620). Lincoln, NE: Buros Institute of Mental Measurements.

Ivnik, R. J., Malec, J. F., Smith, G. E., Tangalos, E. G., Peterson, R. C., Kokmen, E., & Kurkland, L. T. (1992). Mayo's older American normative studies: *WAIS-R* norms for ages 56–97. *Clinical Neuropsychologist, 6* (Suppl.), 1–30.

Iwata, B. A., Pace, G. M., Dorsey, M. F., Zarcone, J. R., Vollmer, T. R., Smith, R. G., et al. (1994). The functions of self-injurious behavior: An experimental-epidemiological analysis. *Journal of Applied Behavior Analysis, 27,* 215–240.

Jackson, D. N. (1994). *Manual for the Jackson Personality Inventory—Revised.* Port Huron, MI: Sigma Assessment Systems.

Jackson, D. N. (1998). *Multidimensional Aptitude Battery—II.* Port Huron, MI: Sigma Assessment System.

Jackson, D. N. (1999). *Jackson Vocational Interest Survey.* Port Huron, MI: Sigma Assessment Systems.

Jacobs, J. (1970). Are we being misled by fifty years of research on our gifted children? *Gifted Child Quarterly, 14,* 120–123.

Janda, L. H. (1998). *Psychological testing: Theory and applications.* Boston: Allyn & Bacon.

Jensen, A. R. (1969). How much can we boost IQ and scholastic achievement? *Harvard Educational Review, 39,* 1–123.

Jensen, A. R. (1980). *Bias in mental testing.* New York: Free Press.

Jensen, A. R. (1985). Compensatory education and the theory of intelligence. *Phi Delta Kappan, 66,* 554–558.

Jeske, P. J. (1985). Review of the *Piers-Harris Self-Concept Scale.* In J. V. Mitchell Jr. (Ed.), *The ninth mental measurements yearbook* (Vol. 2, pp. 1169–1170). Lincoln, NE: Buros Institute of Mental Measurements.

Johannson, C. B. (1984). *Manual for the Career Assessment Inventory: The enhanced version.* Minneapolis: National Computer Systems.

Johannson, C. B. (1986). *Manual for the Career Assessment Inventory* (2nd ed.). Minneapolis: National Computer Systems.

Johns, J. L., & Van Leirsburg, P. (1994). Test review: *Slosson Intelligence Test—Revised (SIT-R).* In D. J. Keyser & R. C. Sweetland (Eds.), *Test critiques* (pp. 672–679). Kansas City, MO: Test Corporation of America.

Johnson, C. (2005). Review of the *Musical Aptitude Profile—Fourth Edition.* In B. S. Plake, J. C. Impara, & R. A. Spies (Eds.), *The sixteenth mental measurements yearbook.* Lincoln, NE: Buros Institute of Mental Measurements.

Johnson, J. (1992). Review of the *Test of Early Mathematics Ability, Second Edition.* In J. J. Kramer & J. C. Conoley (Eds.), *The eleventh mental measurements yearbook* (pp. 940–941). Lincoln, NE: Buros Institute of Mental Measurements.

Johnson, R. W. (1995). Review of the *Adult Career Concerns Inventory.* In J. C. Conoley & J. C. Impara (Eds.), *The twelfth mental measurements yearbook* (pp. 47–48). Lincoln, NE: Buros Institute of Mental Measurements.

Johnson, W. L., Mauzey, E., Johnson, A. M., Murphy, S. D., & Zimmerman, K. J. (2002). A higher order analysis of the factor structure of the *Myers-Briggs Type Indicator. Measurement and Evaluation in Counseling Development, 34,* 96–109.

Johnston, J. A., & Rakes, T. D. (1992). Ten assessment questions to aid with interpreting the *Self-Directed Search.* Unpublished manuscript.

Joinson, A. N., & Buchanan, T. (2001). Doing educational psychology research on the Web. In C. Wolfe (Ed.), *Teaching and learning on the World Wide Web* (pp. 221–242). San Diego, CA: Academic Press.

Joint Committee on Standards for Educational Evaluation (2003). *The student evaluation standards.* Thousand Oaks, CA: Corwin Press and ETS Educational Policy Institute.

Jordan, K. (2001). Family art therapy: The joint family holiday drawing. *The Family Journal: Counseling and Therapy for Couples and Families, 9,* 52–54.

Juhnke, G. A., Coll, K. A., Brunelli, M. A., & Kardatzke, K. N. (2006). Review of the *SASSI-3.* In B. T. Erford (Ed.), *Counselor's guide to clinical, personality and behavioral assessment* (pp. 58–64). Boston: Lahaska/Houghton Mifflin.

Jung, C. G. (1923). *Psychological types.* London: Rutledge & Kegan Paul.

Kamphaus, R. W. (1994). Review of the *Slosson Intelligence Test* [1991 Edition]. In J. J. Kramer & J. C. Conoley (Eds.), *The eleventh mental measurements yearbook* (Vol. 2, pp. 227–229). Lincoln, NE: Buros Institute of Mental Measurements.

Kamphaus, R.W. (2001). Review of the *Metropolitan Readiness Tests—Sixth Edition*. In B. S. Plake & J. C. Impara (Eds.), *The fourteenth mental measurements yearbook* (Vol. 2, pp. 227–229). Lincoln, NE: Buros Institute of Mental Measurements.

Kane, M. (2001). Review of *Hay Aptitude Test Battery*. In B. S. Plake & J. C. Impara (Eds.), *The fourteenth mental measurements yearbook* (pp. 532–534). Lincoln, NE: Buros Institute of Mental Measurements.

Kanfer, R., Eyberg, S. M., & Krahn, G. L. (1992). Interviewing strategies in child assessment. In M. C. Roberts & C. E. Walker (Eds.), *Handbook of clinical child psychology* (2nd ed.). New York: Wiley.

Kapes, J. T., & Whitfield, E. (Eds.). (2002). *A counselor's guide to career assessment instruments* (4th ed.). Tulsa, OK: National Career Development Association.

Kaplan, F. E. (1996). The *WISC-III, TONI-2,* and *WRAT-3*: Are they significantly culturally biased? [Abstract]. Abstract obtained from *Dissertation Abstracts International Section A: Humanities & Social Sciences, 56,* 4370.

Kaplan, P. S. (1998). *The human odyssey: Life span development* (3rd ed.). Pacific Grove, CA: Brooks/Cole.

Kaplan, R. M., & Saccuzzo, D. P. (2001). *Psychological testing: Principles, applications, and issues* (5th ed.). Belmont, CA: Wadsworth/Thomson Learning.

Karlsen, B., & Gardner, E. F. (1996). *Stanford Diagnostic Reading Test* (4th ed.). San Antonio, TX: Harcourt Brace Educational Measurement.

Kaufman, A. S. (1990). *Assessing adolescent and adult intelligence.* Needham Heights, MA: Allyn & Bacon.

Kaufman, A. S. (1994). *Intelligent testing with the WISC-III.* New York: Wiley.

Kaufman, A. S., & Kaufman, N. L. (1983a). *Kaufman Assessment Battery for Children (K-ABC): Administration and scoring manual.* Circle Pines, MN: American Guidance Services.

Kaufman, A. S., & Kaufman, N. L. (1983b). *Kaufman Assessment Battery for Children: Interpretive manual.* Circle Pines, MN: American Guidance Services.

Kaufman, A. S., & Kaufman, N. L. (2004a). *Kaufman Brief Intelligence Test—Second Edition (KBIT-2).* Circle Pines, MN: American Guidance Services.

Kaufman, A. S., & Kaufman, N. L. (2004b). *Manual for the Kaufman Assessment Battery for Children—Second Edition (KABC-II).* Circle Pines, MN: American Guidance Services.

Kaufman, A. S., & Kaufman, N. L. (2005). *Manual for the Kaufman Test of Educational Achievement—Second Edition.* Circle Pines, MN: American Guidance Services.

Kaufman, A. S., & Lichtenberger, E. O. (2000). *Essentials of WISC-III and WPPSI-R assessment.* New York: Wiley.

Kaufman, J., Birmaher, B., Brent, D. A., Rao, U., & Ryan, N. (1996). *Revised Schedule for Affective Disorders and Schizophrenia for School-Aged Children: Present and Lifetime versions (K-SADS-PL).* Pittsburgh, PA: Western Psychiatric Institute and Clinic.

Kavale, K. A. (1995). Setting the record straight on learning disability and low achievement: The tortuous path of ideology. *Learning Disabilities Research and Practice, 10,* 145–152.

Kavan, M. G. (1992). Review of the *Children's Depression Inventory.* In J. J. Kramer & J. C. Conoley (Eds.), *The eleventh mental measurements yearbook* (pp. 174–175). Lincoln, NE: Buros Institute of Mental Measurements.

Kavan, M. G. (1995). Review of the *Personality Assessment Inventory.* In J. C. Conoley & J. C. Impara (Eds.), *The twelfth mental measurements yearbook* (pp. 766–768). Lincoln, NE: Buros Institute of Mental Measurements.

Kazdin, A. E. (1982). *Single-case research designs: Methods for clinical and applied settings.* New York: Oxford University Press.

Keith, T. (2001). Review of the *Wechsler Abbreviated Scale of Intelligence.* In B. S. Plake & J. C.

Impara (Eds.), *The fourteenth mental measurements yearbook*. Lincoln, NE: Buros Institute of Mental Measurements.

Keith, T., Kransler, J. H., & Flanagan, D. P. (2001). What does the *Cognitive Assessment System* (*CAS*) measure? Joint confirmatory factor analysis of the *CAS* and the *Woodcock-Johnson: Tests of Cognitive Ability—Third Edition*. *School Psychology Review, 30,* 89–119.

Kelly, K. R. (2002a). Concurrent validity of the *Kuder Career Search* activity preference scales and career clusters. *Journal of Career Assessment, 10,* 127–144.

Kelly, K. R. (2002b). *Kuder Occupational Interest Survey, Form DD* (*KOIS-DD*) *and Kuder Career Search with Person Match* (*KCS*). In J. T. Kapes & E. A. Whitfield (Eds.). *A counselor's guide to career assessment instruments* (pp. 265–275). Alexandria, VA: National Career Development Association.

Kelly, M. (2005). Review of the *Piers-Harris Children's Self-Concept Scale—Second Edition*. In B. S. Plake, J. C. Impara, & R. A. Spies (Eds.), *The sixteenth mental measurements yearbook*. Lincoln, NE: Buros Institute of Mental Measurements.

Kelly, T., Ruch, G., & Terman, L. (1923). *Stanford Achievement Test*. Stanford, CA: Stanford University.

Kilbride, H. W., Johnson, D. L., & Streissguth, A. P. (1977). Social class, birth order, and newborn experience. *Child Development, 48,* 1686–1688.

Killer's diary reveals plans for Columbine attack. (2001). Retrieved August 9, 2004, from www.usatoday.com/news/nation/2001/12/05/columbine.htm.

King, R. A., & Noshpitz, J. D. (1991). *Pathways of growth: Essentials of child psychiatry*. New York: Wiley.

Kingsbury, G. G. (2001). Review of the *KeyMath Revised: A Diagnostic Inventory of Essential Mathematics 1998 Normative Update* (*KeyMath-R/NU*). In B. S. Plake & J. C. Impara (Eds.), *The fourteenth mental measurements yearbook* (pp. 638–640). Lincoln, NE: Buros Institute of Mental Measurements.

Kinston, W., Loader, P., & Sullivan, J. (1985). *Clinical assessment of family health*. London: Hospital for Sick Children, Family Studies Group.

Kirk, W. D. (1974). *Aids and precautions in administering the Illinois Test of Psycholinguistic Abilities*. Chicago: University of Illinois Press.

Klecker, B. (2001). Review of the *Attention Deficit Disorders Evaluation Scale, Second Edition*. In B. S. Plake & J. C. Impara (Eds.), *The fourteenth mental measurements yearbook* (pp. 90–92). Lincoln, NE: Buros Institute of Mental Measurements.

Knapp, R. R., Knapp, L., & Knapp-Lee, L. (1990). *COPSystem technical manual*. San Diego, CA: EdITS.

Knoff, H. M. (1992). Review of the *Children's Depression Inventory*. In J. J. Kramer & J. C. Conoley (Eds.), *The eleventh mental measurements yearbook* (pp. 175–177). Lincoln, NE: Buros Institute of Mental Measurements.

Knoff, H. M. (1998). Review of the *Children's Apperception Test 1991 Revision*. In J. C. Impara & B. S. Plake (Eds.), *The thirteenth mental measurements yearbook* (pp. 231–233). Lincoln, NE: Buros Institute of Mental Measurements.

Knoff, H. M., & Prout, H. T. (1985). *Kinetic Drawing System for Family and School*. Los Angeles: Western Psychological Services.

Knoop, A. (2004). Test review: *Wide Range Achievement Test-3. Rehabilitation Counseling Bulletin, 47,* 184–185.

Kobal, A., Wrightstone, J. W., & Kunze, K. R. (1943). *Mechanical Aptitude Test: Acorn National Aptitude Tests*. Murfreesboro, TN: Psychometric Affiliates.

Kobal, A., Wrightstone, J. W., & Kunze, K. R. (1944). *Clerical Aptitude Test: Acorn National Aptitude Tests*. Murfreesboro, TN: Psychometric Affiliates.

Koh, T., Abbatiello, A., & McLoughlin, C. S. (1984). Cultural bias in *WISC* subtest items: A response to Judy Grady's suggestion in relation to the PASE case. *School Psychology Review, 13,* 89–94.

Koppitz, E. M. (1975). *The Bender-Gestalt test for young children, Vol. 2.* New York: Grune & Stratton.

Kovacs, M. (1992). *Manual for the Children's Depression Inventory.* North Tonawanda, NY: Multi-Health Systems.

Kozma, A., & Stones, M. J. (1987). Social desirability in measures of subjective well-being: A systematic evaluation. *Journal of Gerontology, 42,* 56–59.

Kraepelin, E. (1895). Der psychologische Versuch in der Psychiatrie. *Psychologische Arbeiten, 1,* 1–91.

Kratochwill, T. R., & Bergan, J. R. (1990). *Behavioral consultation in applied settings: An individual guide.* New York: Plenum.

Kratochwill, T. R., Sheridan, S. M., Carlson, J., & Lasecki, K. L. (1999). Advances in behavioral assessment. In C. R. Reynolds, & T. B. Gutkin (Eds.), *Handbook of school psychology* (3rd ed., pp. 350–382). New York: Wiley.

Kronenberger, W. G., & Meyer, R. G. (1996). *The child clinician's handbook.* Needham Heights, MA: Allyn & Bacon.

Krumboltz, J. D. (1997). *Manual for the Career Beliefs Inventory.* Palo Alto, CA: Consulting Psychologists Press.

Kuder, F. (1939). *The Kuder Preference Record—Vocational.* Chicago: Science Research Associates.

Kuder, F. (1988). *Kuder General Interest Survey, Form E.* Chicago, IL: Science Research Associates.

Kuder, F., & Zytowski, D. G. (1991). *Kuder Occupational Interest Survey Form DD, general manual* (3rd ed.). Adel, IA: National Career Assessment Services.

Kuder, F., & Zytowski, D. G. (1999). *Kuder Career Search with Person Match.* Adel, IA: National Career Assessment Services.

Kuhn, L. R., & Bodkin, A. E. (2006). Review of the *Revised Children's Manifest Anxiety Scale.* In B. T. Erford (Ed.), *The counselor's guide to clinical, personality, and behavioral assessment* (pp. 54–56). Boston: Lahaska/Houghton Mifflin.

Kunen, S., Overstreet, S., & Salles, C. (1996). Concurrent validity study of the *Slosson Intelligence Test—Revised* in mental retardation testing. *Mental Retardation, 34,* 380–386.

Kupermintz, H. (2002). *School reform proposals: The research evidence.* Tempe: Arizona State University, Education Policy Studies Laboratory.

Kwate, N. O. A. (2001). Intelligence or misorientation? Eurocentrism in the *WISC-III. Journal of Black Psychology, 27,* 221–231.

Kwiatkowska, H. Y. (1978). *Family therapy and evaluation through art.* Springfield, IL: Thomas.

L'Abate, L. (1994). *Family evaluation: A psychological approach.* Thousand Oaks, CA: Sage.

L'Abate, L., & Bagarozzi, D. A. (1993). *Sourcebook of marriage and family evaluation.* New York: Brunner/Mazel.

Lachar, B. (1992). Review of the *Minnesota Importance Questionnaire.* In J. J. Kramer & J. C. Conoley (Eds.), *The eleventh mental measurements yearbook* (pp. 542–544). Lincoln, NE: Buros Institute of Mental Measurements.

Lachar, D., & Gruber, C. P. (2001). *Manual for the Personality Inventory for Children—Second Edition* (*PIC-2*). Los Angeles: Western Psychological Services.

Lafayette Instrument. (n.d.a). *Minnesota Manual Dexterity Test.* North Lafayette, IN: Lafayette Instruments.

Lafayette Instrument. (n.d.b). *O'Connor Tweezer Dexterity Test.* Lafayette, IN: Lafayette Instruments.

Lambert, N., Nihira, K., & Leland, H. (1993). *AAMR Adaptive Behavior Scale—School Edition* (Rev.). Austin, TX: PRO-ED.

Lanyon, R. I. (1995). Review of the *Minnesota Multiphasic Personality Inventory—Adolescent*. In J. C. Conoley & J. C. Impara (Eds.), *The twelfth mental measurements yearbook* (pp. 628–629). Lincoln, NE: Buros Institute of Mental Measurements.

Larson, J. H. (2002). *Consumer update: Marriage preparation* [Brochure]. Alexandria, VA: American Association of Marriage and Family Therapists.

Larson, J. H., Newell, K., Topham, G., & Nichols, S. (2002). A review of three comprehensive premarital assessment questionnaires. *Journal of Marital and Family Therapy, 28*, 233–239.

Larson, S., Hammill, D., & Moats, L. (1999). *Manual for the Test of Written Spelling—Fourth Edition (TWS-4)*. Austin, TX: PRO-ED.

Last, C. G., Strauss, C., & Francis, G. (1987). Comorbidity among child and adolescent disorders. *Journal of Nervous and Mental Disease, 175*, 726–730.

Lattimore, R. R., & Borgen, F. H. (1999). Validity of the 1994 *Strong Interest Inventory* with racial and ethnic groups in the United States. *Journal of Counseling Psychology, 46*, 185.

Laurent, J., Swerdlik, M., & Ryburn, M. (1992). Review of validity research on the *Stanford-Binet Intelligence Scale—Fourth Edition. Psychological Assessment, 4*, 102–112.

Lavin, M., & Rifkin, A. (1993). Diagnosis and pharmacotherapy of Conduct Disorder. *Progress in Neuro-psychopharmacology and Biological Psychiatry, 17*, 875–885.

Layton, W. L. (1992). Review of the *Minnesota Importance Questionnaire*. In J. J. Kramer & J. C. Conoley (Eds.), *The eleventh mental measurements yearbook* (pp. 544–546). Lincoln, NE: Buros Institute of Mental Measurements.

Lazowski, L. E., Miller, F. G., Boye, M. W., & Miller, G. A. (1998). Efficacy of the *Substance Abuse Subtle Screening Inventory—3 (SASSI-3)* in identifying substance dependence disorders in clinical settings. *Journal of Personality Assessment, 71*, 114–128.

Leckman, J. F., & Cohen, D. J. (1994). Tic disorders. In M. Rutter, E. Taylor, & L. Hersov (Eds.), *Child and adolescent psychiatry: Modern approaches* (pp. 455–466). Cambridge, MA: Blackwell.

Lee, C. (2001). Culturally responsive school counselors and programs: Addressing the needs of all students. *Professional School Counseling, 4*, 257–261.

Lehmann, I. J. (1998). Review of the *Stanford Diagnostic Mathematics Test, Fourth Edition*. In J. C. Impara & B. S. Plake (Eds.), *The thirteenth mental measurements yearbook* (pp. 932–936). Lincoln, NE: Buros Institute of Mental Measurements.

Lerner, B. (1981). The minimum competence testing movement: Social, scientific, and legal implications. *American Psychologist, 36*, 1056–1066.

Lichtenberg, P. (1999). Depression in geriatric medical and nursing home patients, a treatment manual. Wayne, IN: Wayne State University Press.

Likert, R., & Quasha, W. H. (1995). *Revised Minnesota Paper Form Board Test, Second Edition*. San Antonio, TX: Psychological Corporation.

Lindquist, E. (1936). *Iowa Every-Pupil Tests of Basic Skills*. Itasca, IL: Riverside Publishing.

Linn, L., & Slindle, J. A. (1977). The determination of the significance of change between pre- and posttesting periods. *Review of Educational Research, 47*, 121–150.

Linn, R. L., & Gronlund, N. E. (2000). *Measurement and assessment in teaching* (8th Ed.). Upper Saddle River, NJ: Prentice Hall.

Lock, R. D. (2005). *Taking charge of your career direction: Career planning guide, Book 1* (5th ed.). Belmont, CA: Thomson Brooks/Cole.

Lockhart, E. J. (2003). Students with disabilities. In B. T. Erford (Ed.), *Transforming the school counseling profession* (pp. 357–410). Columbus, OH: Merrill/Prentice Hall.

Lockhart, E. J., & Keys, S. G. (1998). The mental health counseling role of school counselors. *Professional School Counseling, 1*, 3–6.

Loehlin, J. C. (1989) Partitioning environmental and genetic contributions to behavioral development. *American Psychologist, 10*, 1285–1292.

Loehlin, J. C., Lindzey, G., & Spuhler, J. N. (1975). *Race differences in intelligence.* San Francisco, CA: Freeman.

Lohman, D. F., & Hagen, E. P. (2001). *The Cognitive Abilities Test (CogAT), Form 6.* Itasca, IL: Riverside Publishing.

Lord, F. M. (1956). The measurement of growth. *Educational and Psychological Measurement, 16,* 421–437.

Lord, F. M. (1957). Do tests of the same length have the same standard error of measurement? *Educational and Psychological Measurement, 17,* 510–521.

Lord, F. M., & Novick, R. (1968). *Statistical theories of mental test scores.* Reading, MA: Addison-Wesley.

Loyd, B. H. (1985). Review of the *Secondary Level English Proficiency Test.* In J. V. Mitchell (Ed.), *The ninth mental measurements yearbook* (pp. 1335–1336). Lincoln, NE: Buros Institute of Mental Measurements.

Loyer-Carlson, V. L., Busby, D., Holman, T., Klein, D., & Larson, J. (2002). *RELATE: User's guide.* Needham Heights, MA: Allyn & Bacon.

Luftig, R. L. (1989). *Assessment of learners with special needs.* Boston: Allyn & Bacon.

Lukin, L. E. (2005). Review of the *Metropolitan Achievement Test—Eighth Edition.* In B. S. Plake, J. C. Impara, & R. A. Spies (Eds.), *The sixteenth mental measurements yearbook.* Lincoln, NE: Buros Institute of Mental Measurements.

Mace, F. C. (1985). Review of the *Walker Problem Behavior Identification Checklist (WPBIC).* In J. V. Mitchell, Jr. (Ed.), *The ninth mental measurements yearbook* (pp. 479–480). Lincoln, NE: Buros Institute of Mental Measurements.

Magnuson, S., & Shaw, H. E. (2003). Adaptations of the multifaceted genogram in counseling, training, and supervision. *The Family Journal: Counseling and Therapy for Couples and Families, 11,* 45–54.

Mahurin, R. (1992). Review of the *Computer Programmer Aptitude Battery—Third Edition.* In J. J. Kramer & J. C. Conoley (Eds.), *The eleventh mental measurements yearbook* (pp. 225–227). Lincoln, NE: Buros Institute of Mental Measurements.

Maloney, M. P., & Ward, M. P. (1976). *Psychological assessment: A conceptual approach.* New York: Oxford University Press.

Mancini, J. A. (2001). Review of the *Family Environment Scale—Third Edition.* In B. S. Plake & J. C. Impara (Eds.), *The fourteenth mental measurements yearbook* (pp. 480–482). Lincoln, NE: Buros Institute of Mental Measurements.

Manges, K. J. (2001). Review of the *Family Assessment Measure Version III.* In B. S. Plake & J. C. Impara (Eds.), *The fourteenth mental measurements yearbook* (pp. 480–482). Lincoln, NE: Buros Institute of Mental Measurements.

Manuele-Adkins, C. (1995). Review of the *Adult Career Concerns Inventory.* In J. C. Conoley & J. C. Impara (Eds.), *The twelfth mental measurements yearbook* (pp. 48–50). Lincoln, NE: Buros Institute of Mental Measurements.

March, J. S., & Leonard, H. L. (1996). Obsessive-Compulsive Disorder in children and adolescents: A review of the past 10 years. *Journal of the American Academy of Child and Adolescent Psychiatry, 34,* 1265–1273.

Marchant, G. J., & Paulson, S. E. (1998). Review of the *Parent-Child Relationship Inventory.* In J. C. Impara & B. S. Plake (Eds.), *The thirteenth mental measurements yearbook* (pp. 720–721). Lincoln, NE: Buros Institute of Mental Measurements.

Marco, G. L. (2001). Review of the *Leiter International Performance Scale—Revised.* In B. S. Plake & J. C. Impara (Eds.), *The fourteenth mental measurements yearbook* (pp. 683–687). Lincoln, NE: Buros Institute of Mental Measurements.

Marin, G., & Marin B. V. (1991). *Research with Hispanic populations.* Newbury Park, CA: Sage.

Markey, B., Micheletto, M., & Becker, A. (2000). *Facilitating Open Couple Communication, Understanding, and Study* (*FOCCUS*) (3rd ed.). Omaha, NE: FOCCUS.

Markwardt, F. C., Jr. (1998). *Peabody Individual Achievement —Test* (Rev. ed.). Circle Pines, MN: AGS Publishing.

Marsh, J. W., & Holmes, I. W. M. (1990). Multidimensional self-concepts: Construct validation of responses by children. *American Educational Research Journal, 27,* 89–117.

Martinez, M. E. (1999). Cognition and the question of test item format. *Educational Psychologist, 34,* 207–218.

Masling, J. (1960). The influence of situational and interpersonal variables in projective testing. *Psychological Bulletin, 57,* 65–85.

Mather, N., & Jaffe, L. E. (2002). *Woodcock-Johnson III: Reports, recommendations, and strategies.* New York: Wiley.

Mather, N., Wendling, B. J., & Woodcock, R. W. (2001). *Essentials of WJIII Tests of Achievement assessment.* New York: Wiley.

Mather, N., & Woodcock, R. W. (2001). *Woodcock-Johnson: Tests of Achievement* (3rd ed.)*: Examiner's manual.* Itasca, IL: Riverside Publishing.

Matzen, R., & Hoyt, J. (2004). Basic writing placement with holistically scored essays: Research evidence. *Journal of Developmental Education, 28,* 1.

Maxwell, S. E. (1980). Dependent variable reliability and determination of sample size. *Applied Psychological Measurement, 4,* 253–260.

Mayfield, D. G., McLeod, G., & Hall, P. (1974). The CAGE questionnaire: Validation of a new alcoholism screening instrument. *American Journal of Psychiatry, 131,* 1121–1123.

McArthur, D. S., & Roberts, G. E. (1994). *Manual for the Roberts Apperception Test for Children* (2nd ed.).—Los Angeles: Western Psychological Services.

McArthur, D. S., & Roberts, G. E. (2005). *Roberts Apperception Test for Children—Second Edition, Revised.* Los Angeles: Western Psychological Services.

McCall, R. B., Hogarty, P. S., & Hurlburt, N. (1972). Transitions in infant sensorimotor development and the prediction of childhood IQ. *American Psychologist, 27,* 728–748.

McCarney, S. B. (1994). *Attention Deficit Disorders intervention manual* (2nd ed.). Columbia, MO: Hawthorne Educational Services.

McCarney, S. B., & Arthaud, T. J. (2004a). *Attention Deficit Disorders Evaluation Scale—Third Edition—Home Version technical manual.* Columbia, MO: Hawthorne Educational Services.

McCarney, S. B., & Arthaud, T. J. (2004b). *Attention Deficit Disorders Evaluation Scale—Third Edition—School Version technical manual.* Columbia, MO: Hawthorne Educational Services.

McCarney, S. B., & Baker, A. M. (1995). *Parent's guide to Attention Deficit Disorders* (2nd ed.). Columbia, MO: Hawthorne Educational Services.

McClure, E. B., Kubiszyn, T., & Kaslow, J. J. (2002). Advances in the diagnosis and treatment of childhood mood disorders. *Professional Psychology: Research and Practice, 33,* 125–134.

McConaughy, S. H., & Achenbach, T. M. (1994). *Manual for the Semistructured Clinical Interview for Children and Adolescents* (*SCICA*). Burlington, VT: University Associates in Psychiatry.

McCornack, R. L., & McLeod, M. (1988). Gender bias in the prediction of college course performance. *Journal of Educational Measurement, 25,* 321–331.

McCrae, R. R., & Costa, P. T., Jr. (1983). Social desirability scales: More substance than style. *Journal of Consulting and Clinical Psychology, 51,* 882–888.

McCrae, R. R., & Costa, P.T., Jr. (1987). Validation of the five-factor model of personality across instruments and observers. *Journal of Personality and Social Psychology, 52,* 81–90.

McCrae, R. R., & Costa, P. T., Jr. (1989). Reinterpreting the *Myers-Briggs Type Indicator* from the perspective of the five-factor model of personality. *Journal of Personality, 57,* 17–40.

McDivitt, P. J. (2004). Training educators to develop good educational tests. In J. E. Wall & G. R. Walz (Eds.) *Measuring up: Assessment issues for teachers, counselors, and administrators* (pp. 33–52). Greensboro, NC: CAPS Publications.

McDivitt, P. J., & Gibson, D. (2004). Guidelines for selecting appropriate tests. In J. E. Wall & G. R. Walz (Eds.) *Measuring up: Assessment issues for teachers, counselors, and administrators* (pp. 33–52). Greensboro, NC: CAPS Publications.

McGoldrick, M., Gerson, R., & Shellenberger, S. (1999). *Genograms: Assessment and intervention* (2nd ed.). New York: Norton.

McGrew, K. S., & Flanagan, D. P. (1998). *The intelligence test desk reference (ITDR): Gf-Gc cross-battery assessment.* Boston: Allyn & Bacon.

McGrew, K. S., & Woodcock, R. W. (2001). *Technical manual for the Woodcock-Johnson III.* Itasca, IL: Riverside Publishing.

McGue, M., Bouchard, T. J., Jr., Iacono, W. G., & Lykken, D. T. (1993). Behavioral genetics of cognitive ability: A life-span perspective. In R. Ploomin & G. E. McClearn (Eds.), *Nature, nurture, & psychology* (pp. 59–76). Washington, DC: American Psychological Association.

McKechnie, J. A. (2006). Review of the *Disruptive Behavior Rating Scale (DBRS)*. In B. T. Erford (Ed.), *Counselor's guide to clinical, personality, and behavioral assessment* (pp. 141–143). Boston: Lahaska/Houghton Mifflin.

McKechnie, J. A., & Erford, B. T. (2001). Test review: *Slosson Intelligence Test—Revised (SIT-R)*. Retrieved February 15, 2005, from http://aace.ncat.edu/newsnotes/y01win/html.

McLarty, J. R. (1992). Review of the *Test of Early Mathematics Ability, Second Edition.* In J. J. Kramer & J. C. Conoley (Eds.), *The eleventh mental measurements yearbook* (pp. 941–942). Lincoln, NE: Buros Institute of Mental Measurements.

McLellan, M. J. (1995). Review of the *Sixteenth Personality Factor Questionnaire—Fifth Edition.* In J. C. Conoley & J. C. Impara (Eds.), *The twelfth mental measurements yearbook* (pp. 947–948). Lincoln, NE: Buros Institute of Mental Measurements.

McMillan, J. H. (1997). *Classroom assessment: Principles and practice for effective instruction.* Needham Heights, MA: Allyn & Bacon.

McMurtry, L. (1975). *Terms of endearment.* Forge Village, MA: Murray Printing.

McPhatter, A. R. (1991). Assessment revisited: A comprehensive approach to understanding family dynamics. *Families in Society, 72,* 11–21.

McReynolds, P. (1989). Diagnosis and clinical assessment: Current status and major issues. *Annual Review of Psychology, 40,* 83–108.

Mead, M. A., Hohensil, T. H., & Singh, S. (1997). How the *DSM* system is used by clinical counselors: A national study. *Journal of Mental Health Counseling, 19,* 383–395.

Means-Christensen, A. J., Snyder, D. K., & Negy, C. (2003). Assessing nontraditional couples: Validity of the *Marital Satisfaction Inventory—Revised* with gay, lesbian, and cohabiting heterosexual couples. *Journal of Marital and Family Therapy, 29,* 69–83.

Meehl, P. E. (1954). *Clinical versus statistical prediction: A theoretical analysis and a review of the evidence.* Minneapolis: University of Minnesota Press.

Meehl, P. E. (1957). When shall we use our heads instead of the formula? *Journal of Counseling Psychology, 4,* 268–273.

Meehl, P. E. (1965). Seer over sign: The first good example. *Journal of Experimental Research in Personality, 1,* 27–32.

Mehrens, W. A., & Lehmann, I. J. (1991). *Measurement and evaluation in education and psychology* (4th ed.). Fort Worth, TX: Holt, Rinehart, & Winston.

Meikamp, J. (2001). Review of the *Das-Naglieri Cognitive Assessment System.* In B. S. Plake & J. C. Impara (Eds.), *The fourteenth mental measurements yearbook* (pp. 366–367). Lincoln, NE: Buros Institute of Mental Measurements.

Mercer, J. R. (1976). *A System of Multicultural Pluralistic Assessment* (*SOMPA*). In *Proceedings: With bias toward none.* Lexington: Coordinating Office for Regional Resource Centers, University of Kentucky.

Merrell, K. W. (1999). *Behavioral, social, and emotional assessment of children and adolescents.* Mahwah, NJ: Erlbaum.

Meyer, G. J., Finn, S. E., Eyde, L. D., Kay, G. G., Moreland, K. L., Dies, R. R., et al. (2001). Psychological testing and psychological assessment: A review of evidence and issues. *American Psychologist, 56,* 128–165.

Michael, J. (2003). Using the *Myers-Briggs Type Indicator* as a tool for leadership development? Apply with caution. *Journal of Leadership & Organizational Studies, 10,* 68–81.

Miller, G. A. (1997). The SASSI Institute: Newsletter Volume 5, Number 2; June 1997. Retrieved June 15, 2004, from www.sassi.com/docs/news_5_2.htm.

Miller, G. A. (2001). *Manual for the SASSI-A2.* Springville, IN: SASSI Institute.

Miller, G. A., & Lazowski, M. (1999). *Manual for the SASSI-3.* Springville, IN: SASSI Institute.

Miller, J. A., & Barona, A. (1997). Screening for learning disabilities in adult basic education programs. *Adult Basic Education, 7,* 46–58.

Miller, J. O., & Phillips, J. (1966). A *preliminary evaluation of the Head Start and other metropolitan Nashville kindergartens.* Unpublished manuscript, George Peabody College for Teachers, TN.

Miller, L. (1999). *Kaufman Test of Educational Achievement/Normative Update* (*KTEA/NU*). *Diagnostique, 24,* 145–159.

Miller, W. S. (1992). *Miller Analogy Test.* San Antonio, TX: Psychological Corporation.

Millon, T. (1969). *Modern psychopathology: A biosocial approach to maladaptive learning and functioning.* Philadelphia: Saunders.

Millon, T. (1994). *The Million Index of Personality Styles* (*MIPS*). Minneapolis: NCS Pearson.

Millon, T. (2003). *Manual for the Millon Index of Personality Styles—Revised* (*MIPS Revised*). Minneapolis: NCS Pearson.

Millon, T., Davis, R., & Millon, C. (1997). *Manual for the Millon Clinical Multiaxial Inventory* (3rd ed.). Minneapolis: NCS Pearson.

Millon, T., Millon, C., & Davis, R. (1993). *The Millon Adolescent Clinical Inventory* (*MACI*). Minneapolis: NCS Pearson.

Miltenberger, R. G. (2004). *Behavior modification principles and procedures* (3rd ed.). Belmont, CA: Thomson Wadsworth.

Minuchin, S. (1974). *Families and family therapy.* Cambridge, MA: Harvard University Press.

Minuchin, S., & Fishman, H. (1981). *Family therapy techniques.* Cambridge, MA: Harvard University Press.

Mirenda, P. (1995). Review of the *Denver II.* In J. C. Conoley & J. C. Impara (Eds.), *The twelfth mental measurements yearbook* (pp. 265–266). Lincoln, NE: Buros Institute of Mental Measurements.

Mohr, D. C. (1995). Negative outcome in psychotherapy: A critical review. *Clinical Psychology: Science and Practice, 2,* 1–27.

Molloy, D. W, Alemayehu, E., & Roberts, R. (1991). Reliability of a *Standardized Mini-Mental State Examination* compared with the traditional mini-mental state examination. *American Journal of Psychiatry, 140,* 102–105.

Moore, R. D., Bone, L. R., Geller, G., Mamon, J. A., Stokes, E. J., & Levine, D. M. (1989). Prevalence, detection, and treatment of alcoholism in hospitalized patients. *Journal of the American Medical Association, 261,* 403–407.

Moos, R. H., & Moos, B. S. (1994). *Family Environment Scale Manual: Development, applications, research* (3rd ed.). Palo Alto, CA: Consulting Psychologists Press.

Moreno, J. J. (1945). *Group psychotherapy: A symposium.* New York: Beacon House.

Moreno, J. J. (1999). Ancient sources and modern applications: The creative arts in psychodrama. *Arts in Psychotherapy, 27,* 95–101.

Morey, L. C. (1991). *Manual for the Personality Assessment Inventory.* Lutz, FL: Psychological Assessment Resources.

Moum, T. (1998). Mode of administration and interviewer effect in self-reported symptoms of anxiety and depression. *Social Indicators Research, 45*(1–3), 279–318.

Muir, S. P., & Tracy, D. M. (1999). Collaborative essay testing. *College Teaching, 47,* 33.

Multi–Health Systems. (2003). MHS: Helping you to help others. Retrieved June 15, 2004, from https://www.mhs.com/ecom.

Murphy, K. R., & Davidshofer, C. O. (2001). *Psychological testing: Principles and applications* (5th ed.). Upper Saddle River, NJ: Prentice Hall.

Murray, H. A., & Bellak, L. (1973). *Thematic Apperception Test.*(). San Antonio, TX: Harcourt Assessment.

Murray-Ward, M. (1998). Review of the *Nelson-Denny Reading Test, Forms G & H.* In J. C. Impara & B. S. Plake (Eds.), *The thirteenth mental measurements yearbook* (pp. 683–685). Lincoln, NE: Buros Institute of Mental Measurements.

Myers, I. B., Kirby, L. K., & Myers, K. D. (1998). *Introduction to type* (6th ed.). Palo Alto, CA: Consulting Psychologists Press.

Myers, I. B., McCaulley, M. H., Quenk, N. L., & Hammer, A. L. (1998). *MBTI Manual: A guide to the development and use of the Myers-Briggs Type Indicator* (3rd ed.). Palo Alto, CA: Consulting Psychologists Press.

Naglieri, J. A., & Das, J. P. (1996). *Manual for the Das-Naglieri Cognitive Assessment System* (*CAS*). Itasca, IL: Riverside Publishing.

Naglieri, J. A., LeBuffe, P., & Pfeiffer, S. I. (1996). *Manual for the Devereux Scales of Mental Disorders* (*DSMD*). San Antonio, TX: Psychological Corporation.

Nagy, P. (1998). Review of the *Stanford Diagnostic Mathematics Test, Fourth Edition.* In J. C. Impara & B. S. Plake (Eds.), *The thirteenth mental measurements yearbook* (pp. 936–938). Lincoln, NE: Buros Institute of Mental Measurements.

National Association for School Psychologists. (1992). *Principles for professional ethics.* Washington, DC: Author.

National Board of Certified Counselors. (1989). *Code of ethics.* Greensboro, NC: Author.

National Education Goals Panel. (1993). *Promises to keep: Creating high standards for American students.* Washington, DC: Author.

National Institute of Mental Health. (1990). *Research on children and adolescents with mental, behavioral and developmental disorders.* Rockville, MD: Author.

National Institute of Mental Health. (2005). National Institute of Mental Health. Website. Retrieved December 3, 2004, from www.nimh.nih.gov.

National-Institutes of Health. (1998). *NIH consensus statement: Diagnosis and treatment of Attention Deficit Hyperactivity Disorder* (Vol. 16, no. 2). Bethesda, MD: Author.

Neisser, U., Boodoo, G., Bouchard, T. J., Boykin, A. W., Brody, N., Ceci, S. J., et al. (1996). Intelligence: Knowns and unknowns. *American Psychologist, 51,* 77–98.

Nelson, R. O. (1985). Behavioral assessment in the school setting. In T. R. Kratochwill (Ed.), *Advances in school psychology* (Vol. 4, pp. 45–87). Hillsdale, NJ: Erlbaum.

Nettelbeck, T., & Rabbit, P. M. A. (1992). Aging, cognitive performance, and mental speed. *Intelligence, 16,* 189–205.

Nevill, D. D., & Super, D. E. (1989). *The Values Scale theory, application, and research manual* (2nd ed.). Palo Alto, CA: Consulting Psychologists Press.

New Freedom Commission on Mental Health. (2003). Achieving the promise: Transforming mental health care in America. Retrieved on December 17, 2003, from www.mentalhealthcommission.gov/reports/FinalReport/downloads/downloads.html.

Newman, D. L. (1995). Review of the *General Clerical Test*. In J. C. Conoley & J. C. Impara (Eds.), *The twelfth mental measurements yearbook* (pp. 404–405). Lincoln, NE: Buros Institute of Mental Measurements.

Nichols, D. S. (1992). Review of the *Minnesota Multiphasic Personality Inventory—Second Edition*. In J. J. Kramer and J. C. Conoley (Eds.), *The eleventh mental measurements yearbook* (pp. 562–565). Lincoln, NE: Buros Institute of Mental Measurements.

Nichols, M. P., & Schwartz, R. C. (2001). *Family therapy: Concepts and methods* (5th ed.). Needham Heights, MA: Allyn & Bacon.

Nicholson, C. (1999). *Manual for the Slosson Visual-Motor Performance Test* (*S-VMTP*). East Aurora, NY: Slosson Educational Publications.

Nicholson, C., & Hipshman, T. (1990). *Manual for the Slosson Intelligence Test—Revised*. East Aurora, NY: Slosson Educational Publications.

Nicholson, C., & Hibpsham, T. (1997). *Technical manual for the Slosson Intelligence Test—Revised* (*SIT-R*). East Aurora, NY: Slosson Educational Publications.

Niles, S. G., & Harris-Bowlsbey, J. H. (2002). *Career development interventions in the 21st century*. Upper Saddle River, NJ: Merrill/Prentice Hall.

Niles, S. G., & Harris-Bowlsbey, J. H. (2005). *Career development interventions in the 21st century* (2nd ed.). Upper Saddle River, NJ: Merrill/Prentice Hall.

Nitko, A. J. (2001). *Educational assessment of students* (3rd ed.). Upper Saddle River, NJ: Merrill/Prentice Hall.

Nitko, A. J. (2004). *Educational assessment of students* (4th ed.). Upper Saddle River, NJ: Merrill/Prentice Hall.

No Child Left Behind Act of 2001 (NCLB) Public Law 107–110.

Noble, J., & Camera, W. (2003). Issues in college admissions testing. In J. Wall & G. Walz (Eds.), *Measuring up: Assessment issues for teachers, counselors, and administrators* (pp. 283–296). Greensboro, NC: CAPS Press.

Novak, C. (2001). Review of the *Metropolitan Readiness Tests—Sixth Edition*. In B. S. Plake & J. C. Impara, (Eds.), *The fourteenth mental measurements yearbook* (pp. 749–751). Lincoln, NE: Buros Institute of Mental Measurements.

Nunnally, J. C., & Bernstein, I. H. (1994). *Psychometric theory* (3rd ed.). New York: McGraw-Hill.

Nurss, J., & McGauvran, M. (1995). *Metropolitan Readiness Tests—Sixth Edition* (*MRT6*). San Antonio, TX: Psychological Corporation.

Oehrn, A. (1889). Experimentelle Studien zur Individual-Psychologie. Doctoral dissertation, Dorpat University, Tartu, Estonia.

Oetting, E. R., & Beauvais, F. (1990). Adolescent drug use: Findings of national and local surveys. *Journal of Consulting and Clinical Psychology, 58*, 385–394.

O'Hanlon, S., & O'Hanlon, B. (2002). Solution-oriented therapy with families. In J. Carlson & D. Kjos (Eds.), *Theories and strategies of family therapy* (pp. 190–215). Boston: Allyn & Bacon.

Olson, D. H. (1997). Family stress and coping: A multi-system perspective. In S. Dreman (Ed.), *The family on the threshold of the 21st century* (pp. 258–282). Mahwah, NJ: Erlbaum.

Olson, D. H. (2004). *PREPARE/ENRICH counselor's manual*. Minneapolis, MN: Life Innovations.

Olson, D. H., & Gorall, D. M. (2003). Circumplex model of marital and family systems. In F. Walsh (Ed.), *Normal family processes* (3rd ed., pp. 514–547). New York: Guilford.

Olson, D. H., Gorall, D., & Tiesel, J. (2002). *Family inventories package*. Minneapolis: Life Innovations.

Olson, D. H., Larsen, A., & McCubbin, H. I. (1989). Family strengths. In D. H. Olson, H. I. McCubbin, H. Barnes, A. Larsen, M. Muxen, & M. Wilson (Eds.), *Family inventories*. St. Paul: Family Social Science, University of Minnesota.

Olson, D. H., Russell, C., & Sprenkle, D. H. (1989). *Circumplex model: Systematic assessment and treatment of families*. New York: Haworth Press.

O'Rourke, N., & Cappeliez, P. (2001). Marital satisfaction and marital aggrandizement among older adults: Analysis of gender invariance. *Measurement and Evaluation in Counseling and Development, 34,* 66–79.

Orvaschel, H. (1995). *Schedule for Affective Disorders and Schizophrenia for School-Age Children—Epidemiological Version 5 (K-SADS-E5).* Ft. Lauderdale, FL: NOVA Southeastern University.

Osberg, T. M. (1992). Review of the *Salience Inventory.* In J. J. Kramer & J. C. Conoley (Eds.), *The eleventh mental measurements yearbook* (pp. 778–779). Lincoln, NE: Buros Institute of Mental Measurements.

Osborn, D. (2002). Test review: *Self-Directed Search. Rehabilitation Counseling Bulletin, 46,* 57–59.

Osipow, S. H., Carney, C. G., Winer, J., Yanico, B., & Koschier, M. (1980). *Career Decision Scale.* Odessa, FL: Psychological Assessment Resources.

Osman, A., Barrios, F. X., Aukes, D., Osman, J. R., & Markway, K. (1993). *The Beck Anxiety Inventory*: Psychometric properties in a community population. *Journal of Psychopathology and Behavioral Assessment, 15,* 287–297.

Osterlind, S. J. (1989). *Constructing test items.* Boston, MA: Kluwer Academic Publishers.

Otis, A. S., & Lennon, R. T. (2004). *Manual for the Otis-Lennon School Ability Test—Eighth Edition (OLSAT-8).* San Antonio, TX: Psychological Corporation.

Overall, J. E., & Woodward, J. A. (1975). Unreliability of difference scores: A paradox for measurement of change. *Psychological Bulletin, 82,* 85–86.

Overton, T. (1996). *Assessment in special education: An applied approach* (2nd ed.). Upper Saddle River, NJ: Prentice Hall.

Palormo, J. M., Fisher, B., & Saville, P. (1985). *Computer Programmer Aptitude Battery—Third Edition.* Chicago: Pearson Reid London House.

Parsons, F. (1909). *Choosing a vocation.* Boston: Houghton Mifflin.

Patterson, M., Slate, J. R., Jones, C. H., & Steger, H. S. (1995). The effects of practice administrations in learning to administer and score the *WAIS-R:* A partial replication. *Educational and Psychological Measurement, 55(1),* 32–37.

Pauker, J. D. (1985). Review of the *SCL-90-R.* In J. V. Mitchell Jr. (Ed.), *The ninth mental measurements yearbook* (pp. 1325–1326). Lincoln, NE: Buros Institute of Mental Measurements.

Payne, R. (2003). *A framework for understanding poverty* (3rd ed.) Highlands, TX: Aha! Process.

Payne, R. W. (1985). Review of the *SCL-R-90.* In J. V. Mitchell Jr. (Ed.), *The ninth mental measurements yearbook* (pp. 1326–1329). Lincoln, NE: Buros Institute of Mental Measurements.

Pearlman, C. (1998). Review of the *Test of Reading Comprehension—Third Edition (TORC-3).* In J. C. Impara & B. S. Plake (Eds.), *The thirteenth mental measurement yearbook* (pp. 1053–1055). Lincoln, NE: Buros Institute of Mental Measurements.

Pearson, L. C. (2001). Review of the *Revised Minnesota Paper Form Board Test—Second Edition.* In B. S. Plake & J. C. Impara (Eds.), *The fourteenth mental measurements yearbook* (pp. 1011–1012). Lincoln, NE: Buros Institute of Mental Measurements.

Peleg-Popko, O., & Klingman, A. (2002). Family environment, discrepancies between perceived, actual and desirable environment, and children's test and trait anxiety. *British Journal of Guidance & Counseling, 30,* 451–466.

Peterson, C. (1985). Review of *Coopersmith Self-Esteem Inventories.* In J. V. Mitchell (Ed.), *The ninth mental measurements yearbook* (pp. 396–397). Lincoln, NE: Buros Institute of Mental Measurements.

Peterson, C. A. (2001). Review of the *Devereux Scales of Mental Disorders.* In B. S. Plake & J. C. Impara (Eds.), *The fourteenth mental measurements yearbook* (pp. 410–412). Lincoln, NE: Buros Institute of Mental Measurements.

Piaget, J. (1954). *The construction of reality on the child.* New York: Basic.

Piaget, J. (1971). *Biology and knowledge.* Chicago: University of Chicago Press.

Pickering, J. W. (1998). Test review: *Career Thoughts Inventory.* Retrieved September 8, 2004, from http://aac.ncat.edu/newsnotes/y98sp2.html.

Piedmont, R. L. (1994). Validation of the *NEO-PI-R* observer form for college students: Towards a paradigm for studying personality development. *Assessment, 1,* 258–268.

Piedmont, R. L. (1998). *The Revised NEO Personality Interview: Clinical and research applications.* New York: Plenum Press.

Piedmont, R. L. (2006). Review of the *NEO-PI-R.* In B. T. Erford (Ed.), *The counselor's guide to clinical, personality, and behavioral assessment* (pp. 98–100). Boston: Lahaska/Houghton Mifflin.

Piers, E. V., & Herzberg, D. S. (2002). *Manual for the Piers-Harris Children's Self-Concept Scale—Second Edition.* Los Angeles: Western Psychological Services.

Piotrowski, C., & Zalewski, C. (1993). Training in psychodiagnostic testing in APA-approved PsyD and PhD clinical psychology programs. *Journal of Personality Assessment, 61,* 393–404.

Pittenger, D. J. (1998). Review of the *Jackson Personality Inventory—Revised.* In J. C. Impara & B. S. Plake (Eds.), *The thirteenth mental measurements yearbook* (pp. 556–557). Lincoln, NE: Buros Institute of Mental Measurements.

Pittenger, D. J. (2003). Review of the *Substance Abuse Subtle Screening Inventory-3.* In B. S. Plake, J. C. Impara, & R. A. Spies (Eds.), *The fifteenth mental measurements yearbook* (pp. 916–918). Lincoln, NE: Buros Institute of Mental Measurements.

Plake, B. S., Impara, J. C., & Spies, R. A. (Eds.). (2003). *The fifteenth mental measurements yearbook.* Lincoln, NE: Buros Institute of Mental Measurements.

Pledge, D. S., Lapan, R. T., Heppner, P. P., Kivlighan, D., & Roehlke, H. J. (1998). Stability and severity of presenting problems at a university counseling center: A 6-year analysis. *Professional Psychology: Research and Practice, 29,* 396–399.

Pope, M. (2002). *Kuder General Interest Survey, Form E (KGIS-E).* In J. T. Kapes & E. A. Whitfield (Eds.). *A counselor's guide to career assessment instruments* (pp. 257–264). Tulsa, OK: National Career Development Association.

Popham, W. J. (1999). *Classroom assessment: What teachers need to know* (2nd ed.). Boston: Allyn & Bacon.

Popham, W. J. (2002). *Classroom assessment: What teachers need to know* (3rd ed.). Boston, MA: Allyn & Bacon.

Popham, W. J. (2003, April). *Curriculum, instruction, and assessment: Amiable allies or phony friends.* NCME Career Award Address, presented at the annual meeting of the National Council on Measurement in Education.

Prince, D. J., & Heiser, L. J. (2000). *Essentials of career interest assessment.* New York: Wiley.

Proctor, B., & Prevatt, F. (2003). Agreement among four models used for diagnostic learning disabilities. *Journal of Learning Disabilities, 36,* 459–466.

PRO-ED. (2003). *Tests: A comprehensive reference for assessments in psychology, education, and business.* Austin, TX: PRO-ED.

PRO-ED. (2005). *AAMR.* Retrieved January 24, 2005 from www.proedinc.com.

Prouty, A. M., Markowski, E. M., & Barnes, H. L. (2000). Using the *Dyadic Adjustment Scale* in marital therapy: An exploratory study. *The Family Journal: Counseling and Therapy for Couples and Families, 8,* 250–257.

Psychological Assessment Resources. (2004a). *Catalog of professional testing resources.* Lutz, FL: Author.

Psychological Assessment Resources. (2004b). PAR-Psychological Assessment Resources: Innovative solutions and outstanding customer service! *Eating Disorder Inventory-2 (EDI-2).* Retrieved June 15, 2004, from www.parinc.com/product.cfm?ProductID=201.

Psychological Corporation. (1983). *Manual for the Basic Achievement Skills Individual Screener (BASIS)*. San Antonio, TX: Author.

Psychological Corporation. (1988). *General Clerical Test*. San Antonio, TX: Psychological Corporation.

Psychological Corporation. (1991a). *Differential Aptitude Tests, with Career Interest Inventory counselor's manual (1991)*. San Antonio, TX: Author.

Psychological Corporation. (1991b). *Manual for interpreting the Career Interest Inventory* (1991). San Antonio, TX: Author.

Psychological Corporation. (2001). *Technical manual for the Wechsler Individual Achievement Test—Second Edition* (*WIAT-II*). San Antonio, TX: Author.

Psychological Corporation (2002). *Wechsler Individual Achievement Test* (2nd ed.). San Antonio, TX: Author.

Psychological Corporation. (2005a). *Catalog*. San Antonio, TX: Author.

Psychological Corporation. (2005b). *SAT-10* information. Retrieved on January 7, 2005, from www.harcourtassessment.com.

Psychological Corporation. (2005c). *WASI*. Retrieved January 24, 2005, from www.psychcorp.com.

Purdue Research Foundation. (n.d.). *Purdue Pegboard*. Chicago: Pearson Reid London House.

Rapoport, J. L., & Ismond, D. R. (1996). *DSM-IV training guide for diagnosis of childhood disorders*. Levittown, PA: Brunner/Mazel.

Raven, J., Raven, J. C., & Court, J. H. (1998). *Raven's Progressive Matrices*. Oxford, England: Oxford University Press.

Rayman, J. R. (1998). Interpreting Ellenore Flood's *Self-Directed Search*. *The Career Development Quarterly, 46,* 330–337.

Reardon, R., & Lenz, J. (1998). *The Self-Directed Search and related Holland career materials: A practitioner's guide*. Lutz, FL: Psychological Assessment Resources.

Reich, W. (Ed.) (1996). *Diagnostic Interview for Children and Adolescents—Revised (DICA-R) 8.0.* St. Louis: Washington University.

Reid, D. K., Hresko, W. P., & Hammill, D. D. (2001). *Manual for the Test of Early Reading Ability—Third Edition*. Austin, TX: PRO-ED.

Reinehr, R. C. (1998). Review of the *Children's Apperception Test 1991 Revision*. In J. C. Impara & B. S. Plake (Eds.), *The thirteenth mental measurements yearbook* (pp. 233–234). Lincoln, NE: Buros Institute of Mental Measurements.

Renzulli, J. S., Smith, L. H., White, A. J., Callahan, C. M., Hartman, R. K., & Westberg, K. L (2002). *Scales for Rating the Behavior Characteristics of Superior Students (SRBCSS-R): Technical and administration manual* (Rev. ed.). Mansfield, CT: Creative Learning Press.

Retzlaff, P. (1995). Review of the *Millon Adolescent Clinical Inventory*. In J. C. Conoley & J. C. Impara (Eds.), *The twelfth mental measurements yearbook* (pp. 620–622). Lincoln, NE: Buros Institute of Mental Measurements.

Reynolds, C. R., & Brown, R. T. (1984). Bias in mental testing: An introduction to the issues. In C. R. Reynolds & R. T. Brown (Eds.), *Perspectives on bias in mental testing* (pp. 1–39). New York: Plenum Press.

Reynolds, C. R., Chastain, R. L., Kaufman, A. S., & McLean, J. E. (1987). Demographic characteristics and IQ among adults: Analysis of the *WAIS-R* standardization sample as a function of the stratification variables. *Journal of School Psychology, 25,* 323–342.

Reynolds, C. R., & Kamphaus, R. W. (1992). *The Behavior Assessment System for Children*. Circle Pines, MN: American Guidance Services.

Reynolds, C. R., & Kamphaus, R. W. (1998). *Manual for the Behavior Assessment System for Children*. Circle Pines, MN: American Guidance Services.

Reynolds, C. R., & Richmond, B. O. (1994). *Revised Children's Manifest Anxiety Scale*. Los Angeles: Western Psychological Services.

Reynolds, W. M. (1988). *Manual for the Suicide Ideation Questionnaire.* Lutz, FL: Psychological Assessment Resources.

Reynolds, W. M. (1991). *Manual for the Adult Suicide Ideation Questionnaire.* Lutz, FL: Psychological Assessment Resources.

Reynolds, W. M. (2002). *Manual for the Reynolds Adolescent Depression Scale—Second Edition (RADS-2).* Lutz, FL: Psychological Assessment Resources.

Reynolds, W. M., & Mazza, J. J. (1998). Reliability and validity of the *Reynolds Adolescent Depression Scale* with young adolescents. *Journal of School Psychology, 36,* 295–312.

Riddle, J., & Bergin, J. J. (1997). Effects of group counseling on the self-concept of children of alcoholics. *Elementary School Guidance and Counseling, 31,* 192–204.

Riley, S. (1987). The advantages of art therapy in an outpatient clinic. *American Journal of Art Therapy, 26,* 21–29.

Riverside Publishing. (2005a). Online catalog description of the *Das-Naglieri Cognitive Assessment System.* Retrieved January 24, 2005, from www.riverpub.com.

Riverside Publishing. (2005b). *Woodcock-Johnson III (WJ III) Tests of Cognitive Abilities* web page. Retrieved February 7, 2005, from www.riverpub.com/products/clinical/wj3/chart.html.

Rizza, M. G., McIntosh, D. E., & McGunn, A. (2001). Profile analysis of the *Woodcock-Johnson III—Tests of Cognitive Abilities* with gifted students. *Psychology in the Schools, 38,* 447–455.

Robinson, N. W. (1992). *Stanford-Binet IV,* of course! Time marches on! *Roeper Review, 15,* 32–35.

Rogers, M. (1998). Psychoeducational assessment of culturally and linguistically diverse children and youth. In H. B. Vance (Ed.), *Psychological assessment of children: Best practices for school and clinical settings* (2nd ed., pp. 355–384). New York: Wiley.

Roid, G. H. (2003). *The Stanford-Binet Intelligence Scale—Fifth Edition (SB5).* Itasca, IL: Riverside Publishing.

Roid, G. H., & Miller, L. J. (1997). *Manual for the Leiter International Performance Scale—Revised (Leiter-R).* Wood Dale, IL: Stoelting Company.

Rorschach, H. (1921/1942). *Psychodiagnostics: A diagnostic test based on perception* (P. Lemkau & B. Kronenburg, Trans.). Berne: Huber. (First German edition: 1921. Distributed in the United States by Grune & Stratton.)

Rorschach, H. (1921/1998). *The Rorschach Inkblot Test.* Kirkland, WA: Hogrefe & Huber Publishers.

Rorschach, H. (1969). *Rorschach Inkblot Test.* New York: Grune & Stratton.

Rosen-Grandon, J. R., Myers, J. E., & Hattie, J. A. (2004). The relationship between marital characteristics, marital interaction processes, and marital satisfaction. *Journal of Counseling and Development, 82,* 58–68.

Rosenthal, R. (1966). *Experimenter effects in behavioral research.* New York: Appleton-Century-Crofts.

Rosenzwieg, S. (1949). *Rosenzwieg Picture-Frustration Study.* Lutz, FL: Psychological Assessment Resources.

Ross, N. M., & Doherty, W. J. (2001). Validity of the *Global Assessment of Relational Functioning (GARF)* when used by community-based therapists. *American Journal of Family Therapy, 29,* 239–253.

Roszkowski, M. J. (2001). Review of *Revised Minnesota Paper Form Board Test, Second Edition.* In B. S. Plake & J. C. Impara (Eds.), *The fourteenth mental measurements yearbook* (pp. 1012–1015). Lincoln, NE: Buros Institute of Mental Measurements.

Rounds, J. B., Jr. (1990). The comparative and combined utility of work value and interest data in career counseling with adults. *Journal of Vocational Behavior, 37,* 32–45.

Rounds, J. B., Jr., Henly, G. A., Dawis, R. V., Lofquist, L. H., & Weiss, D. J. (1981). *Manual for the Minnesota Importance Questionnaire: A measure of vocational needs and values.* Minneapolis: University of Minnesota, Department of Psychology.

Ruch, W. W., Shub, A. N., Moinat, S. M., & Dye, D. A. (1982). *PSI Basic Skills for Tests for Business, Industry & Government.* Glendale, CA: Psychological Services.

Russell, M., & Karol, D. (1994). *Administration manual for the 16PF.* Champaign, IL: IPAT.

Russo, A., & Warren, S. H. (1999). Collaborative test taking. *College Teaching, 47,* 18.

Ryan, M. (1985). Review of the *Minnesota Clerical Test.* In J. V. Mitchell (Ed.), *The ninth mental measurements yearbook* (pp. 992–993). Lincoln, NE: Buros Institute of Mental Measurements.

Salend, S. J. (1984). Selecting and evaluating educational assessment instruments. *Pointer, 28,* 20–22.

Salvia, J., & Ysseldyke, J. E. (2004). *Assessment in special and inclusive education* (9th ed.). Boston: Houghton Mifflin.

Sampson, J. P., Jr., Peterson, G. W., Lenz, J. G., Reardon, R. L., & Saunders, D. E. (1996). *Career Thoughts Inventory: Professional manual.* Lutz, FL: Psychological Assessment Resources.

Sampson, J. P., Jr., Purgar, M. P., & Shy, J. D. (2003). Computer-based test interpretation in career assessment: Ethical and professional issues. *Journal of Career Assessment, 11,* 22–39.

Sanchez, H. B. (2001). Risk factor model for suicide assessment and intervention. *Professional Psychology: Research and Practice, 32,* 351–358.

Sanders, J. (1993). Science and technology: A new alliance. *Science Scope, 15*(6), 56–60.

Sandoval, J. (1995). Review of the *Wechsler Intelligence Scale for Children—Third Edition.* In J. C. Conoley & J. C. Impara (Eds.), *The twelfth mental measurements yearbook* (pp. 1103–1104). Lincoln, NE: Buros Institute of Mental Measurements.

Sandoval, J. (1998). Review of the *Behavior Assessment System for Children (BASC).* In J. C. Impara & B. S. Plake (Eds.), *The thirteenth mental measurements yearbook* (pp. 128–131). Lincoln, NE: Buros Institute of Mental Measurements.

Sandoval, J. (2003). Review of the *Woodcock-Johnson III.* In B. S. Plake, J. C. Impara, & R. A. Spies (Eds.), *The fifteenth mental measurements yearbook* (pp. 1019–1024). Lincoln, NE: Buros Institute of Mental Measurements.

Sandoval, J., Zimmerman, I. L., & Woo-Sam, J. M. (1983). Cultural differences on *WISC-R* verbal items. *Journal of School Psychology, 21,* 49–55.

SASSI Institute (2004). The SASSI Institute: Product catalog. Retrieved June 15, 2004, from www.sassi.com/sassi/bin/catalog.shtml.

Satir, V. M. (1982). The therapist and family therapy: Process model. In A. M. Horne & M. M. Ohlsen (Eds.), *Family counseling and therapy.* Itasca, IL: Peacock.

Sattler, J. M. (1970). Racial "experimenter effects" in experimentation, testing, interviewing, and psychotherapy. *Psychological Bulletin, 73,* 716–721.

Sattler, J. M. (1973). Examiners' scoring style, accuracy, ability, and personality scores. *Journal of Clinical Psychology, 29,* 38–39.

Sattler, J. M. (1982). *Assessment of children's intelligence and special abilities* (2nd ed.). Boston: Allyn & Bacon.

Sattler, J. M. (1988). *Assessment of children* (3rd ed.). San Diego: Author.

Sattler, J. M. (1992). *Assessment of children: Revised and updated* (3rd ed.). San Diego, CA: Author.

Sattler, J. M. (1998). *Clinical and forensic interviewing of children and families: Guidelines for the mental health, education, pediatric, and child maltreatment fields.* San Diego, CA: Author.

Sattler, J. M. (2001). *Assessment of children: Cognitive applications* (4th ed.). La Mesa, CA: Author.

Sattler, J. M. (2002). *Assessment of children: Behavioral and clinical applications* (4th ed.). La Mesa, CA: Sattler.

Sattler, J. M., & Dumont, R. (2004). *Assessment of children: WISC-IV and WPPSI-III supplement.* San Diego, CA: Sattler.

Savickas, M. L., Brizzi, J. S., Brisbin, L. A., & Pethtel, L. L. (1988). Predictive validity of two medical specialty preference inventories. *Measurement and Evaluation in Counseling and Development, 21,* 106–112.

Sax, G. (1980). *Principles of educational and psychological measurement and evaluation* (2nd ed.). Belmont, CA: Wadsworth.

Sax, G. (1997). *Principles of educational and psychological measurement and evaluation* (4th ed.). Belmont, CA: Wadsworth.

Schafer, W. D. (1992). Review of the *Computer Programmer Aptitude Battery.* In J. J. Kramer & J. C. Conoley (Eds.), *The eleventh mental measurements yearbook* (pp. 227–228). Lincoln, NE: Buros Institute of Mental Measurements.

Schaie, K. W., & Gribbon, K. (1975). Adult development and aging. *Annual Review of Psychology, 26,* 65–96.

Schaie, K. W., & Strother, F. (1968). *Human aging and behavior.* New York: Academic Press.

Schinka, J. (1988). *Mental Status Checklist.* Lutz, FL: Psychological Assessment Resources.

Schinka, J. (1989). *Personal History Checklist.* Lutz, FL: Psychological Assessment Resources.

Schinke, S. (1995). Review of the *Eating Disorder Inventory-2.* In J. C. Conoley & J. C. Impara (Eds.), *The twelfth mental measurements yearbook* (p. 335). Lincoln, NE: Buros Institute of Mental Measurements.

Schoenrade, P. (2002). *Values Scale (VS).* In J. T. Kapes & E. A. Whitfield (Eds.). *A counselor's guide to career assessment instruments* (pp. 298–302). Tulsa, OK: National Career Development Association.

Schueger, J. M. (1992). *The 16 Personality Factor Questionnaire* and its junior versions. *Journal of Counseling and Development, 71,* 231–244.

Science Research Associates. (1947). *SRA Clerical Aptitude Test.* Chicago: Author.

Science Research Associates. (1977). *Office Skills Tests.* Chicago: Pearson Reid London House.

Science Research Associates. (1990) *Computer Operator Aptitude Battery.* Chicago: Pearson Reid London House.

Science Research Associates. (n.d.a). *SRA Mechanical Aptitude Test.* Chicago: Author.

Science Research Associates. (n.d.b). *SRA Test of Mechanical Concepts.* Chicago: Author.

Searight, H. R. (1997). *Family-of-origin therapy and diversity.* Washington, DC: Taylor & Francis.

Seashore, C. E., Lewis, D., & Saetveit, J. G. (1940). *Manual of instructions and interpretations for the Seashore Measures of Musical Talents.* Chicago: Stoelting.

Seguin, E. (1907). *Idiocy: Its treatment by the physiological treatment method.* New York: Bureau of Publications, Teachers College, Columbia University. (Original work published 1866)

Seligman, L. (1998). *Selecting effective treatments: A comprehensive, systematic guide to treating mental disorders* (Rev. ed.). San Francisco: Jossey-Bass.

Sewell, T. E. (1985). Review of *Coopersmith Self-Esteem Inventories.* In J. V. Mitchell (Ed.), *The ninth mental measurements yearbook* (pp. 397–398). Lincoln, NE: Buros Institute of Mental Measurements.

Sexton, T. L., Whiston, S. C., Bleuer, J. C., & Walz, G. R. (1997). *Integrating outcome research into counseling practice and training.* Alexandria, VA: American Counseling Association.

Shaffer, D. (1996). *Diagnostic Interview Schedule for Children-Revised (DISC-R).* New York: New York State Psychiatric Institute.

Shavelson, R. J., & Webb, N. M. (1991). *Generalizability theory: A primer.* Newbury Park, CA: Sage.

Shaw, S. R. (1995). Review of the *Slosson Oral Reading Test—Revised (SORT-R).* In J. C. Conoley & J. C. Impara (Eds.), *The twelfth mental measurements yearbook* (pp. 958–959). Lincoln, NE: Buros Institute of Mental Measurements.

Sheperis, C. J. (2001). *The development of an instrument to measure racial identity in juvenile offenders.* Unpublished doctoral dissertation, University of Florida, Gainesville.

Sheperis, C.J., Doggett, T., & Hennington, C. (2005). Behavioral assessment: Principles and applications. In B. T. Erford (Ed.), *Counselor's guide to clinical, personality, and behavioral assessment.* (pp. 105–124): Boston: Lahaska/Houghton Mifflin.

Sherbon, J. W. (2005). Review of *Musical Aptitude Profile*. In B. S. Plake, J. C. Impara, & R. A. Spies (Eds.), *The sixteenth mental measurements yearbook*. Lincoln, NE: Buros Institute of Mental Measurements.

Shimberg, B. (1985). Review of *Office Skills Test*. In J. V. Mitchell (Ed.), *The ninth mental measurements yearbook* (pp. 1081–1082). Lincoln, NE: Buros Institute of Mental Measurements.

Shock, N. W., Greulick, R. C., Andres, R., et al. (1984). *Normal human aging: The Baltimore longitudinal study of aging* (NIH Publication No. 84–2450). Washington, DC: U.S. Government Printing Office.

Shuey, A. M. (1966). *The testing of Negro intelligence* (2nd ed.). New York: Social Science.

Shute, R. E. (2002). *Jackson Vocational Interest Survey (JVIS)*. In J. T. Kapes & E. A. Whitfield (Eds.), *A counselor's guide to career assessment instruments* (pp. 250–256). Tulsa, OK: National Career Development Association.

Sigman, M., & Caps, L. (1997). *Children with autism: A developmental perspective.* Cambridge, MA: Harvard University Press.

Silverman, L. K. (1986). An interview with Elizabeth Hagen. *Roeper Review, 8,* 168–171.

Silverman, L. K., & Kearney, K. (1992). The case for the *Stanford-Binet L-M* as a supplemental test. *Roeper Review, 15,* 34–38.

Skinner, H. A., Steinhauer, P. D., & Santa-Barbara, J. (1995). *The Family Assessment Measure.* North Tonawanda, NY: Multi-Health Systems.

Slate, J. R., & Hunnicutt, L. C. (1988). Examiner errors on the Wechsler scales. *Journal of Psychoeducational Assessment, 6,* 280–288.

Slosson, R., & Nicholson, C. (1990). *Manual for the Slosson Oral Reading Test—Revised (SORT-R).* East Aurora, NY: Slosson Educational Publications.

Smith, A. L., Jr. (1995). Review of the *General Clerical Test*. In J. C. Conoley & J. C. Impara (Eds.), *The twelfth mental measurements yearbook* (pp. 405–406). Lincoln, NE: Buros Institute of Mental Measurements.

Smith, D. K. (1998). Review of the *Nelson-Denny Reading Test*. In J. C. Impara & B. S. Plake (Eds.), *The thirteenth mental measurements yearbook* (pp. 685–686). Lincoln, NE: Buros Institute of Mental Measurements.

Smith, D. K., Klass, P. D., & Stovall, D. L. (1992, August). Relationship of the *K-BIT* and *SIT-R* in a gifted sample. Paper presented at the American Psychological Association meeting, Washington, DC. (ERIC Document Reproduction Service No. ED364558)

Smith, L. F. (2003). Review of the *Test of Early Reading Ability, Third Edition*. In B. S. Plake, J. C. Impara, & R. A. Spies (Eds.), *The fifteenth mental measurements yearbook* (pp. 943–944). Lincoln, NE: Buros Institute of Mental Measurements.

Snyder, C. R. (1997). *Marital Satisfaction Inventory, Revised manual.* Los Angeles: Western Psychological Services.

Snyderman, M., & Rothman, S. (1986). Science, politics, and the IQ controversy. *The Public Interest, 83,* 79–97.

Sontag, L. W., Baker, C. T., & Nelson, V. L. (1958). Personality as a determinant of performance. *American Journal of Orthopsychiatry, 25,* 555–562.

Spanier, G. B. (1989). *Dyadic Adjustment Scale.* Tonawanda, NY: Multi-Health Systems.

Sparrow, S. S., Balla, D. A., & Cicchetti, D. V. (1984a). *Manual for the Vineland Adaptive Behavior Scales—Comprehensive Interview.* Minnesota: American Guidance Service.

Sparrow, S. S., Balla, D. A., & Cicchetti, D. V. (1984b). *Manual for the Vineland Adaptive Behavior Scales—Parent Interview.* Minnesota: American Guidance Service.

Spearman, C. (1904). The proof and measurement of association between two things. *American Journal of Psychology, 15,* 72–101.

Spearman, C. (1927). *The abilities of man: Their nature and measurement.* New York: Macmillan.

Spielberger, R. (1973). *Preliminary manual for the State-Trait Anxiety Inventory.* Palo Alto, CA: Consulting Psychologists Press.

Spillane, S. A. (2001). Review of the *Family Assessment Measure Version III.* In B. S. Plake & J. C. Impara (Eds.), *The fourteenth mental measurements yearbook* (p. 482). Lincoln, NE: Buros Institute of Mental Measurements.

Spinelli, C. G. (2002). *Classroom assessment for students with special needs in inclusive settings.* Upper Saddle River, NJ: Prentice Hall.

Spitzer, R. L., Gibbon, M., Skodol, A. E., Williams, J. B. W., & First, M. B. (1994). *DSM-IV casebook: A learning companion to the diagnostic and statistical manual of mental disorders* (4th ed., text rev.). Washington, DC: American Psychiatric Association.

Sporakowski, M. J. (1995). Assessment and diagnosis in marriage and family counseling. *Journal of Counseling and Development, 74,* 60–64.

Stahl, M. J. (1985). Review of *PSI Basic Skills Tests for Business, Industry, and Government.* In J. V. Mitchell (Ed.), *The ninth mental measurements yearbook* (pp. 1238–1239). Lincoln, NE: Buros Institute of Mental Measurements.

Stanley, J. C. (1993). Quoted in Bock, G. R., & Ackrill, K. A. *The Origins and Development of High Ability* (Ciba Foundation Symposium). Chichester, UK: Wiley.

Stanley, J. C., Benbow, C. P., Brody, L. E., Dauber, S., & Lupkowski, A. E. (1992). Gender differences on eighty-six nationally standardized aptitude and achievement tests. In N. Colangelo, S. G. Assouline, & D. L. Ambroson (Eds.), *Talent development.* Unionville, NY: Trillium Press.

Steer, R. A., Kumar, G., & Beck, A. T. (1993). Self-reported suicidal ideation in adolescent psychiatric inpatients. *Journal of Consulting and Clinical Psychology, 61,* 1096–1099.

Stelmachers, Z. T. (1995). Assessing suicidal clients. In J. N. Butcher (Ed.), *Clinical personality assessment: Practical approaches* (pp. 367–379). New York: Oxford University Press.

Sternberg, R. J. (1986). *Intelligence applied: Understanding and increasing your intellectual skills.* San Diego: Harcourt Brace Jovanovich.

Sternberg, R. J. (1988). *The triarchic mind.* New York: Penguin Books.

Sternberg, R. J. (1990). T & T is an explosive combination: Technology and testing. *Educational Psychologist, 25,* 216–219.

Sternberg, R. J., Wagner, R. K., Williams, W. M., & Horvath, J. A. (1995). Testing common sense. *American Psychologist, 50,* 912–927.

Stewart, J. R. (1998). Review of the *Beck Scale for Suicide Ideation.* In J. C. Impara & B. S. Plake (Eds.), *The thirteenth mental measurements yearbook* (pp. 126–127). Lincoln, NE: Buros Institute of Mental Measurements.

Stinnett, T. A. (1998). Review of the *AAMR Adaptive Behavior Scale-School, Second Edition.* In J. C. Impara & B. S. Plake (Eds.), *The thirteenth mental measurements yearbook* (pp. 9–14). Lincoln, NE: Buros Institute of Mental Measurements.

Stoelting Company. (2005). *Leiter International Performance Scale Revised (Leiter-R).* Retrieved January 24, 2005, from www.stoeltingco.com/tests/store/ViewLevel3.asp?keyword3=842.

Stone, J. E. (1999). Value-added assessment: An accountability revolution. In M. Kanstoroom & E. Finn Jr. (Eds.) *Better teachers, better schools.* Washington, DC: Thomas B. Fordham Foundation.

Storandt, M. (1994). General principles of assessment of older adults. In M. Storandt & G. R. VandernBos (Eds.), *Neuropsychological assessment of dementia and depression in older adults: A clinician's guide* (pp. 7–32). Washington, DC: American Psychological Association.

Strein, W. (1995). *Assessment of self-concept.* Greensboro, NC: ERIC-CASS. (ERIC Document Reproduction Service No.: ED389962)

Stromberg, E. L. (1985). *Stromberg Dexterity Test.* San Antonio, TX: Psychological Corporation.

Strong, E. K. (1927). *The Vocational Interest Blank.* Stanford, CA: Stanford University Press.

Stuart, R. B. (1992). Review of the *Dyadic Adjustment Scale*. In J. J. Kramer & J. C. Conoley (Eds.), *The eleventh mental measurements yearbook* (pp. 297–298). Lincoln, NE: University of Nebraska Press.

Stuart, R. B. (1995). Review of the *Millon Adolescent Clinical Inventory*. In J. C. Conoley & J. C. Impara (Eds.), *The twelfth mental measurements yearbook* (pp. 622–623). Lincoln, NE: Buros Institute of Mental Measurements.

Stumpf, H. & Jackson, D. (1994). Gender-related differences in cognitive abilities: Evidence from a medical school admissions testing program. *Personality and Individual Differences, 17,* 335–344.

Subkoviak, M. J. (1988). A practitioner's guide to computation and interpretation of reliability indices for mastery tests. *Journal of Educational Measurement, 25*(1), 47–55.

Substance Abuse and Mental Health Services Administration. (1998). *National expenditures for mental health, alcohol, and other drug abuse treatment.* Washington, DC: SAMHSA, Department of Health and Human Services.

Sue, D. W. (1999). Counseling the culturally different: Theory and practice. New York: Wiley.

Sue, D. W., Arredondo, P., & McDavis, R. (1992). Multicultural counseling competencies and standards: A call to the profession. *Journal of Counseling and Development, 70,* 477–486.

Super, D. E., Thompson, A. S., & Lindeman, R. H. (1988). *Adult Career Concerns Inventory.* Palo Alto, CA: Consulting Psychologists Press.

Swanson, J. L., & Fouad, N. A. (1999). *Career theory and practice: Learning through case studies.* Thousand Oaks, CA: Sage.

Swerdlik, M. E., & Bucy, J. E. (1998). Review of the *Stanford Diagnostic Reading Test, Fourth Edition*. In J. C. Impara & B. S. Plake (Eds.), *The thirteenth mental measurements yearbook* (pp. 941–943). Lincoln, NE: Buros Institute of Mental Measurements.

Taylor, R. M., & Morrison, W. L. (1996). *Taylor-Johnson Temperament Analysis test manual.* Los Angeles: Western Psychological Services.

Telzrow, C.F. (1985). Best practices in reducing learning disability qualification. In A. Thomas & J. Grimes (Eds.), *Best practices in school psychology.* Kent, OH: National Association of School Psychologists.

Terman, L. M. (1916a). *The measurement of intelligence.* Boston: Houghton Mifflin.

Terman, L. M. (1916b). *Original translations of the Stanford-Binet.* Stanford, CA: Stanford University Press.

Terman, L. M., et al. (1925). *The mental and physical traits of a thousand gifted children. Vol. 1. Genetic studies of genius.* Stanford, CA: Stanford University Press.

Thayer, P. W. (1985). Review of *Office Skills Tests*. In J. V. Mitchell (Ed.), *The ninth mental measurements yearbook* (pp. 1082–1083). Lincoln, NE: Buros Institute of Mental Measurements.

Thissen, D. (1990). Reliability and measurement precision. In H. Wainer (Ed.), *Computerized adaptive testing: A primer* (pp. 161–185). Hillsdale, NJ: Erlbaum.

Thomas, R. G. (1985). Review of *Minnesota Clerical Test*. In J. V. Mitchell (Ed.), *The ninth mental measurements yearbook* (pp. 993–994). Lincoln, NE: Buros Institute of Mental Measurements.

Thompson, B. (1992). Editorial comment: Misuse of ANCOVA and related "statistical control" procedures. *Reading Psychology: An International Quarterly, 13,* iii–xviii.

Thompson, B. (Ed.) (2003). *Score reliability: Contemporary thinking on reliability issues.* Thousand Oaks, CA: Sage Publications.

Thompson, B., & Vacha-Haase, T. (2000). Psychometrics *is* datametrics: The test is not reliable. *Educational and Psychological Measurement, 60,* 174–195.

Thompson, D. (2001). Review of the *Das-Naglieri Cognitive Assessment System*. In B. S. Plake & J. C. Impara (Eds.), *The fourteenth mental measurements yearbook* (pp. 368–370). Lincoln, NE: Buros Institute of Mental Measurements.

Thompson, J. M., & Blain, M. D. (1992). Presenting feedback on the *Minnesota Importance Questionnaire* and the *Minnesota Satisfaction Questionnaire*. *Career Development Quarterly, 41,* 62–65.

Thompson, P., & Nurse, R. (1999). The *KFD:* Clues to family relationships. In R. Nurse (Ed.), *Family assessment* (pp. 124–134). New York: Wiley.

Thompson, S. J., Johnstone, C. J., & Thurlow, M. L. (2002). *Universal design applied to large-scale assessments* (Synthesis Report 44). Minneapolis, MN: University of Minnesota National Center on Educational Outcomes.

Thorndike, R. L. (1997). *Measurement and evaluation in psychology and education* (6th ed.). Upper Saddle River, NJ: Prentice Hall.

Thorndike, R. L. (2005). *Measurement and evaluation in psychology and education* (7th ed.). Upper Saddle River, NJ: Pearson, Merrill/Prentice Hall.

Thorndike, R. L., & Hagen, E. P. (1977). *Measurement and evaluation in psychology and education* (4th ed.). New York: Wiley.

Thorndike, R. L., & Hagen, E. P. (2001). *The Cognitive Abilities Test (CogAT) Form 5.* Chicago: Riverside Publishing.

Thorndike, R. L., Hagen, E. P., & Sattler, J. M. (1986a). *Guide for administering and scoring the Stanford-Binet Intelligence Scale—Fourth Edition.* Chicago: Riverside Publishing.

Thorndike, R. L., Hagen, E. P., & Sattler, J. M. (1986b). *Technical manual for the Stanford-Binet Intelligence Scale, Fourth Edition.* Chicago: Riverside Publishing.

Thrower, S. M. (1982). The Family Circle method for integrating family systems concepts in family medicine. *Journal of Family Practice, 15,* 451–457.

Tileston, D. W. (2004). *What every teacher should know about student assessment.* Thousand Oaks, CA: Corwin Press.

Tirre, W. C. (2003). Review of the *Coping Inventory for Stressful Situations.* In B. S. Plake, J. C. Impara, & R. A. Spies (Eds.), *The fifteenth mental measurements yearbook* (pp. 260–263). Lincoln, NE: Buros Institute of Mental Measurements.

Tisak, J., & Tisak, M. S. (1996). Longitudinal models of reliability and validity: A latent curve approach. *Applied Psychological Measurement, 20,* 275–288.

Touliatos, J., Perlmutter, B. F., & Straus, M. A. (2001). *Handbook of family measurement techniques: Abstracts* (Vols. I, II, III). Thousand Oaks, CA: Sage.

Townsend, A. E., Baylot, L. M., & Erford, B. T. (2006). Review of the various *Conners' Rating Scales.* In B. T. Erford (Ed.). *Counselor's guide to clinical, personality, and behavioral assessment* (pp. 136–141). Boston: Lahaska/Houghton Mifflin.

Trevisan, M. S. (1998). Review of the *Test of Early Written Language, Second Edition.* In J. C. Impara & B. S. Plake (Eds.), *The thirteenth mental measurements yearbook* (pp. 1030–1031). Lincoln, NE: Buros Institute of Mental Measurements.

Tuddenham, R. D., Blumemkrantz, J., & Wilken, W. R. (1968). Age changes on AGCT: A longitudinal study of average adults. *Journal of Consulting and Clinical Psychology, 32,* 659–663.

Tuttle, F. B., & Becker, A. (1980). *Characteristics and identification of gifted and talented students.* Washington, DC: National Education Association.

Ukrainetz, T. A., & Blomquist, C. (2002). The criterion validity of four vocabulary tests compared with a language sample. *Child Language Teaching and Therapy, 18,* 1–20.

United States Census Bureau (2003). *Census report.* Washington, DC: Author.

United States Department of Health & Human Services. (2003). USDHHS website. Retrieved on December 4, 2004, from www.hhs.gov.

United States Department of Labor. (2005). *O*NET Work Importance Profiler.* Retrieved January 6, 2005, from www.onetcenter.org/WIP.html.

United States Employment Service. (1986). *General Aptitude Test Battery (GATB).* Washington, DC: Author.

United States Employment Service. (2003). *O*NET Work Importance Profiler.* Washington, DC: Author.

United States Military Entrance Processing Command. (1992). *Armed Services Vocational Aptitude Battery (ASVAB).* North Chicago, IL: USMEPCOM.

United States Military Entrance Processing Command. (2005). *Armed Services Vocational Aptitude Battery (ASVAB).* North Chicago, IL: USMEPCOM.

Vacc, N. A., & Newsome, D. W. (2002). *Strong Interest Inventory (SII)* and *Skills Confidence Inventory (SCI).* In J. T. Kapes & E. A. Whitfield (Eds.). *A counselor's guide to career assessment instruments* (pp. 288–297). Tulsa, OK: National Career Development Association.

Vacha-Haase, T., & Thompson, B. (1999). Psychometric properties of scores on a new measure of psychological type. (ERIC Document Reproduction Service No. ED434 119)

Van Hutton, V. (1994). *House-Tree-Person.* Odessa, FL: Psychological Assessment Resources.

Vansickle, T. R., & Conn, S. R. (1996, April). The global factors of the *"16PF Fifth Edition"*: Contribution to career development and guidance. Paper presented at the Annual Meeting of the American Educational Research Association, New York, NY.

Varon, E. J. (1936). Alfred Binet's concept of intelligence. *Psychological Review, 43,* 32–49.

Velander, P. L. (1993). *Premarriage Awareness Inventory.* Inver Grove Heights, MN: Logos Productions.

Venn, J. (1994). *Assessment of students with special needs.* New York: Macmillan.

Verhaeghen, P. (2003). Aging and vocabulary scores. A meta-analysis. *Psychology and Aging, 18,* 332–339.

Vernon, P. E. (1960). *The structure of human abilities* (Rev. ed.). London: Methuen.

Vernon, P. E. (1965). Ability factors and environmental influences. *American Psychologist, 20,* 723–733.

Vocational Psychology Research. (2004). Vocational Psychology Research homepage. Retrieved January 10, 2005, from www.psych.umn.edu/psylabs/vpr/miqinf.htm.

Volpe, R. J., & DuPaul, G. J. (2001). Assessment with brief behavior rating scales. In J. J. W. Andrews, D. H. Shklofske, & H. L. Janzen (Eds.), *Handbook of psychoeducational assessment: Ability, achievement, and behavior in children* (pp. 357–387). San Diego, CA: Academic Press.

Voyer, D., Voyer, S. D., & Bryden, M. P. (1995). Magnitude of sex differences in spatial abilities: A meta-analysis and consideration of critical variables. *Psychological Bulletin, 117,* 250–270.

Walker, H. M. (1983). *The Walker Problem Behavior Identification Checklist* (2nd ed.). Los Angeles: Western Psychological Services.

Walker, J. L., Lahey, B. B., Russo, M. F., Christ, M. A. G., McBurnett, K., Loeber, R., et al. (1991). Anxiety, inhibition and Conduct Disorder in children. I: Relation to social impairment. *Journal of the American Academy of Child and Adolescent Psychiatry, 30,* 187–191.

Waller, N. G. (2001). Review of the *Roberts Apperception Test for Children.* In B. S. Plake & J. C. Impara (Eds.), *The fourteenth mental measurements yearbook* (pp. 1032–1033). Lincoln, NE: Buros Institute of Mental Measurements.

Wasyliw, O. E. (2001). Review of the *Peabody Picture Vocabulary Test.* In B. S. Plake & J. C. Impara (Eds.), *The fourteenth mental measurements yearbook* (pp. 909–911). Lincoln, NE: Buros Institute of Mental Measurements.

Waters, E. (1985). Review of the *Gesell School Readiness Test.* In J. V. Mitchell (Ed.), *The ninth mental measurements yearbook* (pp. 610–611). Lincoln, NE: Buros Institute of Mental Measurements.

Watkins, C. E. (1991). What have surveys taught us about the teaching and practice of psychological assessment? *Journal of Personality Assessment, 56,* 426–437.

Watkins, E., & Campbell, V. (2000). *Testing and assessment in counseling practice* (2nd ed.). Mahwah, NJ: Erlbaum.

Watson, J. C. (2006). Review of the *Walker Problem Behavior Identification Checklist* (*WPBIC*). In B. T. Erford (Ed.), *Counselor's guide to clinical, personality, and behavioral assessment* (pp. 150–153). Boston: Lahaska/Houghton Mifflin.

Watson, T. S. (1994). Review of the *Slosson Intelligence Test—Revised*. In J. J. Kramer & J. C. Conoley (Eds.), *The eleventh mental measurements yearbook* (pp. 956–958). Lincoln, NE: Buros Institute of Mental Measurements.

Webb, N. L. (2002). *Alignment study in language arts, mathematics, science, and social studies of state standards and assessments for four states.* Madison: University of Wisconsin Center for Educational Research.

Wechsler, D. (1939). *The measurement of adult intelligence.* Baltimore: Williams & Wilkins.

Wechsler, D. (1949). *Manual for the Wechsler Intelligence Scale for Children.* San Antonio, TX: Psychological Corporation.

Wechsler, D. (1955). *Manual for the Wechsler Adult Intelligence Scale.* New York: Psychological Corporation.

Wechsler, D. (1967). *Manual for the Wechsler Preschool and Primary Scale of Intelligence.* New York: Psychological Corporation.

Wechsler, D. (1975). Intelligence defined and undefined: A relativistic appraisal. *American Psychologist, 30,* 135–139.

Wechsler, D. (1991). *Wechsler Intelligence Scale for Children—Third Edition.* San Antonio, TX: Psychological Corporation.

Wechsler, D. (1997). *Manual for the Wechsler Adult Intelligence Scale* (3rd ed.). San Antonio, TX: Psychological Corporation.

Wechsler, D. (1999). *Manual for the Wechsler Abbreviated Scale of Intelligence* (*WASI*). San Antonio, TX: Psychological Corporation.

Wechsler, D. (2001a). *Manual for the Wechsler Intelligence Scale for Children—Fourth Edition* (*WISC-IV*). San Antonio, TX: Psychological Corporation.

Wechsler, D. (2001b). *Wechsler Individual Achievement Test—Second Edition* (*WIAT-II*). San Antonio, TX: Psychological Corporation.

Wechsler, D. (2002). *Manual for the Wechsler Preschool and Primary Scale of Intelligence—Third Edition* (*WPPSI-III*). San Antonio, TX: Psychological Corporation.

Weiderholf, J. L., & Bryant, B. R. (2001). *Gray Oral Reading Test—Fourth Edition* (*GORT-4*). Austin, TX: PRO-ED.

Weinberg, R. A. (1989). Review of the *Kinetic Drawing System for Family and School.* In J. C. Conoley & J. J. Kramer (Eds.), *The tenth mental measurements yearbook* (pp. 423–425). Lincoln, NE: Buros Institute of Mental Measurements.

Western Psychological Services. (2003a). *Forer Structured Sentence Completion Test.* Retrieved January 25, 2005, from https://www-secure.earthlink.net/www.wpspublish.com/Inetpub4/catalog/W-28.htm.

Western Psychological Services. (2003b). *House-Tree-Person* (*H-T-P*) *Projective Drawing Technique.* Retrieved January 25, 2005, from https://www-secure.earthlink.net/www.wpspublish.com/Inetpub4/catalog/W-500.htm.

Western Psychological Services. (2003c). *Tennessee Self-Concept Scale—Second Edition.* Retrieved January 25, 2005, from https://www-secure.earthlink.net/www.wpspublish.com/Inetpub4/catalog/W-320.htm.

Westman, A. S. (1995). Review of *Minnesota Manual Dexterity Test.* In J. C. Conoley & J. C. Impara (Eds.), *The twelfth mental measurements yearbook* (pp. 624–625). Lincoln, NE: Buros Institute of Mental Measurements.

Whiston, S. C. (2003a). Outcomes research in school counseling. In B. T. Erford (Ed.), *Transforming the school counseling profession* (pp. 435–448). Columbus, OH: Merrill/Prentice Hall.

Whiston, S. C. (2003b). *School Counseling Program Evaluation Scale (SCoPES)—High School Form.* Bloomington: Indiana University.

Whiston, S. C. (2005). *Principles and applications of assessment in counseling* (2nd ed.). Belmont, CA: Thomson Brooks/Cole.

Whitefield, W., McGrath, P., & Coleman, V. (1992, October). *Increasing multicultural sensitivity and awareness.* Paper presented at the annual conference of the National Organization for Human Services Education, Alexandria, VA.

Whyte, W. (1956). *Organization man.* New York: Doubleday.

Wickwire, P. N. (2002). *COPSystem (COPS, CAPS and COPES).* In J. T. Kapes & E. A. Whitfield (Eds.). *A counselor's guide to career assessment instruments* (pp. 210–217). Tulsa, OK: National Career Development Association.

Widiger, T. A. (2001). Review of the *Millon Clinical Multiaxial Inventory—Third Edition (MCMI-III).* In B. S. Plake & J. C. Impara (Eds.), *The fourteenth mental measurements yearbook* (pp. 767–769). Lincoln, NE: Buros Institute of Mental Measurements.

Widiger, T. A., Hurt, S. W., Frances, A., Clarkin, J. F., & Gilmore, M. (1984). Diagnostic efficiency and *DSM-III. Archives of General Psychiatry, 41,* 1005–1012.

Wilde, S. (2002). *Testing and standards: A brief encyclopedia.* Portsmouth, NH: Heinemann.

Wilder, L. K., & Sudweeks, R. R. (2003). Reliability of ratings across studies of the *BASC. Education and Treatment of Children, 26,* 382–399.

Wilkinson, G. S. (1993). *Manual for the Wide-Range Achievement Test—Third Edition.* Wilmington, DE: Jastak Associates.

Willingham, W. W., & Cole, N. S. (1997). *Gender and fair assessment.* Mahwah, NJ: Lawrence Erlbaum Associates.

Wing, H. (1992). Review of the Bennett Mechanical Comprehension Test. In J. J. Kramer & J. C. Conoley (Eds.), The eleventh mental measurements yearbook (pp. 106–107). Lincoln, NE: Buros Institute of Mental Measurements.

Wise, S. L., & Plake, B. S. (1990). Computer-based testing in higher education. *Measurement and Evaluation in Counseling and Development, 23,* 3–10.

Wissler, C. (1901). The correlations of mental physical tests. *Psychological Review Monograph, 3,* 62.

Witmer, J. M., Bernstein, A. V., & Dunham, R. M. (1971). The effects of verbal approval and disapproval upon the performance of third and fourth grade children of four subtests of the *Wechsler Intelligence Scale for Children. Journal of School Psychology, 9,* 347–356.

Witt, J. C., & Jones, K. (1998). Review of the *Behavior Assessment System for Children (BASC).* In J. C. Impara & B. S. Plake (Eds.), *The thirteenth mental measurements yearbook* (pp. 131–133). Lincoln, NE: Buros Institute of Mental Measurements.

Wollack, J. A. (2001). Review of the *KeyMath Revised (KeyMath R/NU).* In B. S. Plake & J. C. Impara (Eds.), *The fourteenth mental measurements yearbook* (pp. 640–641). Lincoln, NE: Buros Institute of Mental Measurements.

Wolraich, M. L., Hannah, J. N., Pinnock, T. Y., Baumgaertel, A., & Brown, J. (1996). Comparison of diagnostic criteria for Attention Deficit Hyperactivity Disorder in a country-wide sample. *Journal of the American Academy of Child and Adolescent Psychiatry, 35,* 319–324.

Wonderlic Personnel Test. (1998). *Wonderlic Personnel Test user's manual.* Libertyville, IL: Author.

Woodcock, R. W. (1998). *Woodcock Reading Mastery Tests—Revised/Normative Update (WRMT-R/NU).* Circle Pines, MN: American Guidance Service.

Woodcock, R., Mather, N., & McGrew, K. (2001). *Woodcock-Johnson III Tests of Achievement.* Itasca, IL: Riverside Publishing.

Woodcock, R., McGrew, K., & Mather, N. (2001). *Woodcock-Johnson III Tests of Cognitive Ability.* Itasca, IL: Riverside Publishing.

Woodruff, D. (2003). Relationships between EPAS scores and college preparatory course work in high schools. (ACT Rep No. 2003-5). Iowa City, IA: ACT.

Woodworth, R. S. (1920). *Personal data sheet.* Chicago: Stoelting.

Worden, M. (2003). *Family therapy basics* (3rd ed.). Pacific Grove, CA: Brooks/Cole.

World Health Organization. (1993). The *Composite International Diagnostic Interview, Authorized Core Version 1.0 (CIDI-Core).* Washington, DC: American Psychiatric Press.

Worthen, B. R., & Sailor, P. (1995). Review of the *Strong Interest Inventory.* In J. C. Conoley & J. J. Kramer (Eds.), *The twelfth mental measurements yearbook* (pp. 999–1002). Lincoln, NE: Buros Institute of Mental Measurements.

Yee, A., Fairchild, H., Weizmann, F., & Wyatt, G. (1993). Addressing psychology's problems with race. *American Psychologist, 48,* 1132–1142.

Yen, W. M., & Henderson, D. L. (2002). Professional standards related to using large-scale state assessments in decisions for individual students. *Measurement and Evaluation in Counseling and Development, 35,* 132–143.

Yerkes, R. M. (Ed.). (1921). Psychological examining in the United States Army. *Memoirs of the National Academy of Sciences, 15,* 1–890.

Youngjohn, J. R., & Crook, T. H., III (1993). Stability of everyday memory in age-associated memory impairment: A longitudinal study. *Neuropsychology, 7,* 406–416.

Zedeck, S. (1985). Review of *PSI Basic Skills Test for Business, Industry, and Government.* In J. V. Mitchell (Ed.), *The ninth mental measurements yearbook* (pp. 1239–1240). Lincoln, NE: Buros Institute of Mental Measurements.

Zima, J. P. (1983). *Interviewing: Key to effective management.* Chicago: Science Research Associates.

Zimmerman, D. W., & Williams, R. H. (1982). Gain scores in research can be highly reliable. *Journal of Educational Measurement, 19,* 149–154.

Zuckerman, M. (1990). Some dubious premises in research and theory on racial differences. *American Psychologist, 45,* 1297–1303.

Zunker, V. G., & Norris, D. (1998). *Using assessment results for career development* (5th ed.). Pacific Grove, CA: Brooks/Cole.

Zunker, V., & Osborn, D. S. (2002). *Using assessment results for career development* (6th ed.). Pacific Grove, CA: Brooks/Cole.

Zybert, P., Stein, Z., & Belmont, L. (1978). Maternal age and children's ability. *Perceptual and Motor Skills, 47,* 815–818.

Zytowski, D. G. (1992). Three generations: The continuing evolution of Frederic Kuder's interest inventories. *Journal of Counseling and Development, 71,* 245–248.

Zytowski, D. G. (2002). *Super's Work Values Inventory, Revised.* Adel, IA: National Career Assessment Services.

Zytowski, D. G. (2004). *Kuder Career Search with Person Match: User manual, version 1.0.* Retrieved August 6, 2004, from www.kuder.com/custom/user_manual.

Zytowski, D. G., & Luzzo, D. A. (2002). Developing the *Kuder Skills Assessment. Journal of Career Assessment, 10,* 190–199.

Name Index

Subject Index